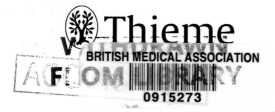
Thieme
BRITISH MEDICAL ASSOCIATION
0915273

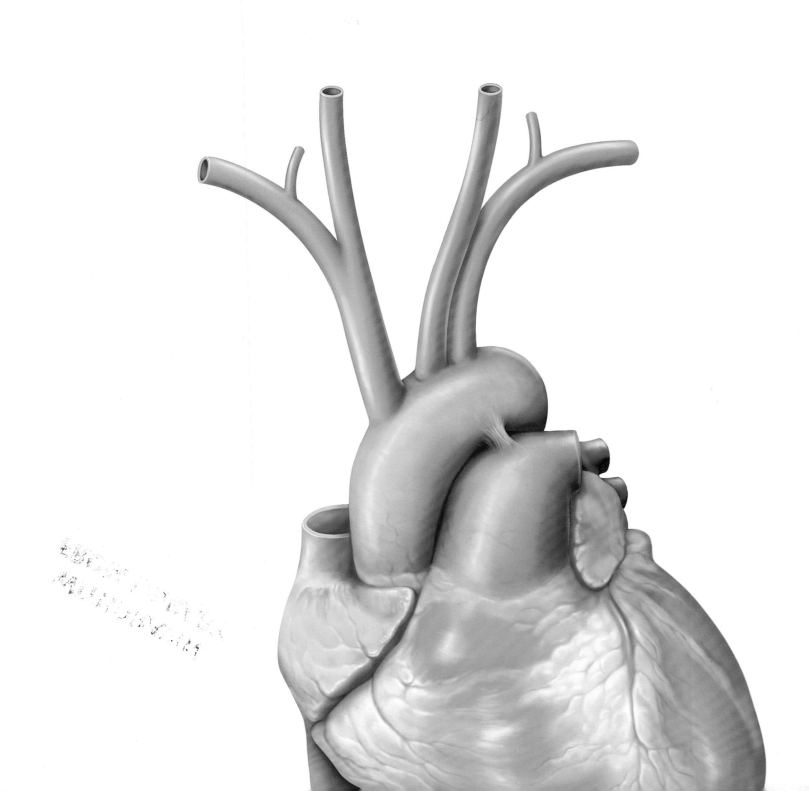

Neck
and Internal Organs

THIEME
Atlas of Anatomy

Consulting Editors

Lawrence M. Ross, M.D., Ph.D.,
The University of Texas Medical School at Houston

Edward D. Lamperti, Ph.D.,
Boston University School of Medicine

Authors

Michael Schuenke, M.D., Ph.D.,
University of Kiel Medical School

Erik Schulte, M.D.,
University of Mainz Medical School

Udo Schumacher, M.D.,
FRCPath, CBiol, FIBiol, DSc,
Hamburg University Medical Center

In collaboration with Juergen Rude

Illustrations by

Markus Voll

Karl Wesker

962 Illustrations
78 Tables

Thieme
Stuttgart · New York

Library of Congress Cataloging-in-Publication Data is available from the publisher.

This book is an authorized and revised translation of the German edition published and copyrighted 2005 by Georg Thieme Verlag, Stuttgart, Germany. Title of the German edition: Schuenke et al.: Hals und Innere Organe: Prometheus Lernatlas der Anatomie.

Illustrators
Markus Voll, Fürstenfeldbruck, Germany;
Karl Wesker, Berlin, Germany (homepage: www.karlwesker.de)

Translator
Terry Telger, Fort Worth, Texas, USA

© 2006 Georg Thieme Verlag
Rüdigerstraße 14
D-70469 Stuttgart
Germany
http://www.thieme.de
Thieme New York, 333 Seventh Avenue,
New York, NY 10001, USA
http://www.thieme.com

We wish to thank the leading manufacturer
of anatomical teaching aids, 3B Scientific
(www.3bscientific.com), for the kind support.

Typesetting by weyhing digital, Ostfildern-Kemnat
Printed in Germany by Appl, Wemding

Softcover
ISBN-10: 1-58890-443-1 (The Americas)
ISBN-13: 978-1-58890-443-0 (The Americas)
ISBN-10: 3-13-142111-8 (Rest of World)
ISBN-13: 978-3-13-142111-8 (Rest of World)

Hardcover
ISBN-10: 1-58890-360-5 (The Americas)
ISBN-13: 978-1-58890-360-0 (The Americas)
ISBN-10: 3-13-142091-X (Rest of World)
ISBN-13: 978-3-13-142091-6 (Rest of World)

Important note: Medicine is an ever-changing science undergoing continual development. Research and clinical experience are continually expanding our knowledge, in particular our knowledge of proper treatment and drug therapy. Insofar as this book mentions any dosage or application, readers may rest assured that the authors, editors, and publishers have made every effort to ensure that such references are in accordance with **the state of knowledge at the time of production of the book**.

Nevertheless, this does not involve, imply, or express any guarantee or responsibility on the part of the publishers in respect to any dosage instructions and forms of applications stated in the book. **Every user is requested to examine carefully** the manufacturers' leaflets accompanying each drug and to check, if necessary in consultation with a physician or specialist, whether the dosage schedules mentioned therein or the contraindications stated by the manufacturers differ from the statements made in the present book. Such examination is particularly important with drugs that are either rarely used or have been newly released on the market. Every dosage schedule or every form of application used is entirely at the user's own risk and responsibility. The authors and publishers request every user to report to the publishers any discrepancies or inaccuracies noticed. If errors in this work are found after publication, errata will be posted at www.thieme.com on the product description page.

1 2 3 4 5 6

Foreword

Our enthusiasm for the THIEME Atlas of Anatomy began when each of us, independently, saw preliminary material from this Atlas. Both of us continue to be captivated by the new approach, the conceptual organization, and by the stunning quality and detail of the images of the Atlas. We were delighted by the ongoing opportunity provided by the editors at Thieme to cooperate with them in making this outstanding resource available to our students and colleagues in North America.

As consulting editors we were asked to review, for accuracy, the English edition of the THIEME Atlas of Anatomy. Our work involved a conversion of nomenclature to terms in common usage and some organizational changes to reflect pedagogical approaches in anatomy programs in North America. This task was eased greatly by the clear organization of the original text. In all of this, we have tried diligently to remain faithful to the intentions and insights of the original authors.

We extend our special thanks to Brian R. MacPherson, Ph. D. for his timely assistance in the role of a Consulting Editor during the emergency illness of one editor (LMR).

We would like to thank the team at Thieme Medical Publishers who worked with us: Kelly Wright, Developmental Editor, and Cathrin E. Schulz M.D., Executive Editor, for checking and correcting our work and for their constant availability and encouragement.

We would also like to extend our heartfelt thanks to Stefanie Langner, Production Manager, for preparing this volume with care and speed.

Lawrence M. Ross,
Edward D. Lamperti

Preface

As it started planning this Atlas, the publisher sought out the opinions and needs of students and lecturers in both the United States and Europe. The goal was to find out what the "ideal" atlas of anatomy should be—ideal for students wanting to learn from the atlas, master the extensive amounts of information while on a busy class schedule, and, in the process, acquire sound, up-to-date knowledge. The result of this work is this Atlas. The THIEME Atlas of Anatomy, unlike most other atlases, is a comprehensive educational tool that combines illustrations with explanatory text and summarizing tables, introducing clinical applications throughout, and presenting anatomical concepts in a step-by-step sequence that allows for the integration of both system-by-system and topographical views.

Since the THIEME Atlas of Anatomy is based on a fresh approach to the underlying subject matter itself, it was necessary to create for it an entirely new set of illustrations—a task that took eight years. Our goal was to provide illustrations that would compellingly demonstrate anatomical relations and concepts, revealing the underlying simplicity of the logic and order of human anatomy without sacrificing detail or aesthetics.

With the THIEME Atlas of Anatomy, it was our intention to create an atlas that would guide students in their initial study of anatomy, stimulate their enthusiasm for this intriguing and vitally important subject, and provide a reliable reference for experienced students and professionals alike.

"If you want to attain the possible, you must attempt the impossible"
(Rabindranath Tagore).

Michael Schünke, Erik Schulte, Udo Schumacher,
Markus Voll, and Karl Wesker

Acknowledgments

First we wish to thank our families. This atlas is dedicated to them.

We also thank Prof. Reinhard Gossrau, M.D., for his critical comments and suggestions. We are grateful to several colleagues who rendered valuable help in proofreading: Mrs. Gabriele Schünke, Jakob Fay, M.D., Ms. Claudia Dücker, Ms. Simin Rassouli, Ms. Heinke Teichmann, and Ms. Sylvia Zilles. We are also grateful to Dr. Julia Jürns-Kuhnke for helping with the figure labels.

We extend special thanks to Stephanie Gay and Bert Sender, who composed the layouts. Their ability to arrange the text and illustrations on facing pages for maximum clarity has contributed greatly to the quality of the Atlas.

We particularly acknowledge the efforts of those who handled this project on the publishing side:

Jürgen Lüthje, M.D., Ph.D., executive editor at Thieme Medical Publishers, has "made the impossible possible." He not only reconciled the wishes of the authors and artists with the demands of reality but also managed to keep a team of five people working together for years on a project whose goal was known to us from the beginning but whose full dimensions we came to appreciate only over time. He is deserving of our most sincere and heartfelt thanks.

Sabine Bartl, developmental editor, became a touchstone for the authors in the best sense of the word. She was able to determine whether a beginning student, and thus one who is not (yet) a professional, could clearly appreciate the logic of the presentation. The authors are indebted to her.

We are grateful to Antje Bühl, who was there from the beginning as project assistant, working "behind the scenes" on numerous tasks such as repeated proofreading and helping to arrange the figure labels.

We owe a great dept of thanks to Martin Spencker, Managing Director of Educational Publications at Thieme, especially to his ability to make quick and unconventional decisions when dealing with problems and uncertainties. His openness to all the concerns of the authors and artists established conditions for a cooperative partnership.

Without exception, our collaboration with the entire staff at Thieme Medical Publishers was consistently pleasant and cordial. Unfortunately we do not have room to list everyone who helped in the publication of this atlas, and we must limit our acknowledgments to a few colleagues who made a particularly notable contribution: Rainer Zepf and Martin Waletzko for support in all technical matters; Susanne Tochtermann-Wenzel and Manfred Lehnert, representing all those who were involved in the production of the book; Almut Leopold for the Index; Marie-Luise Kürschner and her team for creating the cover design; to Birgit Carlsen and Anne Döbler, representing all those who handled marketing, sales, and promotion.

The Authors

Table of Contents

Neck

Thorax

Abdomen and Pelvis

Neurovascular Supply to the Organs

Appendix

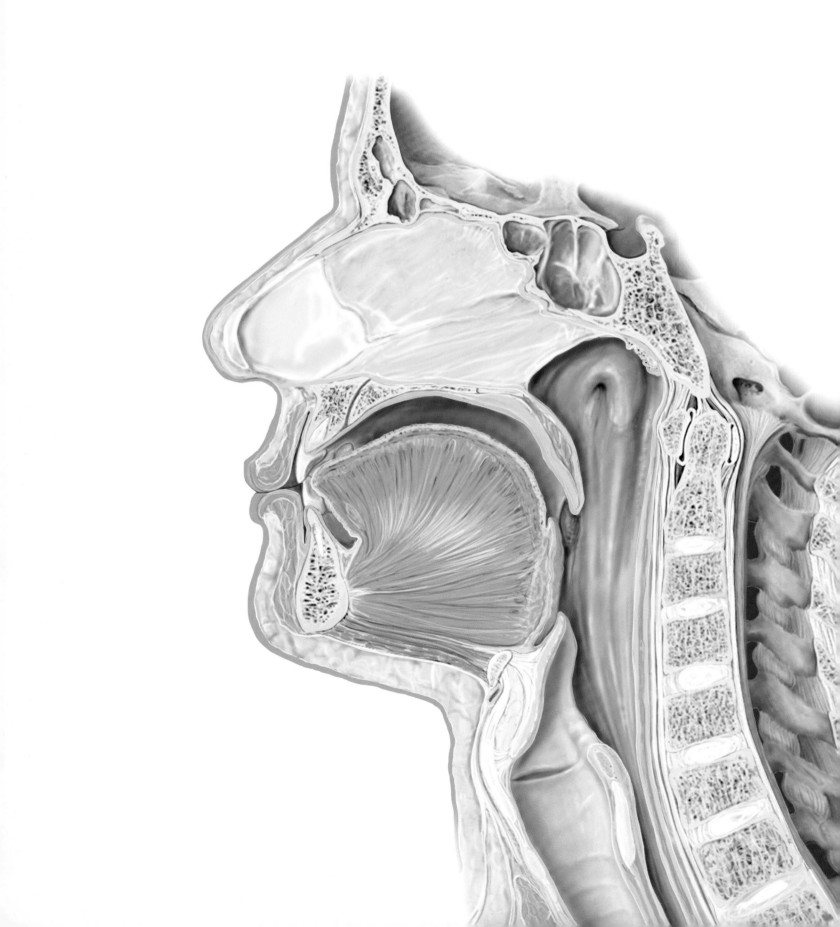

Neck

1.1 The Neck: General Aspects

The neck is the region of the body betweeen the head and trunk. Its skeletal foundation is the vertebral column. Its anterior surface anatomy is defined by muscles and viscera (e.g., the larynx), and it is traversed by a number of closely related neurovascular structures. The muscles, viscera, and neurovascular structures are all enveloped by cervical fasciae (see **B**), which subdivide the neck into compartments. In the sections that follow, these fascial spaces (see **B** and **D**) will provide a basis for discussing the neck muscles by functional groups. This will be followed by a description of the arteries, veins, lymphatics, and nerves (including the peripheral autonomic nervous system) and then the cervical viscera. The usual order of presentation, in which viscera are discussed before nerves and vessels, has been altered in order to emphasize the unique importance of the neurovascular pathways in the neck. The closing sections on topographical and sectional anatomy will explore the interrelationships of the muscles, neurovascular structures, and viscera.

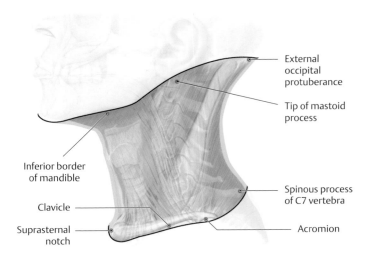

A Sequence of topics in this chapter

Neck muscles
- Superficial muscles
- Nuchal muscles
- Suprahyoid muscles
- Infrahyoid muscles
- Prevertebral muscles
- Lateral (deep) neck muscles

Neurovascular structures
- Arteries
- Veins
- Lymphatic system
- Nerves

Cervical viscera
- Embryology of the cervical viscera
- Thyroid and parathyroid glands
- Larynx
- Pharynx
- Parapharyngeal space

Topographical anatomy
- Surface anatomy and regions
- Anterior cervical region
- Lateral cervical regions
- Posterior cervical and occipital regions
- Cross-sectional anatomy

C Superficial and inferior boundaries of the neck
Left lateral view. The following palpable structures define the superior and inferior boundaries of the neck:

- Superior boundaries: inferior border of the mandible, tip of the mastoid process, and external occipital protuberance
- Inferior boundaries: suprasternal notch, clavicle, acromion, and spinous process of the C 7 vertebra

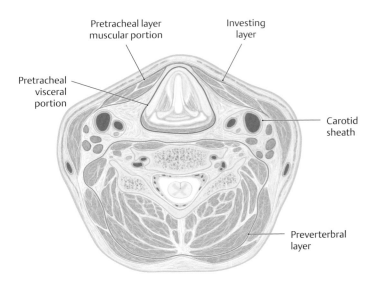

B Cervical fascia
Deep to the skin is the superficial cervical fascia (subcutaneous tissue) which contains the platysma muscle anterolaterly. Deep to the superficial fascia are the following layers of deep cervical fascia:

1. Investing layer: envelops the entire neck, and splits to enclose the sternocleidomastoid and trapezius muscles.
2. Pretracheal layer: the muscular portion encloses the infrahyoid muscles, while the visceral portion surrounds the thyroid gland, larynx, trachea, pharynx, and esophagus.
3. Prevertebral layer: surrounds the cervical vertebral column, and the muscles associated with it.
4. Carotid sheath: encloses the common carotid artery, internal jugular vein, and vagus nerve.

D Relationships of the deep fascia in the neck. Transverse section at the level of the C 5 vertebra
The full extent of the cervical fascia is best appreciated in a transverse section of the neck:

- The *muscle fascia* splits into three layers:
  – Superficial lamina (yellow)
  – Pretracheal lamina (light green)
  – Prevertebral lamina (violet)
- There is also a neurovascular fascia, called the *carotid sheath* (light blue), and
- a *visceral fascia* (dark green).

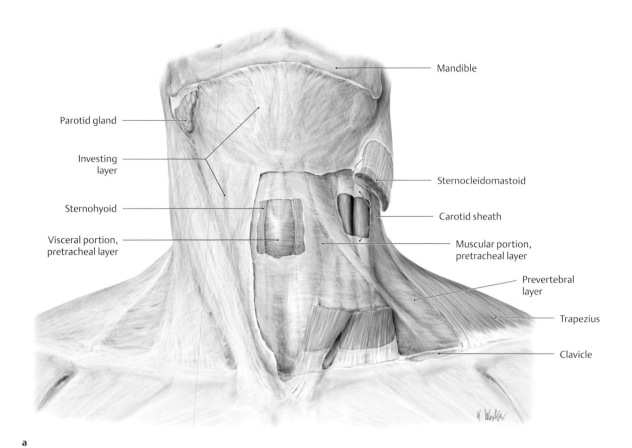

Mandible

Parotid gland

Investing layer

Sternocleidomastoid

Sternohyoid

Carotid sheath

Visceral portion, pretracheal layer

Muscular portion, pretracheal layer

Prevertebral layer

Trapezius

Clavicle

a

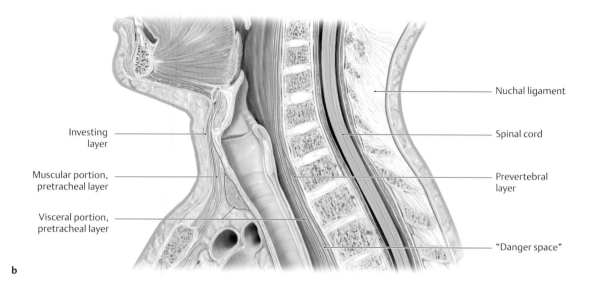

Investing layer

Nuchal ligament

Spinal cord

Muscular portion, pretracheal layer

Prevertebral layer

Visceral portion, pretracheal layer

"Danger space"

b

E Fascial relationships in the neck

a Anterior view. The cutaneous muscle of the neck, the platysma, is highly variable in its development and is subcutaneous in location, overlying the superficial cervical fascia. In the dissection shown, the platysma has been removed at the level of the inferior mandibular border on each side. The cervical fasciae form a fibrous sheet that encloses the muscles, neurovascular structures, and cervical viscera (see **B** for further details). These fasciae subdivide the neck into spaces, some of which are open superiorly and inferiorly for the passage of neurovascular structures. The *investing layer* of the deep cervical fascia has been removed at left center in this dissection. Just deep to the investing layer is the *muscular portion of the pretreacheal layer*, part of which has been removed to display the *visceral portion of the pretracheal layer*. The neurovascular structures are surrounded by a condensation of the cervical fascia called the *carotid sheath*. The

deepest layer of the deep cervical fascia, called the *prevertebral layer*, is visible posteriorly on the left side. These fascia-bounded connective-tissue spaces in the neck are important clinically because they provide routes for the spread of inflammatory processes, although the inflammation may (at least initially) remain confined to the affected compartment.

b Left lateral view. This midsagittal section shows that the deepest layer of the deep cervical fascia, the prevertebral layer, directly overlies the vertebral column in the median plane and is split into two parts. With tuberculous osteomyelitis of the cervical spine, for example, a gravitation abscess may develop in the "danger space" along the prevertebral fascia (retropharyngeal abscess). This fascia encloses muscles laterally and posteriorly (see **D**). The carotid sheath is located farther laterally and does not appear in the midsagittal section.

1.2 Overview and Superficial Neck Muscles

A Scheme used for classifying the neck muscles into groups
The next few sections follow the outline below, which is based on the topographical anatomy of the neck. Various schemes may be used, however: While the nuchal muscles are classified as neck muscles from a topographical standpoint, they belong functionally to the category of intrinsic back muscles (which are not described here).

Superficial neck muscles
- Platysma
- Sternocleidomastoid
- Trapezius*

Suprahyoid muscles
- Digastric
- Geniohyoid
- Mylohyoid
- Stylohyoid

Infrahyoid muscles
- Sternohyoid
- Sternothyroid
- Thyrohyoid
- Omohyoid

* Not a neck muscle in the strict sense, but included here owing to its topographical importance

Prevertebral muscles (deep strap muscles)
- Longus capitis
- Longus colli
- Rectus capitis anterior
- Rectus capitis lateralis

Lateral (deep) neck muscles
- Scalenus anterior
- Scalenus medius
- Scalenus posterior

Nuchal muscles (intrinsic back muscles)
- Semispinalis capitis
- Semispinalis cervicis
- Splenius capitis
- Splenius cervicis
- Longissimus capitis
- Iliocostalis cervicis
- Suboccipital muscles

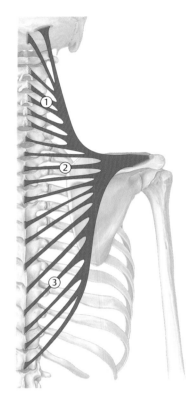

C Schematic of the trapezius

Origin:	① Descending part: • Occipital bone (superior nuchal line and external occipital protuberance) • The spinous processes of all cervical vertebrae via the nuchal ligament ② Transverse part: Broad aponeurosis at the level of the T1–T4 spinous processes ③ Ascending part: Spinous processes of T5–T12
Insertion:	• Lateral third of the clavicle (descending part) • Acromion (transverse part) • Scapular spine (ascending part)
Actions:	• Descending part: – Draws the scapula obliquely upward and rotates it externally (acting with the inferior part of the serratus anterior) – Tilts the head to the same side and rotates it to the opposite side (with the shoulder girdle fixed) • Transverse part: draws the scapula medially • Ascending part: draws the scapula medially downward (supports the rotating action of the descending part) • Entire muscle: stabilizes the scapula on the thorax
Innervation:	Accessory nerve (CN XI) and cervical plexus (C2–C4)

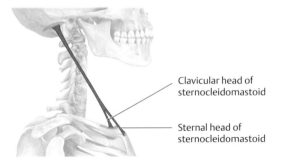

Clavicular head of sternocleidomastoid

Sternal head of sternocleidomastoid

B Schematic of the sternocleidomastoid

Origin:	• Sternal head: manubrium sterni • Clavicular head: medial third of the clavicle
Insertion:	Mastoid process and superior nuchal line
Actions:	• Unilateral: – Tilts the head to the same side – Rotates the head to the opposite side • Bilateral: – Extends the head – Assists in respiration when the head is fixed
Innervation:	Accessory nerve (cranial nerve XI [CN XI]) and direct branches from the cervical plexus (C1–C4)

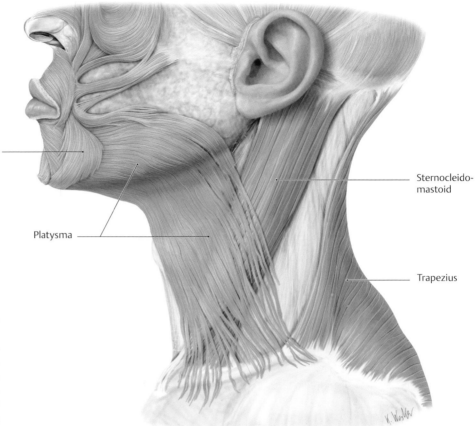

Depressor
anguli oris

Platysma

Sternocleido-
mastoid

Trapezius

D Cutaneous muscle of the neck (platysma)

Left lateral view. The platysma is a broad, flat, subcutaneous muscular sheet located superficial to the investing layer of the deep cervical fascia. Unlike most muscles, it is not enveloped in its own fascial sheath (see classification scheme in **A**), but is instead directly associated with (and in part inserts into) the skin. This characteristic, which it shares with the muscles of facial expression, makes the platysma difficult to dissect. It also shares with those craniofacial muscles its source of innervation: the facial nerve. The platysma is highly variable in size—its fibers may reach from the lower part of the face to the upper thorax.

E Superficial neck muscles: sternocleidomastoid and cervical part of trapezius, anterior view

Torticollis (from L. tortus = "*twisted*" and collum = "*neck*") is a contraction or shortening of the neck muscles causing the head to remain tilted to the affected side, and rotated to the other (contralateral) side. The condition is also called wryneck. It can also be caused by damage to the innervation of the sternocleidomastoid (see p. 19). Congenital torticollis can involve degenerative scarring and shortening of the sternocleidomastoid on one side (see p. 43).

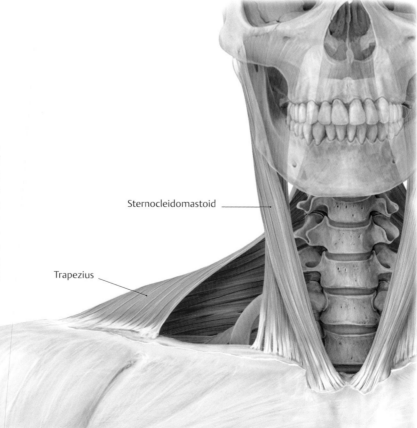

Sternocleidomastoid

Trapezius

1.3   Suprahyoid and Infrahyoid Muscles

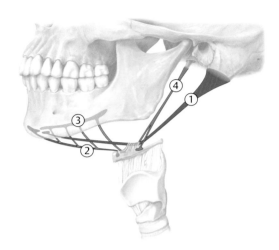

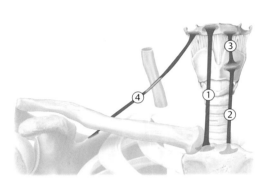

A Overview of the suprahyoid muscles

B Schematic of the infrahyoid muscles

① Digastric muscle

Origin:	• Anterior belly: digastric fossa of the mandible
	• Posterior belly: medial to the mastoid process (mastoid notch)
Insertion:	Body of the hyoid bone via an intermediate tendon with a fibrous loop
Actions:	• Elevates the hyoid bone (during swallowing)
	• Assists in opening the mandible
Innervation:	• Anterior belly: Mylohyoid nerve (from the mandibular nerve, a division of CN V)
	• Posterior belly: fascial nerve (CN VII)

② Geniohyoid muscle

Origin:	Inferior mental spine of the mandible
Insertion:	Body of the hyoid bone
Actions:	• Draws the hyoid bone forward (during swallowing)
	• Assists in opening the mandible
Innervation:	Ventral ramus of C 1

③ Mylohyoid muscle

Origin:	Mylohyoid line of the mandible
Insertion:	Body of the hyoid bone by a median tendon of insertion (mylohyoid raphe)
Actions:	• Tightens and elevates the oral floor
	• Draws the hyoid bone forward (during swallowing)
	• Assists in opening the mandible and moving it from side to side (mastication)
Innervation:	Mylohyoid nerve (from the mandibular nerve, a division of CN V)

④ Stylohyoid muscle

Origin:	Styloid process of the temporal bone
Insertion:	Body of the hyoid bone by a split tendon
Actions:	• Elevates the hyoid bone (during swallowing)
	• Assists in opening the mandible
Innervation:	Facial nerve (CN VII)

① Sternohyoid muscle

Origin:	Posterior surface of the manubrium sterni and sternoclavicular joint
Insertion:	Body of the hyoid bone
Actions:	• Depresses (fixes) the hyoid bone
	• Depresses the larynx and hyoid bone (for phonation and the terminal phase of swallowing)
Innervation:	Ansa cervicalis of the cervical plexus (C 1–C 3)

② Sternothyroid muscle

Origin:	Posterior surface of the manubrium sterni
Insertion:	Thyroid cartilage
Actions:	• Draws the larynx and hyoid bone downward (fixes the hyoid bone)
	• Depresses the larynx and hyoid bone (for phonation and the terminal phase of swallowing)
Innervation:	Ansa cervicalis of the cervical plexus (C 1–C 3)

③ Thyrohyoid muscle

Origin:	Thyroid cartilage
Insertion:	Body of the hyoid bone
Actions:	• Depresses and fixes the hyoid bone
	• Raises the larynx during swallowing
Innervation:	Ventral ramus of C 1

④ Omohyoid muscle

Origin:	Superior border of the scapula
Insertion:	Body of the hyoid bone
Actions:	• Depresses (fixes) the hyoid bone
	• Draws the larynx and hyoid bone downward (for phonation and the terminal phase of swallowing)
	• Tenses the cervical fascia with its intermediate tendon and maintains patency of the internal jugular vein
Innervation:	Ansa cervicalis of the cervical plexus (C 1–C 3)

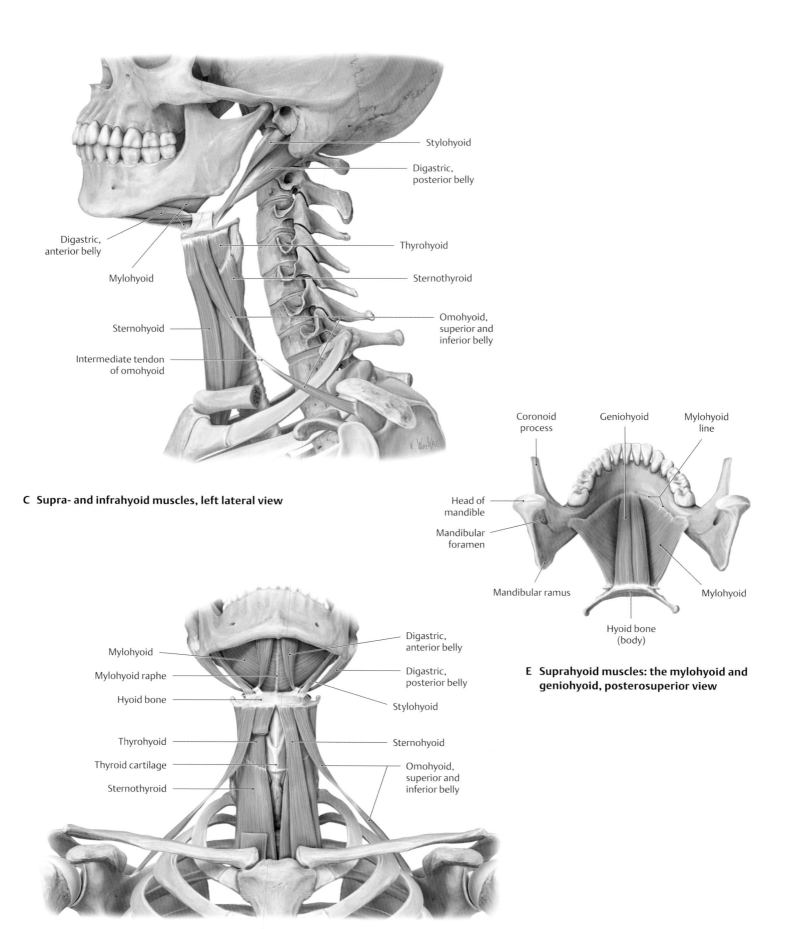

C Supra- and infrahyoid muscles, left lateral view

Labels in image C:
- Stylohyoid
- Digastric, posterior belly
- Digastric, anterior belly
- Mylohyoid
- Thyrohyoid
- Sternothyroid
- Sternohyoid
- Omohyoid, superior and inferior belly
- Intermediate tendon of omohyoid

Labels in image E:
- Coronoid process
- Geniohyoid
- Mylohyoid line
- Head of mandible
- Mandibular foramen
- Mandibular ramus
- Mylohyoid
- Hyoid bone (body)

E Suprahyoid muscles: the mylohyoid and geniohyoid, posterosuperior view

Labels in image D:
- Mylohyoid
- Mylohyoid raphe
- Hyoid bone
- Thyrohyoid
- Thyroid cartilage
- Sternothyroid
- Digastric, anterior belly
- Digastric, posterior belly
- Stylohyoid
- Sternohyoid
- Omohyoid, superior and inferior belly

D Supra- and infrahyoid muscles, anterior view
Part of the sternohyoid muscle has been removed on the right side.

7

1.4 Prevertebral and Lateral (Deep) Neck Muscles

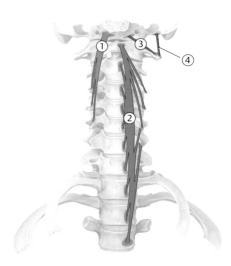

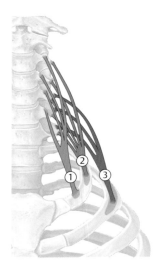

A Schematic of the prevertebral muscles

B Schematic of the lateral (deep) neck muscles

① **Longus capitis muscle**

Origin:	Anterior tubercles of the transverse processes of the C3–C6 vertebrae
Insertion:	Basilar part of the occipital bone
Actions:	• Unilateral: tilts and slightly rotates the head to the same side • Bilateral: flexes the head
Innervation:	Direct branches from the cervical plexus (C1–C3)

② **Longus colli muscle**

Origin:	• Vertical (intermediate) part: anterior surfaces of the C5–C7 and T1–T3 vertebral bodies • Superior oblique part: anterior tubercles of the transverse processes of the C3–C5 vertebrae • Inferior oblique part: anterior surfaces of the T1–T3 vertebral bodies
Insertion:	• Vertical part: anterior surfaces of the C2–C4 vertebrae • Superior oblique part: anterior tubercle of the atlas • Inferior oblique part: anterior tubercles of the transverse processes of the C5 and C6 vertebrae
Actions:	• Unilateral: tilts and rotates and cervical spine to the same side • Bilateral: flexes the cervical spine
Innervation:	Direct branches from the cervical plexus (C2–C6)

③ **Rectus capitis anterior**

Origin:	Lateral mass of the atlas
Insertion:	Basilar part of the occipital bone
Actions:	• Unilateral: lateral flexion at the atlanto-occipital joint • Bilateral: flexion at the atlanto-occipital joint
Innervation:	Ventral rami of C1 and C2

④ **Rectus capitis lateralis**

Origin:	Transverse process of the atlas
Insertion:	Basilar part of the occipital bone (lateral to the occipital condyles)
Actions:	• Unilateral: lateral flexion at the atlanto-occipital joint • Bilateral: flexion at the atlanto-occipital joint
Innervation:	Ventral rami of C1 and C2

Scalene muscles

Origin:	① Scalenus anterior: anterior tubercles of the transverse processes of the C3–C6 vertebrae ② Scalenus medius: transverse processes of atlas and axis (not depicted here: see page 9); posterior tubercles of the transverse processes of the C3–C7 vertebrae ③ Scalenus posterior: posterior tubercles of the transverse processes of the C5–C7 vertebrae
Insertion:	• Scalenus anterior: scalene tubercle on the first rib • Scalenus medius: first rib (posterior to the groove for the subclavian artery) • Scalenus posterior: outer surface of the second rib
Actions:	• With the ribs mobile: inspiration (elevates the upper ribs) • With the ribs fixed: bends the cervical spine to the same side (with unilateral contraction) • Flexes the neck (with bilateral contraction)
Innervation:	Direct branches from the cervical plexus and brachial plexus (C3–C8)

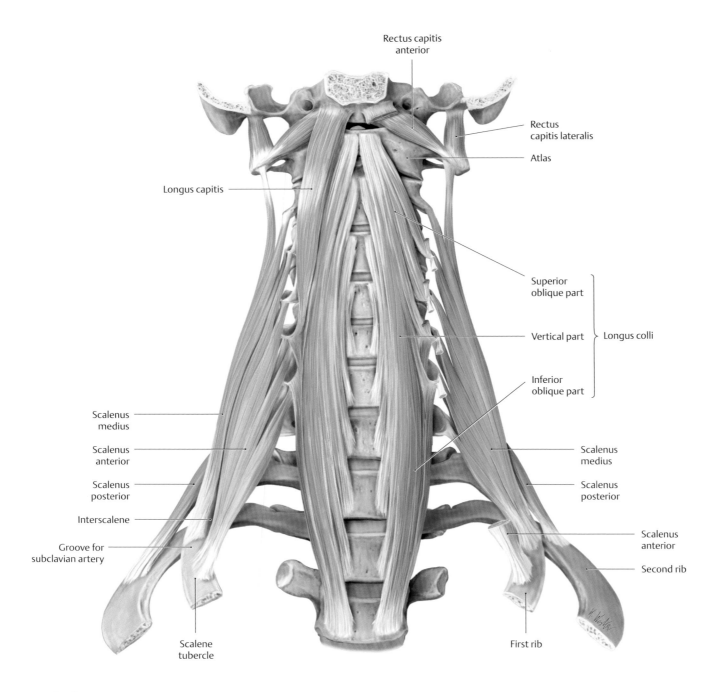

Rectus capitis anterior

Rectus capitis lateralis

Atlas

Longus capitis

Superior oblique part

Vertical part — Longus colli

Inferior oblique part

Scalenus medius

Scalenus anterior

Scalenus posterior

Interscalene

Groove for subclavian artery

Scalenus medius

Scalenus posterior

Scalenus anterior

Second rib

Scalene tubercle

First rib

C Prevertebral and lateral (deep) neck muscles, anterior view
The longus capitis and scalenus anterior muscles have been partially removed on the left side. The prevertebral muscles stretch between the cervical spine and skull, acting upon both. The three overlapping scalene muscles (the scaleni) are classified as lateral (deep) neck muscles. As they pass between the cervical spine and the upper two ribs, they also assist in respiration. The scalenus anterior and scalenus medius are separated by the *interscalene space*—a topographically important interval that is traversed by the brachial plexus and subclavian artery.

2.1   Arteries

Anterior branches
- Superior thyroid artery
  - Infrahyoid branch
  - Superior laryngeal artery
  - Cricothyroid branch
  - Sternocleidomastoid branch
  - Glandular branches
- Lingual artery*
- Facial artery*
- Ascending pharyngeal artery

Posterior branches
- Occipital artery*
- Posterior auricular artery*

Terminal branches
- Maxillary artery*
- Superficial temporal artery*

* Not visible in the dissection in **A**

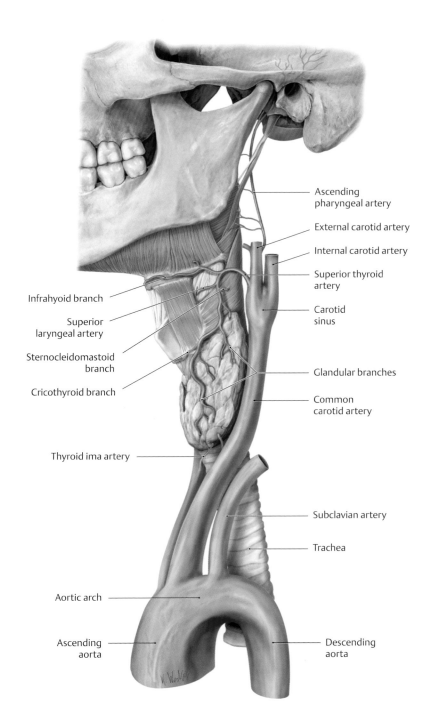

Ascending
pharyngeal artery

External carotid artery

Internal carotid artery

Superior thyroid
artery

Carotid
sinus

Glandular branches

Common
carotid artery

Subclavian artery

Trachea

Descending
aorta

Infrahyoid branch

Superior
laryngeal artery

Sternocleidomastoid
branch

Cricothyroid branch

Thyroid ima artery

Aortic arch

Ascending
aorta

C Branches of the subclavian artery

Internal thoracic artery
- Mediastinal branches
- Thymic branches
- Pericardiacophrenic branch
- Mammary branches
- Anterior intercostal branches
- Musculophrenic artery
- Superior epigastric artery

Vertebral artery
- Spinal branches
- Meningeal branch
- Posterior spinal arteries
- Anterior spinal artery
- Posterior inferior cerebellar artery
- Basilar artery

Thyrocervical trunk
- Inferior thyroid artery
  - Ascending cervical artery
- Transverse cervical artery
  - Superficial branch (superficial cervical artery)
  - Deep branch (dorsal scapular artery)
- Suprascapular artery

Costocervical trunk
- Deep cervical artery
- Supreme intercostal artery

A Common carotid and external carotid arteries and their branches in the neck

Left lateral view. Each side of the neck is traversed by two major arteries which function as "thoroughfares" to carry blood from the aortic arch to the head and brain: the common carotid artery (and the internal carotid artery arising from it) and the nevertebral artery (see **D**). The right common carotid artery arises from the brachiocephalic trunk, while the left common carotid artery branches directly from the aorta. The common carotid artery bi-furcates at approximately the level of the C 4 vertebral body into the internal and external carotid arteries. The *internal* carotid artery ascends directly to the base of the skull and enters the cranial cavity, giving off *no* branches in the neck. The *external* carotid artery gives off numerous branches in the head and neck (see **B**). The cervical part of this artery mainly supplies anterior structures in the neck, including the cervical viscera. Both carotid arteries are enclosed in a fibrous expansion of the cervical fascia, the carotid sheath (see p. 2).

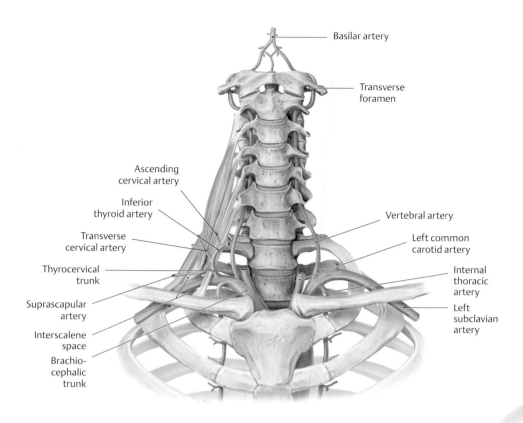

D Subclavian artery and its branches

Anterior view. The subclavian artery distributes a number of branches to structures located at the base of the neck and about the thoracic inlet. Two branches of special importance are the thyrocervical trunk, which gives origin to the transverse cervical artery, and the costocervical trunk (see **C** and **E**).

Note that the branches of the subclavian artery may arise in a variable sequence.

After emerging from the thoracic inlet, the subclavian artery passes through the interscalene space (between the scalenus anterior and medius muscles, see p. 8) to the arm. The *vertebral artery* arises from the posterior aspect of the subclavian artery on each side and ascends through the foramina in the transverse processes of the cervical vertebrae. After entering the skull, both vertebral arteries unite with the two internal carotid arteries, forming anastomoses (circle of Willis) that have major clinical importance in supplying blood to the brain.

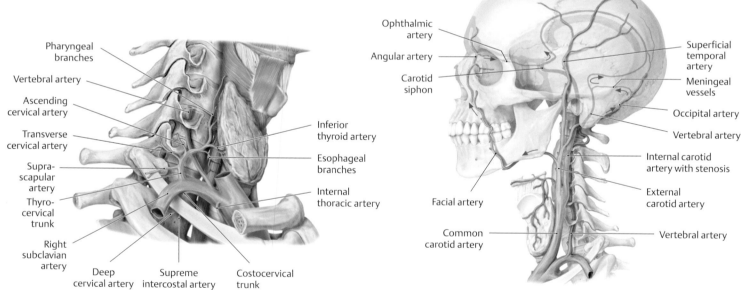

E Thyrocervical trunk and costocervical trunk and their branches

Right lateral view. The thyrocervical trunk arises from the subclavian artery and divides into the inferior thyroid artery, transverse cervical artery, and suprascapular artery. It mainly supplies structures located at the lateral base of the neck and is variable in its development.

The costocervical trunk arises posteriorly from the subclavian artery at the level of the scalenus anterior muscle. It divides into the deep cervical artery and supreme intercostal artery, supplying blood to the posterior neck muscles and the first intercostal space.

F Collateral pathways that develop in response to internal carotid artery stenosis

Atherosclerosis of the internal carotid artery is a frequent clinical problem. Narrowing of the carotid lumen (stenosis) eventually results in decreased blood flow to the brain. If the lumen is occluded suddenly, the result is a stroke. But if the stenosis develops over time, blood can still reach the brain through the gradual recruitment of collateral channels. As this occurs, the direction of blood flow may become reversed in anastomotic areas close to the brain (see arrows). As long as an adequate collateral circulation is maintained, the stenosis does not produce clinical manifestations.

The principal collateral pathways are as follows:

- Ophthalmic collaterals: external carotid artery → facial artery → angular artery → ophthalmic artery → carotid siphon
- Occipital anastomosis: external carotid artery → occipital artery → small meningeal arteries → vertebral artery

11

2.2 Veins

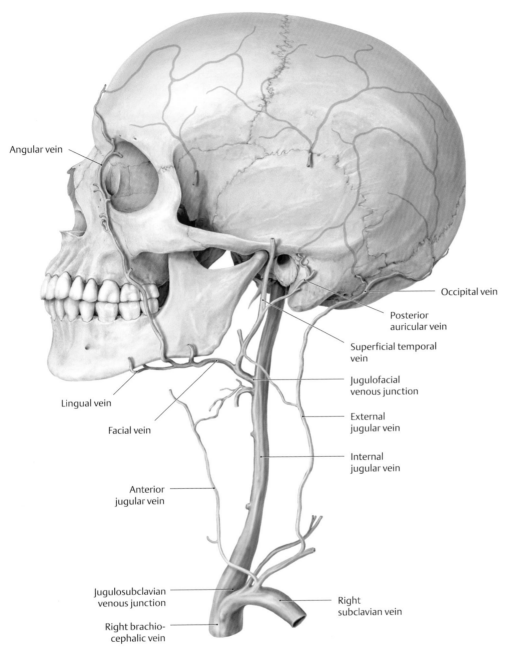

Labels on figure:
- Angular vein
- Occipital vein
- Posterior auricular vein
- Superficial temporal vein
- Jugulofacial venous junction
- Lingual vein
- External jugular vein
- Facial vein
- Internal jugular vein
- Anterior jugular vein
- Jugulosubclavian venous junction
- Right subclavian vein
- Right brachio-cephalic vein

A Principal venous trunks in the neck
Left lateral view. Three jugular veins return blood to the superior vena cava from the head and neck region:

- The large internal jugular vein (located in the carotid sheath) drains blood from the cranial cavity (brain!), face, and thyroid gland to the subclavian vein.
- The external jugular vein (smaller than the internal jugular vein, runs superficial to the investing layer of the deep cervical fascia but deep to the platysma) typically opens into the subclavian vein and drains superficial areas located behind the ear.
- The anterior jugular vein (smallest of the three jugular veins, not always present) begins below the hyoid bone and usually terminates at the external jugular vein. It drains the superficial anterior wall of the neck.

The internal jugular vein and subclavian vein on each side unite to form the brachiocephalic vein (see **D**). The veins on the right and left sides may communicate via the jugular venous arch (see **D**).

B Principal veins in the neck, their tributaries and anastomoses
In addition to the veins listed below, there are a number of smaller veins that drain blood from adjacent structures. Since they are highly variable in their development, they are not listed here.

The cervical veins are interconnected by extensive anastomoses (not all of which are shown here, in some cases because they are too small). As a result, the ligation of one vein will not cause a serious impairment of venous return. A *venous junction* is a site where two larger veins join at an approximately 90° angle. The two principal venous junctions in the neck are the jugulofacial and the jugulosubclavian. The jugulofacial venous junction is smaller than the jugulosubclavian venous junction, which also marks the termination of the thoracic duct (see p. 48).

Tributaries of the superior vena cava
- Right brachiocephalic vein
- Left brachiocephalic vein

Tributaries of the brachiocephalic vein
- Internal jugular vein
- Subclavian vein
  - External jugular vein
- Thyroid venous plexus (usually drains to left brachiocephalic vein)
- Vertebral vein
- Internal thoracic veins

Tributaries of the internal jugular vein
- Dural sinuses
- Lingual vein
- Superior thyroid vein
- Facial vein
  - Angular vein (anastomosis with ophthalmic vein)
  - Retromandibular vein
  - Superficial temporal veins (anastomoses with pterygoid plexus)
- Posterior auricular vein

Tributaries of the external jugular vein
- Occipital vein

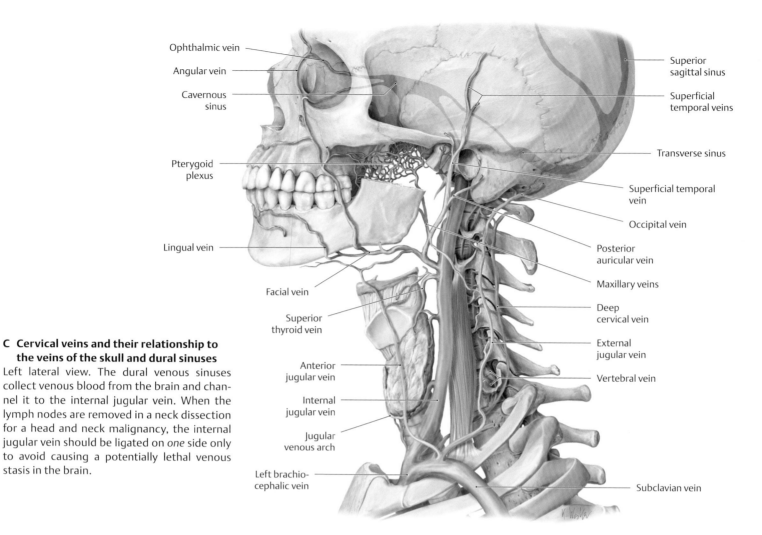

C Cervical veins and their relationship to the veins of the skull and dural sinuses

Left lateral view. The dural venous sinuses collect venous blood from the brain and channel it to the internal jugular vein. When the lymph nodes are removed in a neck dissection for a head and neck malignancy, the internal jugular vein should be ligated on *one* side only to avoid causing a potentially lethal venous stasis in the brain.

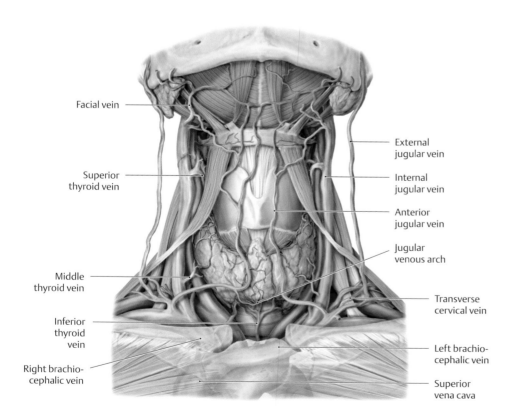

D Cervical veins

Anterior view. Most veins in the neck are valveless "thoroughfares" that drain blood from the head. They are minimally distended and not readily visible above the plane of the heart in both the standing and sitting positions. In the supine position, however, the veins become engorged and are visible even in a healthy individual. Visible distention of cervical veins, specifically the jugular veins, in the standing position is a sign of right-sided heart failure, in which blood collects proximal to the right heart, generally due to improper functioning of the right ventricle. The internal jugular vein is a large and is frequently used as an access site for the placement of a central venous catheter in intensive care medicine, making it possible to infuse greater fluid volumes than with a peripheral venous line. The jugular venous arch forms a connecting trunk between the anterior jugular veins on each side, which creates a potential hazard for hemorrhage in tracheostomies.

2.3 Lymphatic System

Lymphatic system of the head and neck

A distinction is made between regional lymph nodes, which are associated with a particular organ or region and constitute their primary filtering stations, and collecting lymph nodes, which usually receive lymph from multiple regional lymph node groups. Lymph from the head and neck region, gathered in scattered regional nodes, flows through its system of deep cervical collecting lymph nodes, into the right and left jugular trunks, each closely associated with its corresponding internal jugular vein. The jugular trunk on the right side drains into the right lymphatic duct, which terminates at the right jugulosubclavian junction. The jugular trunk on the left side terminates at the thoracic duct, which empties into the left jugulosubclavian junction (see **D**).

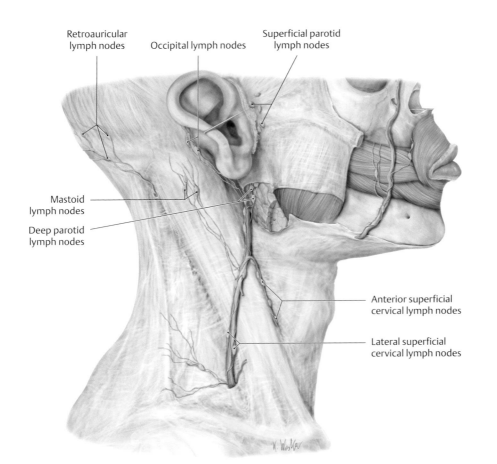

Retroauricular lymph nodes
Occipital lymph nodes
Superficial parotid lymph nodes
Mastoid lymph nodes
Deep parotid lymph nodes
Anterior superficial cervical lymph nodes
Lateral superficial cervical lymph nodes

A Superficial lymph nodes in the neck

Right lateral view. It is extremely important to know the distribution of the lymph nodes in the neck because enlarged cervical lymph nodes are a common finding at physical examination. The enlargement of cervical lymph nodes may be caused by inflammation (usually a *painful* enlargement) or neoplasia (usually a *painless* enlargement) in the area drained by the nodes. The superficial cervical lymph nodes are primary drainage locations for lymph from adjacent areas or organs.

B Deep cervical lymph nodes

Right lateral view. The deep lymph nodes in the neck consist mainly of collecting nodes. They have major clinical importance as potential sites of metastasis from head and neck tumors (see **D** and **E**). Affected deep cervical lymph nodes may be surgically removed (neck dissection) or may be treated by regional irradiation. For this purpose the American Academy of Otolaryngology, Head and Neck Surgery has grouped the deep cervical lymph nodes into six levels (Robbins 1991):

I   Submental and submandibular lymph nodes
II–IV Deep cervical lymph nodes distributed along the internal jugular vein (lateral jugular lymph nodes):
  – **II**   Deep cervical lymph nodes (upper lateral group)
  – **III** Deep cervical lymph nodes (middle lateral group)
  – **IV** Deep cervical lymph nodes (lower lateral group)
V   Lymph nodes in the posterior cervical triangle
VI Anterior cervical lymph nodes (anterior group of cervical nodes)

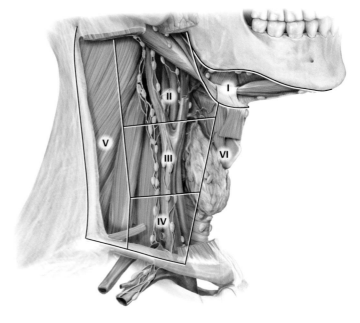

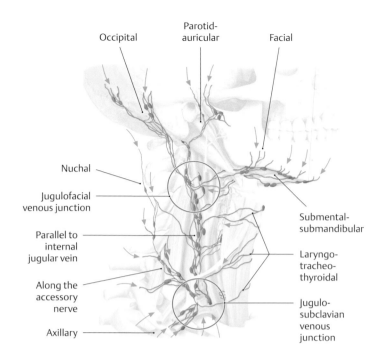

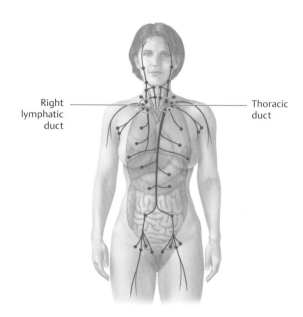

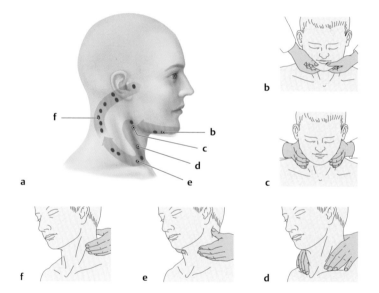

C Directions of lymphatic drainage in the neck

Right lateral view. The principal pattern of lymphatic flow in the neck is depicted. Understanding this pattern is critical to identifying the location of a potential cause of enlarged cervical lymph nodes. There are two main sites in the neck where the lymphatic pathways intersect:

- The jugulofacial venous junction: Lymphatics from the head pass obliquely downward to this site, where the lymph is redirected vertically downward in the neck.
- The jugulosubclavian venous junction: The main lymphatic trunk, the thoracic duct, terminates at this central location, where lymph collected from the left side of the head and neck region is combined with lymph draining from the rest of the body.

If only peripheral nodal groups are affected, this suggests a localized disease process. If the central groups (e.g., those at the venous junctions) are affected, this usually signifies an extensive disease process. Central lymph nodes can be obtained for diagnostic evaluation by prescalene biopsy.

D Relationship of the cervical nodes to the systemic lymphatic circulation

Anterior view. The cervical lymph nodes may be involved by diseases that are not primary to the head and neck region, because lymph from the entire body is channeled to the left and right jugulosubclavian junctions (red circles, see p. 129). This can lead to retrograde involvement of the cervical nodes. The *right lymphatic duct* terminates at the right jugulosubclavian junction, the *thoracic duct* at the left jugulosubclavian junction. Besides cranial and cervical tributaries, the lymph from thoracic lymph nodes (mediastinal and tracheobronchial) and from abdominal and caudal lymph nodes may reach the cervical nodes by way of the thoracic duct. As a result, diseases in those organs may lead to cervical lymph node enlargement.

Note: Gastric carcinoma may metastasize to the left supraclavicular group of lymph nodes, producing an enlarged *sentinel node* that suggests an abdominal tumor. Systemic lymphomas may also spread to the cervical lymph nodes by this pathway.

E Systematic palpation of the cervical lymph nodes

The cervical lymph nodes are systematically palpated during the physical examination to ensure the detection of any enlarged nodes (see **D** for the special diagnostic significance of cervical lymph nodes).

Panel **a** shows the sequence in which the various nodal groups are successively palpated, and panels **b–f** illustrate how each of the groups are palpated. The examiner usually palpates the submental-submandibular group first (**b**), including the mandibular angle (**c**), then proceeds along the anterior border of the sternocleidomastoid muscle (**d**). The supraclavicular lymph nodes are palpated next (**e**), followed by the lymph nodes along the accessory nerve and the nuchal group of nodes (**f**).

2.4 Overview of the Nervous System in the Neck and the Distribution of Spinal Nerve Branches

A Overview of the nervous system in the neck

The following structures of the peripheral nervous system are present in the neck: spinal nerves, cranial nerves, and nerves of the autonomic nervous system. The table below reviews the most important structures, following the sequence in which they are discussed in the next sections.

The spinal nerves that supply the neck arise from the C1–C4 segments of the cervical spinal cord. The spinal nerves divide into dorsal rami and ventral rami:

- The dorsal rami of the spinal nerves arising from the C1–C3 spinal cord segments (suboccipital nerve, greater occipital nerve, third occipital nerve) supply motor innervation to the intrinsic nuchal muscles and sensory innervation to the C2 and C3 dermatomes on the back of the neck and the occiput (see **B**).
- The ventral rami of the spinal nerves arising from the C1–C4 spinal cord segments supply motor innervation to the deep neck muscles (short, direct branches from the ventral rami) and finally unite in the neck to form the cervical plexus (see **C**). This plexus supplies the skin and musculature of the anterior and lateral neck (all but the nuchal region).

The neck contains the following cranial nerves, which arise from the brainstem:

- Glossopharyngeal nerve (CN IX)
- Vagus nerve (CN X)
- Accessory nerve (CN XI)
- Hypoglossal nerve (CN XII)

These nerves supply motor and sensory innervation to the pharynx and larynx (CN IX and X) and motor innervation to the trapezius and sternocleidomastoid muscles (CN XI), lingual muscles (CN XII), and floor of the mouth.

The **sympathetic trunk** is part of the autonomic nervous system, consisting of a nerve cord with three ganglia that extends along the vertebral column on each side. The postganglionic fibers course with the carotid arteries to their territories in the head and neck region.

Another part of the autonomic nervous system, the **parasympathetic system**, is represented in the neck by the vagus nerve.

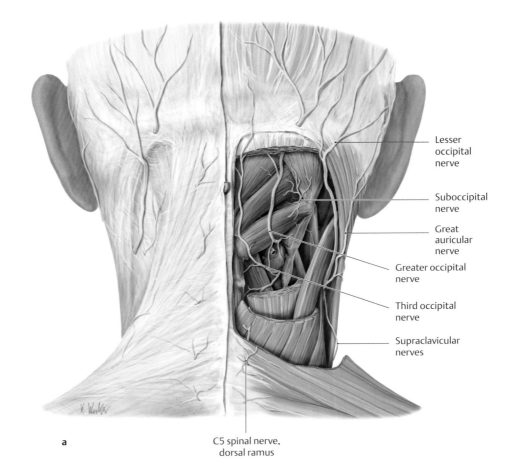

Lesser occipital nerve

Suboccipital nerve

Great auricular nerve

Greater occipital nerve

Third occipital nerve

Supraclavicular nerves

a

C5 spinal nerve, dorsal ramus

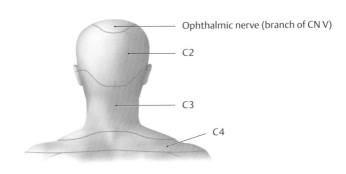

Ophthalmic nerve (branch of CN V)

C2

C3

C4

b

B Motor and sensory innervation of the nuchal region

Posterior view. **a** Spinal nerve branches in the nuchal region. **b** Segmental distribution.

The nuchal region receives most of its motor and sensory innervation from *dorsal* rami of the cervical spinal nerves arising from the C1–C3 cord segments:

- Suboccipital nerve (C1)
- Greater occipital nerve (C2)
- Third occipital nerve (C3)

Note their subcutaneous course on the left side (**a**). The following nerves are derived from *ventral* rami of the cervical spinal nerves and enter the nuchal region from the lateral side:

- Lesser occipital nerve
- Great auricular nerve

Note: The dorsal ramus of the first cervical spinal nerve (the suboccipital nerve) is purely motor (see **a**), and consequently there is no C1 dermatome.

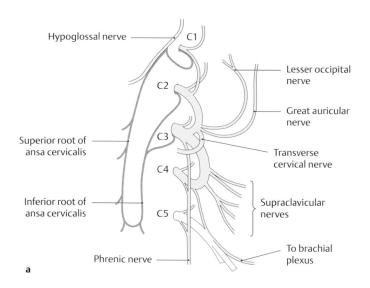

a

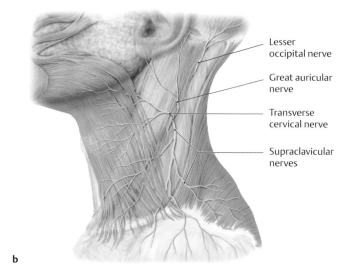

b

C Motor and sensory innervation of the anterior and lateral neck
The anterolateral portions of the neck, unlike the nuchal region and occiput, are supplied entirely by *ventral* rami of the C1–C4 cervical spinal nerves. These rami distribute short branches to the deep neck muscles (see **c**). They also give off branches that form the cervical plexus, which consists of a sensory part and a motor part supplying the skin and muscles of the neck.

a Branching pattern of the cervical plexus (viewed from the left side). The motor fibers from C1–C3 form the ansa cervicalis, which innervates the infrahyoid muscles (see **c**). The fibers from C1 course briefly with the hypoglossal nerve, without exchanging fibers with it, before they separate to form the *superior root* of the ansa cervicalis, which supplies the omohyoid, sternothyroid and sternohyoid muscles. Only the fibers for the thyrohyoid and geniohyoid muscles continue to course with the hypoglossal nerve. Other fibers from C2 unite with the fibers from C3 to form the *inferior root* of the ansa cervicalis. The bulk of the fibers from C4 descend in the phrenic nerve to the diaphragm (see **D**).

b Sensory innervation of the anterior and lateral neck (viewed from the left side). Erb's point is located approximately at the mid-posterior border of the sternocleidomastoid muscle, and is the site where the following nerves of the cervical plexus emerge to supply sensory innervation to the anterior and lateral neck (the *sensory part* of the cervical plexus):

- Lesser occipital nerve
- Great auricular nerve with its anterior and posterior branches
- Transverse cervical nerve
- Supraclavicular nerves

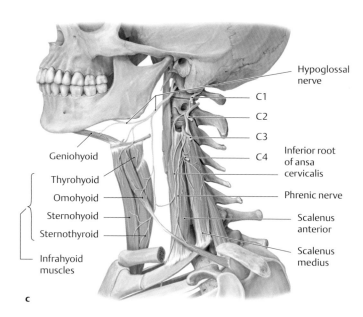

c

c Motor innervation of the anterior and lateral neck. Most of the anterior and lateral neck muscles are supplied by ventral rami of the spinal nerves. Their motor fibers either pass directly as short fibers from the ventral rami to the deep neck muscles or combine to form the *motor root* of the cervical plexus.

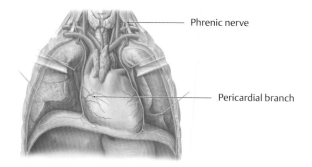

D Phrenic nerve
Anterior view. The phrenic nerve arises from the C3, 4, and 5 ventral roots ("C3, 4 and 5 keep the diaphragm alive"), with the major contribution from C4. It descends through the cervical region in front of the scalenus anterior, behind the sternocleidomastoid, through the thoracic inlet to the diaphragm, which it provides with motor innervation. Although this is an unusual anatomical relation between nerve origin and target location in the adult, the embryonic diaphragm develops from a precursor (the septum transversum) at the cervical level, and carries its innervation with it as it migrates. If the C4 segment of the spinal cord (the main root of the phrenic nerve) sustains bilateral injury in an accident, the victim will usually die at the scene from asphyxiation brought on by paralysis of the diaphragm.

17

2.5 Cranial Nerves and Autonomic Nervous System in the Neck

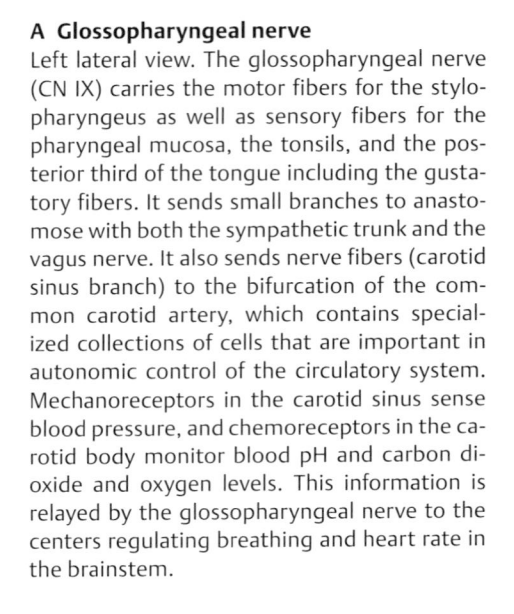
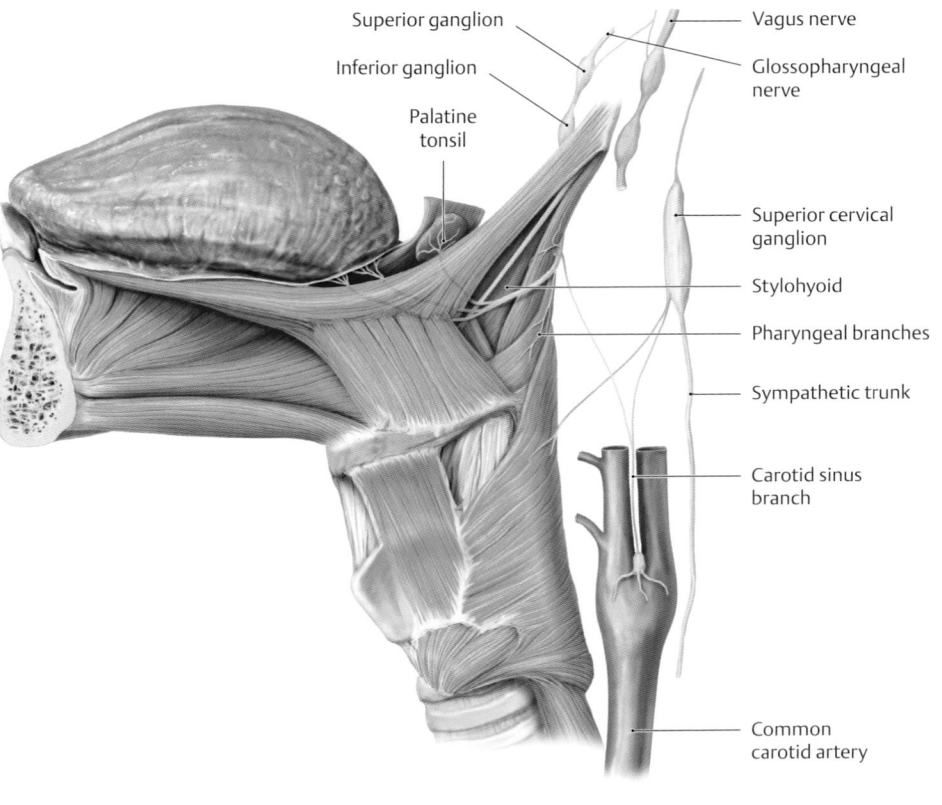

A Glossopharyngeal nerve
Left lateral view. The glossopharyngeal nerve (CN IX) carries the motor fibers for the stylopharyngeus as well as sensory fibers for the pharyngeal mucosa, the tonsils, and the posterior third of the tongue including the gustatory fibers. It sends small branches to anastomose with both the sympathetic trunk and the vagus nerve. It also sends nerve fibers (carotid sinus branch) to the bifurcation of the common carotid artery, which contains specialized collections of cells that are important in autonomic control of the circulatory system. Mechanoreceptors in the carotid sinus sense blood pressure, and chemoreceptors in the carotid body monitor blood pH and carbon dioxide and oxygen levels. This information is relayed by the glossopharyngeal nerve to the centers regulating breathing and heart rate in the brainstem.

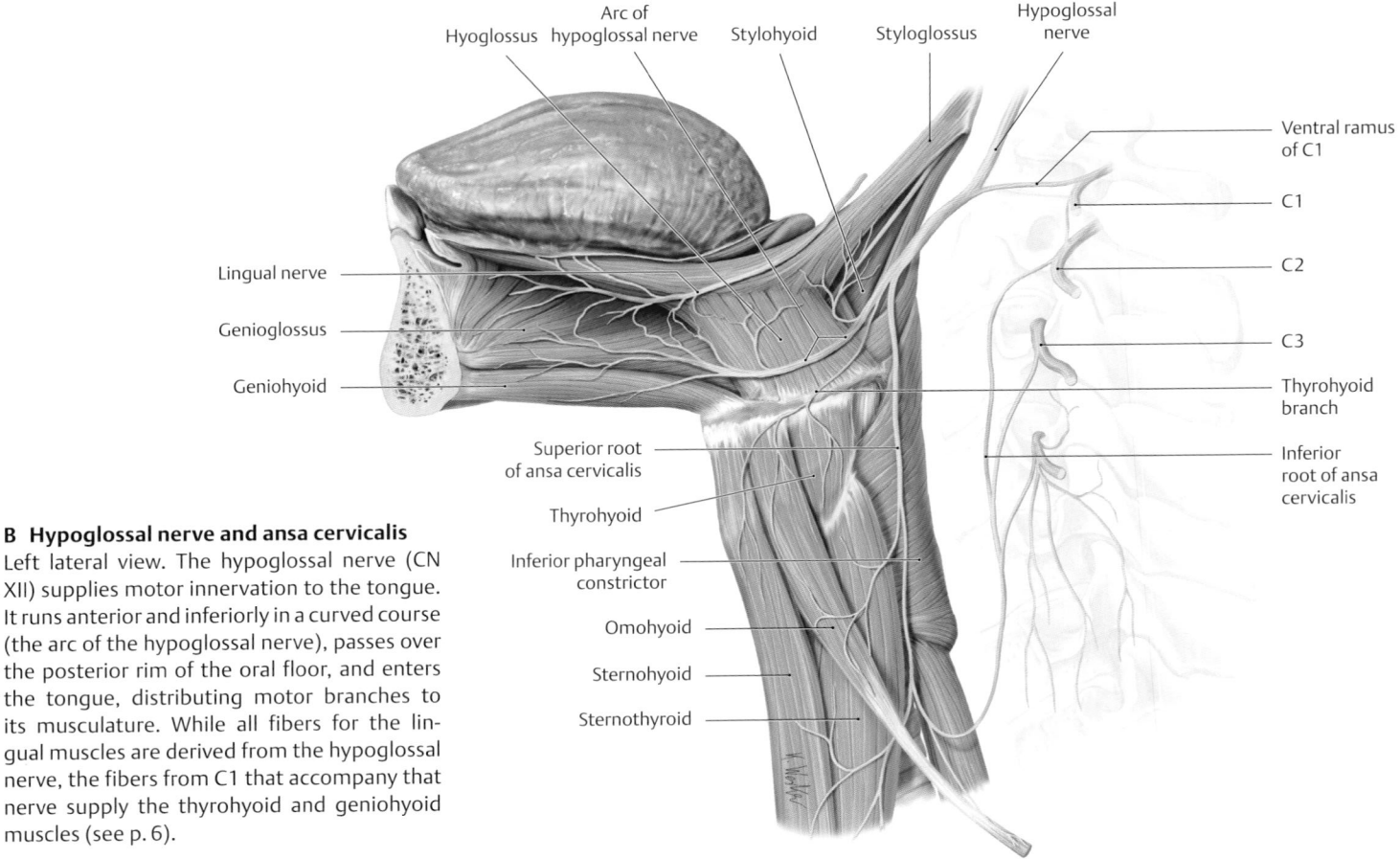

B Hypoglossal nerve and ansa cervicalis
Left lateral view. The hypoglossal nerve (CN XII) supplies motor innervation to the tongue. It runs anterior and inferiorly in a curved course (the arc of the hypoglossal nerve), passes over the posterior rim of the oral floor, and enters the tongue, distributing motor branches to its musculature. While all fibers for the lingual muscles are derived from the hypoglossal nerve, the fibers from C1 that accompany that nerve supply the thyrohyoid and geniohyoid muscles (see p. 6).

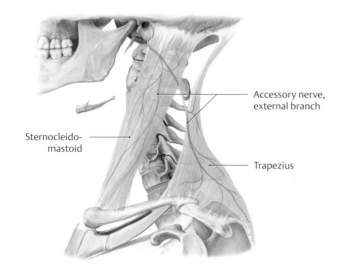

C Accessory nerve in the neck

Left lateral view. The accessory nerve (CN XI) is purely motor. Some of its fibers enter the sternocleidomastoid muscle from behind while others continue on to the trapezius. A deep (prescalene) lymph node biopsy may injure the accessory nerve in the neck. Damage to the fibers supplying the trapezius results in lateral rotation of the scapula and some shoulder drop. Damage to the fibers supplying the sternocleidomastoid leads to weakness in turning the head to the opposite side.

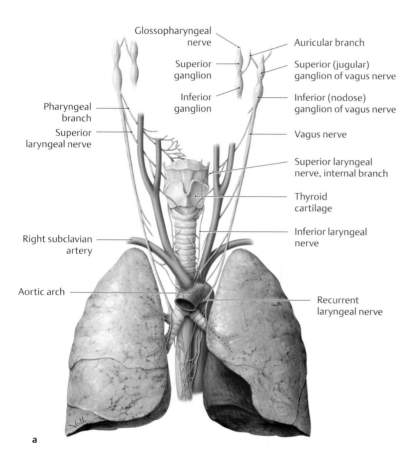

a

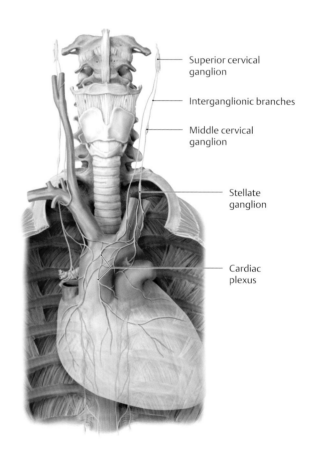

b

D Vagus nerve in the neck and the cervical sympathetic trunk

a Anterior view. The vagus nerve (CN X) conveys the fibers of the cranial portion of the parasympathetic nervous system (part of the autonomic nervous system) that supply the neck, thorax, and parts of the abdominal cavity. It passes down the neck in the carotid sheath (see topographical anatomy, p. 47), giving off only a few branches in the head and neck:

- The auricular branch, a sensory branch that supplies the posterior surface of the ear and the external auditory canal
- The pharyngeal branch, which supplies motor innervation to the muscles of the pharynx and soft palate
- The superior laryngeal nerve, a mixed sensory and somatomotor nerve that supplies the cricothyroid muscle and the surrounding mucosa

- The recurrent laryngeal nerve and its terminal branch, the inferior laryngeal nerve, which supplies the somatomotor pharyngeal muscles and the surrounding mucosa (see p. 30). The recurrent laryngeal nerve winds around the subclavian artery on the right side and around the aortic arch on the left side.

b Anterior view. The paravertebral chain of sympathetic ganglia terminates in the cervical region in the superior cervical ganglion, approximately 2 cm below the base of the skull, deep to the bifurcation of the common carotid artery. Postganglionic fibers from this ganglion follow both the internal and external carotid arteries to provide sympathetic innervation to the entire cranial vasculature, to the iris, and to glands and mucosa in the head. The lowest of the cervical ganglia in the paravertebral chain is often fused with the first thoracic sympathetic ganglion to form a stellate ganglion.

19

3.1 Embryology

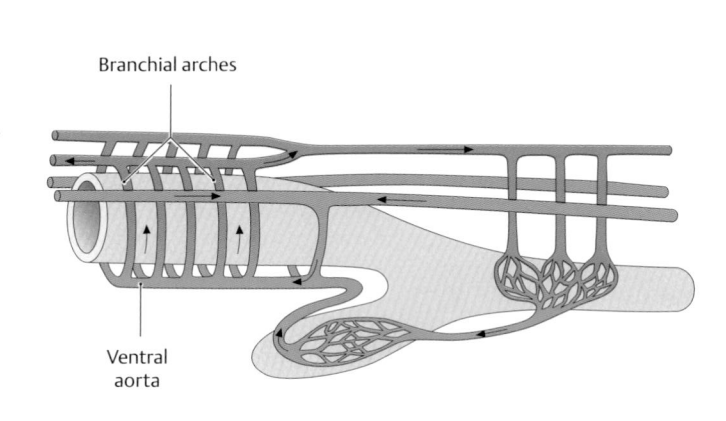

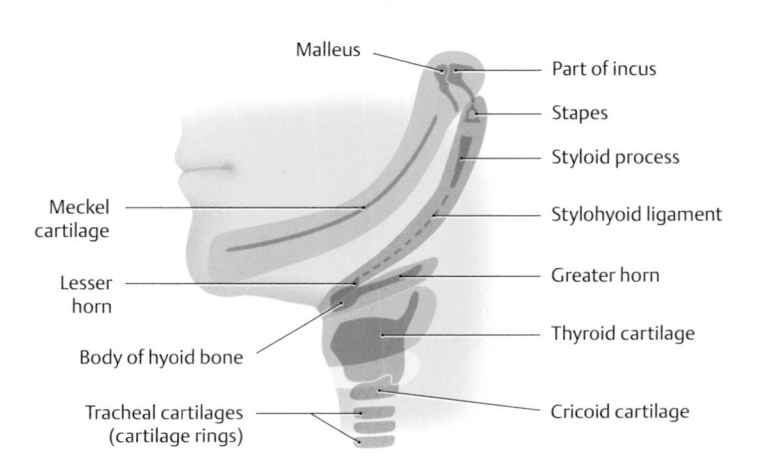

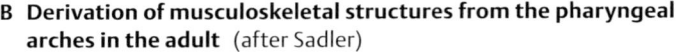

A The branchial arches of the lancelet
(after Romer, Parsons, and Frick)

Left lateral view. This simplified schematic of the circulatory system of a lancelet fish illustrates the basic relation between the vascular tree and the branchial arches in chordates, including the vertebrates. Oxygen-depleted blood (in blue) is pumped rostrally (toward the head) through a ventral aorta to a series of branchial arches, where it passes through gills, picks up oxygen (red), and then is distributed to the body (compare this paired, segmental arterial arch with the thoracic segment in humans). A similar anatomical organization and circulatory pattern is seen in the human embryo, where the gills and branchial arches are transformed into pharyngeal arches which develop into various structures in the head and neck. Errors during this developmental process give rise to a series of relatively common anatomical anomalies in the neck (see **G**).

B Derivation of musculoskeletal structures from the pharyngeal arches in the adult (after Sadler)

Left lateral view. Besides the cartilaginous rudiments of the skeleton (see labels), the muscles and their associated nerves can be traced embryologically to specific pharyngeal arches. The first pharyngeal arch gives rise to the masticatory muscles, the mylohyoid muscle, the anterior belly of the digastric muscle, the tensor veli palatini, and the tensor tympani. The second pharyngeal arch gives origin to the muscles of facial expression, the posterior belly of the digastric, the stylohyoid muscle, and the stapedius. The stylopharyngeus muscle is derived from the third pharyngeal arch. The fourth and sixth pharyngeal arches give rise to the cricothyroid muscle, levator levi palatini, constrictor pharyngis, and the intrinsic muscles of the larynx. The nerve supply to the muscles can also be explained in terms of their embryologic origins (see **D**).

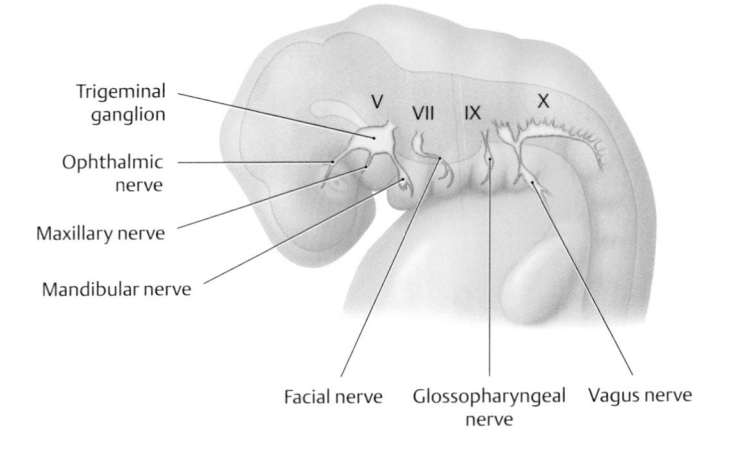

C Pharyngeal arches and pharyngeal clefts of a 4-week-old embryo (after Sadler)

Left lateral view. The human embryo has four pharyngeal arches separated by intervening pharyngeal clefts. The cartilages of the four pharyngeal arches are shown in different colors. Like other tissues of the pharyngeal arches, they migrate with further development to form various skeletal and ligamentous elements in the adult (see **B**).

D Innervation of the pharyngeal arches

Left lateral view. Each of the pharyngeal arches is associated with a cranial nerve (see *Thieme Atlas* Vol. I, General Anatomy and Musculoskeletal System):

First pharyngeal arch	Trigeminal nerve (CN V) (mandibular nerve)
Second pharyngeal arch	Facial nerve (CN VII)
Third pharyngeal arch	Glossopharyngeal nerve (CN IX)
Fourth and sixth pharyngeal arches	Vagus nerve (CN X) (superior and inferior laryngeal nerve)

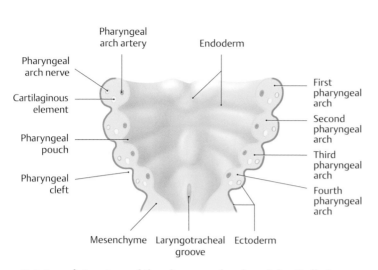

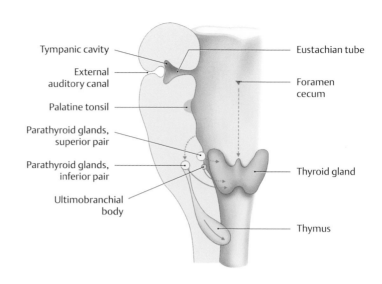

E Internal structure of the pharyngeal arches (after Sadler)

Anterior view (plane of section shown in **C**). The pharyngeal arches are covered externally by ectoderm and internally by endoderm. Each pharyngeal arch contains an arch artery, an arch nerve, and a cartilaginous element, all of which are surrounded by mesodermal and muscular tissue. The external furrows are called the pharyngeal clefts, and the internal furrows are called the pharyngeal pouches. The endodermal lining of the pharingeal pouches develops into endocrine glands of the neck, a process which may involve significant migration of cells from their site of origin.

F Migratory movements of the pharyngeal arch tissues (after Sadler)

Anterior view. During embryonic development, the epithelium from which the thyroid gland is formed migrates from its site of origin on the basal midline of the tongue to the level of the first tracheal cartilage, where the thyroid gland is located in postnatal life. As the thyroid tissue buds off from the tongue base, it leaves a vestigial depression on the dorsum of the tongue, the foramen cecum. The parathyroid glands are derived from the fourth pharyngeal arch (superior pair) or third pharyngeal arch (inferior pair), which also gives origin to the thymus (see p. 132). The ultimobranchial body, whose cells migrate into the thyroid gland to form the calcitonin-producing C cells or parafollicular cells, is derived from the fifth, vestigial, pharyngeal arch. The latter arch is the last to develop and is usually considered part of the fourth pharyngeal arch. The external auditory canal is derived from the first pharyngeal cleft, the tympanic cavity and eustachian tube from the first pharyngeal pouch, and the palatine tonsil from the second pharyngeal pouch.

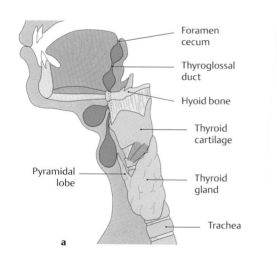

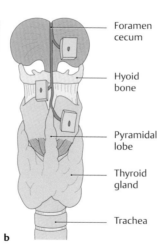

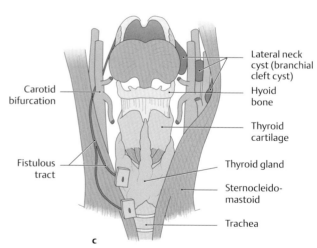

G Location of cysts and fistulas in the neck

a Median cysts, **b** median fistulas, **c** lateral fistulas and cysts.

Median cysts and fistulas in the neck (**a, b**) are remnants of the thyroglossal duct. Failure of this duct to regress completely may lead to the formation of a mucus-filled cavity (cyst), which presents clinically as a firm neck mass.

Lateral cysts and fistulas in the neck are anomalous remnants of the ductal portions of the cervical sinus, which forms as a result of tissue migrations during embryonic development. If epithelium-lined remnants persist, neck cysts (right) or fistulas (left) may appear in postnatal life (**c**). A complete fistula opens into the pharynx and onto the surface of the skin, whereas an incomplete (blind) fistula is open at one end only. The external orifice of a lateral cervical fistula is typically located at the anterior border of the sternocleidomastoid muscle.

3.2 Thyroid Gland and Parathyroid Glands

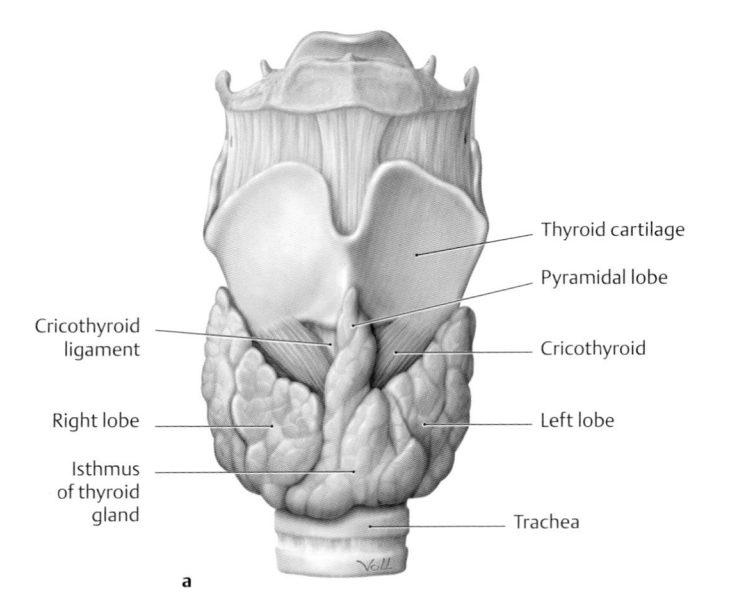

a

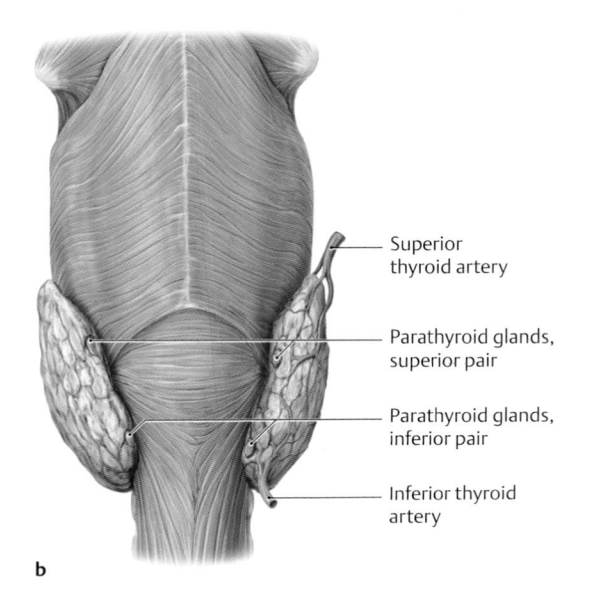

b

A Thyroid gland and parathyroid glands

a Thyroid gland, anterior view. The thyroid gland consists of two laterally situated lobes and a central narrowing or isthmus. In place of the isthmus there is often a pyramidal lobe, whose apex points cranially to the embryonic origin of the thyroid at the base of the tongue (see p. 21).

b Thyroid gland and parathyroid glands, posterior view. The parathyroid glands may show considerable variation in their number (generally four) and location.

Note: Because the parathyroid glands are usually contained within the capsule of the thyroid gland, there is a considerable risk of removing them during thyroid surgery (see **B**).

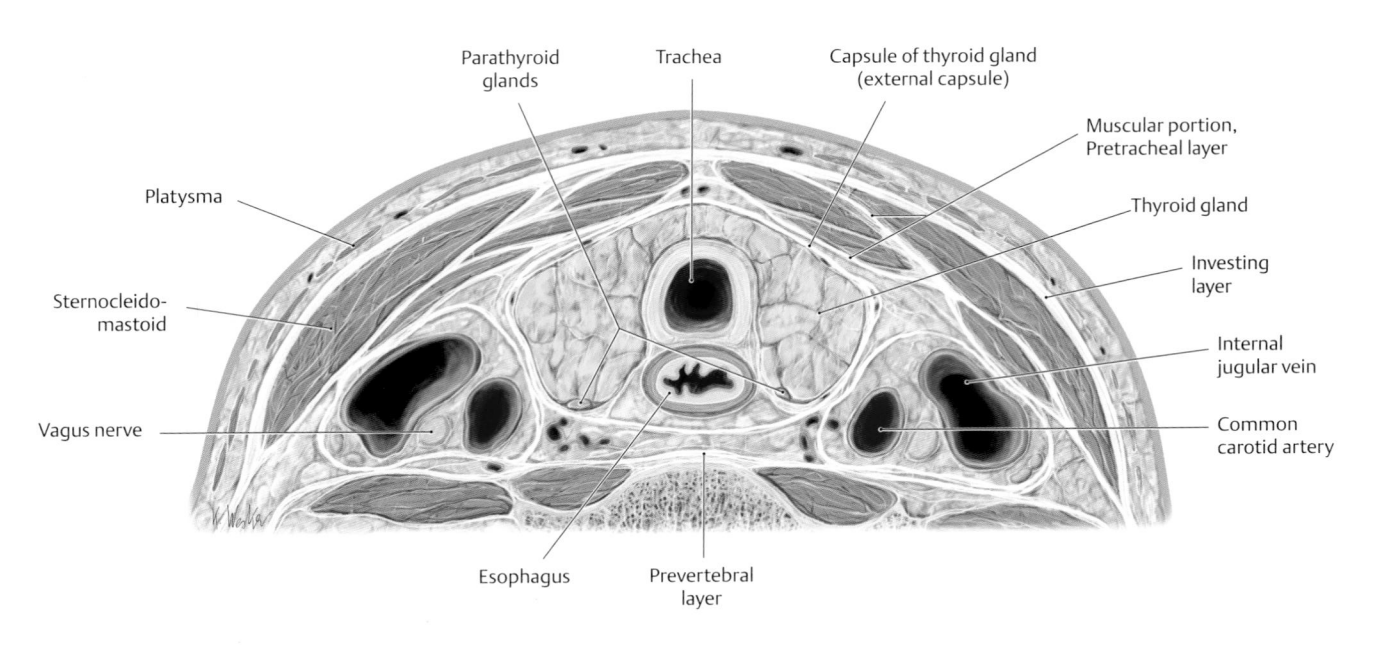

B Relationship of the thyroid gland to the trachea and neurovascular structures

Transverse section through the neck at the T 1 level, superior view. The thyroid gland partially surrounds the trachea and is bordered posterolaterally by the neurovascular bundle. When the thyroid gland is pathologically enlarged (e. g., due to iodine-deficiency goiter), it may gradually compress and narrow the tracheal lumen, causing respiratory distress.

Note the arrangement of the fasciae: The thyroid gland is surrounded by a fibrous capsule composed of an internal and external layer. The delicate internal layer (*internal capsule*, not shown here) directly invests the thyroid gland and is fused with its glandular parenchyma. Vascularized fibrous slips extend from the internal capsule into the substance of the gland, subdividing it into lobules. The internal capsule is covered by the tough *external capsule*, which is part of the pretracheal layer of the deep cervical fascia. This capsule invests the thyroid gland and parathyroid glands and is also called the "surgical capsule" because it must be opened to gain surgical access to the thyroid gland. Between the external and internal capsules is a potential space that is traversed by vascular branches and is occupied by the parathyroid glands.

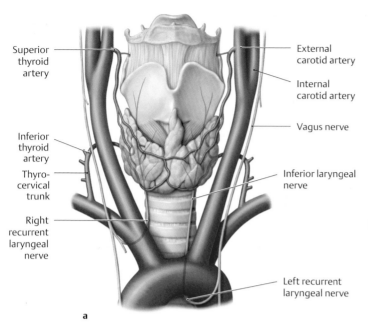

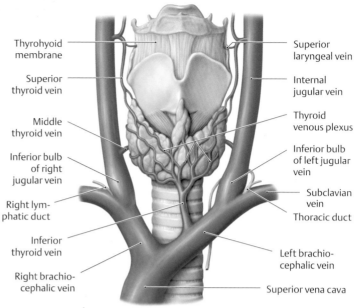

a

b

C Blood supply and innervation of the thyroid gland
Anterior view.

a **Arterial supply:** The thyroid gland derives most of its arterial blood supply from the superior thyroid artery (the first branch of the external carotid artery), which runs forward and downward to supply the gland. It is supplied from below by the inferior thyroid artery, which branches from the thyrocervical trunk (see p. 48). All of these arteries, which course on the right and left sides of the organ, must be ligated during surgical removal of the thyroid gland.
Note: Operations on the thyroid gland carry a risk of injury to the recurrent (inferior) laryngeal nerve, which is closely related to the posterior surface of the gland. Because it supplies important laryngeal muscles, unilateral injury to the nerve will cause postoperative hoarseness while bilateral injury may additionally result in dyspnea (difficulty in breathing). Prior to thyroid surgery, therefore, an otolaryngologist should confirm the integrity of the nerve supply to the laryngeal muscles and exclude any preexisting nerve lesion.

b **Venous drainage:** The thyroid gland is drained anteroinferiorly by a well-developed *thyroid venous plexus*, which usually drains through the inferior thyroid vein to the left brachiocephalic vein. Blood from the thyroid gland also drains to the internal jugular vein via the superior and middle thyroid veins.

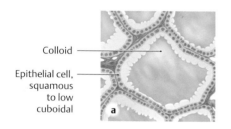

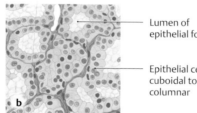

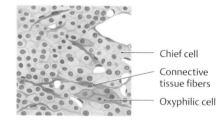

D Histology of the thyroid gland
The thyroid gland absorbs iodide from the blood and uses it to make the thyroid hormones, thyroxine (T 4, tetraiodothyronine) and triiodothyronine (T 3). These hormones are stored at extracellular sites in the gland, bound to protein, and when needed they are mobilized from the thyroid follicles and secreted into the bloodstream. A special feature of the thyroid gland is the appearance of its epithelium, which varies depending on whether it is storing hormones or releasing them into the blood. The epithelial cells are flattened or squamous when in their resting or "storage state" (**a**), but they are columnar when in their active or "secretory state" (**b**). The epithelial morphology thus indicates the current functional state of the cells. Iodine deficiency causes an enlargement of the colloidal follicular lumen, which eventually results in a gross increase in the size of the thyroid (goiter). With prolonged iodine deficiency there is a reduction in body metabolism, and concomitant lethargy, fatigue, and mental depression. Conversely, hyperactivity of the thyroid, as in Graves' disease (an autoimmune disorder), causes a generalized metabolic acceleration, with irritability and weight loss. In the midst of the thyroid follicles are parafollicular cells (C cells), which secrete calcitonin. Calcitonin inhibits bone resorption and reduces the calcium concentration in the blood.

E Histology of the parathyroid gland
The principal cell type in the parathyroid gland is the *chief cell*, which responds directly to low blood calcium levels by secreting parathyroid hormone (PTH, parathormone). Parathyroid hormone increases calcium concentration in the blood by various means, including the stimulation of bone resorption by osteoclasts and the renal tubular reabsorption of calcium. Parathyroid hormone thus acts antagonistically against calcitonin produced by the thyroid's C cells. Inadvertent removal of the parathyroid glands during thyroid surgery can cause a dramatic fall in serum calcium, with catastrophic consequences. Such a *hypocalcemic* condition causes neuromuscular irritability and, potentially, generalized fatal seizures involving respiratory muscles. Conversely, pathological hyperactivity of the parathyroid can lead to chronic *hypercalcemia*, often associated with bone loss (osteoporosis) and abnormal calcium deposition in the circulatory and urinary systems. Chronic hyperparathyroidism with hypertrophy of chief cells and elevated serum calcium is a common consequence of end-stage renal failure, by a mechanism not clearly established.

3.3 Larynx: Location, Shape, and Laryngeal Cartilages

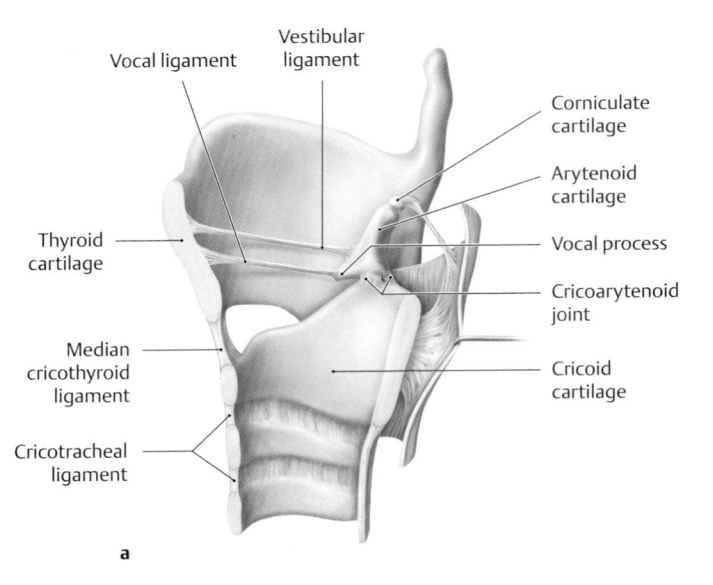

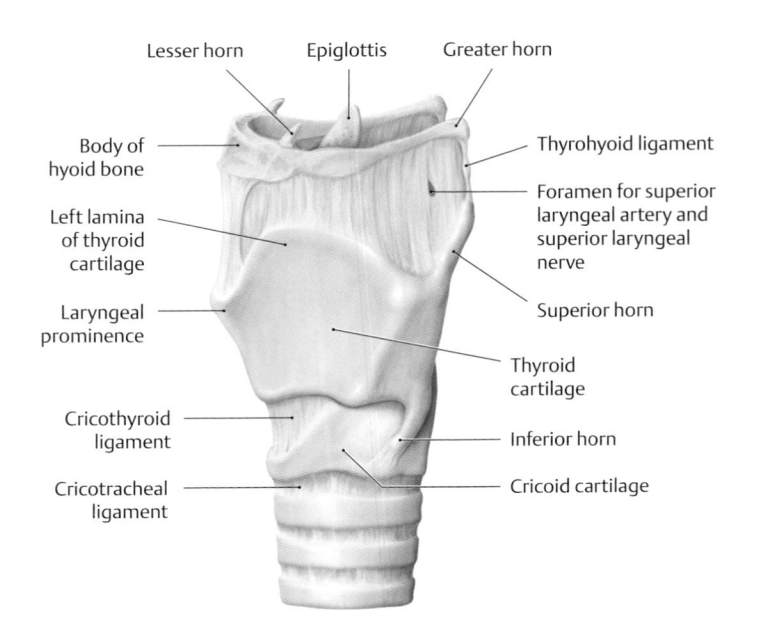

A Location of the larynx in the neck
Anterior view. In the adult male, when the head is upright and the larynx is centered in the neck:

- The hyoid bone is at the level of the C 3 vertebra.
- The superior border of the thyroid cartilage is at the C 4 level.
- The laryngotracheal junction is at the C 6–C 7 level.

These structures are located approximately one-half vertebra higher in women and children. The upper part of the larynx (the thyroid cartilage, see **B**) is especially prominent in the male, forming the laryngeal prominence or "Adam's apple."

B General features of the larynx
Left anterior oblique view. The following cartilaginous structures of the larynx can be identified in this view:

- Epiglottis (see **D**)
- Thyroid cartilage (see **E**)
- Cricoid cartilage (see **F**)

These cartilages are connected to one another and to the trachea and hyoid bone by elastic ligaments, which allow some degree of laryngeal motion during swallowing (see p. 37). The arytenoid cartilages and corniculate cartilage are not visible in this view (see **G**).

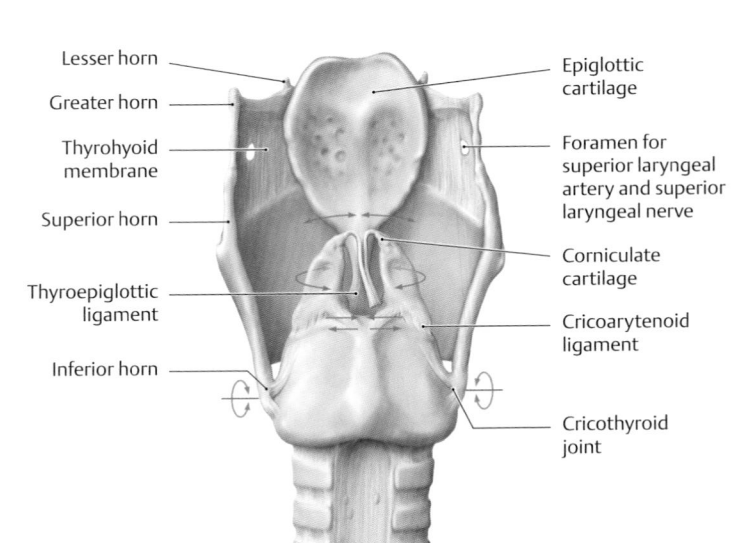

C Laryngeal cartilages and ligaments
a Sagittal section, viewed from the left medial aspect. The thyroid cartilage encloses most of the laryngeal cartilages, its inferior part articulating with the cricoid cartilage (cricothyroid joint).
b Posterior view. Arrows indicate the directions of movement in the various joints. The thyroid cartilage can tilt relative to the cricoid car-

tilage in the cricothyroid joint. The base of the arytenoid cartilage on each side can translate or rotate relative to the upper edge of the cricoid cartilage at the cricoarytenoid joint. The arytenoid cartilages move during phonation.

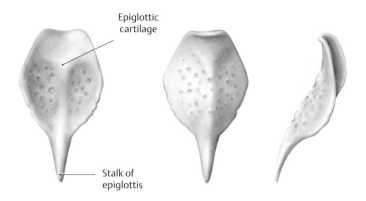

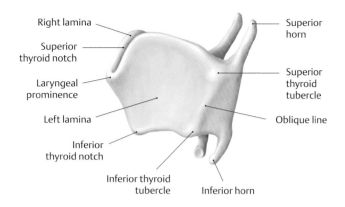

D Epiglottic cartilage

Laryngeal, lingual, and left lateral views. The internal skeleton of the epiglottis is composed of the elastic cartilage shown here (the epiglottic cartilage). This cartilage enables the epiglottis to return spontaneously to its initial position at the end of swallowing (when muscular traction is lost). If the epiglottis is removed as part of a tumor resection, the patient must go through an arduous process of learning how to swallow effectively without an epiglottis, avoiding aspiration of ingested material into the trachea.

E Thyroid cartilage

Left oblique view. This hyaline cartilage consists of two quadrilateral plates, the right and left laminae, which are joined in the midline to form a keel-shaped projection. At the upper end of this junction is the laryngeal prominence, called the "Adam's apple" in the male. The posterior ends of the laminae are prolonged to form the superior and inferior horns, which serve as anchors for ligaments (see **B**).

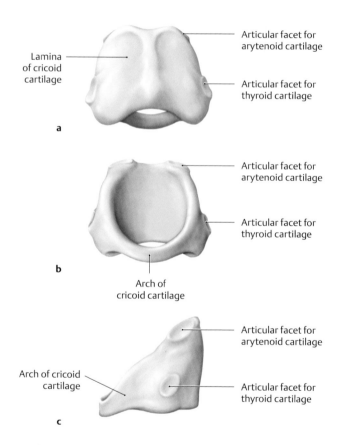

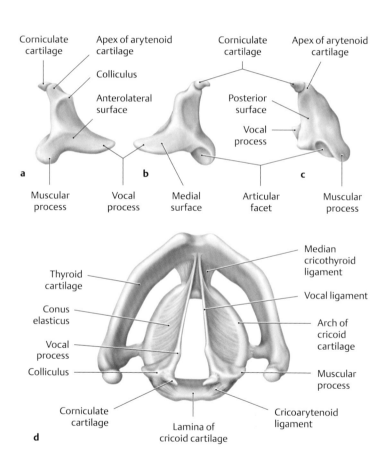

F Cricoid cartilage

Posterior view (**a**), anterior view (**b**), left lateral view (**c**). This hyaline cartilage is shaped like a signet ring. It consists posteriorly of an expanded cartilaginous plate, the lamina of the cricoid cartilage. The upper end of the plate bears an articular facet for the arytenoid cartilage, and the lower end bears a facet for the thyroid cartilage. The inferior border of the cricoid cartilage is connected to the highest tracheal cartilage by the cricotracheal ligament (see **B** and **C**).

G Arytenoid cartilage and corniculate cartilage

Right cartilages, viewed from the lateral (**a**), medial (**b**), posterior (**c**), and superior (**d**) aspects. The function of the arytenoid cartilage ("arytenoid" literally means "ladle-shaped") is to alter the position of the vocal cords during phonation (see p. 29). The pyramid-shaped, hyaline arytenoid cartilage has three surfaces (anterolateral, medial, and posterior), a base with two processes (vocal and muscular), and an apex. The apex articulates with the tiny corniculate cartilage, which is composed of elastic fibrocartilage.

25

3.4 Larynx: Internal Features and Neurovascular Structures

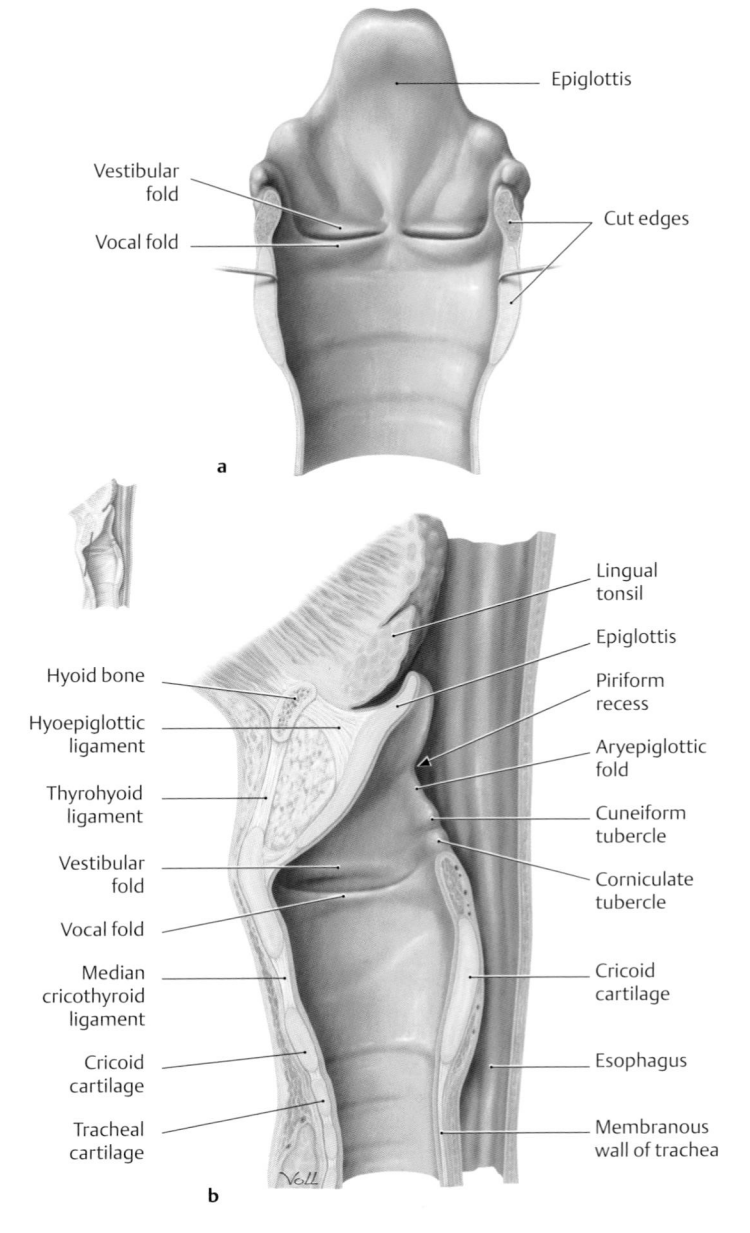

a

Epiglottis

Vestibular fold

Vocal fold

Cut edges

Lingual tonsil

Epiglottis

Piriform recess

Aryepiglottic fold

Cuneiform tubercle

Corniculate tubercle

Cricoid cartilage

Esophagus

Membranous wall of trachea

Hyoid bone

Hyoepiglottic ligament

Thyrohyoid ligament

Vestibular fold

Vocal fold

Median cricothyroid ligament

Cricoid cartilage

Tracheal cartilage

b

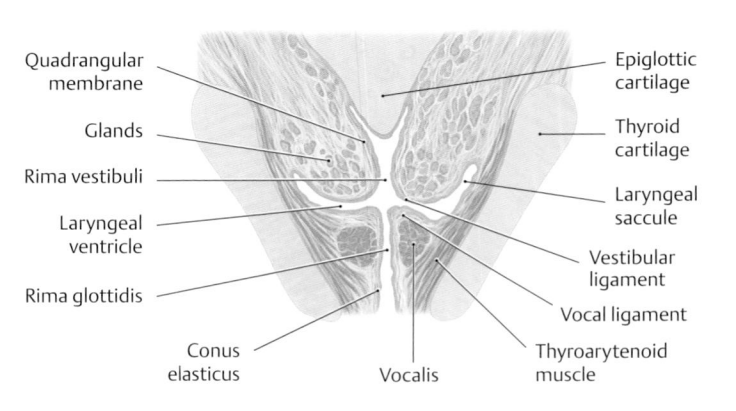

Quadrangular membrane

Glands

Rima vestibuli

Laryngeal ventricle

Rima glottidis

Conus elasticus

Vocalis

Epiglottic cartilage

Thyroid cartilage

Laryngeal saccule

Vestibular ligament

Vocal ligament

Thyroarytenoid muscle

B Vestibular folds and vocal folds
The vestibular folds ("false vocal cords") are clearly displayed in this coronal section. They contain the vestibular ligament, which is the free inferior end of the quadrangular membrane. The fissure between the vestibular folds is the rima vestibuli. Below the vestibular folds are the vocal folds ("true vocal cords"), which contain the vocal ligament and the vocalis muscle. The fissure between the vocal folds is the rima glottidis (glottis), which is narrower than the rima vestibuli.
Note: The loose connective tissue of the laryngeal inlet may become markedly swollen in response to an insect bite or inflammatory process, obstructing the rima vestibuli. This laryngeal edema (often incorrectly called "glottic edema") presents clinically with dyspnea and a risk of asphyxiation.

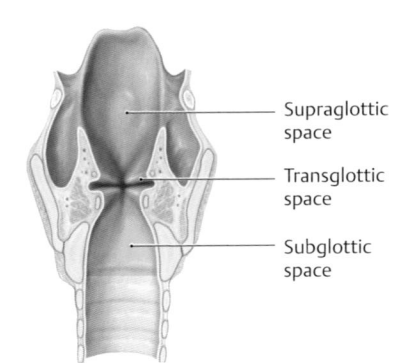

Supraglottic space

Transglottic space

Subglottic space

A Cavity of the larynx: mucosal surface anatomy and division into levels

a **Posterior view.** The muscular tube of the pharynx and esophagus has been incised posteriorly and spread open (cut edges). Mucous membrane completely lines the interior of the larynx and, except at the vocal folds, is loosely applied to its underlying tissue (creating the potential for laryngeal edema, see **B**). The aryepiglottic folds are located on each side of the laryngeal cavity between the arytenoid cartilages and epiglottis, and lateral to those folds are pear-shaped mucosal fossae, the piriform recesses.
Note: These recesses have an important role in food transport. The airway and foodway intersect in this region, and the piriform recesses channel food past the larynx and into the esophagus. The epiglottis seals off the laryngeal inlet during swallowing (see p. 37).

b **Midsagittal section viewed from the left side.** The cavity of the larynx can be divided into three levels or spaces to aid in describing the precise location of a laryngeal lesion (see **C**).

C Levels of the larynx and their boundaries
Posterior view. The larynx is divided into three levels from above downward to aid in describing the precise location of abnormalities. These three levels are also important in terms of lymphatic drainage.

Levels of the larynx	Extent
Level I: supraglottic space (laryngeal vestibule)	From the laryngeal inlet (aditus laryngis) to the vestibular folds
Level II: transglottic space (intermediate laryngeal cavity)	from the vestibular folds across the laryngeal ventricle (lateral evagination of mucosa) to the vocal folds
Level III: subglottic space (infraglottic cavity)	From the vocal folds to the inferior border of the cricoid cartilage

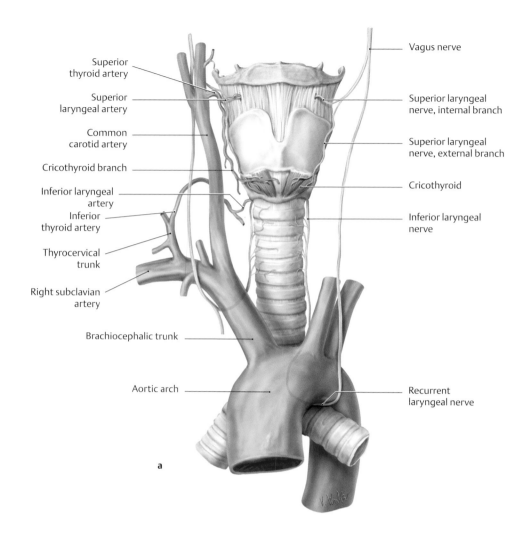

Superior thyroid artery

Superior laryngeal artery

Common carotid artery

Cricothyroid branch

Inferior laryngeal artery

Inferior thyroid artery

Thyrocervical trunk

Right subclavian artery

Brachiocephalic trunk

Aortic arch

Vagus nerve

Superior laryngeal nerve, internal branch

Superior laryngeal nerve, external branch

Cricothyroid

Inferior laryngeal nerve

Recurrent laryngeal nerve

a

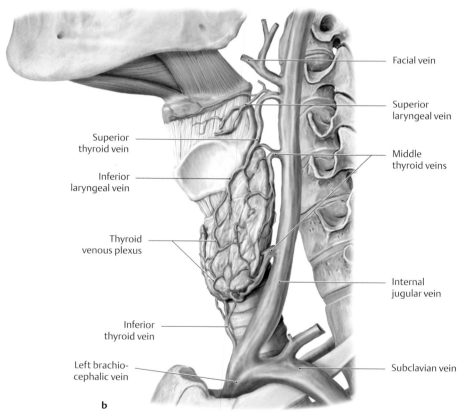

Superior thyroid vein

Inferior laryngeal vein

Thyroid venous plexus

Inferior thyroid vein

Left brachio-cephalic vein

Facial vein

Superior laryngeal vein

Middle thyroid veins

Internal jugular vein

Subclavian vein

b

D Blood supply and innervation

a Arterial and nerve supply. Anterior view. The larynx derives its *blood supply* from two major arteries: (1) the superior laryngeal artery from superior thyroid branches of the external carotid artery and (2) the inferior laryngeal artery from the subclavian artery (via the thyrocervical trunk). Thus the arterial supply of the larynx is analogous to that of the thyroid gland. The larynx is *innervated* by the superior and inferior laryngeal nerves, both of which arise from the vagus nerve (see p. 19).
Note: Owing to the close proximity of the nerves and arteries, a left-sided aortic aneurysm may cause recurrent laryngeal nerve palsy resulting in hoarseness (the pathophysiology is explored more fully on p. 31).

b Venous drainage. Left lateral view. The superior laryngeal vein drains into the superior thyroid vein, which terminates at the internal jugular vein. The inferior laryngeal vein drains into the thyroid venous plexus, which usually drains into the left brachiocephalic vein via the inferior thyroid vein.

3.5   Larynx: Muscles

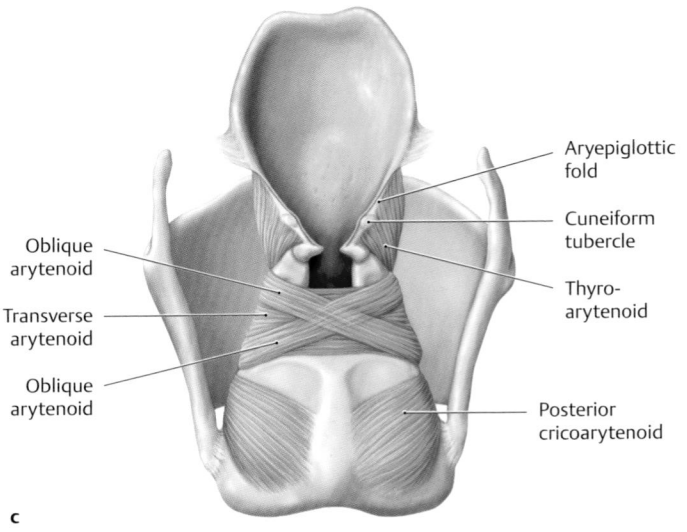

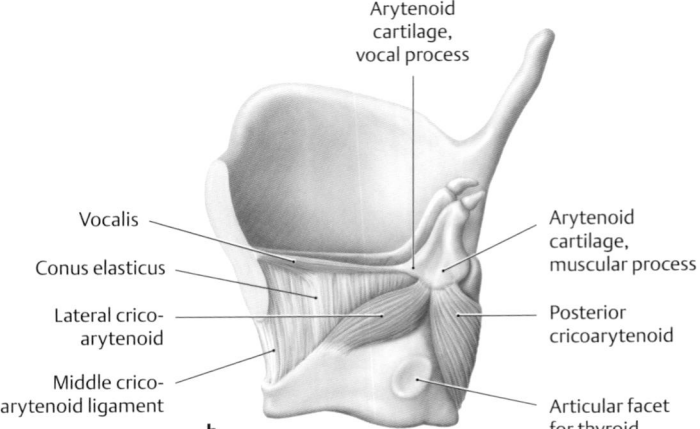

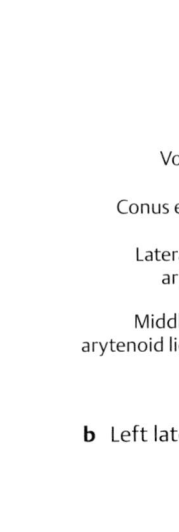

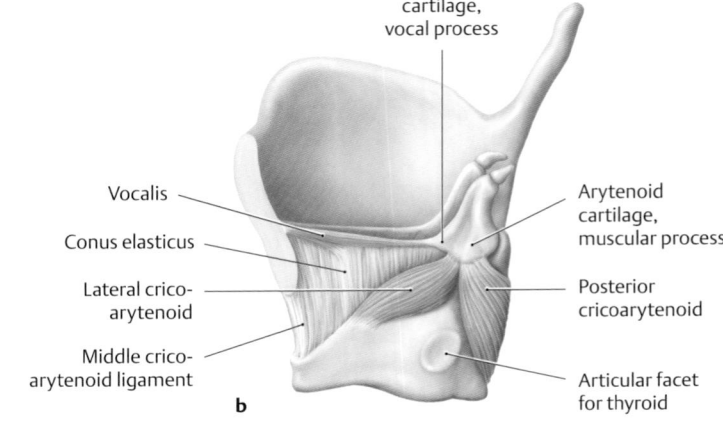

a Left lateral oblique view

b Left lateral view with the left half of the thyroid cartilage removed

c Posterior view

d Left lateral view. Almost the entire left half of the thyroid cartilage has been removed to demonstrate the epiglottis and the external part of the thyroarytenoid muscle.

A Laryngeal muscles*

a Extrinsic laryngeal muscles. The cricothyroid (or anterior cricothyroid) is the only laryngeal muscle that attaches to the external surface of the larynx. Contraction of the cricothyroid muscle tilts the cricoid cartilage posteriorly, acting with the *vocalis muscle* (see **b**) to increase tension on the vocal folds. The cricothyroid is the only muscle innervated by the superior laryngeal nerve (external branch).

b–d Intrinsic laryngeal muscles (the posterior and lateral cricoarytenoids and the thyroarytenoid). These muscles insert on the arytenoid cartilage and can alter the position of the vocal folds. Contraction of the *posterior cricoarytenoid* rotates the arytenoid cartilage outward and slightly to the side; thus it is the only laryngeal muscle that abducts the vocal cords. The *lateral cricoarytenoid* adducts the cords. Because this mechanism initiates speech production, this intrinsic laryngeal muscle is also called the *muscle of phonation*. Besides the vocalis muscle, the *transverse arytenoid* and *thyroarytenoid* muscles produce *complete* closure of the rima glottidis (see **c**).

Note: All of the *intrinsic* laryngeal muscles receive their motor innervation from the inferior laryngeal nerve, the terminal branch of the recurrent laryngeal nerve. Unilateral loss of the recurrent laryngeal nerve (e. g., on the left side due to nodal metastases from a hilar bronchial carcinoma) leads to ipsilateral palsy of the posterior cricoarytenoid muscle. This prevents complete abduction of the vocal folds, resulting in hoarseness. Bilateral loss of the recurrent laryngeal nerve (e. g., due to thyroid surgery) leads to dominance of the muscles that close the rima glottidis, causing adduction of the vocal folds with a risk of asphyxiation, but speech is not completely lost (see page 31).

* The muscles described here move the laryngeal cartilages relative to one another and affect the tension and / or position of the vocal folds. The muscles that move the larynx *as a whole* (infra- and suprahyoid muscles, constrictor pharyngis inferior) are described on p. 6.

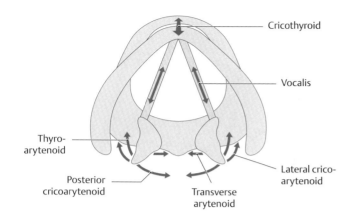

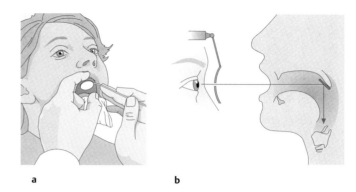

a   b

B The laryngeal muscles and their actions
(arrows indicate directions of pull)

Posterior cricoarytenoid muscle	Abduct the vocal folds (open the rima glottidis)
Lateral cricoarytenoid muscle	Adduct the vocal folds (close the rima glottidis)
Transverse arytenoid muscle, thyroarytenoid muscle	Adduct the vocal folds (close the rima glottidis)
Cricothyroid muscle, vocalis muscle	Tighten the vocal folds

C Indirect laryngoscopy

a **Mirror examination of the larynx** from the perspective of the examiner. The larynx is not accessible to direct inspection but can be viewed with the aid of a small mirror. The examiner depresses the tongue with one hand while introducing the laryngeal mirror (or endoscope) with the other hand.

b Optical path: The laryngeal mirror is held in front of the uvula, directing light from the examiner's head mirror down toward the larynx. The image seen by the examiner is shown in **D**.

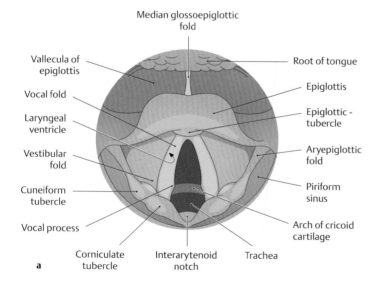

a

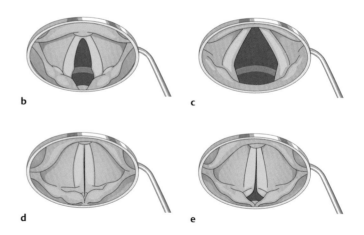

b   c

d   e

D Appearance of the larynx on indirect laryngoscopy
(after Berghaus, Rettinger, and Böhme)

The mirror produces a virtual image of the larynx with an anatomically correct portrayal of the right and left sides, i.e., the right vocal fold appears on the right side of the mirror image. Anatomically anterior structures (e.g., the tongue base, valleculae, and epiglottis) appear at the top of the image, while posterior structures (e.g., the interarytenoid notch) appear at the bottom. The vocal folds appear as smooth-edged bands that are markedly lighter in color than the surrounding mucosa. Reason: There are no blood vessels or submucosa below the stratified, nonkeratinized squamous epithelium of the vocal folds; this contrasts with the adjacent mucosa, which has a rich blood supply. The glottis is evaluated in both the closed (respiratory) and open (phonation) posi-

tions by having the patient alternately inhale and sing "heee." The evaluation is based on pathoanatomical changes (e.g., redness, swelling, ulceration) as well as functional changes (e.g., vocal fold position).

a Depiction of the laryngoscopic mirror image.

b–e Indirect laryngoscopic findings. *Respiratory positions:* opening of the rima glottidis during normal (**b**) and vigorous respiration (**c**). *Phonation position* with the vocal folds completely adducted (**d**). During whispered speech, the vocal folds are slightly abducted in their posterior third (**e**).

3.6 Larynx: Topographical and Clinical Anatomy

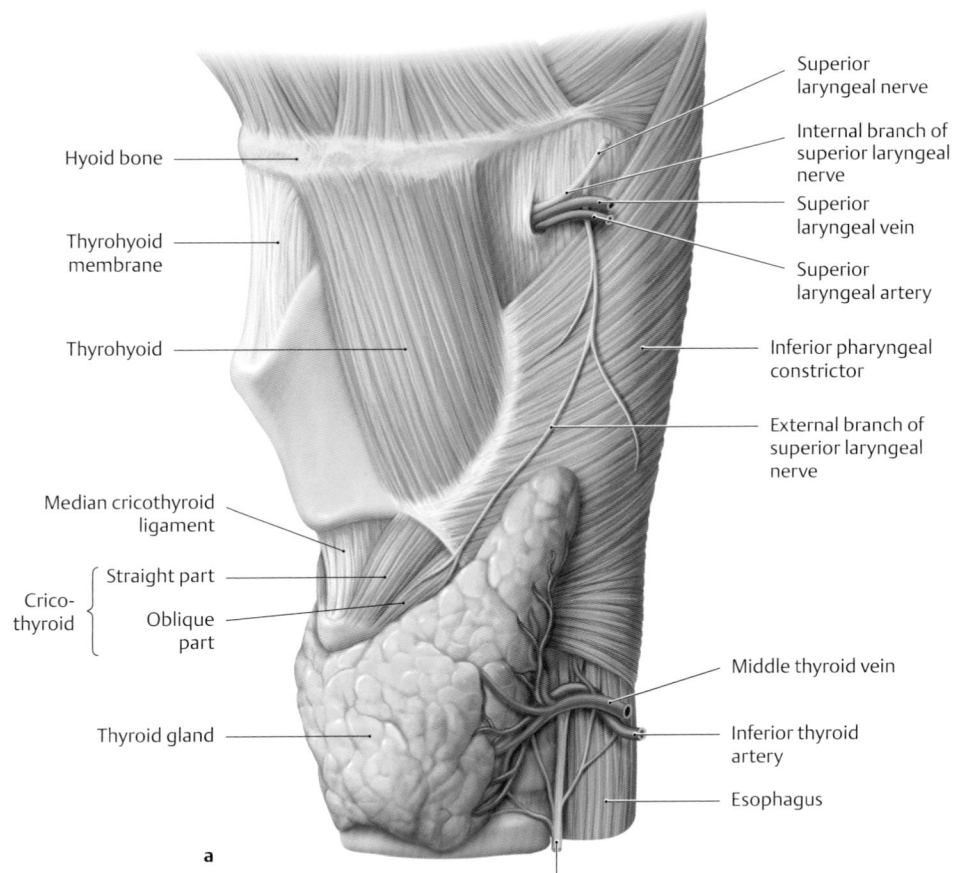

Hyoid bone

Thyrohyoid membrane

Thyrohyoid

Median cricothyroid ligament

Crico-thyroid {
Straight part
Oblique part
}

Thyroid gland

Superior laryngeal nerve

Internal branch of superior laryngeal nerve

Superior laryngeal vein

Superior laryngeal artery

Inferior pharyngeal constrictor

External branch of superior laryngeal nerve

Middle thyroid vein

Inferior thyroid artery

Esophagus

a

Inferior laryngeal nerve

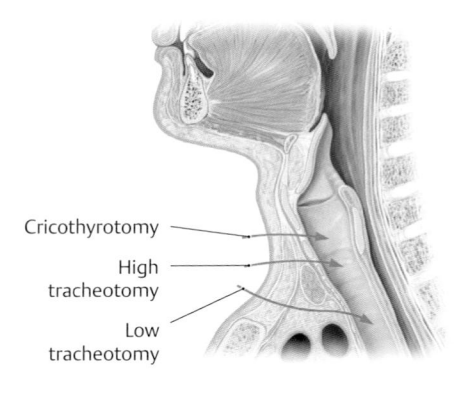

Cricothyrotomy

High tracheotomy

Low tracheotomy

B Approaches to the larynx and trachea

Midsagittal section, left lateral view. When an acute edematous obstruction of the larynx (e. g., due to an allergic reaction) poses an acute risk of asphyxiation, the following surgical approaches are available for creating an emergency airway:

- Division of the median cricothyroid ligament (cricothyrotomy)
- Incision of the trachea (tracheotomy) at a level just below the cricoid cartilage (high tracheostomy) or just superior to the jugular notch (low tracheostomy).

A Topographical anatomy of the larynx: blood supply and innervation

Left lateral view. **a** Superficial layer, **b** deep layer. The cricothyroid muscle and left lamina of the thyroid cartilage have been removed, and the pharyngeal mucosa has been mobilized and retracted. Arteries and veins enter the larynx mainly from the posterior side.

Note: The motor (external) branch of the superior laryngeal nerve supplies the cricothyroid muscle, and its sensory (internal) branch supplies the laryngeal mucosa down to the level of the vocal folds. By contrast, the inferior laryngeal nerve supplies motor innervation to *all* other (intrinsic) laryngeal muscles and sensory innervation to the laryngeal mucosa below the vocal folds.

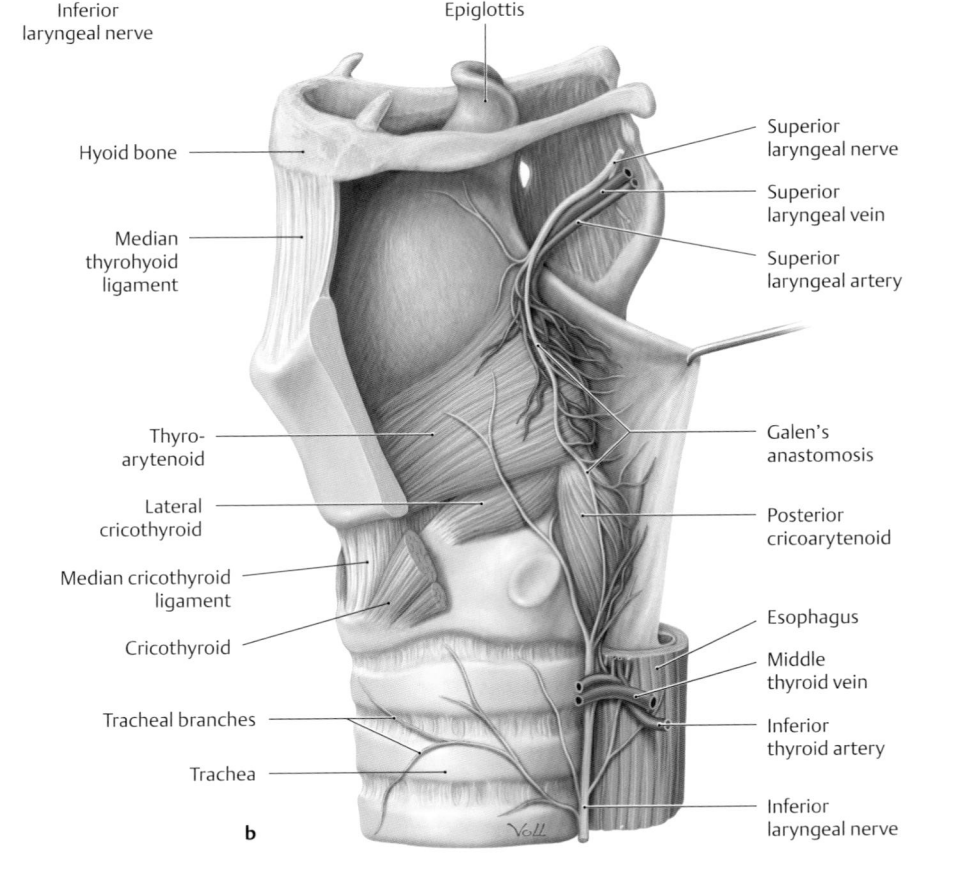

Hyoid bone

Median thyrohyoid ligament

Thyro-arytenoid

Lateral cricothyroid

Median cricothyroid ligament

Cricothyroid

Tracheal branches

Trachea

Epiglottis

Superior laryngeal nerve

Superior laryngeal vein

Superior laryngeal artery

Galen's anastomosis

Posterior cricoarytenoid

Esophagus

Middle thyroid vein

Inferior thyroid artery

Inferior laryngeal nerve

b

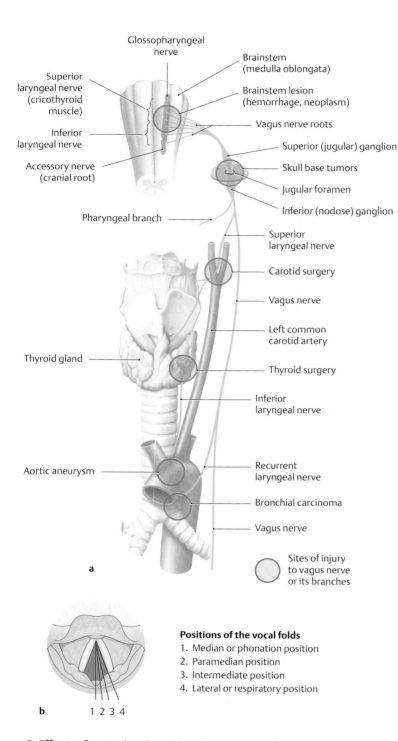

a

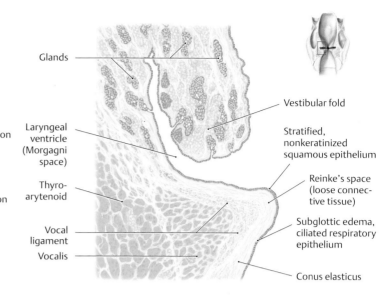

Positions of the vocal folds
1. Median or phonation position
2. Paramedian position
3. Intermediate position
4. Lateral or respiratory position

b   1 2 3 4

C Effects of central and peripheral vagus nerve lesions on the position of the vocal folds

The vagus nerve provides motor innervation to the pharyngeal and laryngeal muscles (see page 37). This innervation originates in the *nucleus ambiguus* in the brainstem, which contains motor neurons that contribute axons to three cranial nerves, arranged in a somatotopic order: the most rostral neurons send axons into the glossopharyngeal nerve; neurons in the middle of the group, to the vagus; the most caudal neurons, to the accessory nerve. The vagus also receives sensory information from the larynx, transmitted by primary sensory neurons with cell bodies in the inferior (nodose) ganglion.

Lesions affecting the vagus nerve can interrupt central control of the nucleus ambiguus, leaving its muscle targets in spastic paralysis. Lesions that destroy the motor neurons themselves or transect their axons will denervate the muscles, causing flaccid paralysis and eventual muscle atrophy. This muscle paralysis alters the position of the vocal folds.

D Structure of the vocal fold

Schematic coronal histologic section, posterior view. Exposed to severe mechanical stresses, the vocal fold (see image inset navigator for more information) is covered by nonkeratinized squamous epithelium. Degenerative changes in vocal fold mucosa may lead to thickening, loss of elasticity, and, potentially, to squamous cell carcinoma. The adjacent subglottic space is covered by ciliated respiratory epithelium. The mucosa of the vocal folds and subglottic space (Reinke's space) overlies loose connective tissue, and so chronic irritation from cigarette smoke in a heavy smoker may cause chronic edema in the Reinke space, resulting in a harsh voice ("smoker's voice").

- *Central lesions in the brainstem or higher* involving the nucleus ambiguus (e. g., caused by a tumor or hemorrhage → an intermediate or paramedian position of the vocal fold on the affected side (see **b**).
- Peripheral lesions of the vagus nerve have variable effects, depending on the site of the lesion:
  - Skull base lesions at the level of the jugular foramen (e. g., caused by a nasopharyngeal tumor) → an intermediate or paramedian position of the affected vocal fold due to a flaccid paralysis of all intrinsic and extrinsic laryngeal muscles (see **b**) → inability to close the glottis with severe hoarseness. Sensation is lost in the larynx on the affected side.
  - Superior laryngeal nerve in the midcervical region (e. g., as a complication of carotid surgery) → hypotonicity of the cricothyroid muscle → mild hoarseness with a weak voice, especially at higher frequencies. Sensation is lost above the vocal fold.
  - Inferior (recurrent) laryngeal nerve in the lower neck (e. g., lesion caused by thyroid surgery, bronchial carcinoma, or an aortic aneurysm) → paralysis of all intrinsic laryngeal muscles on the affected side → a median or paramedian position of the vocal fold, mild hoarseness, poor tonal control, rapid voice fatigue, no dyspnea. Sensation is lost below the vocal fold.

Other motor deficits with high peripheral lesions include drooping of the soft palate on the affected side and deviation of the uvula to the unaffected side. Gag and cough reflexes may be diminished, with swallowing difficulty (dysphagia) and hypernasal speech due to deficient closure of the oronasal cavity. Sensory defects may include a foreign-body sensation in the throat. Bilateral lesions have more severe effects. Transection of both recurrent laryngeal nerves leaves the vocal cords fixed in paramedian position and can cause significant dyspnea and inspiratory stridor (high-pitched noise indicating obstruction), necessitating tracheotomy in acute cases.

3.7 Pharynx: Muscles

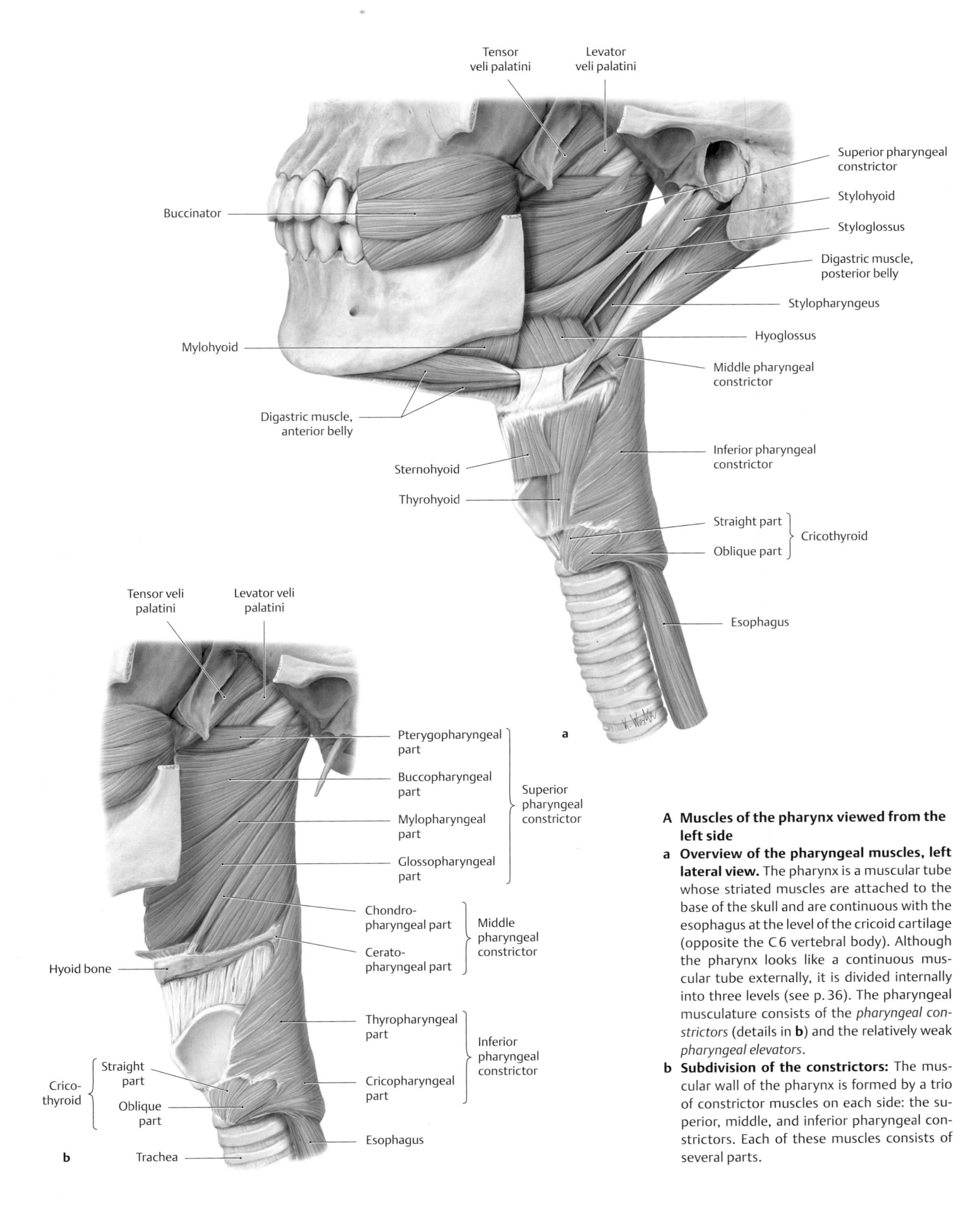

Tensor veli palatini

Levator veli palatini

Buccinator

Mylohyoid

Digastric muscle, anterior belly

Sternohyoid

Thyrohyoid

Superior pharyngeal constrictor

Stylohyoid

Styloglossus

Digastric muscle, posterior belly

Stylopharyngeus

Hyoglossus

Middle pharyngeal constrictor

Inferior pharyngeal constrictor

Straight part
Oblique part } Cricothyroid

Esophagus

a

Tensor veli palatini

Levator veli palatini

Pterygopharyngeal part

Buccopharyngeal part

Mylopharyngeal part

Glossopharyngeal part

} Superior pharyngeal constrictor

Chondro-pharyngeal part

Cerato-pharyngeal part

} Middle pharyngeal constrictor

Hyoid bone

Thyropharyngeal part

Cricopharyngeal part

} Inferior pharyngeal constrictor

Crico-thyroid {
Straight part
Oblique part

Esophagus

b

Trachea

A Muscles of the pharynx viewed from the left side

a Overview of the pharyngeal muscles, left lateral view. The pharynx is a muscular tube whose striated muscles are attached to the base of the skull and are continuous with the esophagus at the level of the cricoid cartilage (opposite the C6 vertebral body). Although the pharynx looks like a continuous muscular tube externally, it is divided internally into three levels (see p. 36). The pharyngeal musculature consists of the *pharyngeal constrictors* (details in **b**) and the relatively weak *pharyngeal elevators*.

b Subdivision of the constrictors: The muscular wall of the pharynx is formed by a trio of constrictor muscles on each side: the superior, middle, and inferior pharyngeal constrictors. Each of these muscles consists of several parts.

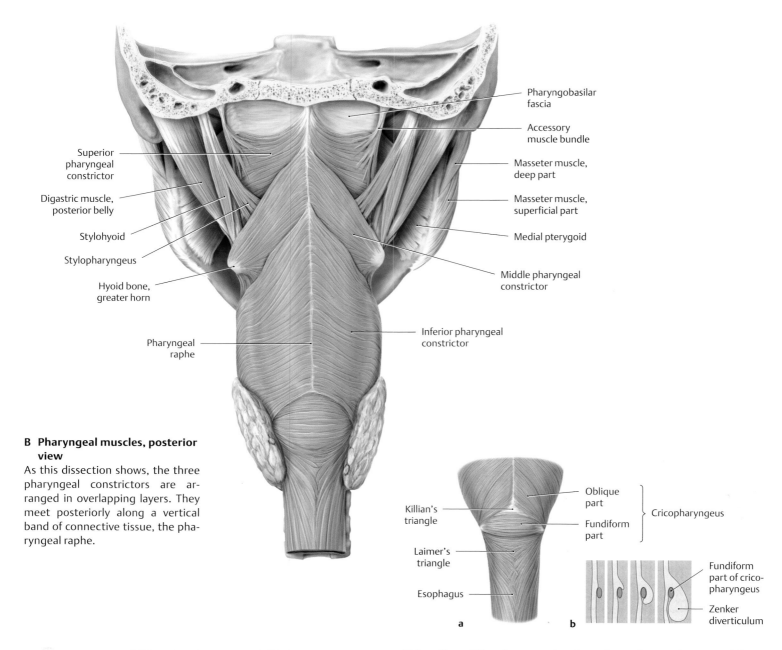

Pharyngobasilar fascia

Accessory muscle bundle

Masseter muscle, deep part

Masseter muscle, superficial part

Medial pterygoid

Middle pharyngeal constrictor

Superior pharyngeal constrictor

Digastric muscle, posterior belly

Stylohyoid

Stylopharyngeus

Hyoid bone, greater horn

Pharyngeal raphe

Inferior pharyngeal constrictor

B Pharyngeal muscles, posterior view

As this dissection shows, the three pharyngeal constrictors are arranged in overlapping layers. They meet posteriorly along a vertical band of connective tissue, the pharyngeal raphe.

Killian's triangle

Oblique part

Fundiform part

Cricopharyngeus

Laimer's triangle

Esophagus

Fundiform part of cricopharyngeus

Zenker diverticulum

a   **b**

D Junction of the pharyngeal and esophageal musculature and the development of Zenker diverticula

a Posterior view, **b** left lateral view.

The cricopharyngeal part of the inferior pharyngeal constrictor muscle is further subdivided into an oblique part and a fundiform part. Between these two parts is an area of muscular weakness known as *the Killian triangle*. At the inferior border of the fundiform part, the muscle fibers form a V-shaped area called *the Laimer triangle*. The weak spot at Killian's triangle may allow the mucosa of the hypopharynx to bulge outward through the fundiform part of the cricopharyngeus muscle (**b**). This can result in a *Zenker diverticulum*, a saclike protrusion in which food residues may collect and gradually expand the sac (with risk of obstructing the esophageal lumen by extrinsic pressure from the diverticulum). The diagnosis is suggested by the regurgitation of trapped food residues. Zenker diverticula are most common in middle-aged and elderly individuals. In older patients who are not optimal surgical candidates, treatment consists of dividing the fundiform part of the inferior constrictor endoscopically.

Note: Because a Zenker diverticulum is located at the junction of the hypopharynx with the esophagus, it is known also as a pharyngoesophageal diverticulum (the term "esophageal diverticulum," while common, is incorrect).

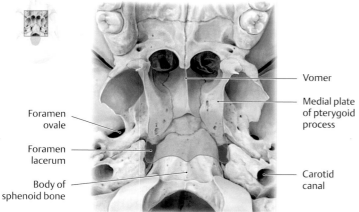

Vomer

Medial plate of pterygoid process

Foramen ovale

Foramen lacerum

Body of sphenoid bone

Carotid canal

C Pharyngobasilar fascia at the base of the skull

Inferior view. The pharyngeal musculature arises from the base of the skull by a thick sheet of connective tissue, the pharyngobasilar fascia (shown in red). It may be considered the tendon of origin for the musculature.

33

3.8 Pharynx:
Surface Anatomy of the Mucosa and its Connections with the Skull

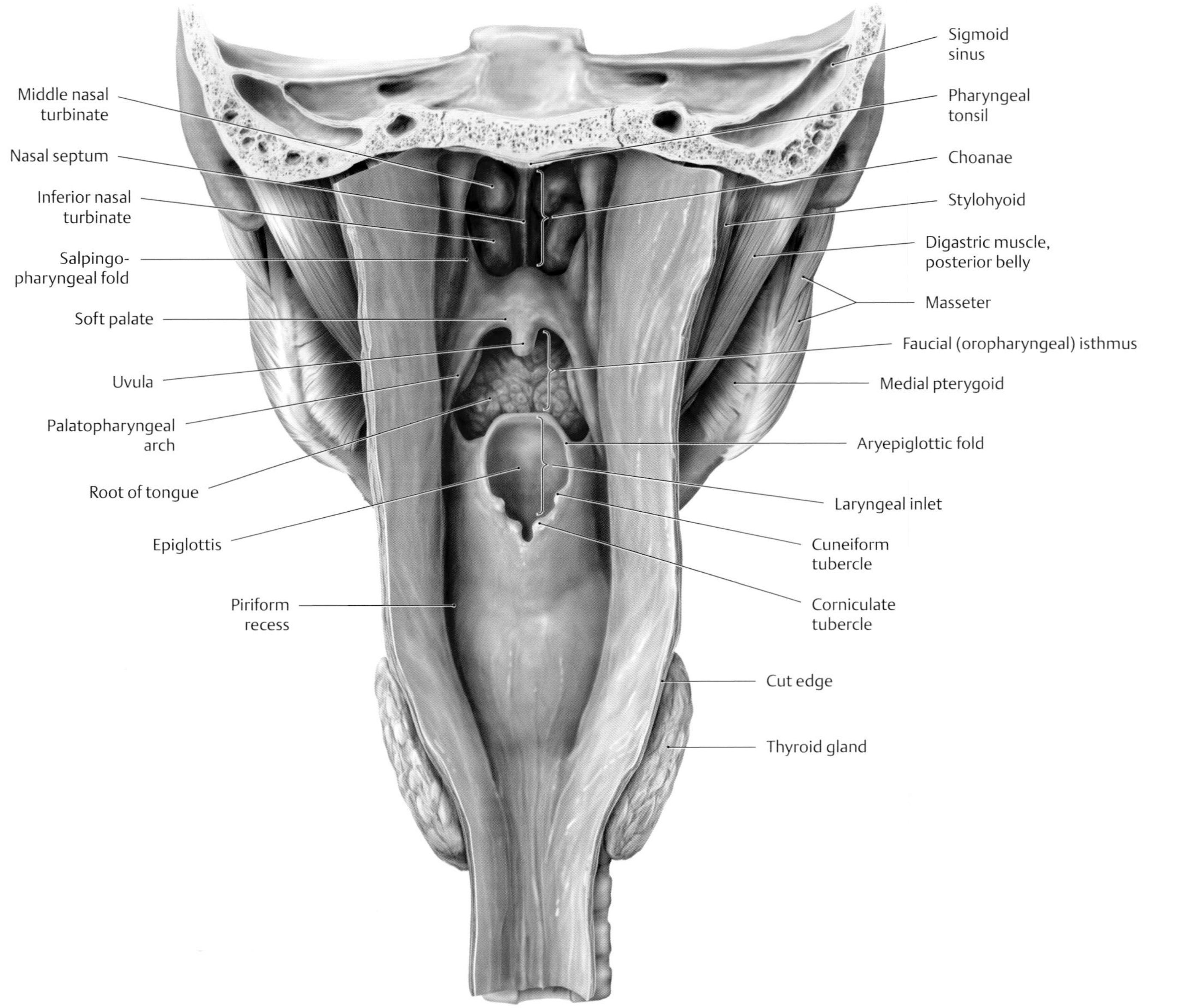

Middle nasal turbinate

Nasal septum

Inferior nasal turbinate

Salpingo- pharyngeal fold

Soft palate

Uvula

Palatopharyngeal arch

Root of tongue

Epiglottis

Piriform recess

Sigmoid sinus

Pharyngeal tonsil

Choanae

Stylohyoid

Digastric muscle, posterior belly

Masseter

Faucial (oropharyngeal) isthmus

Medial pterygoid

Aryepiglottic fold

Laryngeal inlet

Cuneiform tubercle

Corniculate tubercle

Cut edge

Thyroid gland

A Surface anatomy of the pharyngeal mucosa
Posterior view. The muscular posterior wall of the pharynx is closed posteriorly. In this dissection it has been divided and spread open in the
midline to demonstrate its mucosal anatomy. The anterior part of the
muscular tube is interrupted by three openings:

- To the nasal cavity (choanae)
- To the oral cavity (faucial [oropharyngeal] isthmus)
- To the laryngeal inlet (aditus)

The pharynx is divided accordingly into a naso-, ovo-, and laryngopharynx (see p. 36).

B Posterior rhinoscopy
The nasopharynx can be visually inspected by posterior rhinoscopy.

a Technique of holding the tongue blade and mirror. The angulation of
   the mirror is continually adjusted to permit complete inspection of
   the nasopharynx (see **b**).
b Composite posterior rhinoscopic image acquired at various mirror angles. The eustachian tube orifice and pharyngeal tonsil can be
   identified (see p. 35).

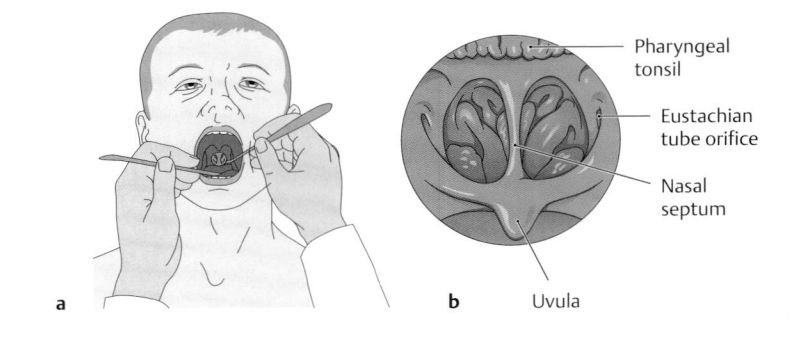

Pharyngeal tonsil

Eustachian tube orifice

Nasal septum

a

b   Uvula

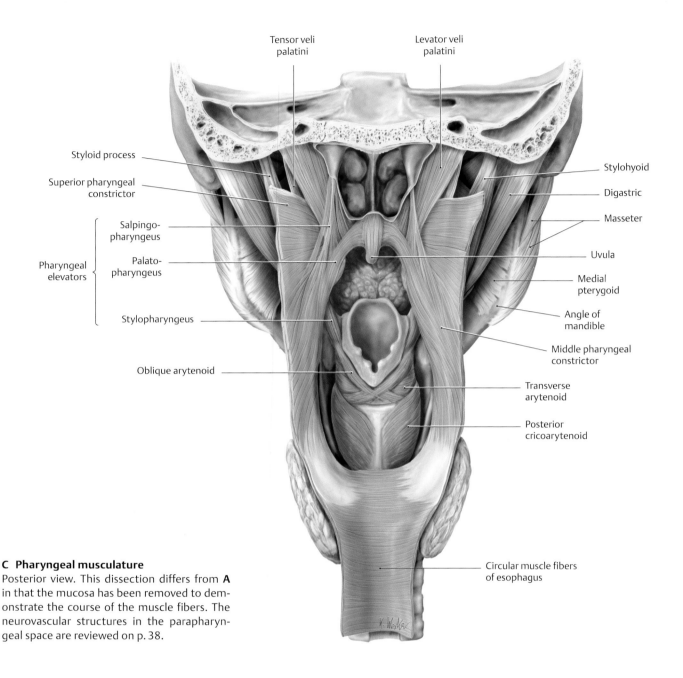

Tensor veli palatini

Levator veli palatini

Styloid process

Superior pharyngeal constrictor

Salpingo-pharyngeus

Palato-pharyngeus

Pharyngeal elevators

Stylopharyngeus

Oblique arytenoid

Stylohyoid

Digastric

Masseter

Uvula

Medial pterygoid

Angle of mandible

Middle pharyngeal constrictor

Transverse arytenoid

Posterior cricoarytenoid

Circular muscle fibers of esophagus

C Pharyngeal musculature
Posterior view. This dissection differs from **A** in that the mucosa has been removed to demonstrate the course of the muscle fibers. The neurovascular structures in the parapharyngeal space are reviewed on p. 38.

Levator veli palatini

Salpingo-pharyngeus

Superior pharyngeal constrictor

Uvula

Palato-pharyngeus

Pharyngeal tonsil

Cartilaginous part of eustachian tube

Tubal orifice

Tensor veli palatini

Medial plate of pterygoid process

Pterygoid hamulus

D Muscles of the soft palate and eustachian tube
Posterior view. The sphenoid bone has been sectioned posterior to the choanal opening in the coronal plane, and the following muscles have been resected on the right side: levator veli palatini, salpingopharyngeus, palatopharyngeus, and superior pharyngeal constrictor. These muscles are part of the throat (space between the soft palate, palatine arches, and lingual dorsum) that forms the posterior boundary of the oral cavity. They are shown here to help explain the muscular foundation of the mucosal features that are seen at posterior rhinoscopy (see **B**).

3.9 Pharynx: Topographical Anatomy and Innervation

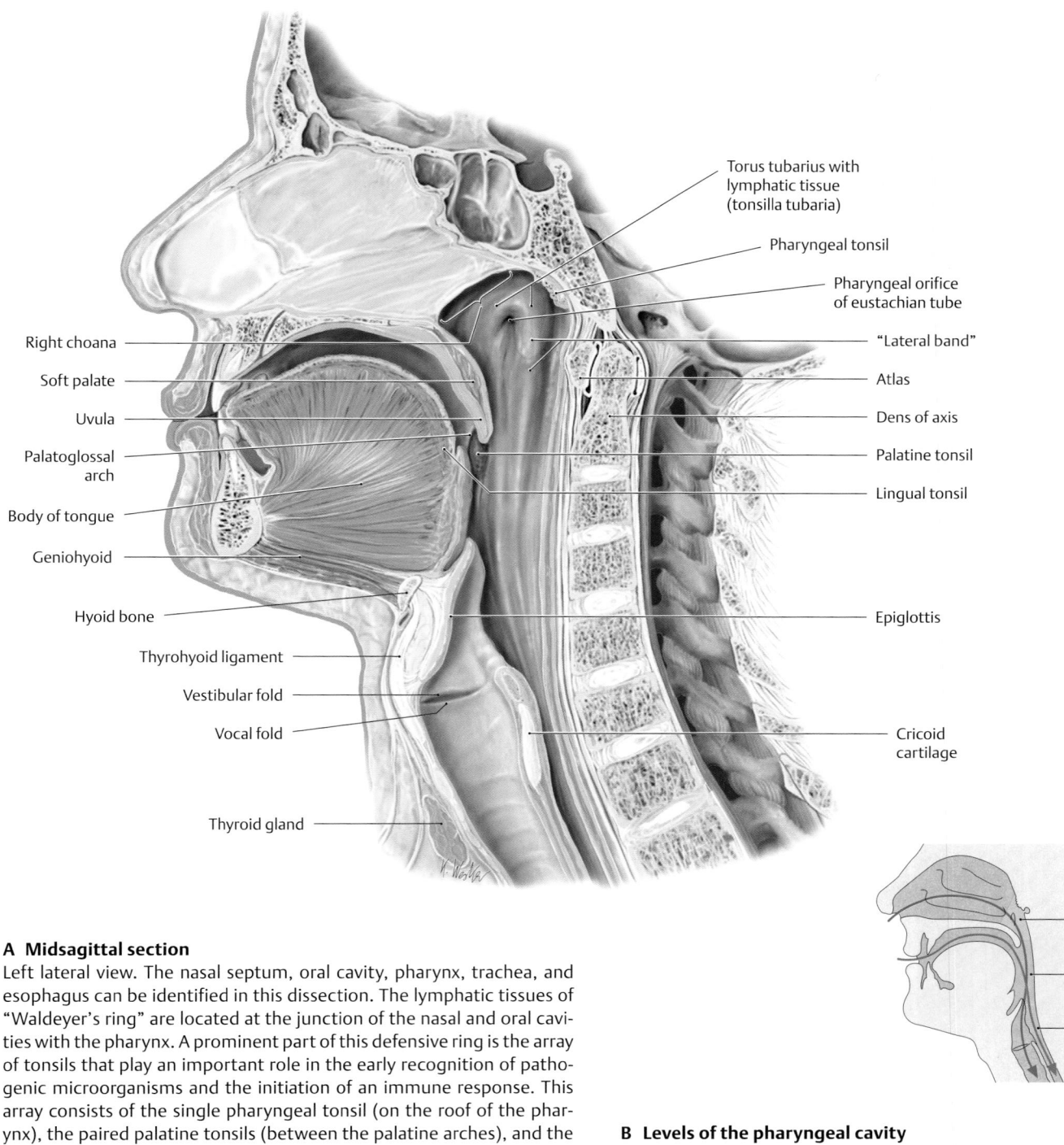

A Midsagittal section

Left lateral view. The nasal septum, oral cavity, pharynx, trachea, and esophagus can be identified in this dissection. The lymphatic tissues of "Waldeyer's ring" are located at the junction of the nasal and oral cavities with the pharynx. A prominent part of this defensive ring is the array of tonsils that play an important role in the early recognition of pathogenic microorganisms and the initiation of an immune response. This array consists of the single pharyngeal tonsil (on the roof of the pharynx), the paired palatine tonsils (between the palatine arches), and the paired lingual tonsils (at the base of the tongue). Additional masses of lymphatic tissue are located around the pharyngeal orifice of each eustachian tube (tonsilla tubaria) and are continued inferiorly as the "lateral bands."

The eustachian tube connects the pharynx with the tympanic cavity and serves to equalize the air pressure in the middle ear. Swelling about the eustachian tube orifice (tonsilla tubaria), which may occur even with a mild inflammation, may occlude the orifice and prevent pressure equalization in the middle ear. This restricts the mobility of the tympanic membrane, causing a mild degree of hearing loss. Enlargement of the pharyngeal tonsil (e. g., polyps in small children) may also obstruct the lumen of the eustachian tube.

B Levels of the pharyngeal cavity

Left lateral view. The pharyngeal cavity is divided into the nasopharynx, oropharynx, and laryngopharynx. The upper airway and lower foodway intersect in the oropharynx. The following synonyms for the three pharyngeal levels are in common use:

Upper level:	Nasal part of pharynx	Nasopharynx	Epipharynx
Middle level:	Oral part of pharynx	Oropharynx	Mesopharynx
Lower level:	Laryngeal part of pharynx	Laryngopharynx	Hypopharynx

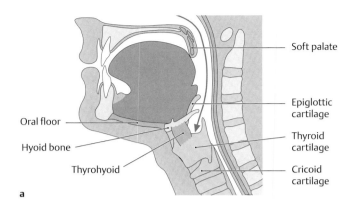

a   b

C Anatomy of swallowing

As part of the airway, the larynx in the adult is located at the inlet to the digestive tract (**a**). During swallowing (**b**), therefore, the airway must be briefly occluded to keep food from entering the trachea. The act of swallowing consists of three phases:

1. Voluntary initiation of swallowing
2. Reflex closure of the airway

3. Reflex transport of the food bolus down the pharynx and esophagus

During the second phase of swallowing, the oral floor muscles (mylohyoid and digastric) and the thyrohyoid muscles elevate the larynx and the epiglottis covers the laryngeal inlet, sealing off the lower airway. Meanwhile the soft palate is tightened, elevated, and apposed to the posterior pharyngeal wall, sealing off the upper airway.

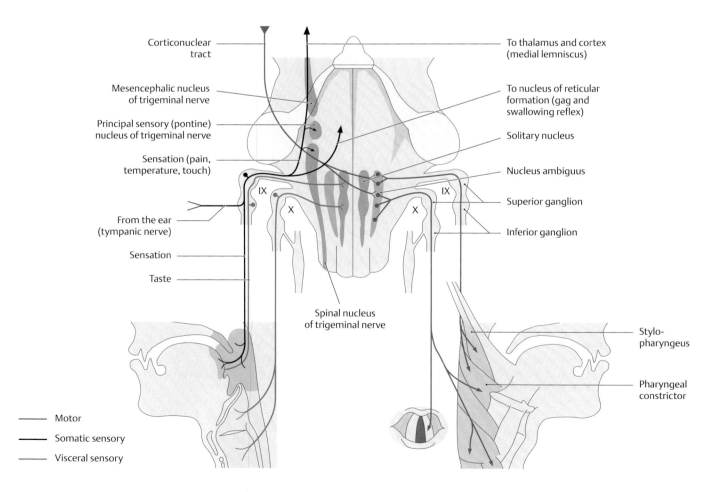

D Vagus nerve and glossopharyngeal nerve: their peripheral distribution and brainstem nuclei (after Duus)

Posterior view. Both the glossopharyngeal nerve (cranial nerve IX) and the vagus nerve (CN X) originate from nuclei in the brainstem. In this simplified schematic, motor pathways are depicted on the right and sensory pathways on the left.

Note that both nerves contribute to the sensory and motor supply of the pharynx. Together they form the pharyngeal plexus.

37

3.10 Pharynx: Neurovascular Structures in the Parapharyngeal Space

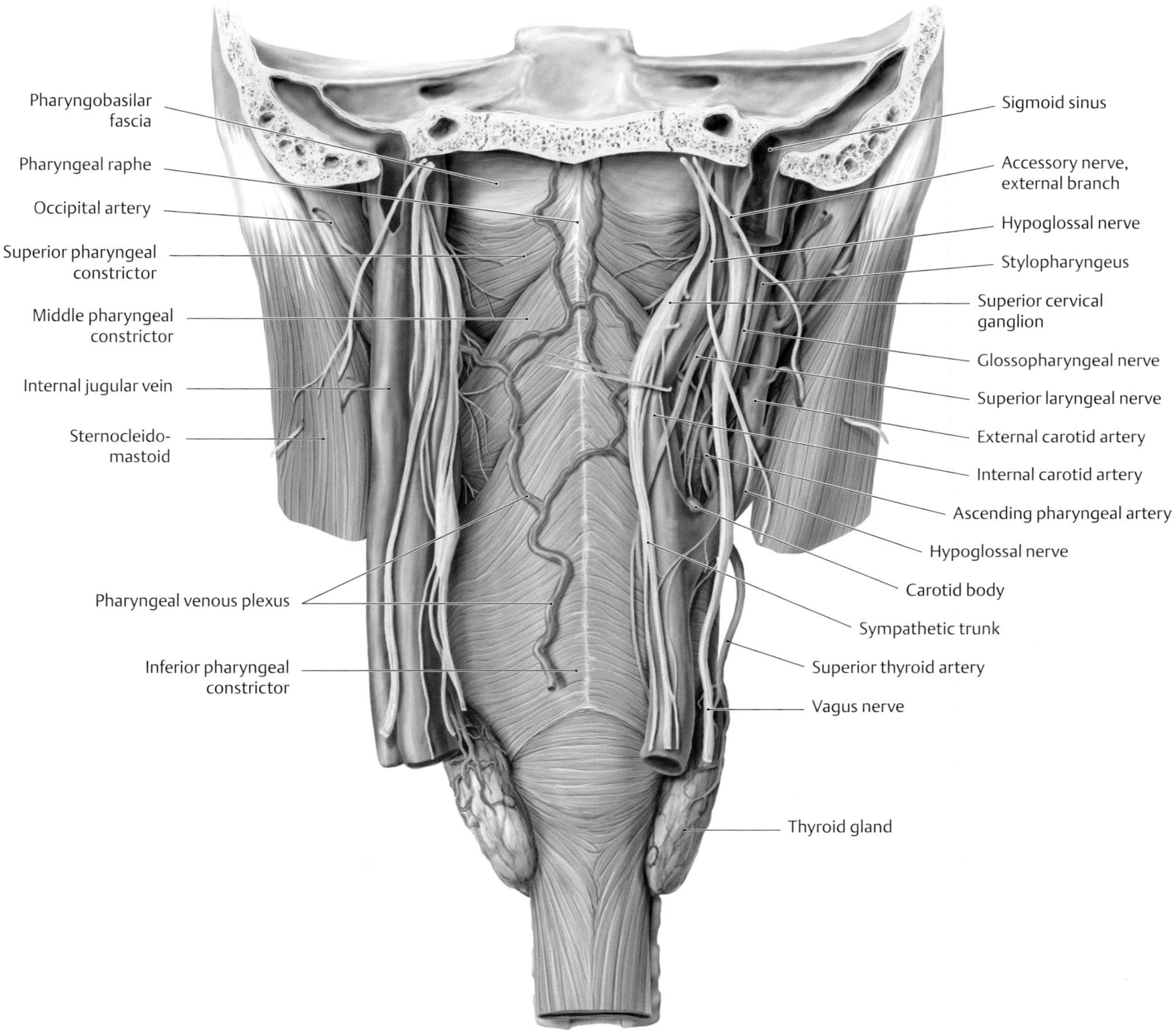

Pharyngobasilar fascia

Pharyngeal raphe

Occipital artery

Superior pharyngeal constrictor

Middle pharyngeal constrictor

Internal jugular vein

Sternocleido- mastoid

Pharyngeal venous plexus

Inferior pharyngeal constrictor

Sigmoid sinus

Accessory nerve, external branch

Hypoglossal nerve

Stylopharyngeus

Superior cervical ganglion

Glossopharyngeal nerve

Superior laryngeal nerve

External carotid artery

Internal carotid artery

Ascending pharyngeal artery

Hypoglossal nerve

Carotid body

Sympathetic trunk

Superior thyroid artery

Vagus nerve

Thyroid gland

A Parapharyngeal space, posterior view
The vertebral column and all structures posterior to it have been completely removed to display the posterior outer wall of the pharynx from the posterior aspect. The neurovascular structures on the left side are intact, while the right internal jugular vein has been removed to demonstrate neurovascular structures lying anterior to the jugular vein. The

internal carotid artery, vagus nerve, and sympathetic trunk on the right side have been retracted medially into the parapharyngeal and lateropharyngeal space.
Note the exposed carotid body, which is innervated by the vagus nerve and sympathetic trunk.

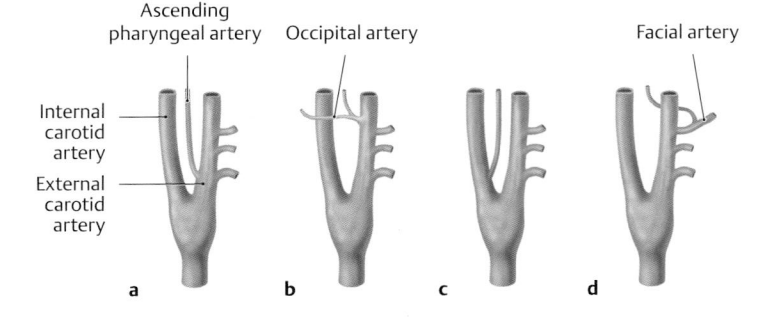

Ascending pharyngeal artery

Occipital artery

Facial artery

Internal carotid artery

External carotid artery

a   b   c   d

B Ascending pharyngeal artery: typical anatomy and variants
    (after Tillmann, Lippert, and Pabst)
Left lateral view. The main arterial vessel supplying the upper and middle pharynx is the ascending pharyngeal artery. In 70 % of cases (**a**) it arises from the posteroinferior surface of the external carotid artery. In approximately 20 % of cases it arises from the occipital artery (**b**). Occasionally (8 %) it originates from the internal carotid artery or carotid bifurcation (**c**), and in 2 % of cases it arises from the facial artery (**d**).

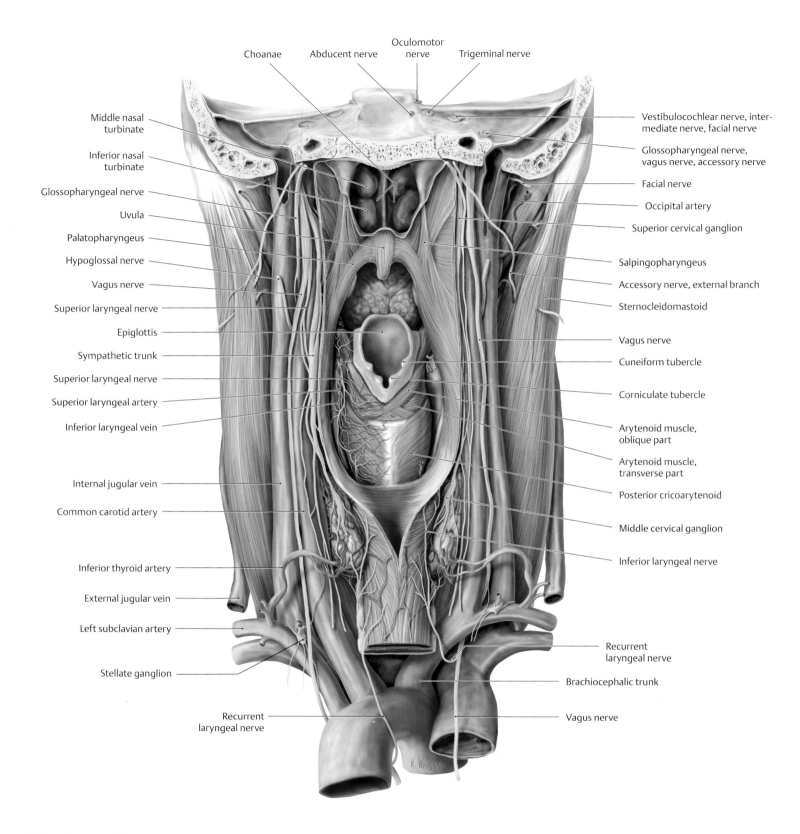

Choanae | Abducent nerve | Oculomotor nerve | Trigeminal nerve

Middle nasal turbinate
Inferior nasal turbinate
Glossopharyngeal nerve
Uvula
Palatopharyngeus
Hypoglossal nerve
Vagus nerve
Superior laryngeal nerve
Epiglottis
Sympathetic trunk
Superior laryngeal nerve
Superior laryngeal artery
Inferior laryngeal vein
Internal jugular vein
Common carotid artery
Inferior thyroid artery
External jugular vein
Left subclavian artery
Stellate ganglion
Recurrent laryngeal nerve

Vestibulocochlear nerve, intermediate nerve, facial nerve
Glossopharyngeal nerve, vagus nerve, accessory nerve
Facial nerve
Occipital artery
Superior cervical ganglion
Salpingopharyngeus
Accessory nerve, external branch
Sternocleidomastoid
Vagus nerve
Cuneiform tubercle
Corniculate tubercle
Arytenoid muscle, oblique part
Arytenoid muscle, transverse part
Posterior cricoarytenoid
Middle cervical ganglion
Inferior laryngeal nerve
Recurrent laryngeal nerve
Brachiocephalic trunk
Vagus nerve

C Parapharyngeal space
Posterior view. The neurovascular structures in the parapharyngeal space are fully displayed from the posterior cranial fossa to the thoracic inlet. Also, the posterior wall of the pharynx has been longitudinally incised and spread open to demonstrate the cavity of the pharynx from the choanae down to the esophagus.

Note: The major neurovascular structures in the neck course along the pharynx in a tightly clustered configuration. Stab injuries that perforate the lumen (from accidentally ingested bones, for example) may lead to inflammation of the parapharyngeal space, causing significant damage (see p. 40). Even minor injuries may incite a purulent bacterial inflammation that spreads rapidly within this connective-tissue space (cellulitis).

3.11 Pharynx:
Parapharyngeal Space and Its Clinical Significance

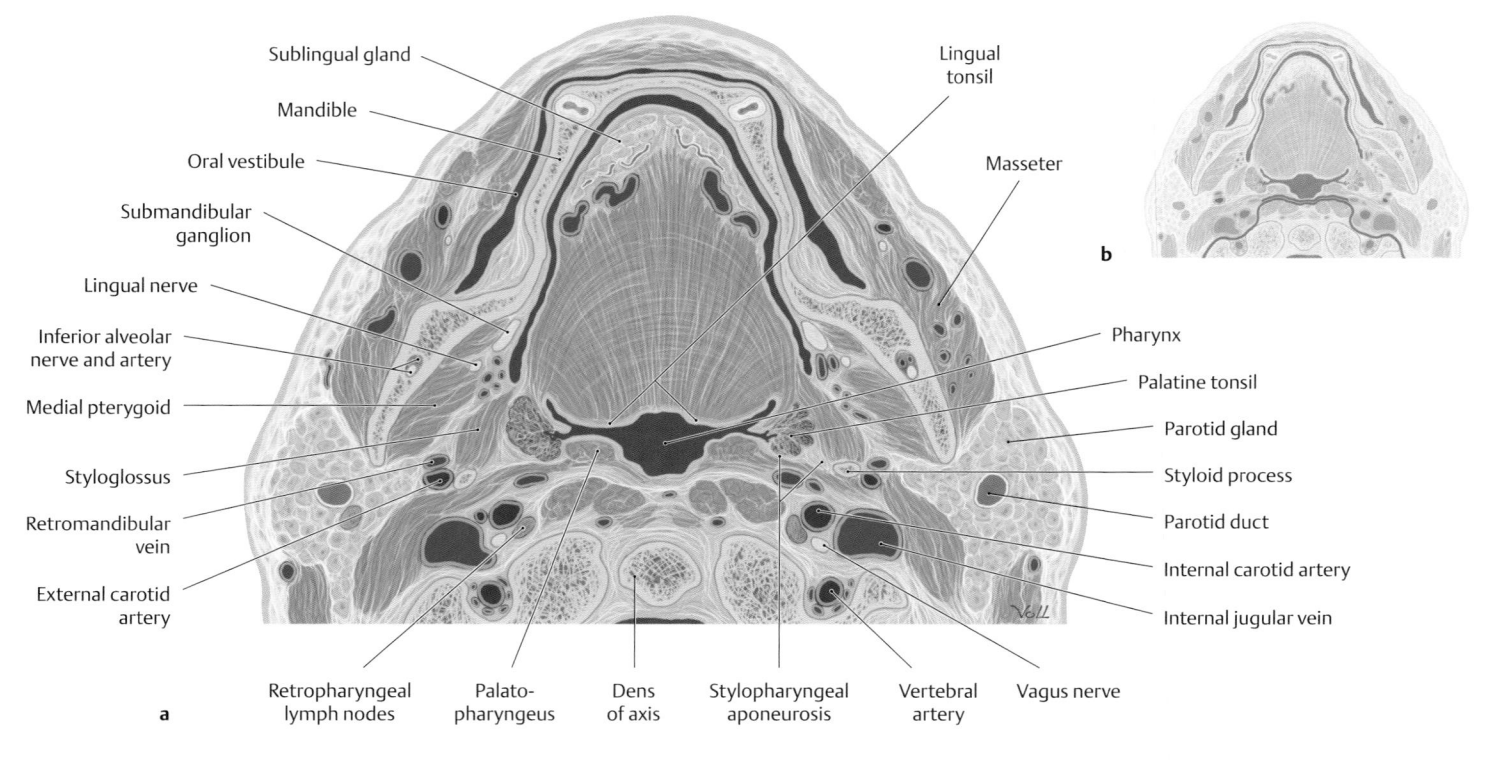

Sublingual gland
Mandible
Oral vestibule
Submandibular ganglion
Lingual nerve
Inferior alveolar nerve and artery
Medial pterygoid
Styloglossus
Retromandibular vein
External carotid artery

Lingual tonsil
Masseter
Pharynx
Palatine tonsil
Parotid gland
Styloid process
Parotid duct
Internal carotid artery
Internal jugular vein

b

Retropharyngeal lymph nodes   Palato-pharyngeus   Dens of axis   Stylopharyngeal aponeurosis   Vertebral artery   Vagus nerve

a

A Parapharyngeal space, superior view
(after Fritsch and Kühnel)

a Transverse section of the neck at the level of the tonsillar fossa. The pharynx is surrounded laterally and posteriorly by a layer of connective tissue (parapharyngeal space), which is traversed by neurovascular structures. It is further subdivided into a *retropharyngeal* and *lateropharyngeal* space.

b The retropharyngeal space (green) is only a thin connective-tissue space directly bordering the deep layer of the cervical fascia (prevertebral lamina, red). The lateropharyngeal space is subdivided by a sheet of connective tissue, the stylopharyngeal aponeurosis, into an anterior part (yellow) and a posterior part (orange). The stylopharyngeus muscle borders this fibrous sheet, which originates from the styloid process of the temporal bone.

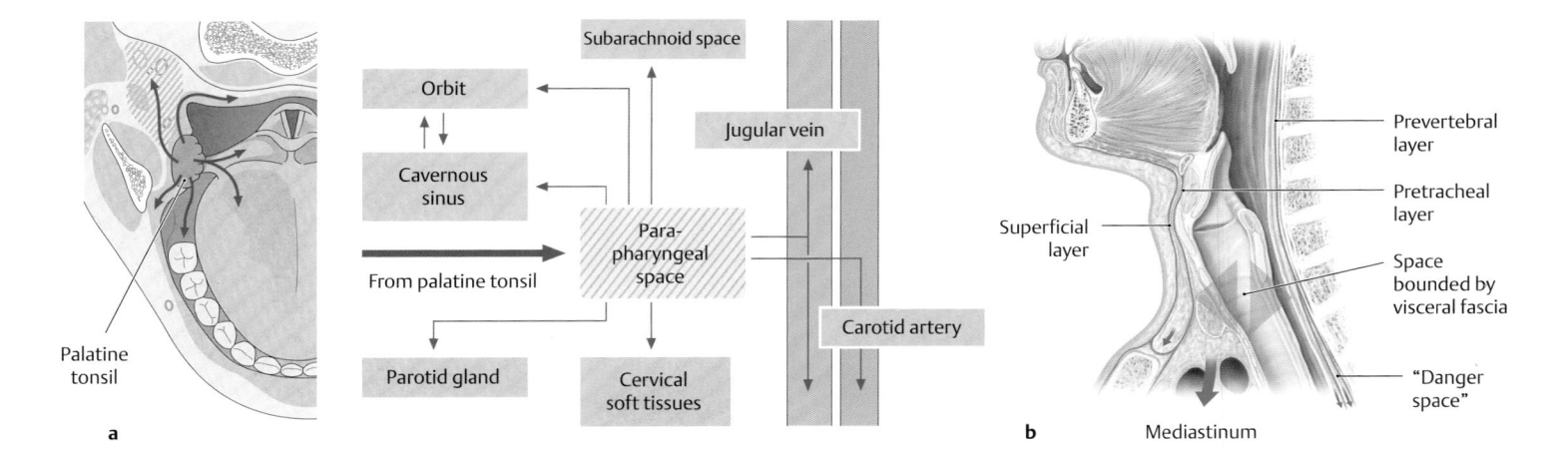

Subarachnoid space
Orbit
Cavernous sinus
Jugular vein
From palatine tonsil
Para-pharyngeal space
Carotid artery
Palatine tonsil
Parotid gland
Cervical soft tissues

a

Prevertebral layer
Pretracheal layer
Superficial layer
Space bounded by visceral fascia
"Danger space"

b   Mediastinum

B Clinical significance of the parapharyngeal space
(after Becker, Naumann, and Pfaltz)

a The parapharyngeal space has major clinical importance because bacteria and inflammatory cells may invade this space from the palatine tonsil and spread in various directions:

  • Invasion of the jugular vein may lead to bacteremia and sepsis.
  • Invasion of the subarachnoid space poses a risk of meningitis.

b An inflammatory process may also track downward from the neck and invade the mediastinum (gravitation abscess), inciting an inflammation of that region (mediastinitis). Similar gravitation abscesses may develop between the anterior and middle layers of the cervical fascia and along the carotid sheath. Infections may also spread directly into the posterior mediastinum through the slit-like "danger space" formed by the prevertebral layer of the deep cervical fascia.

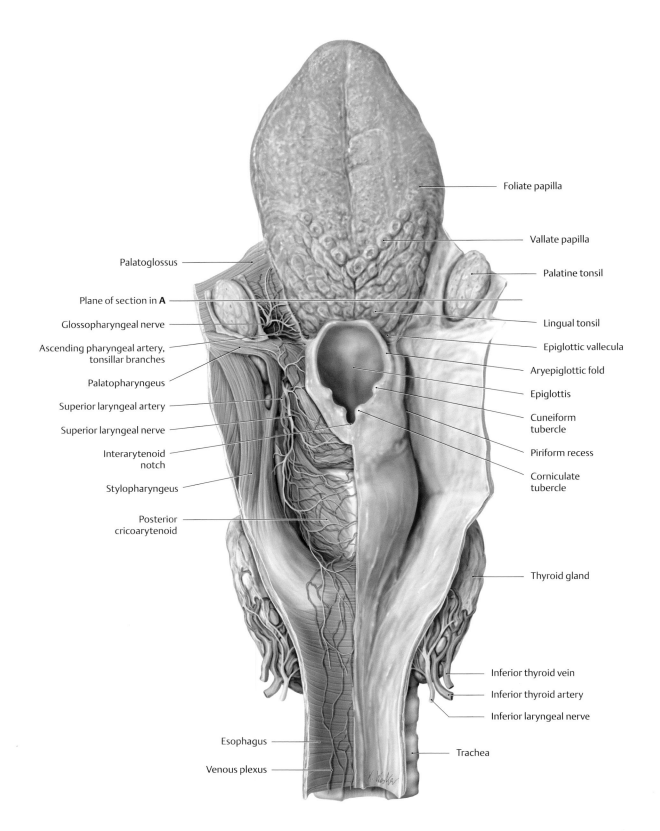

Foliate papilla

Vallate papilla

Palatoglossus

Palatine tonsil

Plane of section in **A**

Glossopharyngeal nerve

Lingual tonsil

Ascending pharyngeal artery,
tonsillar branches

Epiglottic vallecula

Aryepiglottic fold

Palatopharyngeus

Superior laryngeal artery

Epiglottis

Superior laryngeal nerve

Cuneiform
tubercle

Interarytenoid
notch

Piriform recess

Stylopharyngeus

Corniculate
tubercle

Posterior
cricoarytenoid

Thyroid gland

Inferior thyroid vein

Inferior thyroid artery

Inferior laryngeal nerve

Esophagus

Trachea

Venous plexus

C Neurovascular structures of the parapharyngeal space
(after Platzer)
Posterior view of an en-bloc specimen composed of the tongue, larynx, esophagus, and thyroid gland, as it would be resected at autopsy for pathologic evaluation of the neck. This dissection clearly demonstrates the branching pattern of the neurovascular structures that occupy the plane between the pharyngeal muscles.
Note the vascular supply to the palatine tonsil and its proximity to the neurovascular bundle, which creates a risk of hemorrhage during tonsillectomy.

4.1 Surface Anatomy and Triangles of the Neck

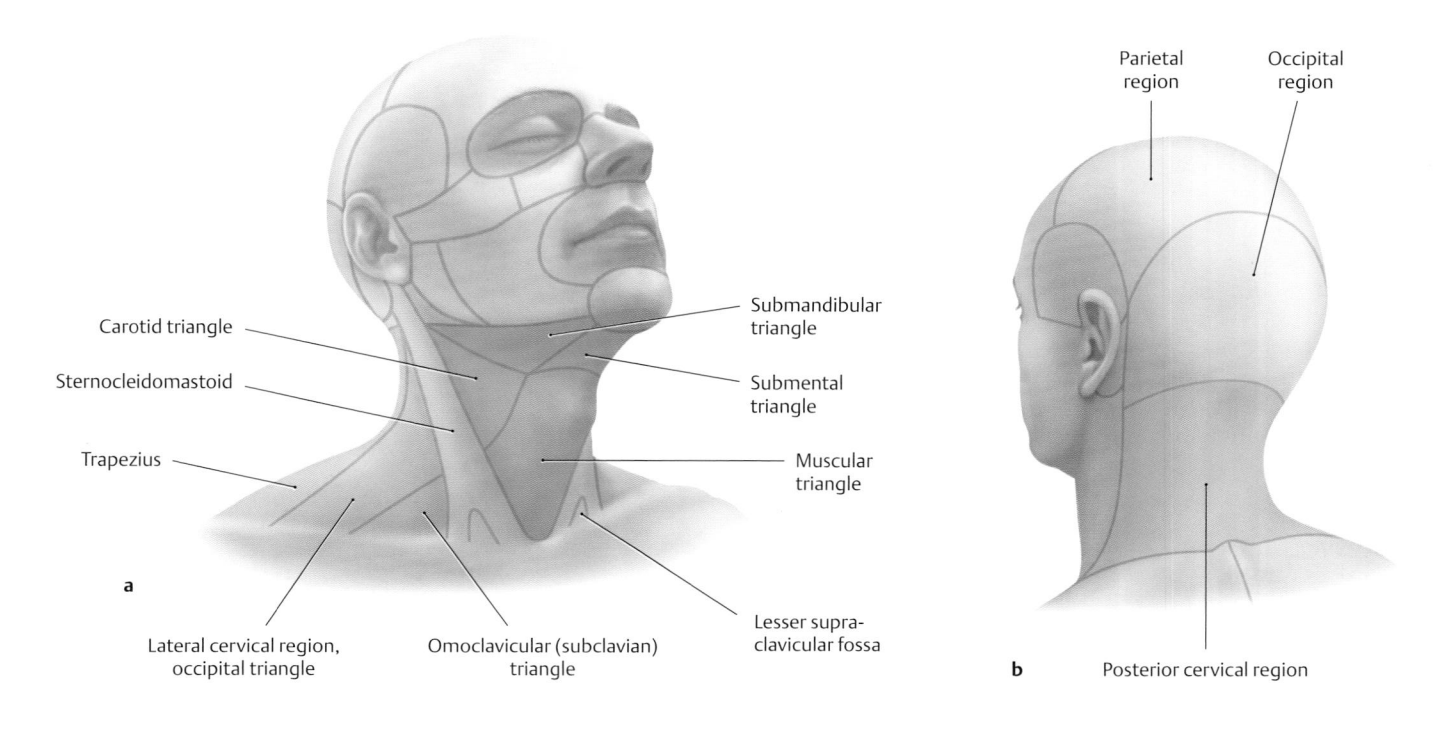

a

Carotid triangle

Sternocleidomastoid

Trapezius

Lateral cervical region, occipital triangle

Omoclavicular (subclavian) triangle

Submandibular triangle

Submental triangle

Muscular triangle

Lesser supra-clavicular fossa

Parietal region

Occipital region

b Posterior cervical region

A Regions of the neck (cervical regions)
a Right lateral view, **b** right posterior oblique view.
For descriptive purposes, the anterior and lateral neck are divided into two triangles which share the sternocleidomastoid as a boundary. Each is further subdivided into smaller triangles (listed in **C**). The clinician should know the boundaries and contents of the cervical triangles in order to perform an organized physical examination of structures within each triangle (see **D**).

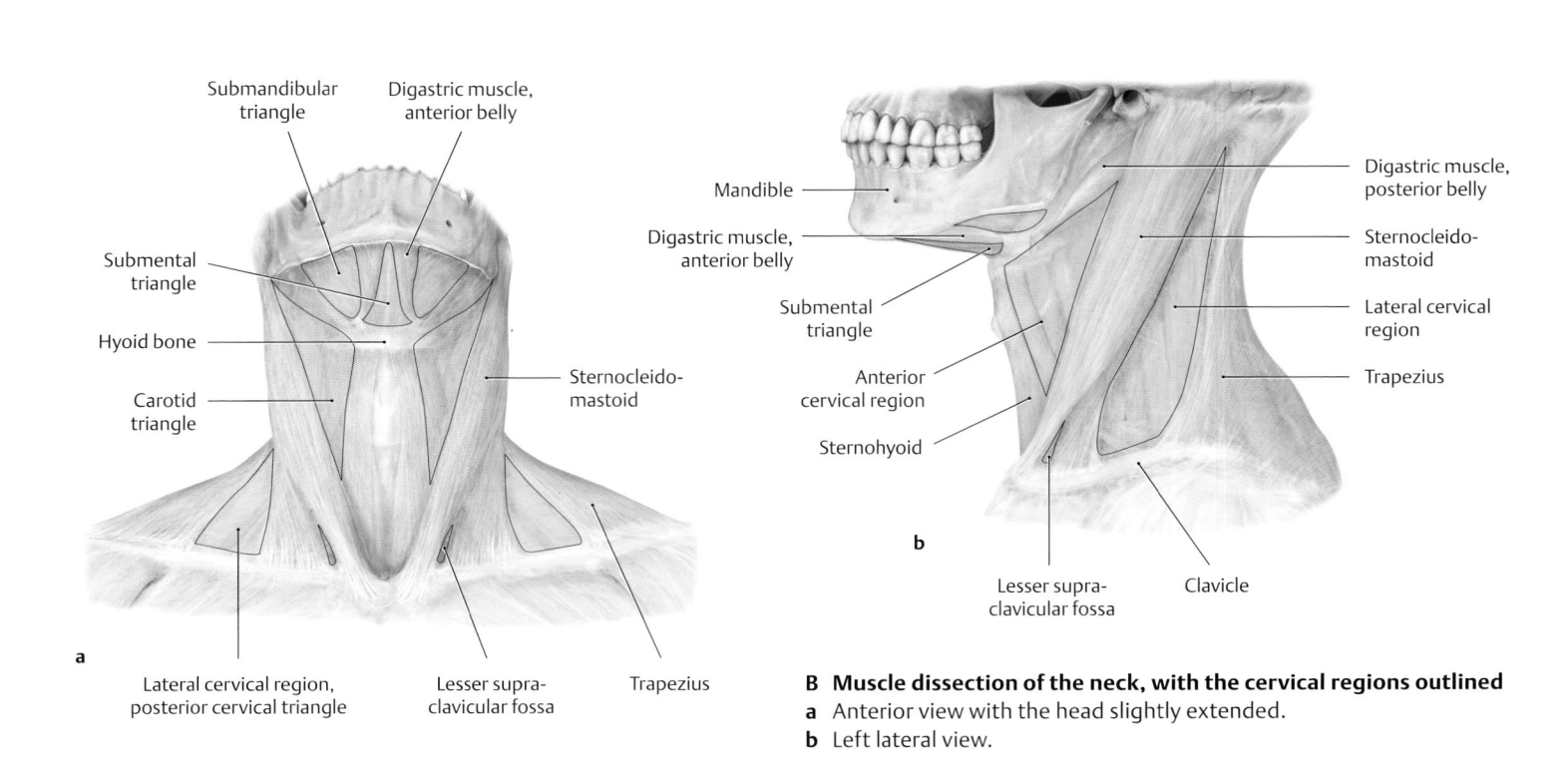

a

Submandibular triangle

Digastric muscle, anterior belly

Submental triangle

Hyoid bone

Carotid triangle

Sternocleido-mastoid

Lateral cervical region, posterior cervical triangle

Lesser supra-clavicular fossa

Trapezius

Mandible

Digastric muscle, anterior belly

Submental triangle

Anterior cervical region

Sternohyoid

Digastric muscle, posterior belly

Sternocleido-mastoid

Lateral cervical region

Trapezius

b

Lesser supra-clavicular fossa

Clavicle

B Muscle dissection of the neck, with the cervical regions outlined
a Anterior view with the head slightly extended.
b Left lateral view.

C Regions of the neck (cervical regions)

Anterior cervical region
- Submandibular triangle
- Carotid triangle
- Muscular triangle
- Submental triangle

Sternocleidomastoid region
- Lesser supraclavicular fossa

Lateral cervical region
- Omoclavicular (subclavian) triangle
- Occipital triangle

Posterior cervical region

D Distribution of anatomically important structures by cervical regions (after Anschütz)

Certain deep structures in the neck have their surface projections in specific cervical regions. Conversely, pathology that is noted in one region can be referred to an underlying anatomical structure. Glomus tumors, for example, are located in the carotid triangle. All of the regions in **C** are not listed because some regions are rarely affected by disease.

Anterior cervical region	
• Submandibular triangle	Submandibular lymph nodes, submandibular gland, hypoglossal nerve, parotid gland (posterior)
• Carotid triangle	Carotid bifurcation, carotid body, hypoglossal nerve
• Muscular triangle	Thyroid gland, larynx, trachea, esophagus
• Submental triangle	Submental lymph nodes
Sternocleidomastoid region	Sternocleidomastoid muscle, carotid artery, internal jugular vein, vagus nerve, jugular lymph nodes
Lateral cervical region	Lateral lymph nodes, accessory nerve, cervical plexus, brachial plexus

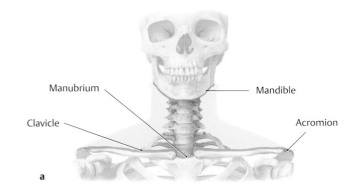

a

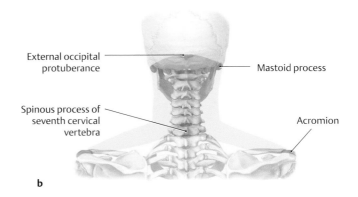

b

E Palpable bony prominences in the neck

a Anterior view, **b** posterior view. These points provide useful anatomical landmarks for physical examination of the neck, and they help to define the boundaries of the cervical regions.

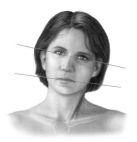

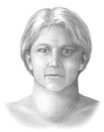

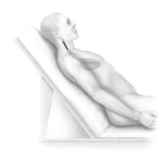

F Left-sided muscular torticollis
(after Anschütz)

Torticollis and goiter (see **B**) are examples of cervical disorders that can be readily diagnosed by visual inspection. Muscular torticollis is caused by unilateral shortening of the sternocleidomastoid muscle, often a postnatal complication of abnormal fetal position in the womb. The head is tilted toward the affected side and is slightly rotated toward the opposite side. Unless corrected by physical therapy or surgery, this condition leads secondarily to asymmetrical growth of the spinal column and facial skeleton. The effects of the cranial asymmetry may include a convergence of the facial planes toward the affected side (red lines).

G Retrosternal goiter (after Hegglin)

A goiter that arises from the inferior poles (see p. 22) of the thyroid gland may extend to the thoracic inlet and compress the cervical veins at that level. The result of this is venous congestion and dilation in the head and neck region (see **H**).

H Assessing the central venous pressure in the neck in a semi-upright position.

Normally the cervical veins are collapsed in the sitting position. But in a patient with right-sided heart failure, there is diminished venous return to the right heart, causing distention of the jugular veins. The extent of the venous congestion is indicated by the level of pulsations in the external jugular vein (the "venous pulse," upper end of the blue line). The higher the level of jugular pulsation, the greater the backup of blood into the vein. This provides a means of assessing the severity of right-sided heart failure.

4.2   Posterior Cervical Triangle

A Lateral view of the neck, subcutaneous layer

The posterior cervical triangle is a topographically important region bounded by the clavicle, the anterior border of the trapezius, and the posterior border of the sternocleidomastoid muscle.

This and the following drawings show progressively deeper dissections of the lateral cervical region. The adjacent sternocleidomastoid region and the anterior cervical region are also exposed. The skin and subcutaneous fat have been removed to display the subcutaneous, purely sensory cutaneous nerves from the cervical plexus in the lateral cervical region. They perforate the investing layer of the deep cervical fascia at the punctum nervosum (Erb's point) to supply the anterior and lateral neck. Specifically these nerves are the lesser occipital nerve, great auricular nerve, transverse cervical nerve, and supraclavicular nerves (medial, intermediate, and lateral).

Note: The transverse cervical nerve passes beneath the external jugular vein and forms an anastomosis with the cervical branch of the facial nerve. This mixed loop contains motor fibers from the facial nerve and sensory fibers for the neck from the transverse cervical nerve.

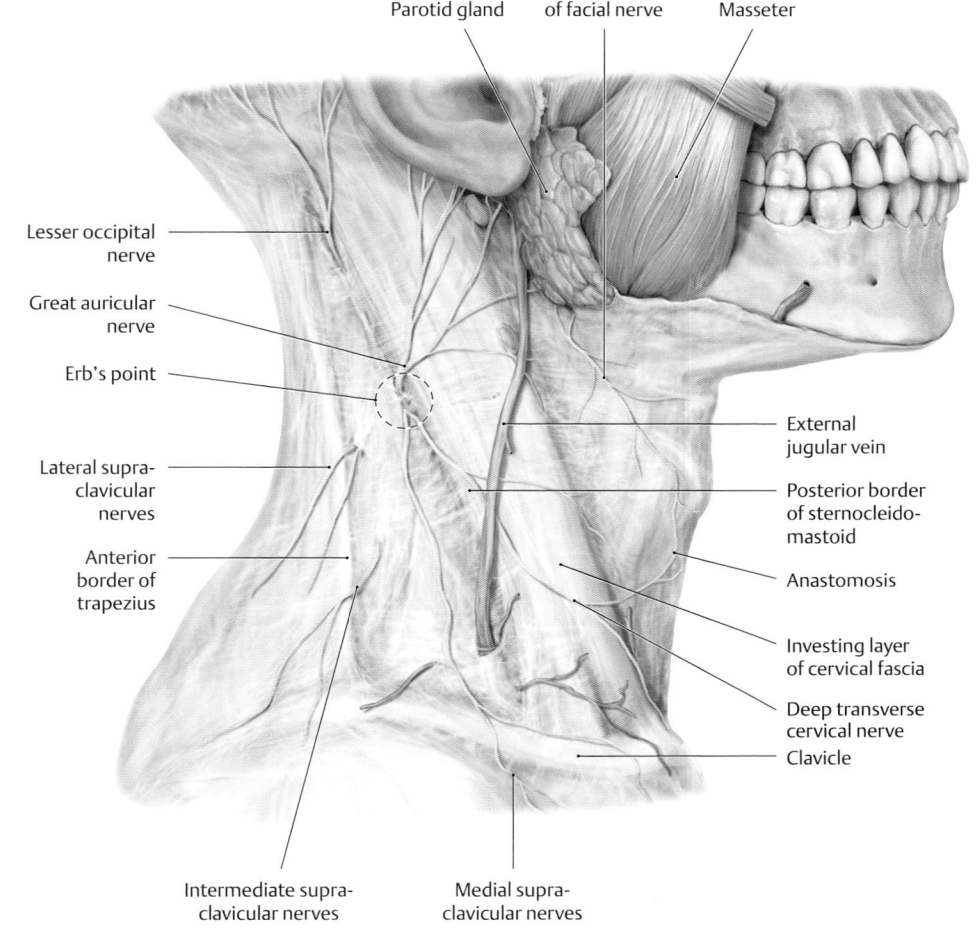

B Lateral cervical region (posterior cervical triangle), subfascial layer

Right lateral view. The investing layer of the deep cervical fascia has been removed over the posterior cervical triangle to expose the prevertebral layer of the cervical fascia, which is fused to the pretracheal lamina at the level of omohyoid muscle (see p. 3). The cutaneous nerves from the cervical plexus perforate the investing layer of the deep cervical fascia at approximately the mid-posterior border of the sternocleidomastoid muscle (Erb's point) and are distributed in the subcutaneous plane.

Note the external branch of the accessory nerve, which passes to the trapezius muscle. A surgeon taking a lymph node biopsy at may accidentally sever the external branch. This injury restricts the mobility of the scapula, and the patient may be unable to elevate the arm beyond 90°.

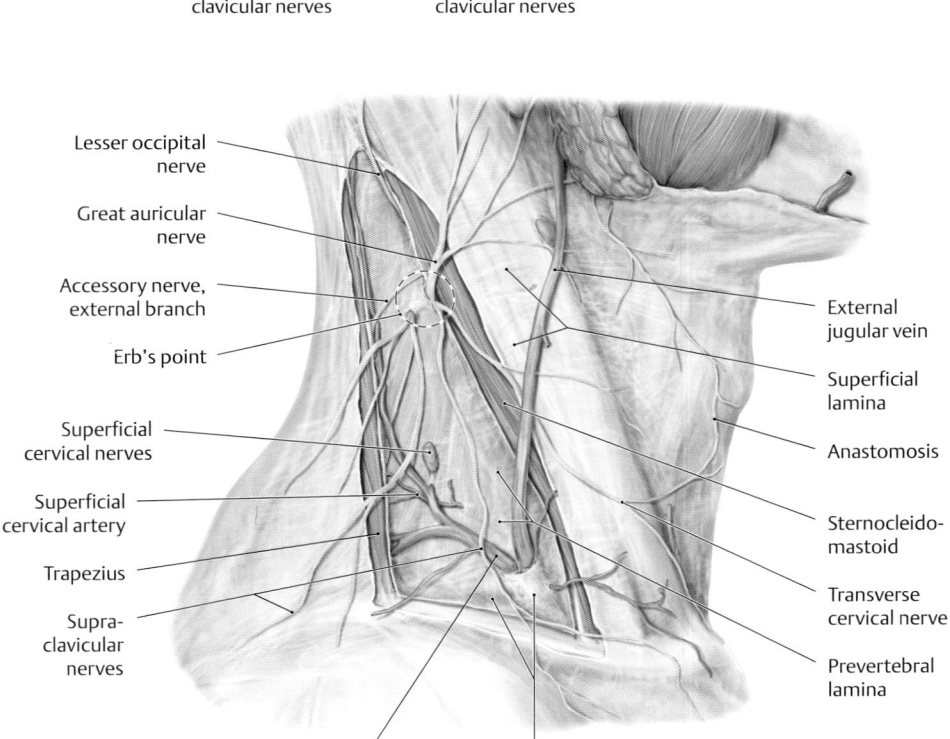

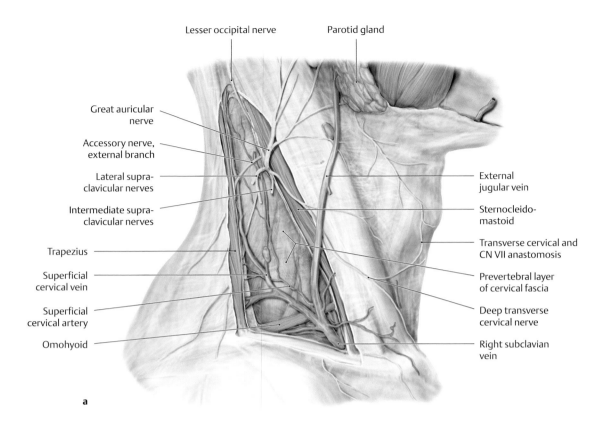

Lesser occipital nerve
Parotid gland
Great auricular nerve
Accessory nerve, external branch
Lateral supra-clavicular nerves
Intermediate supra-clavicular nerves
Trapezius
Superficial cervical vein
Superficial cervical artery
Omohyoid

External jugular vein
Sternocleido-mastoid
Transverse cervical and CN VII anastomosis
Prevertebral layer of cervical fascia
Deep transverse cervical nerve
Right subclavian vein

a

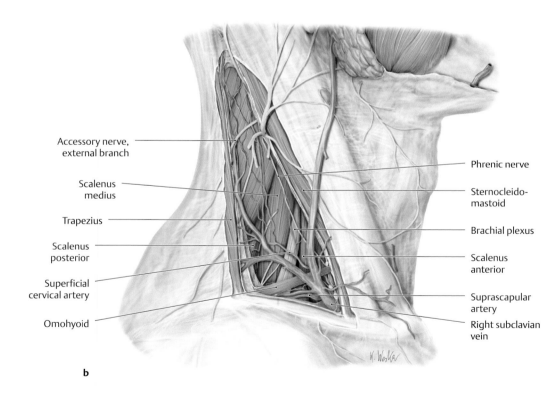

Accessory nerve, external branch
Scalenus medius
Trapezius
Scalenus posterior
Superficial cervical artery
Omohyoid

Phrenic nerve
Sternocleido-mastoid
Brachial plexus
Scalenus anterior
Suprascapular artery
Right subclavian vein

b

C Posterior cervical triangle

a Deeper layer, right lateral view. In this dissection, the pretracheal layer of the deep cervical fascia has additionally been removed to display the omohyoid muscle, which is enveloped by that fascia.

b Deepest layer with a view of the brachial plexus. The prevertebral layer has been removed to expose the scalene muscles.
Note the phrenic nerve, which runs obliquely over the scalenus anterior muscle to the thoracic inlet.

45

4.3   Anterior Cervical Triangle

A   The neck, superficial layer
Anterior view. The subcutaneous platysma has been removed on the right side, and the investing layer of the deep cervical fascia (see p. 2 for cervical fascial structure) has been split in the midline and partially removed, exposing the sternal head of the right sternocleidomastoid muscle. The anterior cervical triangle, which is bounded posteriorly by the sternocleidomastoid muscle and superiorly by the lower border of the mandible, is particularly well delineated on the right side. The anterior jugular vein and arch of the jugular vein can be identified. The inferior pole of the parotid gland projects inferior to the mandible. When the parotid gland is inflamed (mumps), it causes conspicuous facial swelling and deformity in this region ("hamster cheeks" with prominent earlobes). *Note* also the cutaneous nerves of the cervical plexus (great auricular, transverse cervical, supraclavicular), which radiate from Erb's point (see p. 44).

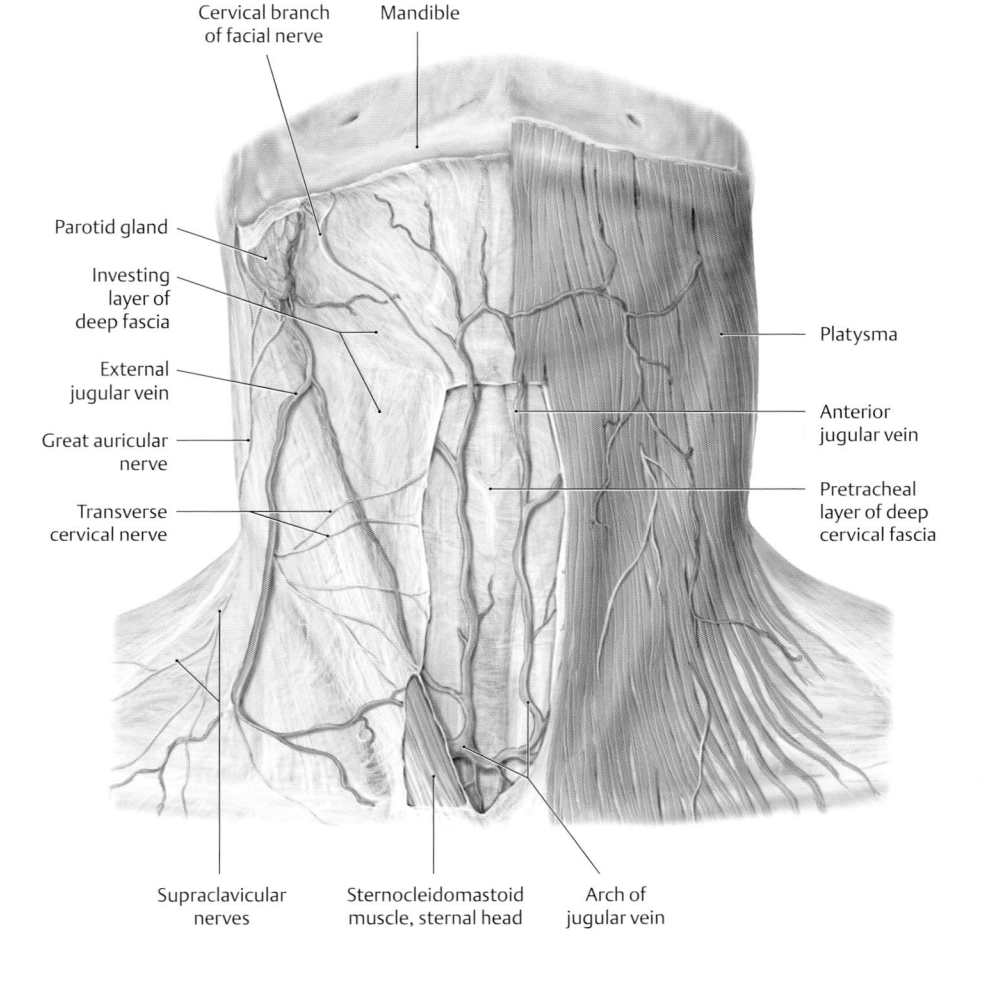

B   The neck, deep layer
Anterior view. The pretracheal lamina (middle layer of cervical fascia) has been removed. The infrahyoid muscles inserting on the pretracheal lamina have been resected and the visceral fascia has been removed to expose the thyroid gland, which is posterior to the infrahyoid muscles. The superior thyroid artery, the first branch of the external carotid artery, can be identified. The external branch of the superior laryngeal nerve, a branch of the vagus nerve, courses with the superior thyroid artery to the cricothyroid muscle. The internal branch of the superior laryngeal nerve passes through the thyrohyoid membrane with the superior laryngeal artery to supply the larynx.

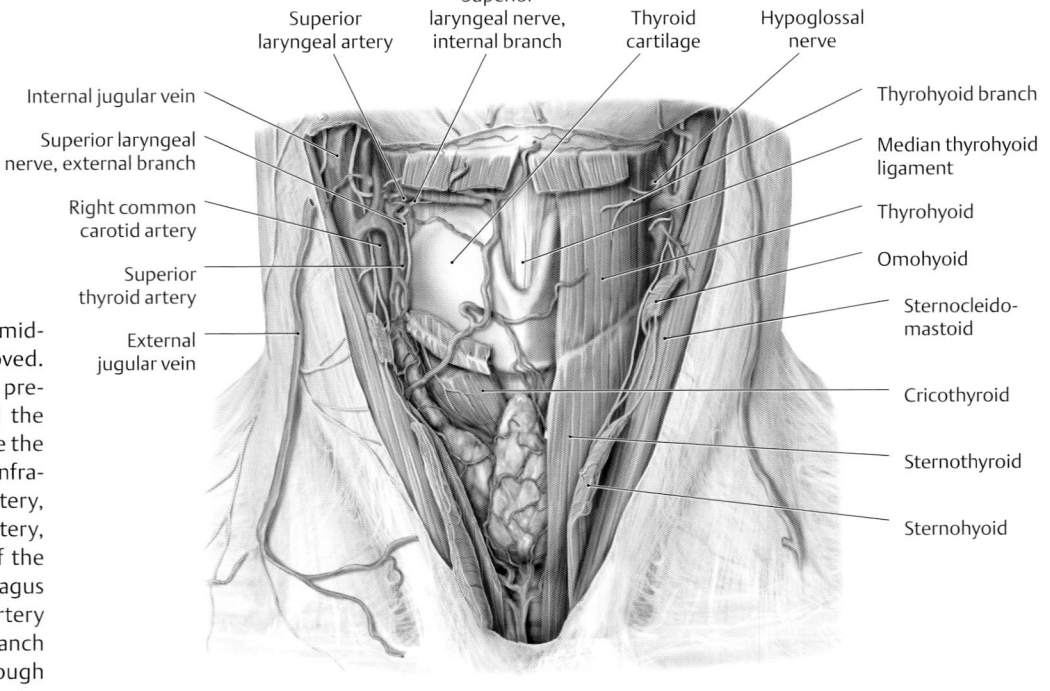

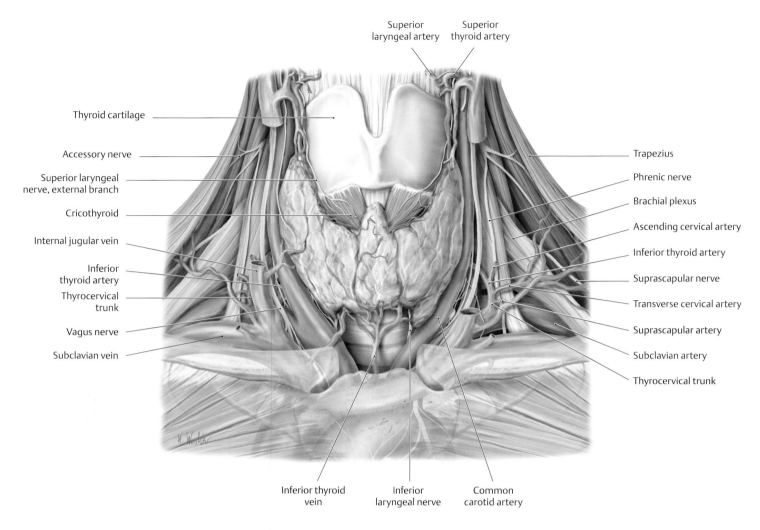

Superior laryngeal artery

Superior thyroid artery

Thyroid cartilage

Accessory nerve

Superior laryngeal nerve, external branch

Cricothyroid

Internal jugular vein

Inferior thyroid artery

Thyrocervical trunk

Vagus nerve

Subclavian vein

Trapezius

Phrenic nerve

Brachial plexus

Ascending cervical artery

Inferior thyroid artery

Suprascapular nerve

Transverse cervical artery

Suprascapular artery

Subclavian artery

Thyrocervical trunk

Inferior thyroid vein

Inferior laryngeal nerve

Common carotid artery

C Deep anterior cervical region with the thyroid gland
Anterior view. The following neurovascular structures are clearly visible in their course through the thoracic inlet: the common carotid artery, subclavian artery, subclavian vein, internal jugular vein, inferior thyroid vein, vagus nerve, phrenic nerve, and inferior laryngeal nerve. It can be seen that a retrosternal goiter enlarging the inferior pole of the thyroid gland can easily compress neurovascular structures at the thoracic inlet (see Fig. **G**, p. 43).

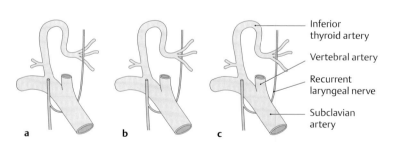

Inferior thyroid artery

Vertebral artery

Recurrent laryngeal nerve

Subclavian artery

a   b   c

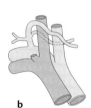

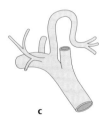

a   b   c

D Course of the right recurrent laryngeal nerve
(after von Lanz and Wachsmuth)
Anterior view. The recurrent laryngeal nerve is a somatomotor and sensory branch of the vagus nerve, which innervates all the muscles of the larynx except the cricothyroid muscle. Unilateral damage to this nerve supply results in hoarseness, while bilateral damage leads to a closed glottis with severe dyspnea. The recurrent laryngeal nerve may pass in front of (**a**), behind (**b**), or between (**c**) the branches of the inferior thyroid artery. Its course should be noted during operations on the thyroid gland.

E Variations in the branching pattern of the right inferior thyroid artery (after Platzer)
The course of the inferior thyroid artery is highly variable. It may run medially behind the vertebral artery (**a**), it may divide immediately after arising from the thyrocervical trunk (**b**), or it may arise as the first branch of the subclavian artery (**c**).

4.4 Deep Lateral Cervical Region, Carotid Triangle, and Thoracic Inlet

A Base of neck and thoracic inlet on the left side

Anterior view. The sternal end of the clavicle, the anterior end of the first rib, the manubrium sterni, and the thyroid gland have been removed to expose the thoracic inlet. The subclavian artery and thyrocervical trunk can be identified.

Note the course of the following structures: The internal thoracic artery descends parallel to the sternum. It is of special clinical interest. In patients with coronary heart disease, the internal thoracic artery can be mobilized and anastomosed to the coronary artery past the point of the stenosis. The sympathetic trunk, vagus nerve, phrenic nerve, and portions of the brachial plexus are visible, the latter passing through the interscalene space (see **C**).

Note also the termination of the thoracic duct at the jugulosubclavian venous junction and the left recurrent laryngeal nerve. This branch of the vagus nerve winds around the aortic arch and ascends to the larynx.

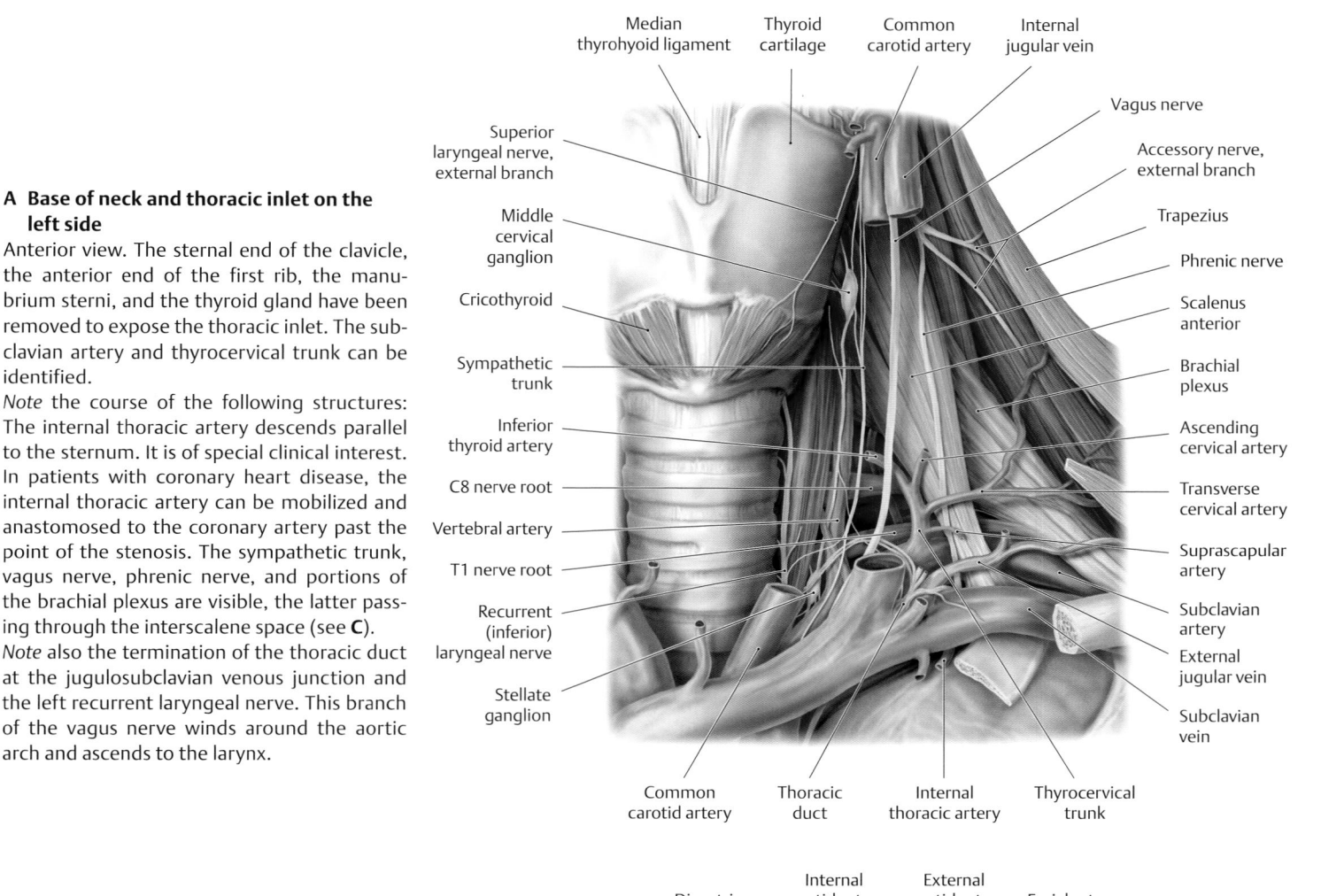

B Carotid triangle

Right lateral view. The carotid triangle is a subregion of the anterior cervical triangle. It is bounded by the sternocleidomastoid muscle, the posterior belly of the digastric muscle, and the superior belly of the omohyoid muscle. The submandibular gland can be seen at the inferior border of the chin, and the sternocleidomastoid muscle has been retracted posterolaterally. The following structures are located in the carotid triangle:

- Internal and external carotid arteries (the superior thyroid and lingual arteries branch from the latter)
- Hypoglossal nerve
- Vagus nerve
- Accessory nerve
- Sympathetic trunk with associated ganglia

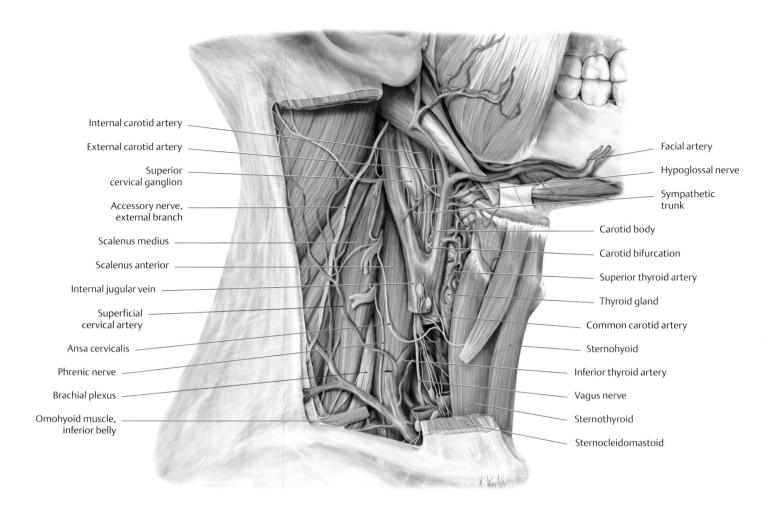

Internal carotid artery
External carotid artery
Superior cervical ganglion
Accessory nerve, external branch
Scalenus medius
Scalenus anterior
Internal jugular vein
Superficial cervical artery
Ansa cervicalis
Phrenic nerve
Brachial plexus
Omohyoid muscle, inferior belly

Facial artery
Hypoglossal nerve
Sympathetic trunk
Carotid body
Carotid bifurcation
Superior thyroid artery
Thyroid gland
Common carotid artery
Sternohyoid
Inferior thyroid artery
Vagus nerve
Sternothyroid
Sternocleidomastoid

C Deep lateral cervical region

Right lateral view. The sternocleidomastoid region and carotid triangle have been dissected along with adjacent portions of the posterior and anterior cervical triangles. The carotid sheath has been removed in this dissection along with the cervical fasciae, sternocleidomastoid muscle, and omohyoid muscle to demonstrate all important neurovascular structures in the neck:

- Common carotid artery with its division into the internal and external carotid arteries
- Superior and inferior thyroid arteries
- Internal jugular vein
- Deep cervical lymph nodes along the internal jugular vein
- Sympathetic trunk including its ganglia

- Vagus nerve
- Hypoglossal nerve
- Accessory nerve
- Brachial plexus
- Phrenic nerve.

The phrenic nerve originates from the C3–C5 segments and therefore is part of the cervical plexus. The muscular landmark for locating the phrenic nerve is the scalenus anterior, along which the nerve descends in the neck. The (posterior) interscalene space is located between the scalenus anterior and medius and the first rib and is traversed by the brachial plexus and subclavian artery. The subclavian vein passes deeply through the interval formed by the scalenus anterior, the sternocleidomastoid muscle (resected), and the first rib (the anterior interscalene space).

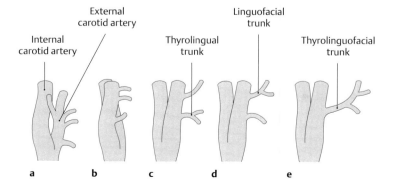

Internal carotid artery
External carotid artery
Thyrolingual trunk
Linguofacial trunk
Thyrolinguofacial trunk

a   b   c   d   e

D Variable position of the external and internal carotid arteries and variants in the anterior branches of the external carotid artery (after Faller and Poisel-Golth)

a, b   The internal carotid artery may arise from the common carotid artery posterolateral (49%) or anteromedial (9%) to the external carotid artery, or at other intermediate sites.
c–e   The external carotid artery may give origin to a thyrolingual trunk (4%), linguofacial trunk (23%), or thyrolinguofacial trunk (0.6%).

49

4.5 Posterior Cervical Region and Occipital Region

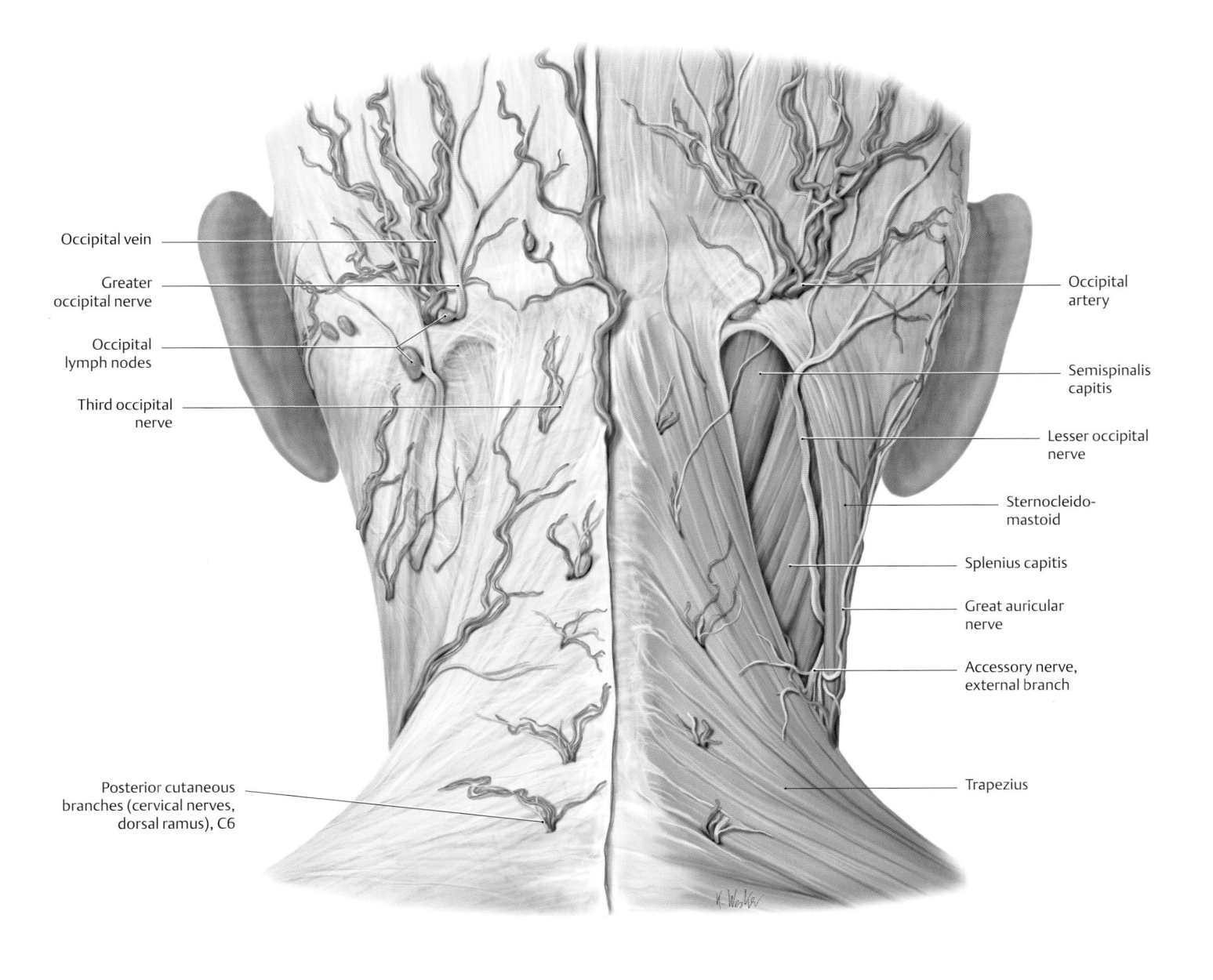

Occipital vein

Greater
occipital nerve

Occipital
lymph nodes

Third occipital
nerve

Posterior cutaneous
branches (cervical nerves,
dorsal ramus), C6

Occipital
artery

Semispinalis
capitis

Lesser occipital
nerve

Sternocleido-
mastoid

Splenius capitis

Great auricular
nerve

Accessory nerve,
external branch

Trapezius

A Posterior cervical region and occipital region
Posterior view of the subcutaneous layer on the left side and the subfascial layer on the right side. Although the occipital region is part of the head, it is discussed here because it borders on the posterior cervical region. The principal arterial vessel in this region is the occipital artery, the second branch arising from the posterior side of the external carotid artery. The medially situated greater occipital nerve is a *dorsal* ramus of the C 2 spinal nerve, while the laterally situated lesser occipital nerve is a *ventral* ramus of C 2 that arises from the cervical plexus (see p. 17). The lymph nodes are located at the sites where the nerves and veins emerge through the cervical fascia.

Note the external branch of the accessory nerve, which crosses the lateral cervical triangle at a relatively superficial level.

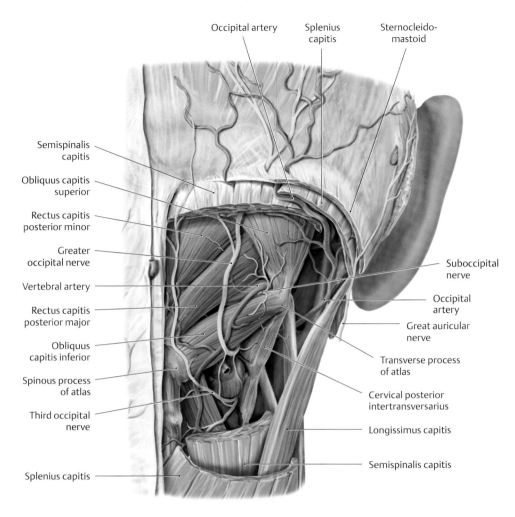

Occipital artery · Splenius capitis · Sternocleido-mastoid

Semispinalis capitis

Obliquus capitis superior

Rectus capitis posterior minor

Greater occipital nerve

Vertebral artery

Rectus capitis posterior major

Obliquus capitis inferior

Spinous process of atlas

Third occipital nerve

Splenius capitis

Suboccipital nerve

Occipital artery

Great auricular nerve

Transverse process of atlas

Cervical posterior intertransversarius

Longissimus capitis

Semispinalis capitis

B Right suboccipital triangle

Posterior view. The suboccipital triangle is bounded superiorly by the rectus capitis posterior major, laterally by the obliquus capitis superior, and inferiorly by the obliquus capitis inferior. This muscular triangle can be seen only after the trapezius, splenius capitis, and semispinalis capitis muscles have been removed. A short, free segment of the vertebral artery runs through the deep part of the triangle after leaving the transverse foramen and before exiting the triangle by perforating the atlanto-occipital membrane (not visible here). That segment of the vertebral artery gives off branches to the surrounding short nuchal muscles. Both vertebral arteries unite intracranially to form the basilar artery, which is a major contributor to cerebral blood flow.

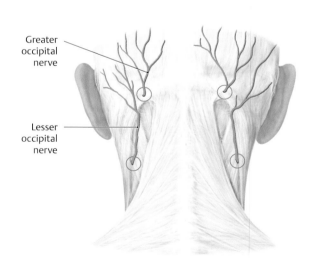

Greater occipital nerve

Lesser occipital nerve

Ophthalmic nerve

C2

C3

C4

a

Ophthalmic nerve

Greater occipital nerve

Lesser occipital nerve

Dorsal rami

Great auricular nerve

Supraclavicular nerves

b

C Clinically important sites of emergence of the occipital nerves

Posterior view. The sites where the lesser and greater occipital nerves emerge from the fascia into the subcutaneous connective tissue are clinically important because they are tender to palpation in certain diseases (e. g., meningitis). The examiner tests the sensation of these nerves by pressing lightly on the circled points with the thumb. If these points (but not their surroundings) are painful, the finding is described, logically, as "tenderness over the occipital nerves."

D Cutaneous innervation of the neck

Posterior view. The pattern of segmental innervation is illustrated on the left, and the territorial assignments of specific cutaneous nerves on the right. The occiput and neck derive most of their segmental innervation from the second and third cervical segments. The ophthalmic nerve supplying the area above the C 2 level is the first branch of the trigeminal nerve (CN V).

Note that in the peripheral innervation pattern, the greater occipital nerve is a *dorsal* spinal nerve ramus while the lesser occipital nerve is a *ventral* ramus (see p. 16).

51

4.6 Cross-sectional Anatomy of the Neck from the T2/T1 to C7/C6 Levels

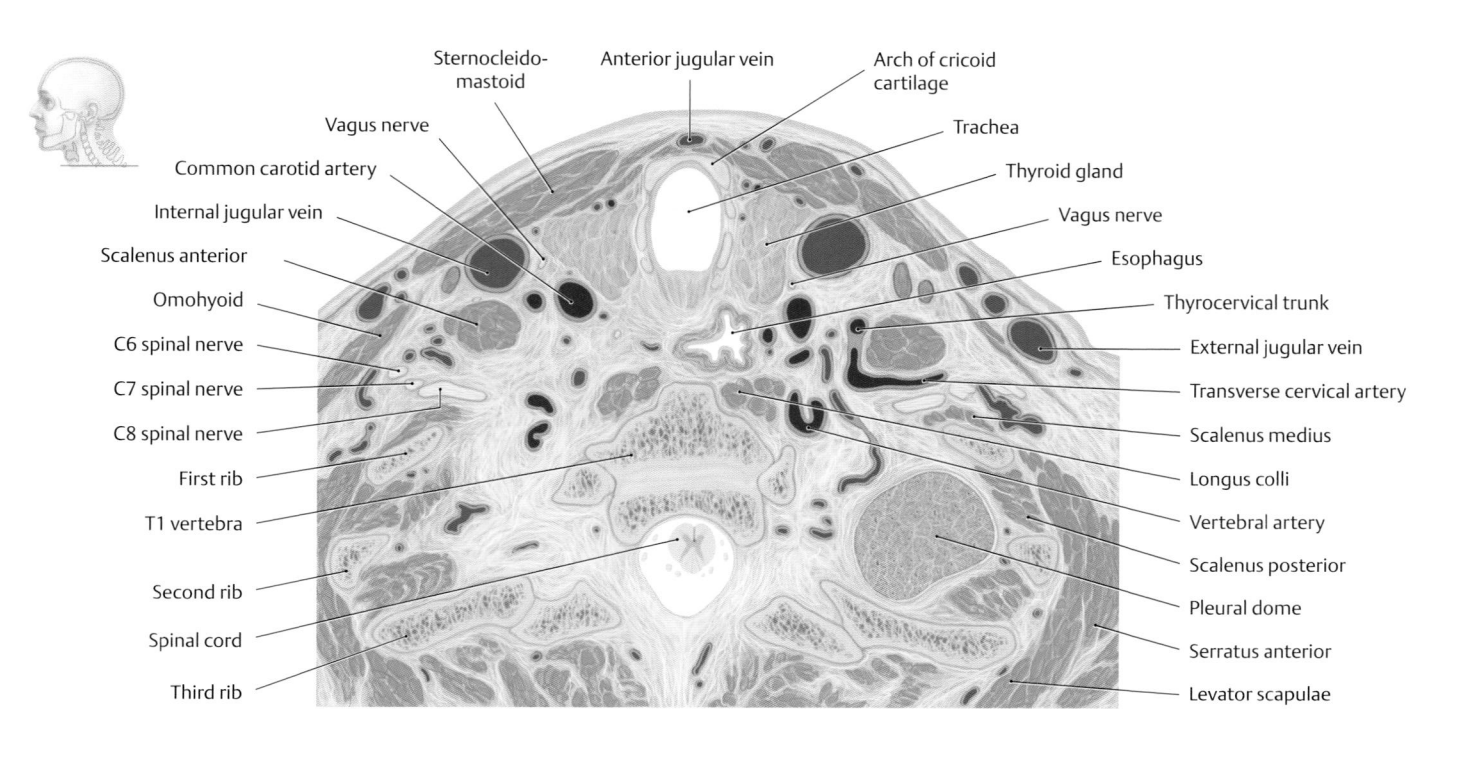

Labels (clockwise/around the image):
Sternocleido-mastoid — Anterior jugular vein — Arch of cricoid cartilage — Vagus nerve — Common carotid artery — Internal jugular vein — Scalenus anterior — Omohyoid — C6 spinal nerve — C7 spinal nerve — C8 spinal nerve — First rib — T1 vertebra — Second rib — Spinal cord — Third rib — Trachea — Thyroid gland — Vagus nerve — Esophagus — Thyrocervical trunk — External jugular vein — Transverse cervical artery — Scalenus medius — Longus colli — Vertebral artery — Scalenus posterior — Pleural dome — Serratus anterior — Levator scapulae

A Transverse cross-section of the neck at a level that just cuts the left pleural dome (level of the T2/T1 vertebral bodies)
Inferior view. Due to the curvature of the neck in this specimen, the section also cuts the intervertebral disk between T1 and T2.
Note that the cross-section is viewed from below like a CT scan or MRI slice. The illustrations that follow are transverse cross-sections through the neck at progressively higher (more cranial) levels (Tiedemann series).

The section in **A** includes cross-sections of the C6–C8 nerve roots of the brachial plexus and a small section of the left pleural dome. The proximity of the pulmonary apex to the brachial plexus shows why the growth of an apical lung tumor may damage the brachial plexus roots.
Note also the thyroid gland and its proximity to the trachea and neurovascular bundle in the carotid sheath (a thin fibrous sheet which is not clearly discernible in these views).

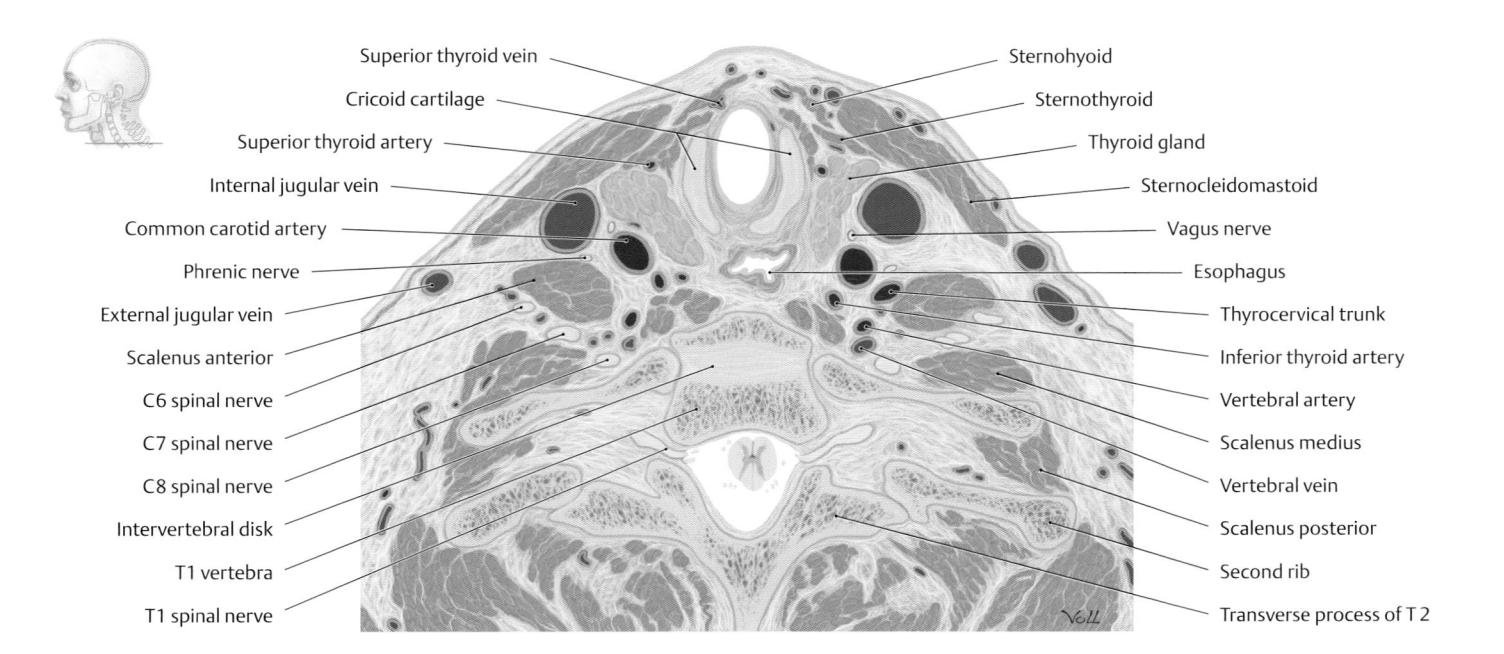

Labels (around the image):
Superior thyroid vein — Cricoid cartilage — Superior thyroid artery — Internal jugular vein — Common carotid artery — Phrenic nerve — External jugular vein — Scalenus anterior — C6 spinal nerve — C7 spinal nerve — C8 spinal nerve — Intervertebral disk — T1 vertebra — T1 spinal nerve — Sternohyoid — Sternothyroid — Thyroid gland — Sternocleidomastoid — Vagus nerve — Esophagus — Thyrocervical trunk — Inferior thyroid artery — Vertebral artery — Scalenus medius — Vertebral vein — Scalenus posterior — Second rib — Transverse process of T2

B Transverse cross-section through the lower third of the thyroid cartilage (junction of the T1/C7 vertebral bodies)
This cross-section clearly displays the scalenus anterior and medius muscles and the interval between them, which is traversed by the

C6–C8 roots of the brachial plexus. *Note* the neurovascular structures in the carotid sheath (common carotid artery, internal jugular vein, vagus nerve).

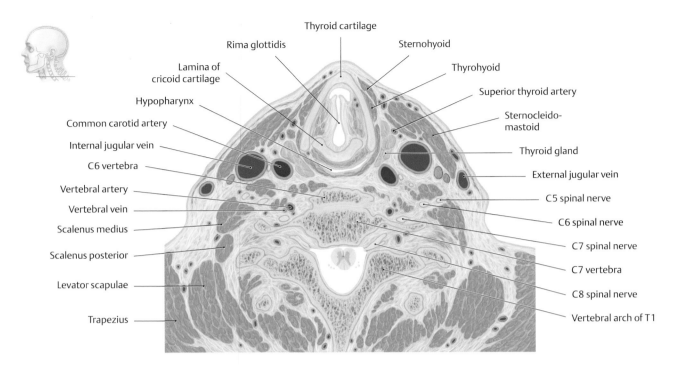

C Transverse cross-section at the level of the vocalis muscle in the larynx (junction of the C 7 / C 6 vertebral bodies)
This cross-section passes through the larynx at the level of the vocal folds. The thyroid gland appears considerably smaller at this level than in views **A** and **B**.

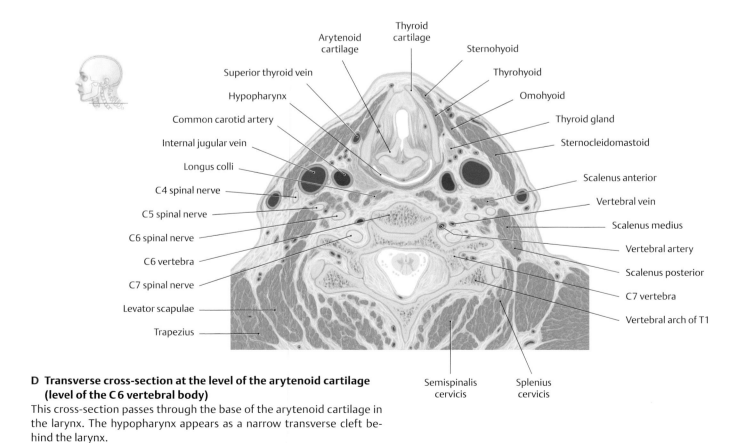

D Transverse cross-section at the level of the arytenoid cartilage (level of the C 6 vertebral body)
This cross-section passes through the base of the arytenoid cartilage in the larynx. The hypopharynx appears as a narrow transverse cleft behind the larynx.

4.7 Cross-sectional Anatomy at the Level of the C6/C5 Vertebral Bodies

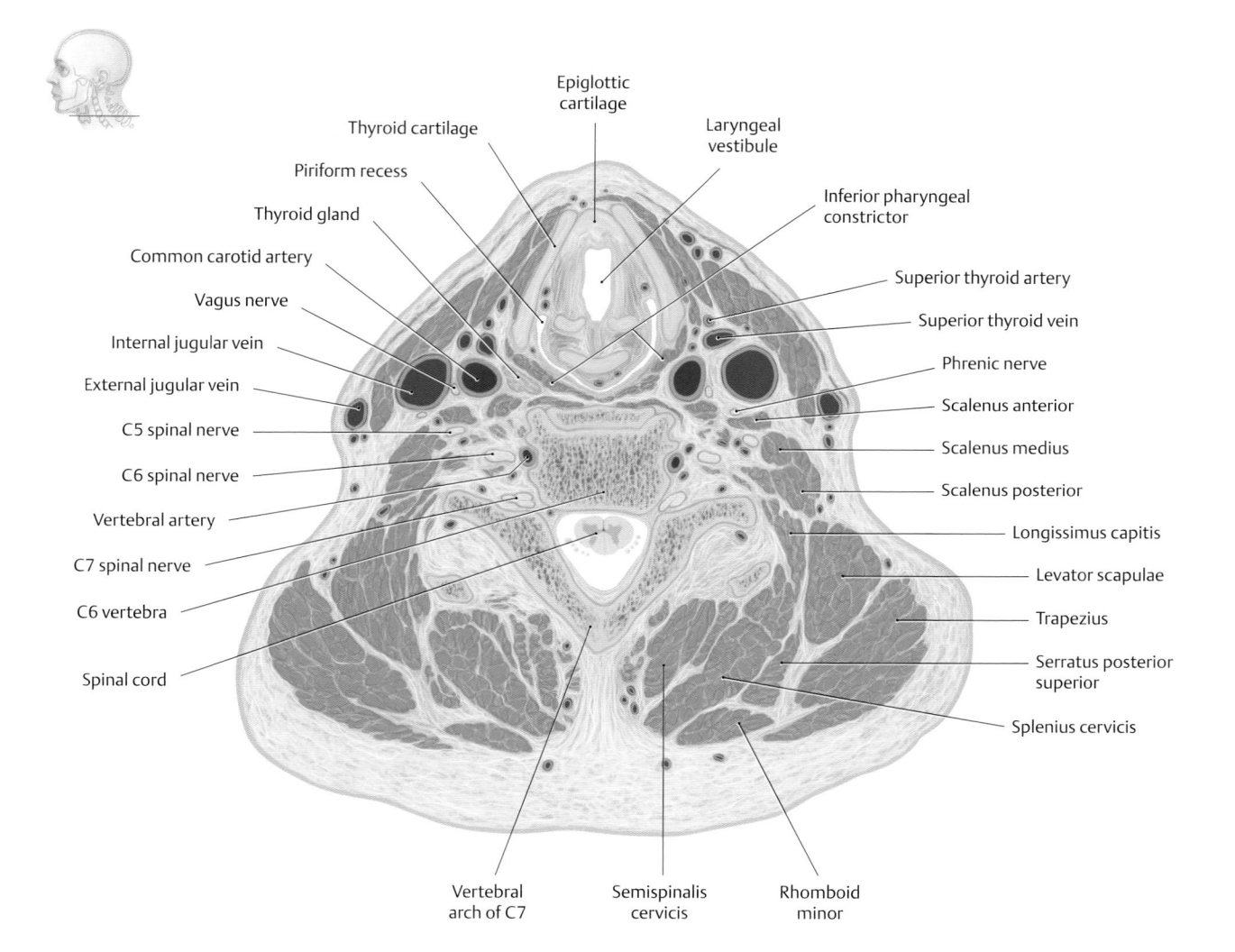

Epiglottic cartilage

Thyroid cartilage

Laryngeal vestibule

Piriform recess

Inferior pharyngeal constrictor

Thyroid gland

Common carotid artery

Superior thyroid artery

Vagus nerve

Superior thyroid vein

Internal jugular vein

Phrenic nerve

External jugular vein

Scalenus anterior

C5 spinal nerve

Scalenus medius

C6 spinal nerve

Scalenus posterior

Vertebral artery

Longissimus capitis

C7 spinal nerve

Levator scapulae

C6 vertebra

Trapezius

Spinal cord

Serratus posterior superior

Splenius cervicis

Vertebral arch of C7

Semispinalis cervicis

Rhomboid minor

A Transverse cross-section at the level of the laryngeal vestibule, demonstrating the epiglottis (C6 vertebral body)

The piriform recess can be identified at this level, and the vertebral artery is visible in its course along the vertebral body. The vagus nerve lies in a posterior angle between the common carotid artery and internal jugular vein. This view shows the profile of the phrenic nerve on the scalenus anterior muscle on the left side.

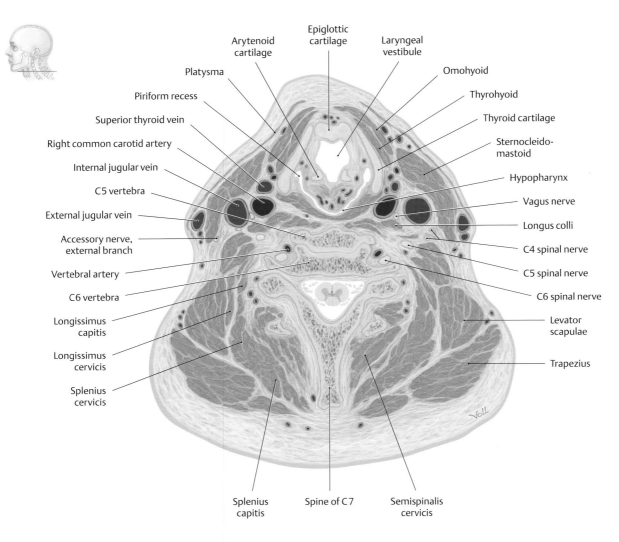

B Transverse cross-section at the level of the C 5 vertebral body
The elongated spinous process of the C 7 vertebra (vertebra prominens) is also visible at this level owing to the lordotic curvature of the neck. The triangular shape of the arytenoid cartilage is clearly demonstrated in the laryngeal cross-section. The laryngeal vestibule can also be identified. This view also shows the external branch of the accessory nerve medial to the sternocleidomastoid muscle.

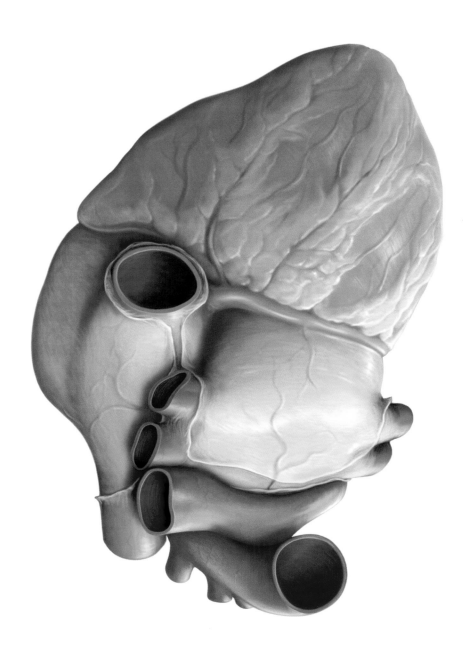

Thorax

1.1 Overview of the Thoracic Skeleton and its Landmarks

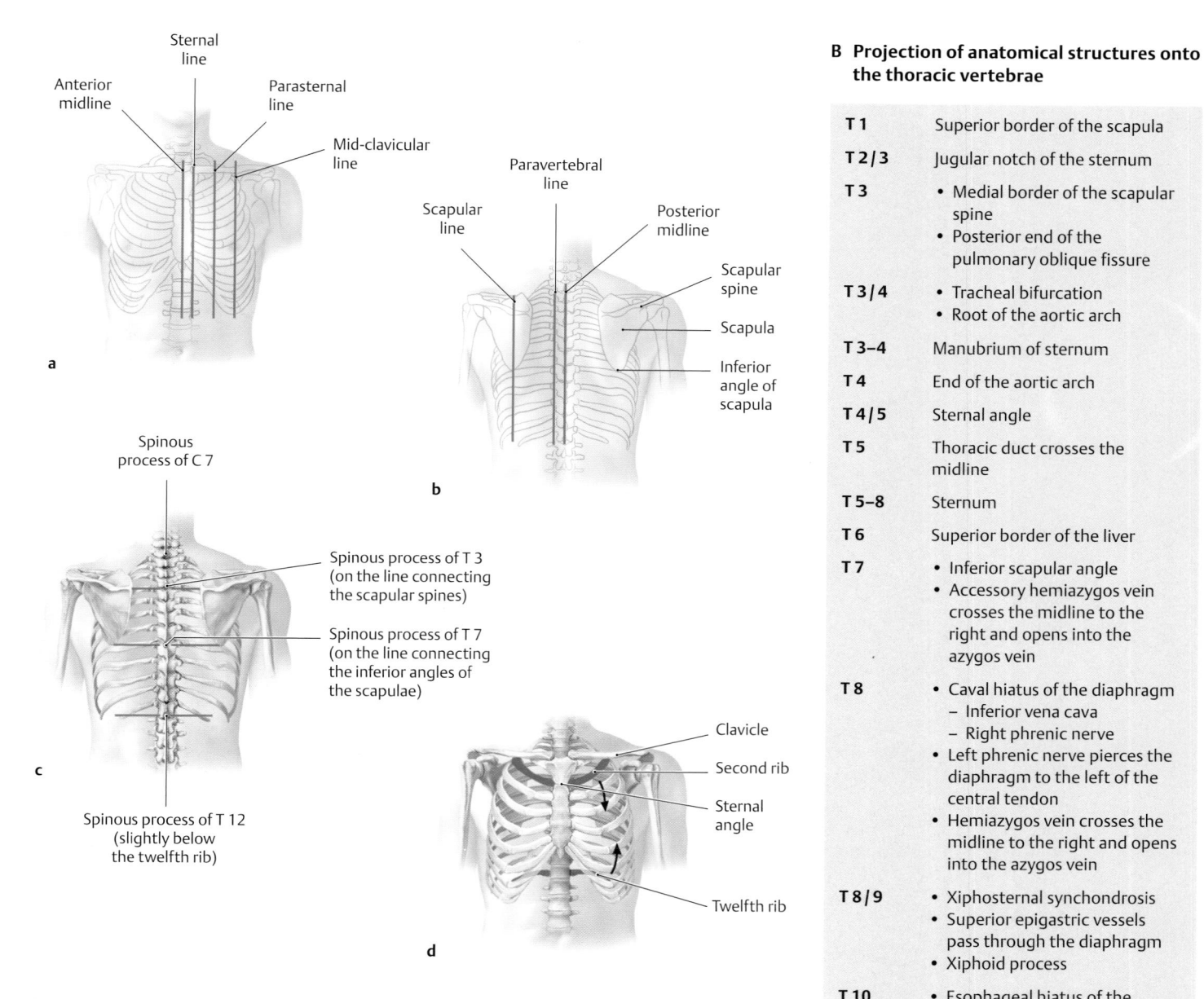

B Projection of anatomical structures onto the thoracic vertebrae

T 1	Superior border of the scapula
T 2/3	Jugular notch of the sternum
T 3	• Medial border of the scapular spine • Posterior end of the pulmonary oblique fissure
T 3/4	• Tracheal bifurcation • Root of the aortic arch
T 3–4	Manubrium of sternum
T 4	End of the aortic arch
T 4/5	Sternal angle
T 5	Thoracic duct crosses the midline
T 5–8	Sternum
T 6	Superior border of the liver
T 7	• Inferior scapular angle • Accessory hemiazygos vein crosses the midline to the right and opens into the azygos vein

T 8	• Caval hiatus of the diaphragm
	  – Inferior vena cava
	  – Right phrenic nerve
	• Left phrenic nerve pierces the diaphragm to the left of the central tendon
	• Hemiazygos vein crosses the midline to the right and opens into the azygos vein

T 8/9	• Xiphosternal synchondrosis • Superior epigastric vessels pass through the diaphragm • Xiphoid process

T 10	• Esophageal hiatus of the diaphragm:
	  – Esophagus
	  – Anterior vagal trunk
	  – Posterior vagal trunk

T 12	• Aortic hiatus of the diaphragm:
	  – Aorta
	  – Azygos and hemiazygos veins
	  – Thoracic duct
	• Origin of the celiac trunk (inferior border of T 12)
	• Splanchnic nerves pass through the crura of the diaphragm
	• Sympathetic trunk passes below the medial arcuate ligament: transpyloric plane (= line in abdomen, see p. 150)

A Anatomical landmarks of the thoracic skeleton

The thoracic skeleton presents a number of visible and palpable landmarks that are accessible to physical and radiographic examination (see **B**). These landmarks can be used to define reference lines for describing and evaluating the location and extent of organs based on their relationship to the lines:

- Longitudinal reference lines (**a, b**) are defined by visible or palpable anterior (**a**) and posterior (**b**) bony structures and provide information on the location and extent of specific thoracic organs (e.g., the apical heartbeat is palpable in the left mid-clavicular line).
- Most horizontal reference lines (**c**) are defined by the position of specific thoracic vertebrae. The seventh cervical vertebra (C 7) is

easily identified by palpating its very prominent spinous process. It provides a starting point from which the examiner can locate all 12 thoracic vertebrae (T 1–T 12). The levels of the T 3 and T 7 vertebrae correspond respectively to the medial end of the scapular spine and the inferior angle of the scapula.

- The ribs as anatomical landmarks (**d**). The levels of intrathoracic organs also correlate with specific ribs and intercostal spaces, particularly on the anterior side. The first rib is usually difficult to palpate because it is behind the clavicle. The second, however, is attached to the palpable sternal angle (where the body and manubrium of the sternum join). Past the second rib, the examiner should have no difficulty counting down the remaining ribs.

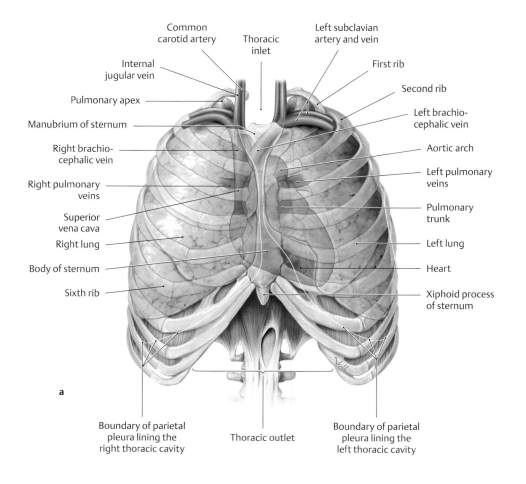

Common carotid artery
Thoracic inlet
Left subclavian artery and vein
Internal jugular vein
First rib
Pulmonary apex
Second rib
Manubrium of sternum
Left brachio-cephalic vein
Right brachio-cephalic vein
Aortic arch
Right pulmonary veins
Left pulmonary veins
Superior vena cava
Pulmonary trunk
Right lung
Left lung
Body of sternum
Heart
Sixth rib
Xiphoid process of sternum

a

Boundary of parietal pleura lining the right thoracic cavity
Thoracic outlet
Boundary of parietal pleura lining the left thoracic cavity

C Overview of the thorax

a Anterior view. The intercostal muscles, fasciae, and abdominal organs have been removed. **b** Simplified schematic view from the posterior side. The scapulae and several abdominal organs have been outlined for clarity. The thoracic cavity is one of the three main body cavities, along with the abdominal and pelvic cavities. The wall surrounding the thoracic cavity consists of:

- bones: 12 thoracic vertebrae, 12 pairs of ribs, and the sternum
- connective tissue: internal fasciae of the thorax, muscle fasciae
- muscles: chiefly the intercostal muscles, internal muscles, and diaphragm

The thoracic cavity is divided into the centrally-located unpaired mediastinum, which contains the *mediastinal organs,* and the paired pleural cavities. The mediastinum contains the central motor of the circulatory system, the heart, and the thoracic part of the digestive system, the esophagus. The pleural cavities enclose the major organs of respiration, the lungs. Also, a number of neurovascular structures pass through or terminate within the thorax.

The bony thoracic cage is open at its apex at the superior thoracic aperture (thoracic inlet), which is closely bounded and protected by muscles and connective tissue but communicates structures from the neck. The inferior aperture of the thoracic cage (thoracic outlet) is almost completely sealed from the abdominal cavity by the diaphragm and its fasciae (shown most clearly in **a**).

Note: The diaphragm is normally in the shape of a high dome, with a substantial superior convexity that places part of the abdominal cavity above the thoracic outlet (see the abdominal organs shadowed in **b**). A perforating injury perpendicular to the trunk wall, as from a gunshot or stab wound, may thus simultaneously breach both the abdominal and thoracic cavities ("multicavity injury").

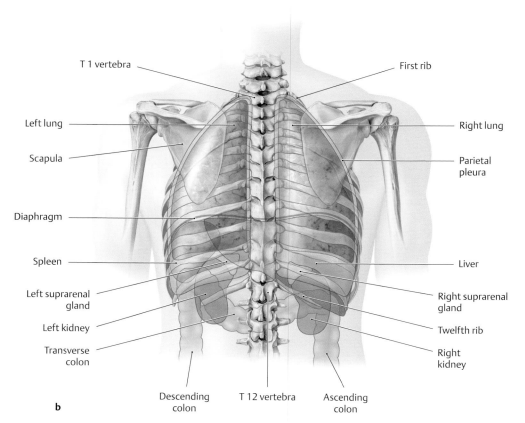

T 1 vertebra
First rib
Left lung
Right lung
Scapula
Parietal pleura
Diaphragm
Spleen
Liver
Left suprarenal gland
Right suprarenal gland
Left kidney
Twelfth rib
Transverse colon
Right kidney

b

Descending colon
T 12 vertebra
Ascending colon

1.2 Divisions of the Thoracic Cavity and Mediastinum

Thoracic inlet

Superior mediastinum

Right pleural cavity (right lung)

Left pleural cavity (left lung)

Inferior mediastinum

Diaphragm

a   Thoracic outlet

Thoracic vertebra   Descending aorta

Right lung

Left lung

Esophagus

Posterior mediastinum

Middle mediastinum

b   Sternum (body)   Anterior mediastinum

A Divisions of the thoracic cavity and mediastinum
a Coronal section, anterior view. **b** Transverse section, superior view.
The thoracic cavity is divided into three large spaces (see **b**):

- The **mediastinum**, in the midline, is divided into an upper, smaller *superior mediastinum* and a lower, larger *inferior mediastinum* (**a**). The inferior mediastinum is further subdivided, from front to back, into the *anterior, middle,* and *posterior mediastinum*. The anterior mediastinum is an extremely narrow space between the sternum and pericardium, containing only small vascular components (see table, **C**).
- The **paired pleural cavities** on the left and right sides of the mediastinum are lined by serosa (= parietal pleura) and contain the left and right lungs. They are completely separated from each other by the mediastinum. The mediastinum extends further to the left than to the right owing to the asymmetrical position of the heart and pericardium. Because of this, the pleural cavity (and lung) is smaller on the left side than on the right. The pleural cavities terminate blindly at their upper end, but the mediastinum is continuous with the connective tissue of the neck.

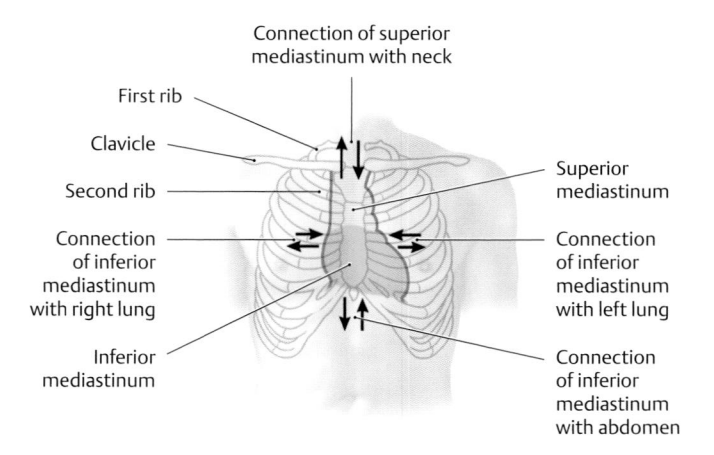

Connection of superior mediastinum with neck

First rib

Clavicle

Second rib

Superior mediastinum

Connection of inferior mediastinum with right lung

Connection of inferior mediastinum with left lung

Inferior mediastinum

Connection of inferior mediastinum with abdomen

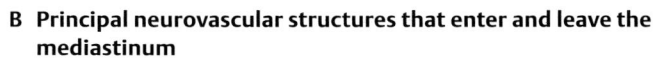

B Principal neurovascular structures that enter and leave the mediastinum

Superior mediastinum (borders the neck, yellow):
- The vagus and phrenic nerves, veins (tributaries of the superior vena cava), esophagus, and trachea enter the superior mediastinum from the neck.
- Arterial branches from the aortic arch and the cervical part of the sympathetic trunk leave the superior mediastinum to enter the neck.

Inferior mediastinum (borders the abdomen and pleural cavities, red):
- The thoracic duct and ascending abdominal lumbar veins (the azygos vein on the right side, the hemiazygos vein on the left side) pass through the diaphragm to enter the inferior mediastinum.
- The vagus and phrenic nerves, portions of the sympathetic nervous system, the aorta, and the esophagus descend from the inferior mediastinum and pass through the diaphragm to enter the abdomen.

C Contents of the mediastinum (for divisions see **A**)

Superior mediastinum	Inferior mediastinum

• Aortic arch
• Brachiocephalic trunk
• Proximal portions of left common carotid artery and left subclavian artery
• Superior vena cava (upper portion)
• Brachiocephalic veins
• Thymus (in older adults: retrosternal fat pad)
• Vagus nerves
• Left recurrent laryngeal nerve
• Cardiac nerves
• Phrenic nerves
• Trachea, esophagus, and thoracic duct
	• *Anterior mediastinum:*
	  – Lymphatic vessels and lymph nodes
	  – Smaller blood vessels
	
	• *Middle mediastinum:*
	  – Heart and pericardium
	  – Ascending aorta
	  – Terminal segment of superior vena cava and azygos vein
	  – Pulmonary trunk and its branches
	  – Pulmonary veins
	  – Phrenic nerves with pericardiacophrenic vessels
	
	• *Posterior mediastinum:*
	  – Esophagus with vagus nerves
	  – Thoracic aorta and its branches
	  – Thoracic duct
	  – Azygos and hemiazygos veins
	  – Sympathetic trunk and greater and lesser splanchnic nerves

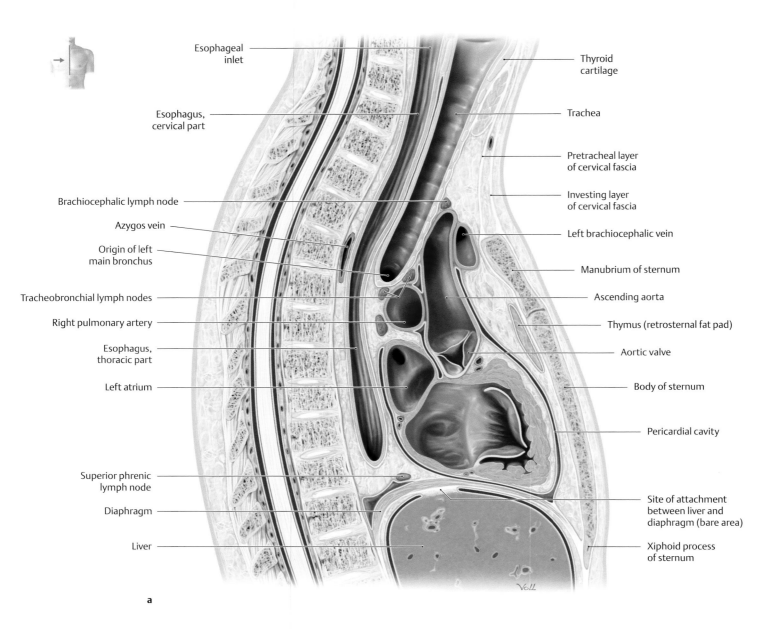

Esophageal inlet

Esophagus, cervical part

Brachiocephalic lymph node

Azygos vein

Origin of left main bronchus

Tracheobronchial lymph nodes

Right pulmonary artery

Esophagus, thoracic part

Left atrium

Superior phrenic lymph node

Diaphragm

Liver

Thyroid cartilage

Trachea

Pretracheal layer of cervical fascia

Investing layer of cervical fascia

Left brachiocephalic vein

Manubrium of sternum

Ascending aorta

Thymus (retrosternal fat pad)

Aortic valve

Body of sternum

Pericardial cavity

Site of attachment between liver and diaphragm (bare area)

Xiphoid process of sternum

a

D Subdivisions of the mediastinum

Midsagittal sections viewed from the right side.

a **Detailed view:** simplified drawing of the pericardium, heart, trachea, and esophagus in midsagittal section. This lateral view demonstrates how the left atrium of the heart narrows the posterior mediastinum and abuts the anterior wall of the esophagus. Because of this proximity, abnormal enlargement of the left atrium may cause narrowing of the esophageal lumen that is detectable by radiographic examination with oral contrast medium. Radiologists call the area between the images of the heart and vertebral column the *retrocardiac space*.

b **Schematic view:** subdivisions of the mediastinum (described in **A**, with contents listed in **C**).

Note: Single diagrams cannot adequately show the components and configuration of the mediastinum, because of is asymmetry and extensions in all three axes. The anatomical relations in this space are best appreciated when viewed from multiple directions, at different planes (see pp. **62** and **63**).

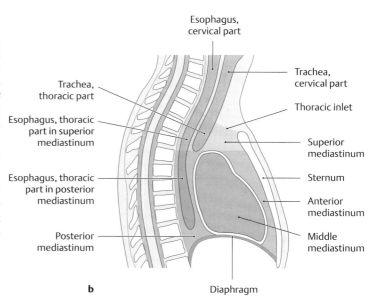

Esophagus, cervical part

Trachea, thoracic part

Esophagus, thoracic part in superior mediastinum

Esophagus, thoracic part in posterior mediastinum

Posterior mediastinum

Trachea, cervical part

Thoracic inlet

Superior mediastinum

Sternum

Anterior mediastinum

Middle mediastinum

Diaphragm

b

1.3   Overview of the Mediastinum

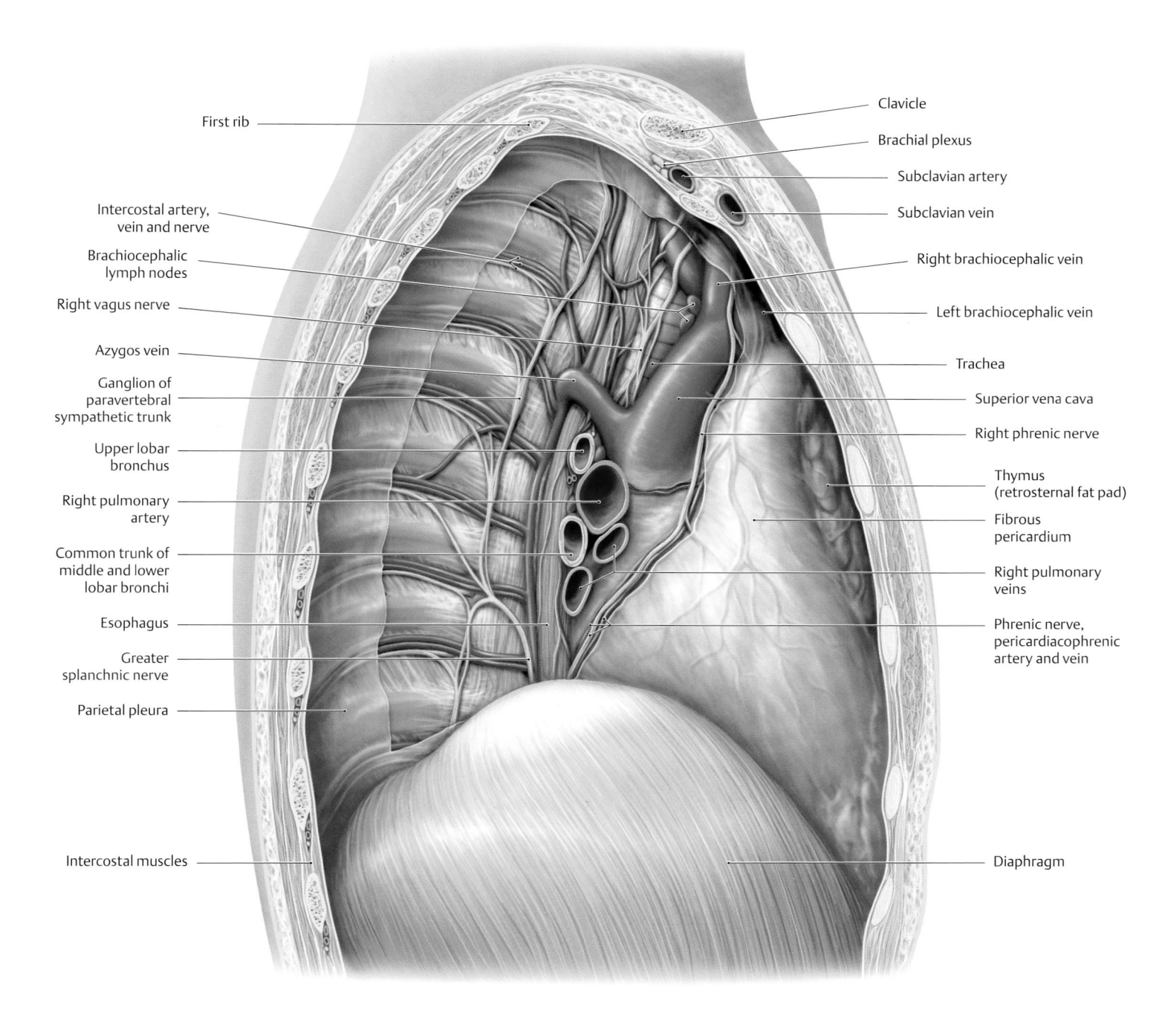

First rib

Clavicle

Brachial plexus

Subclavian artery

Intercostal artery, vein and nerve

Subclavian vein

Brachiocephalic lymph nodes

Right brachiocephalic vein

Right vagus nerve

Left brachiocephalic vein

Azygos vein

Trachea

Ganglion of paravertebral sympathetic trunk

Superior vena cava

Right phrenic nerve

Upper lobar bronchus

Thymus (retrosternal fat pad)

Right pulmonary artery

Fibrous pericardium

Common trunk of middle and lower lobar bronchi

Right pulmonary veins

Esophagus

Phrenic nerve, pericardiacophrenic artery and vein

Greater splanchnic nerve

Parietal pleura

Intercostal muscles

Diaphragm

A   Mediastinum viewed from the right side
Parasagittal section. The entire right lung and most of the wall of the pleural cavity have been removed (parietal pleura, see pp. 64 and 68) to display the structures of the *posterior mediastinum* adjacent to the vertebrae, most notably the sympathetic trunk, and the azygos vein opening into the superior vena cava. In the *middle mediastinum*, the (right) phrenic nerve and the (right) pericardiacophrenic artery and vein are visible on the pericardium. The (right) vagus nerve is directly visible on the lateral wall of the esophagus. The trachea, which descends in the median plane, is largely obscured by other structures; profiles of the lobar bronchi of the right lung can be identified in this view. The thymus, relatively prominent here, is large in early postnatal life (see p. 133), but regresses in adulthood, eventually replaced in old age by a small retrosternal fat pad (involuted thymus).

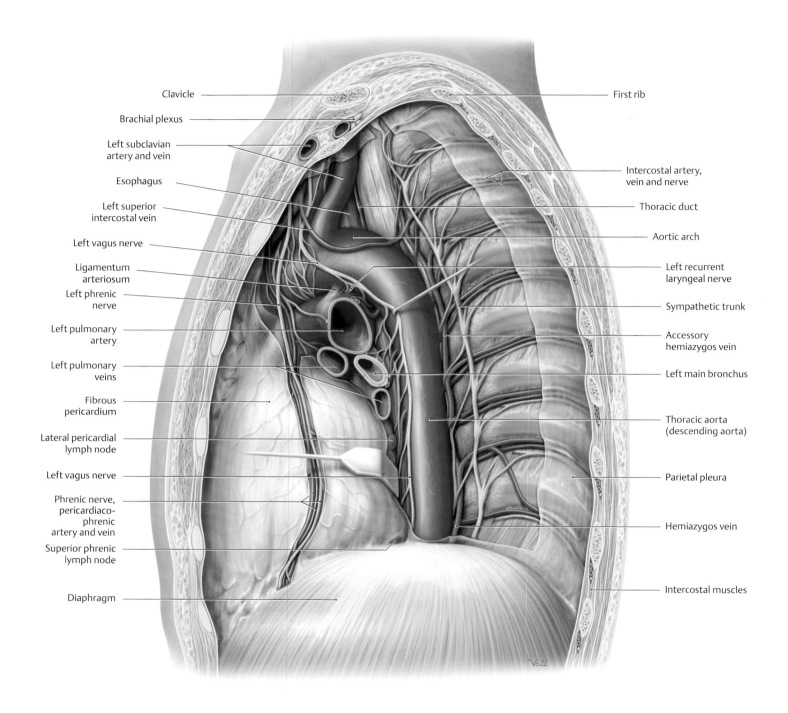

Clavicle

Brachial plexus

Left subclavian
artery and vein

Esophagus

Left superior
intercostal vein

Left vagus nerve

Ligamentum
arteriosum

Left phrenic
nerve

Left pulmonary
artery

Left pulmonary
veins

Fibrous
pericardium

Lateral pericardial
lymph node

Left vagus nerve

Phrenic nerve,
pericardiaco-
phrenic
artery and vein

Superior phrenic
lymph node

Diaphragm

First rib

Intercostal artery,
vein and nerve

Thoracic duct

Aortic arch

Left recurrent
laryngeal nerve

Sympathetic trunk

Accessory
hemiazygos vein

Left main bronchus

Thoracic aorta
(descending aorta)

Parietal pleura

Hemiazygos vein

Intercostal muscles

B Mediastinum viewed from the left side

Parasagittal section. The entire left lung and most of the parietal pleura of the left pleural cavity have been removed, but the pericardium remains intact. The left-sided elements of paired mediastinal structures (sympathetic trunk, vagus nerve, phrenic nerve, pericardiacophrenic vessels) can be identified. Visible unpaired structures include the hemiazygos vein and the (inconstant) accessory hemiazygos vein. The dominant vessel in this field is the aorta, of which the aortic arch and descending aorta can be seen anterior and lateral to the esophagus. Both left pulmonary veins have been transected near their terminations in the left atrium of the heart, again demonstrating the close topographical relationship between the left atrium and esophagus (retrocardiac space, see p. 98). The trachea is also obscured in a left parasagittal section, but the profile of the left main bronchus (surrounded by pulmonary vessels) can be seen clearly (compare with **A**).

1.4   Contents of the Mediastinum

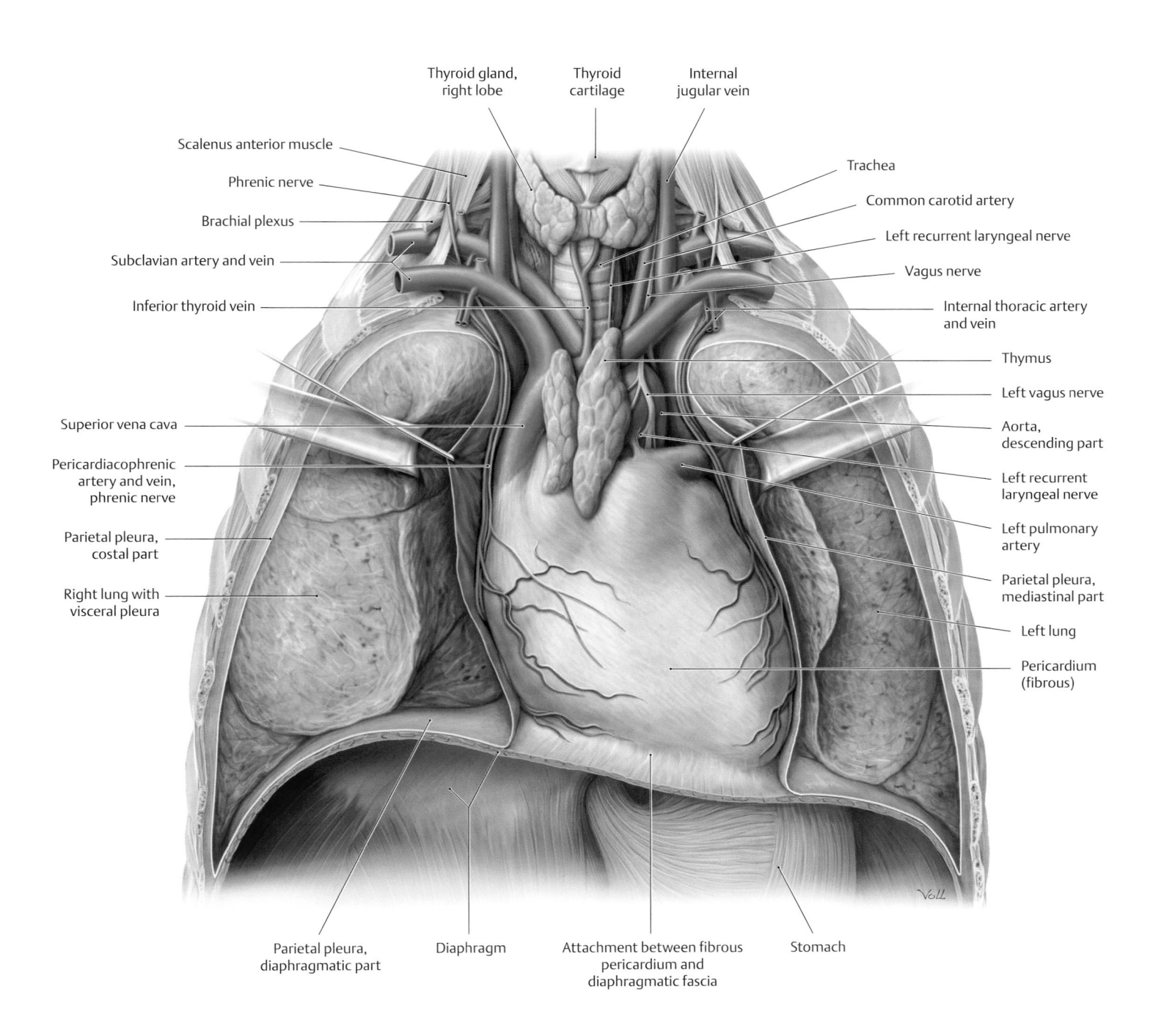

Thyroid gland, right lobe

Thyroid cartilage

Internal jugular vein

Scalenus anterior muscle

Phrenic nerve

Brachial plexus

Subclavian artery and vein

Inferior thyroid vein

Trachea

Common carotid artery

Left recurrent laryngeal nerve

Vagus nerve

Internal thoracic artery and vein

Thymus

Left vagus nerve

Superior vena cava

Pericardiacophrenic artery and vein, phrenic nerve

Parietal pleura, costal part

Right lung with visceral pleura

Aorta, descending part

Left recurrent laryngeal nerve

Left pulmonary artery

Parietal pleura, mediastinal part

Left lung

Pericardium (fibrous)

Parietal pleura, diaphragmatic part

Diaphragm

Attachment between fibrous pericardium and diaphragmatic fascia

Stomach

A Mediastinum, anterior view with the anterior thoracic wall removed
Coronal section through the thorax. All connective tissue has been removed from the *anterior mediastinum.* This dissection displays a prominent thymus, occupying the superior mediastinum and extending inferiorly into the anterior mediastinum. Visible structures that are continued from the superior mediastinum into the neck or upper limb include branches of the aortic arch, the superior vena cava, and the trachea, although the latter is mostly obscured by the vessels surrounding the heart. The *middle mediastinum,* visible in this coronal section, is dominated by the heart and pericardium (fused to the diaphragm) and the associated neurovascular structures—the phrenic nerve and pericardiacophrenic vessels. These vessels descend along the pericardium toward the diaphragm while giving off pericardial branches.

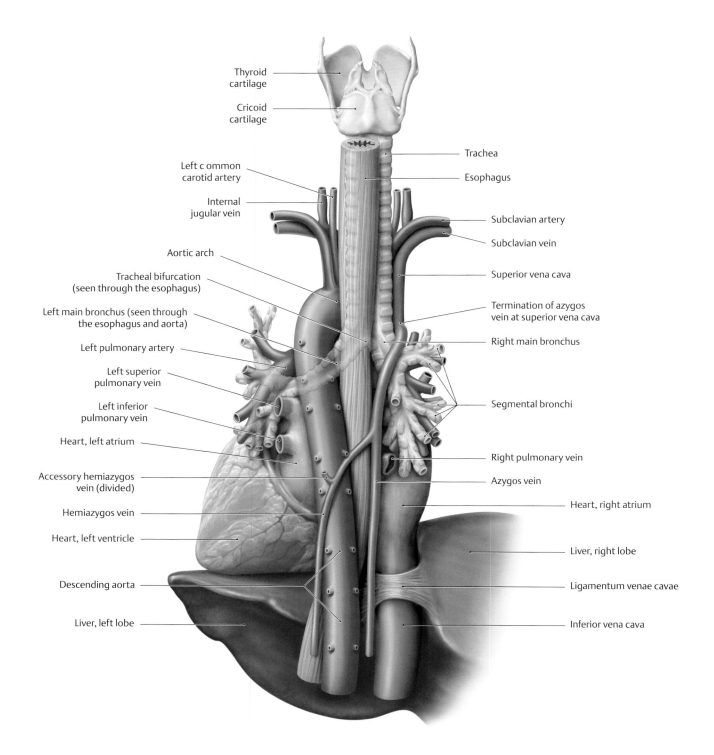

Thyroid cartilage

Cricoid cartilage

Trachea

Left c ommon carotid artery

Esophagus

Internal jugular vein

Subclavian artery

Subclavian vein

Aortic arch

Superior vena cava

Tracheal bifurcation (seen through the esophagus)

Termination of azygos vein at superior vena cava

Left main bronchus (seen through the esophagus and aorta)

Right main bronchus

Left pulmonary artery

Left superior pulmonary vein

Segmental bronchi

Left inferior pulmonary vein

Heart, left atrium

Right pulmonary vein

Accessory hemiazygos vein (divided)

Azygos vein

Hemiazygos vein

Heart, right atrium

Heart, left ventricle

Liver, right lobe

Descending aorta

Ligamentum venae cavae

Liver, left lobe

Inferior vena cava

B Contents of the mediastinum, posterior view
The structures in the *posterior mediastinum* are depicted in this view. Note particularly the course of the descending aorta, the azygos and hemiazygos veins, and the esophagus, which is posterior to the trachea and partially obscures it. (An anterior view of the posterior mediastinum is shown on p. 118.) The topographical relations of the aorta change several times along its course. The proximal part of the aorta ascends in the *middle mediastinum*, which is a subdivision of the inferior mediastinum. At that level the aorta lies anterior to the trachea and esophagus. It then ascends into the superior mediastinum, where it curves posteriorly and to the left to form the aortic arch. This curve lies to the left of the esophagus and trachea, and it arches over the left main bronchus (the aorta "rides" upon that bronchus). In its further course the aorta turns back slightly medially and posteriorly and descends behind the esophagus in the posterior mediastinum, where it is closely related to the azygos and hemiazygos veins. Note also the very close proximity of the liver to the right side of the heart.

1.5   Pericardium

A Location of the pericardium in the thorax, anterior view

The chest has been opened to display the pericardium, which is the dominant structure in the inferior mediastinum. It is attached inferiorly to the diaphragmatic fascia by connective tissue. Anteriorly, it is separated from the posterior surface of the sternum only by connective tissue of the anterior mediastinum (removed here, see p. 60; see **B**). The pericardium is bounded laterally by the pleural cavities, from which it is separated by mediastinal pleura.

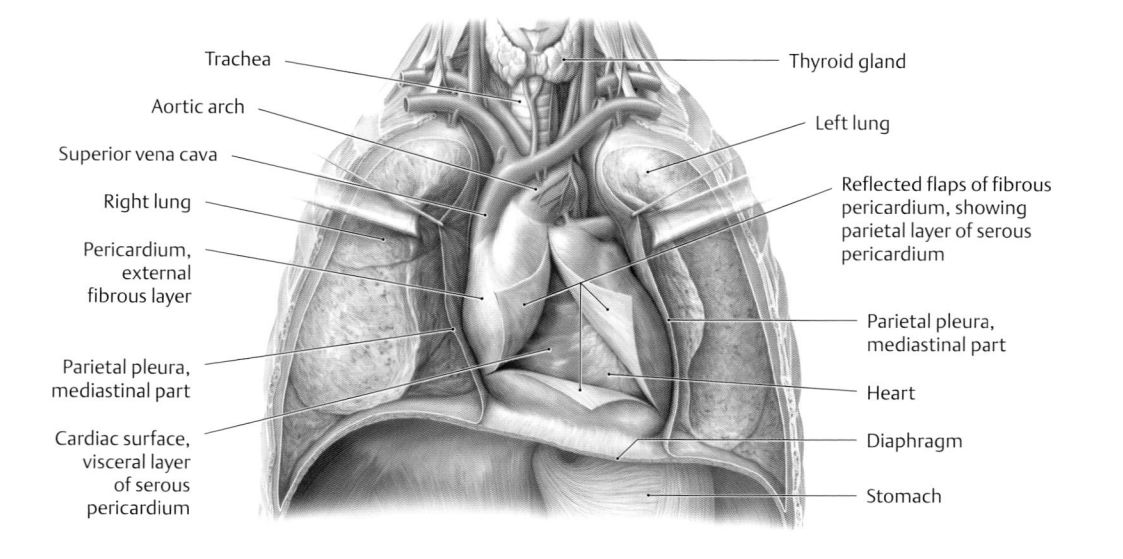

Trachea
Aortic arch
Superior vena cava
Right lung
Pericardium, external fibrous layer
Parietal pleura, mediastinal part
Cardiac surface, visceral layer of serous pericardium

Thyroid gland
Left lung
Reflected flaps of fibrous pericardium, showing parietal layer of serous pericardium
Parietal pleura, mediastinal part
Heart
Diaphragm
Stomach

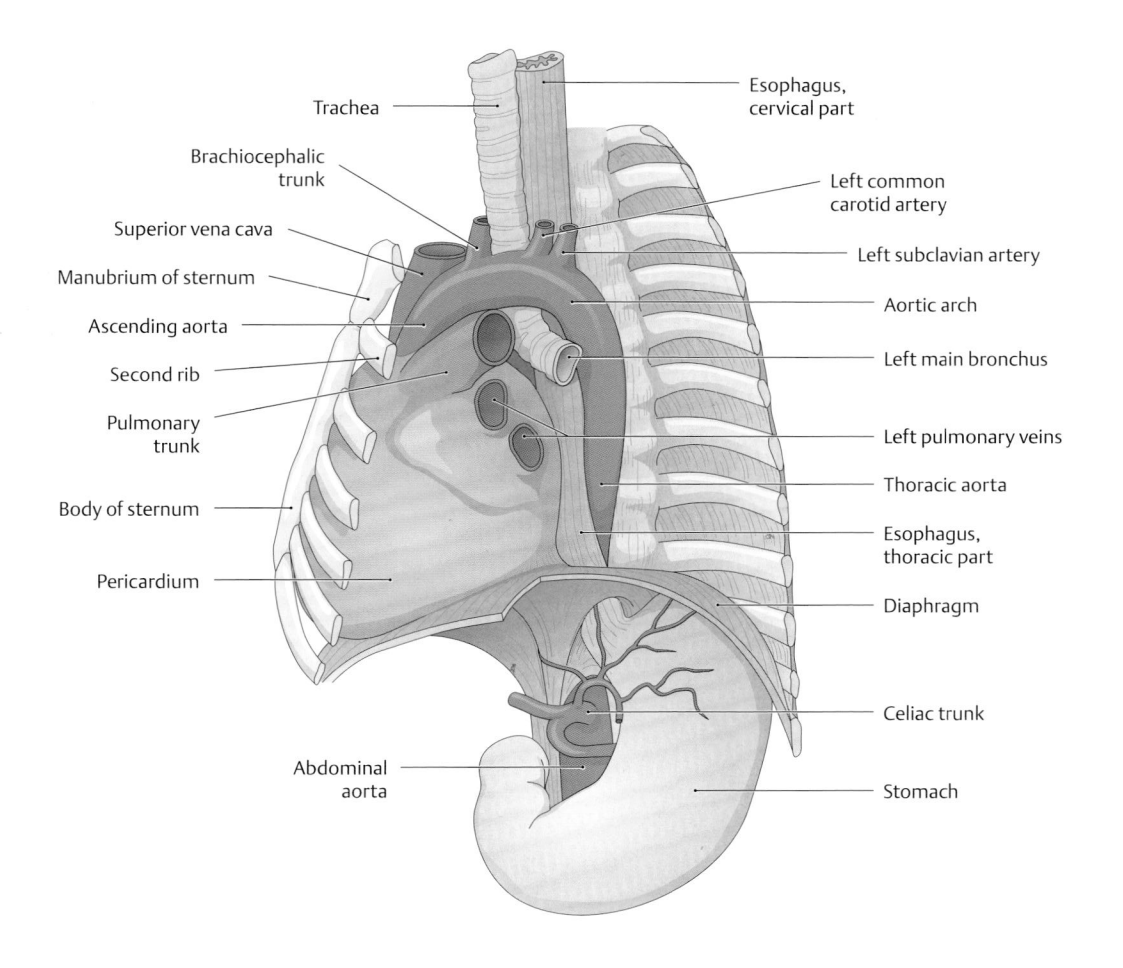

Trachea
Brachiocephalic trunk
Superior vena cava
Manubrium of sternum
Ascending aorta
Second rib
Pulmonary trunk
Body of sternum
Pericardium
Abdominal aorta

Esophagus, cervical part
Left common carotid artery
Left subclavian artery
Aortic arch
Left main bronchus
Left pulmonary veins
Thoracic aorta
Esophagus, thoracic part
Diaphragm
Celiac trunk
Stomach

B Location of the pericardium in the thorax, left anterior oblique view

This view demonstrates the very close proximity of the pericardium to the sternum, to which it may be attached by sternopericardial ligaments (not shown). Only the anterior mediastinum (not shown, see p. 60) separates the pericardium from the posterior surface of the sternum. The pericardium is related posteriorly to the esophagus, especially at the left atrium (marked by the terminations of the left pulmonary veins), and varying degrees of attachments may be present between the pericardium and esophagus. It might be said that the esophagus is "wedged" between the pericardium and descending aorta.

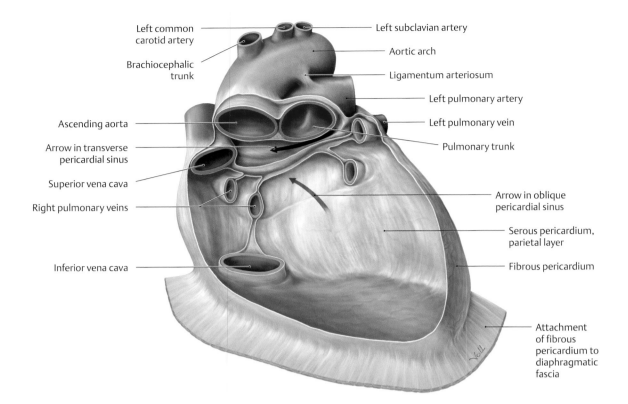

Left common carotid artery
Brachiocephalic trunk
Ascending aorta
Arrow in transverse pericardial sinus
Superior vena cava
Right pulmonary veins
Inferior vena cava

Left subclavian artery
Aortic arch
Ligamentum arteriosum
Left pulmonary artery
Left pulmonary vein
Pulmonary trunk
Arrow in oblique pericardial sinus
Serous pericardium, parietal layer
Fibrous pericardium
Attachment of fibrous pericardium to diaphragmatic fascia

C Pericardial cavity and structure of the pericardium
Anterior view of the empty pericardial sac. The pericardium consists of two **layers**, one within the other, that enclose and protect the heart:

- Parietal layer. The parietal pericardium forms a sac with an outer surface, the *fibrous pericardium*, composed of tough and indistensible connective tissue which is partially attached to the diaphragm. Its inner surface, facing the heart, is lined with a serous membrane.
- Visceral layer (*epicardium*). This is a thin serous membrane which covers, and is firmly adherent to, the heart itself and the proximal parts of the great vessels.

The two serous membranes of the parietal and visceral layers are closely apposed, but move freely over one another, allowing a gliding motion during the heartbeat. These two serous membranes are referred to together as the *serous pericardium*.

In the locations where the parietal layer is folded back onto the visceral layer covering the vessels, two **sinuses** are formed (see arrows):

- The *transverse* pericardial sinus located between the arteries and veins
- The *oblique* pericardial sinus located between the left and right pulmonary veins

Note: Because the pericardium cannot expand significantly, bleeding into the pericardial cavity (e. g., from a ruptured myocardial aneurysm) will place increasing pressure on the heart as the blood accumulates within the sac. This condition, called cardiac tamponade, seriously compromises the ability of the ventricles to fill and pump blood, creating a threat of cardiac arrest. Similar problems may arise from inflammation of the pericardium (pericarditis).

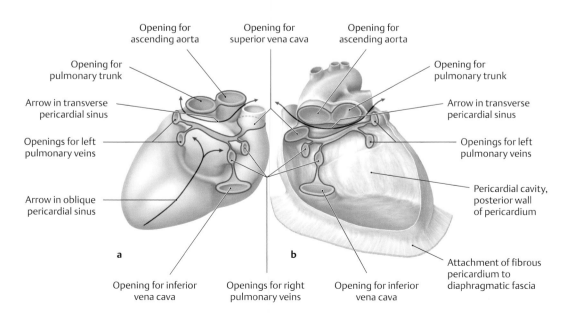

Opening for ascending aorta
Opening for superior vena cava
Opening for ascending aorta
Opening for pulmonary trunk
Opening for pulmonary trunk
Arrow in transverse pericardial sinus
Arrow in transverse pericardial sinus
Openings for left pulmonary veins
Openings for left pulmonary veins
Arrow in oblique pericardial sinus
Pericardial cavity, posterior wall of pericardium

a   b

Opening for inferior vena cava
Openings for right pulmonary veins
Opening for inferior vena cava
Attachment of fibrous pericardium to diaphragmatic fascia

D Openings in the pericardium
a Posterior view of the heart with the epicardium. **b** Anterior view of the "empty" pericardial cavity. An empty pericardium typically has eight openings by which vessels enter and leave the heart:

- One opening for the ascending aorta
- One opening for the pulmonary trunk
- Two openings for the two venae cavae
- Up to four openings for the four pulmonary veins

1.6 Pleural Cavity

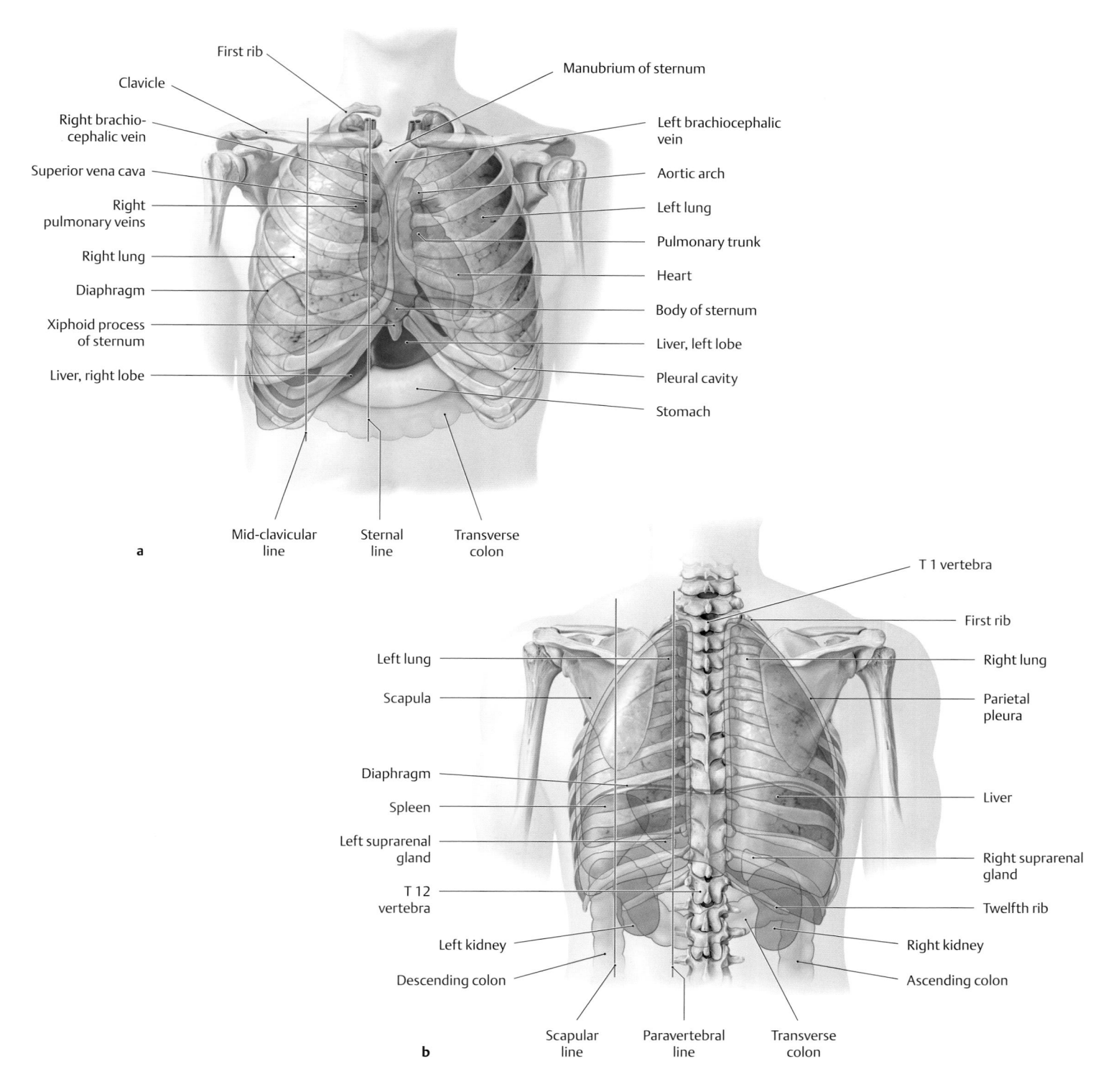

A Projection of the pleural cavities onto the thoracic skeleton
a Anterior view, **b** posterior view.

The pleural cavities are paired like the lungs they enclose. The left pleural cavity is slightly smaller than the right, especially anteriorly, due to the asymmetrical position of the heart in the mediastinum. The pleural cavities have a greater total extent than the lungs, resulting in the presence of recesses (see **D**). Like the peritoneal and pericardial cavities, the pleural cavity is bounded by two serous layers: the *visceral pleura* (pulmonary pleura), which is attached to the surface of the lung, and the *parietal pleura*, which lines the thoracic cavity and is attached to the endothoracic fasccia of the chest wall (see **D**). The parietal pleura extends to the lateral margins of the diaphragm. Because of the convex domed configuration of the diaphragm, the parietal pleura thus extends down to the same thoracic vertebral level (T 12) as the liver, spleen, kidneys, and parts of the colon. In these lateral recesses the visceral pleura is not in contact with the parietal layer. Over most of the extent of the lungs, however, the two pleurae are closely apposed, separated only by a thin layer of clear serous fluid which allows free sliding motion of the lungs in the pleural cavities. This fluid layer also serves to hold the pleural layers together by capillary action, thus transmitting the force of changes in volume of the thoracic cage, caused by the respiratory muscles including the diaphragm, directly to the lungs themselves (see pp. 92–93).

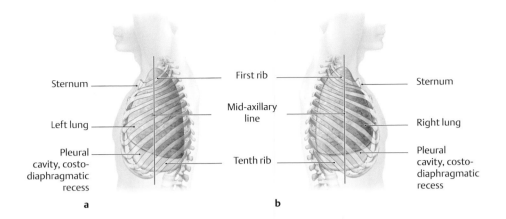

Sternum

First rib

Mid-axillary line

Left lung

Pleural cavity, costo-diaphragmatic recess

Tenth rib

a

Sternum

Right lung

Pleural cavity, costo-diaphragmatic recess

b

B Projection of the parietal pleura onto the thoracic skeleton

Viewed from the left side (**a**) and right side (**b**). The diagrams show the boundaries of the parietal pleura. The positions of the lungs are also depicted (see **C**).

C Relations of the lungs and pleural boundaries to landmarks on the thoracic skeleton

The parietal pleura, which lines much of the inner surface of the thoracic cage, bears specific spatial relationships with palpable or visible landmarks of the thoracic skeleton, as tabulated below. These landmarks can be used in radiographs to determine the extent of pleural inflammations with effusion, etc. Reference lines on the anterior and posterior chest wall, as shown in **A**, and the lateral chest wall, in **B**, are used here for orientation.

Note: The asymmetrical position of the heart, with greater mass on the left side, makes the pleural cavity slightly smaller on the left than on the right. This causes a lateral shift of some of the boundaries of the parietal pleura on the left side at the level of the heart.

Reference line (see also p. 58)	Right lung	Right parietal pleura	Left lung	Left parietal pleura
Sternal line	Intersects the 6th rib	Intersects the 7th rib	Intersects the 4th rib	Intersects the 4th rib
Mid-clavicular line	Runs parallel to the 6th rib	Runs parallel to the 7th rib	Intersects the 6th rib	Intersects the 7th rib
Mid-axillary line	Intersects the 8th rib	Intersects the 9th rib	Same as right lung	Intersects the 7th rib
Scapular line	Intersects the 10th rib	Intersects the 11th rib	Same as right lung	Intersects the 7th rib
Paravertebral line	Intersects the 11th rib	Extends to the T12 vertebra	Same as right lung	Intersects the 7th rib

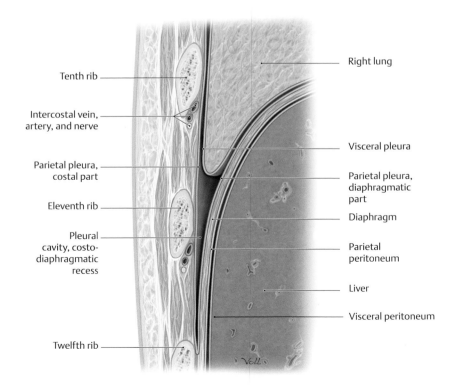

Tenth rib

Intercostal vein, artery, and nerve

Parietal pleura, costal part

Eleventh rib

Pleural cavity, costo-diaphragmatic recess

Twelfth rib

Right lung

Visceral pleura

Parietal pleura, diaphragmatic part

Diaphragm

Parietal peritoneum

Liver

Visceral peritoneum

D Recesses of the parietal pleura

Detail from a parasagittal section through the right side of the thorax and abdomen, viewed from the lateral side. Portions of the right pleural and peritoneal cavities can be seen. Because the *visceral* pleura directly invests the lung, its extent is identical to that of the underlying lung. The *parietal* pleura, on the other hand, completely lines the inner surface of the chest wall and therefore has a greater extent than the lungs. This arrangement creates two major recesses within the pleural cavity:

- The costodiaphragmatic recess, located over the side of the diaphragm facing the ribs
- The costomediastinal recess, located anterior to the pericardium on the left and right sides of the anterior mediastinum (see p. 99)

The internal fasciae of the thorax (endothoracic fascia, phrenicopleural fascia) to which the parietal pleura is attached are not depicted here.

69

2.1 Esophagus: Location, Divisions, and Special Features

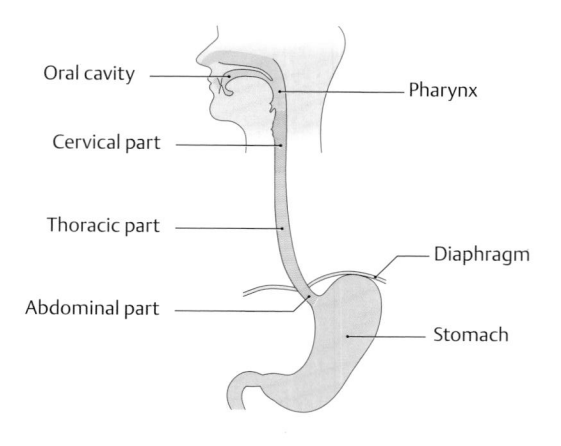

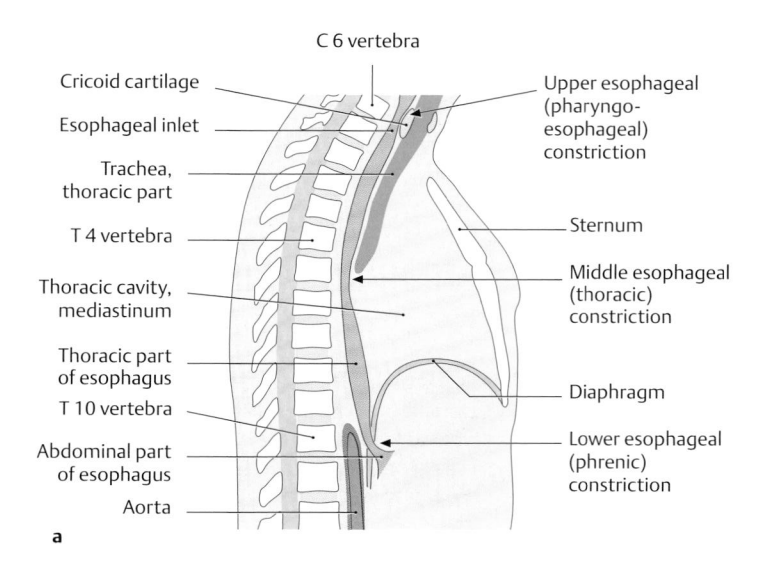

A Projection onto the thoracic skeleton
Anterior view. The esophagus is located slightly to the right of the midline, especially in its course through the thorax, where it descends along the right side of the aorta. It pierces the diaphragm just below the xiphoid process of the sternum. The arrows mark the sites of the three normal anatomical constrictions of the esophagus (see **C**).

B Divisions of the esophagus
Anterior view with the head turned to the right. The esophagus is approximately 23–27 cm long, 1–2 cm in diameter, and is divided into three parts:

- Cervical part: just anterior to the vertebral column in the neck, extends from C 6 to T 1.
- Thoracic part: the longest part, located in the superior and posterior mediastinum, extends from T 1 to the esophageal hiatus of the diaphragm (at approximately T 11).
- Abdominal part: the shortest part, located in the peritoneal cavity, extends from the diaphragm to the cardiac orifice of the stomach.

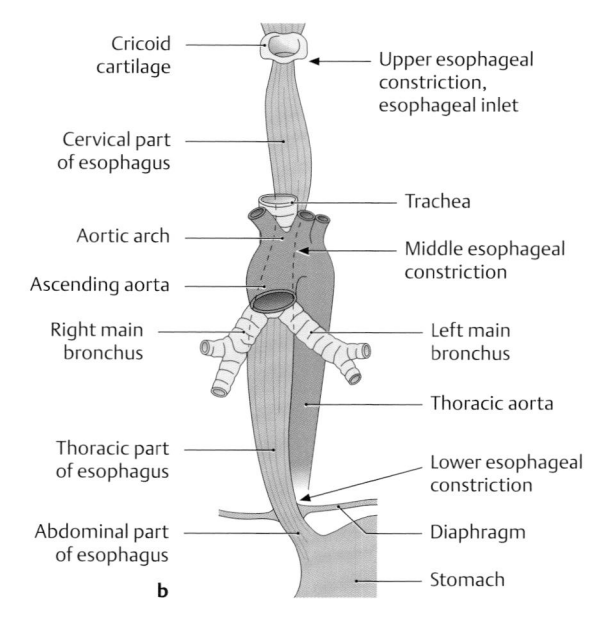

C Constrictions and curves of the esophagus
Right lateral view (**a**), anterior view (**b**).
The esophagus has three normal anatomical **constrictions**, which are projected at the levels of specific vertebrae (**a**). The constrictions are caused by adjacent structures that indent the esophagus and by functional closure mechanisms (lower constriction, see p. 75). These constrictions are visible during gastroscopy, and the scope must be carefully maneuvered past them (normal width of the esophagus is approximately 20 mm):

- Upper constriction (pharyngoesophageal constriction, 14–16 cm from the incisor teeth), corresponds to the esophageal inlet in the cervical part of the esophagus (see p. 74). It is located where the esophagus passes behind the cricoid cartilage (C 6) and has a maximum width of approximately 14 mm.
- Middle constriction (thoracic constriction, 25–27 cm from the incisors), located where the esophagus passes to the right of the aortic arch and thoracic aorta (at T 4 / T 5). Maximum width is 14 mm.

- Lower constriction (phrenic constriction, 36–38 cm from the incisors), located at the start of the abdominal part of the esophagus, where it pierces the diaphragm (T 10 / T 11). Functional closure of the esophagus by muscles and veins of the esophageal wall. The abdominal part is normally occluded except during swallowing (see p. 75). Maximum width is 14 mm.

Besides its constrictions, the esophagus also presents characteristic **curves** (**b**): an upper curve to the left (in the cervical part), a mid-level curve to the right (in the thoracic part, caused by the adjacent thoracic aorta), and a lower curve to the left (in the abdominal part). Additionally, the esophagus is slightly concave anteriorly in the sagittal plane, following the curvature of the vertebral column (thoracic kyphosis, **a**).

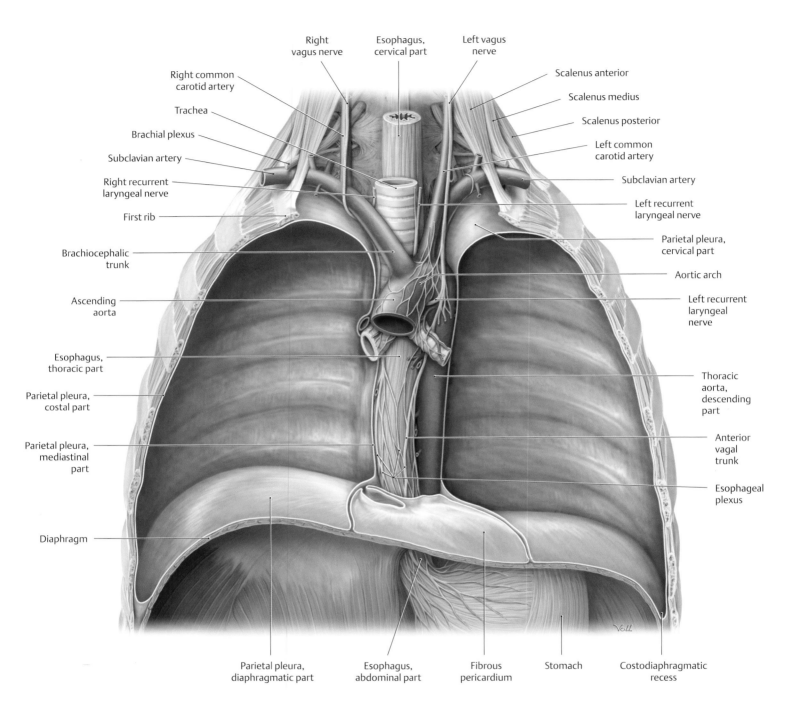

Right vagus nerve

Esophagus, cervical part

Left vagus nerve

Right common carotid artery

Scalenus anterior

Trachea

Scalenus medius

Brachial plexus

Scalenus posterior

Subclavian artery

Left common carotid artery

Right recurrent laryngeal nerve

Subclavian artery

First rib

Left recurrent laryngeal nerve

Brachiocephalic trunk

Parietal pleura, cervical part

Aortic arch

Ascending aorta

Left recurrent laryngeal nerve

Esophagus, thoracic part

Thoracic aorta, descending part

Parietal pleura, costal part

Parietal pleura, mediastinal part

Anterior vagal trunk

Esophageal plexus

Diaphragm

Parietal pleura, diaphragmatic part

Esophagus, abdominal part

Fibrous pericardium

Stomach

Costodiaphragmatic recess

D The esophagus in situ

Anterior view. The chest has been opened and the heart, pericardium, and lungs have been removed, leaving most of the parietal pleura in place. A small portion of the abdominal cavity is shown, and the stomach has been retracted slightly downward to display the gastroesophageal junction. The **cervical part** of the esophagus is vertical, lying directly in front of the vertebral column in the median plane. The **thoracic part** descends behind the trachea to the tracheal bifurcation (covered here by the descending aorta), and past the bifurcation it lies

directly behind the pericardium (see p. 98 for its important relations to the heart and pericardium). Because the esophagus runs alongside the descending aorta, its thoracic part often "curves" slightly to the right as shown in this dissection (the other esophageal curves are described in **C**). Just above the diaphragm the esophagus lies anterior to the aorta before passing through the esophageal hiatus (covered here by pericardium) accompanied by the branches of both vagus nerves. The **abdominal part** of the esophagus in the peritoneal cavity curves to the left after emerging from the diaphragm and joins with the stomach.

2.2 Esophagus: Location and Wall Structure

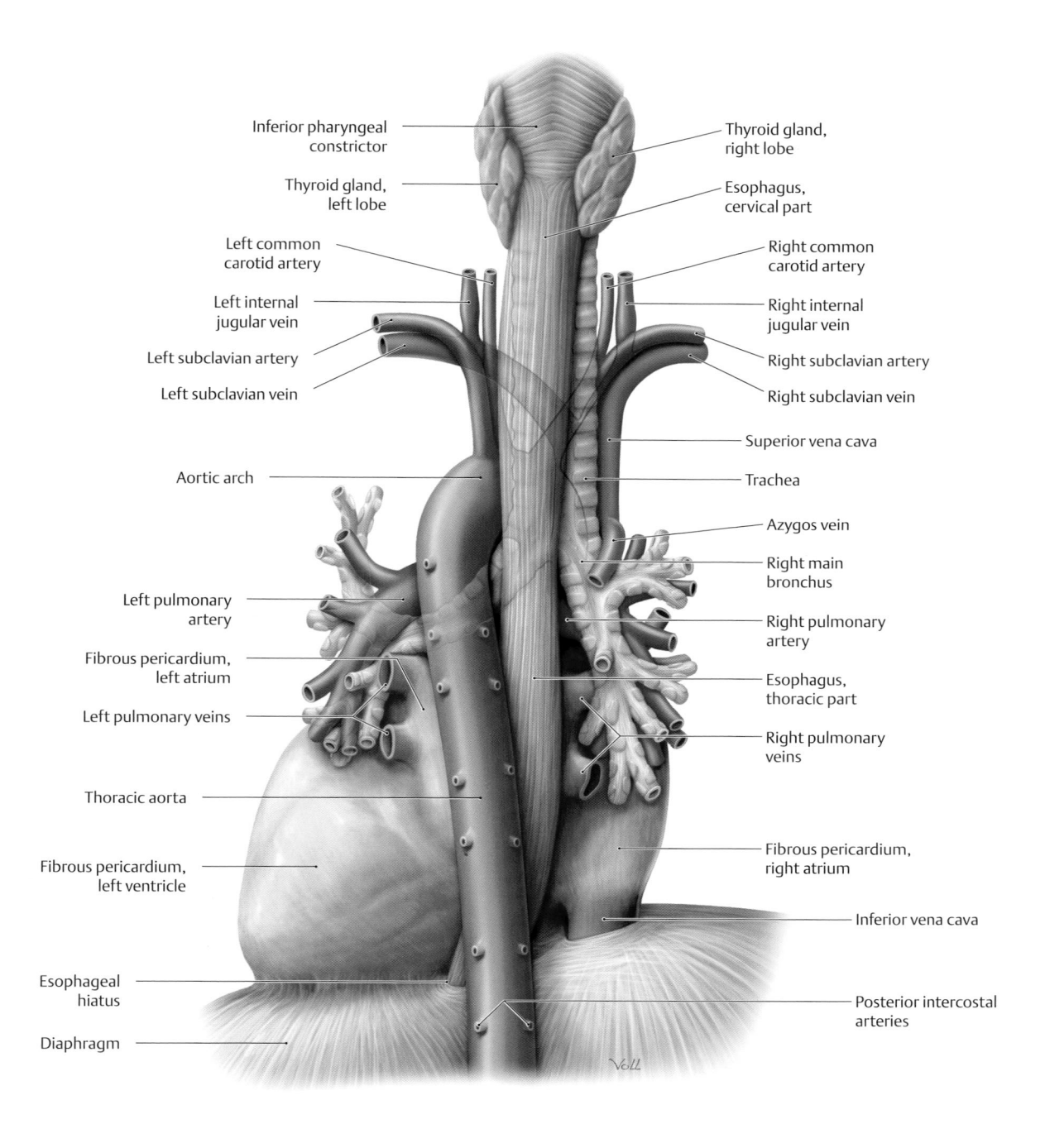

Inferior pharyngeal constrictor

Thyroid gland, right lobe

Thyroid gland, left lobe

Esophagus, cervical part

Left common carotid artery

Right common carotid artery

Left internal jugular vein

Right internal jugular vein

Left subclavian artery

Right subclavian artery

Left subclavian vein

Right subclavian vein

Superior vena cava

Aortic arch

Trachea

Azygos vein

Right main bronchus

Left pulmonary artery

Right pulmonary artery

Fibrous pericardium, left atrium

Esophagus, thoracic part

Left pulmonary veins

Right pulmonary veins

Thoracic aorta

Fibrous pericardium, left ventricle

Fibrous pericardium, right atrium

Inferior vena cava

Esophageal hiatus

Posterior intercostal arteries

Diaphragm

A Topographical relations of the esophagus, posterior view
The relations of the esophagus to the pericardium, great vessels, and trachea are depicted here. The close proximity of the esophagus to the left atrium and thoracic aorta can be seen (see also p. 98). Due to the asymmetrical position of the heart in the thorax, the right pulmonary veins are closer to the esophagus than the left pulmonary veins. The esophagus initially descends to the right of the aorta, but just above the diaphragm it crosses in front of the aorta before piercing the diaphragm to enter the abdominal cavity (see Constrictions, p. 70). The esophagus is loosely attached by its own connective tissue (adventitia) to the connective tissue of the mediastinum (important for swallowing). It is stabilized somewhat by the attachment of its anterior wall to the back of the trachea, again by numerous slips of connective tissue.

Note: The trachea develops as an outgrowth from the esophagus during early embryonic development, at which time a communication exists between the two structures. Normally this communication closes, but its persistence results in a tracheoesophageal fistula, which may allow food to enter the trachea and reach the lung, causing recurrent episodes of pneumonia.

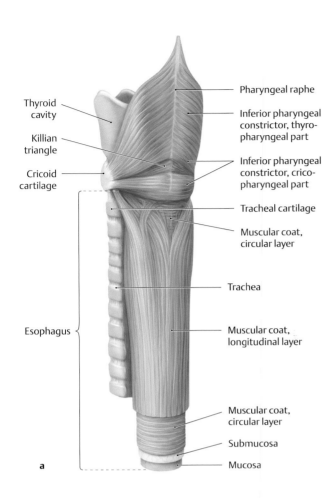

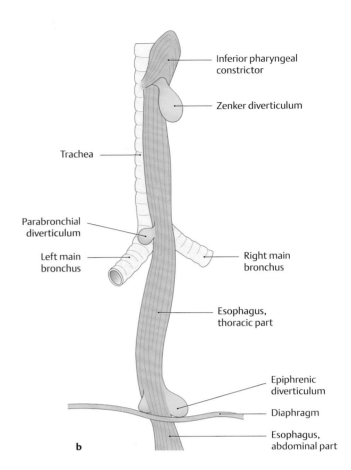

a

b

B Structure of the esophageal wall and the development of diverticula

Viewed from the posterior and left sides.

a Portions of the pharynx, larynx, and trachea are also shown. The outermost layer (adventitia) has been removed, and the remaining layers of the esophageal wall have been telescoped to display both layers of the muscular coat (the circular and longitudinal layers). They are connected to the pharyngeal muscles at the esophageal inlet (hidden here by the pharynx). The muscles of the esophagus can generate powerful peristaltic movements directed toward the stomach (actively propelling a food bolus to the stomach in 5–8 seconds), and they can reverse the direction of these movements during vomiting (antiperistalsis).

b Esophageal *diverticula* (abnormal outpouchings or sacs) most commonly develop at a weak spot like that located above the esophageal hiatus of the diaphragm (parahiatal or epiphrenic diverticulum, 10 %

of cases). These are "false" *pulsion diverticula* in which the mucosa and submucosa herniate through weak spots in the muscular coat due to a rise of pressure in the esophagus (e.g., during normal swallowing). A Zenker diverticulum, often described as the most common esophageal diverticulum (70 % of cases), is actually a *hypopharyngeal* diverticulum occurring at the junction of the pharynx and esophagus (the "Killian triangle"). This wall protrusion, called also a *pharyngoesophageal diverticulum*, is discussed under the heading of the pharynx (see p. 33). The remaining 20 % of esophageal diverticula do not occur at typical weak spots and are characterized by the protrusion of all wall layers ("true" diverticula, *traction diverticula*). They usually result from an inflammatory process such as lymphangitis, in which case they occur at the site where the esophagus closely approaches the bronchi and bronchial lymph nodes (thoracic or parabronchial diverticulum).

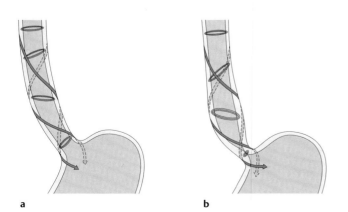

a   b

C Functional architecture of the esophageal muscles

During the act of swallowing, the esophageal outlet at the cardiac end of the stomach opens (**a**) and then immediately closes (**b**). The longitudinal and circular layers of the muscular wall of the esophagus (see **Ba**) contain numerous fibers that wind *obliquely* around the organ (see the circles in the figure). The musculature is additionally "twisted" due to the embryonic rotation of the gut (see p. 178). Owing to the presence of longitudinal, circular, and oblique fibers, the esophagus can be narrowed and closed as needed (by the action of the circular fibers) at its inlet and outlet (see p. 75), but it can also be simultaneously narrowed and shortened by the combined action of the longitudinal, circular and oblique fibers to generate peristaltic motion toward the stomach during swallowing.

73

2.3 Esophagus: Inlet and Outlet, Opening and Closure

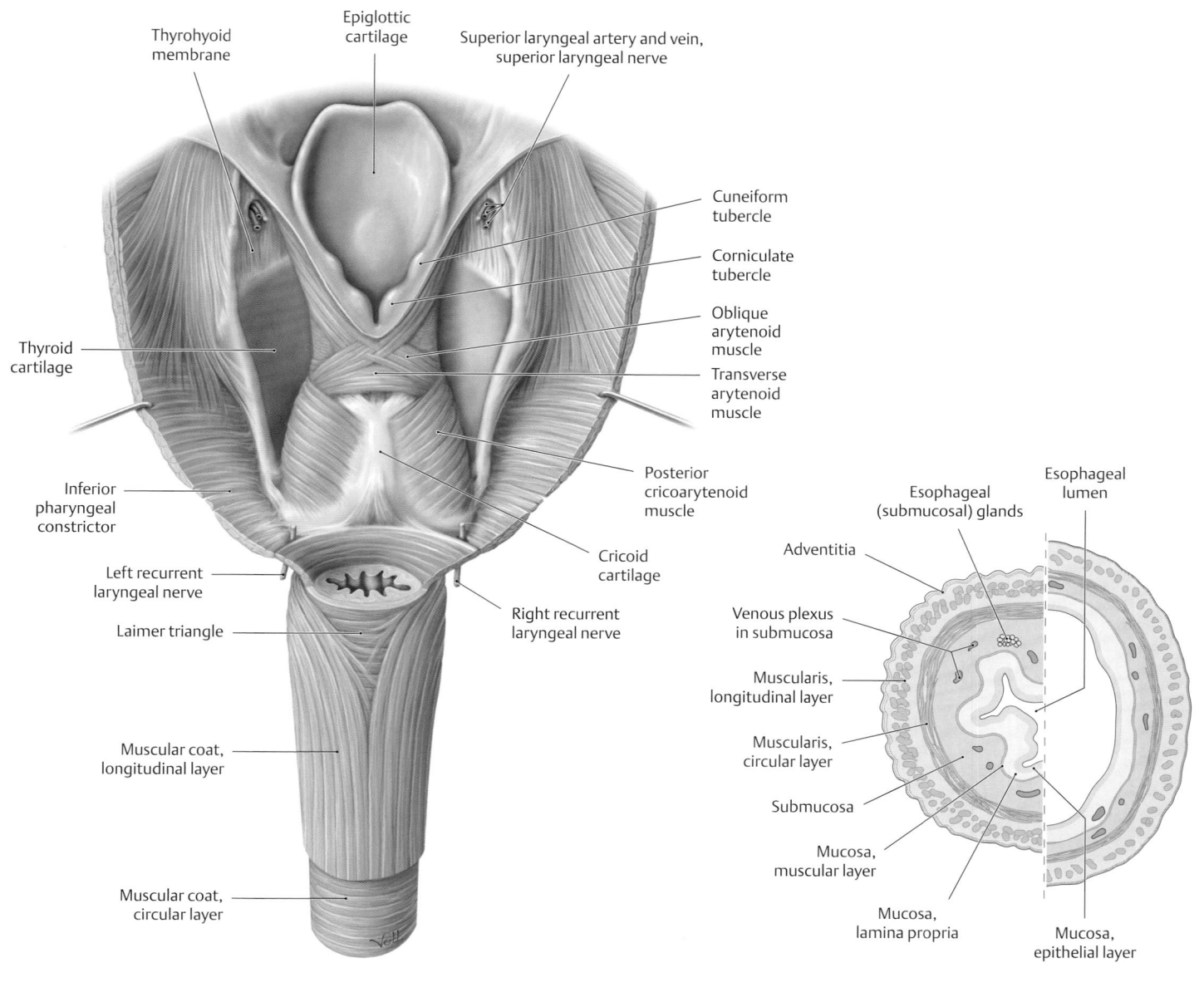

Thyrohyoid membrane

Epiglottic cartilage

Superior laryngeal artery and vein, superior laryngeal nerve

Cuneiform tubercle

Corniculate tubercle

Oblique arytenoid muscle

Thyroid cartilage

Transverse arytenoid muscle

Posterior cricoarytenoid muscle

Inferior pharyngeal constrictor

Cricoid cartilage

Left recurrent laryngeal nerve

Laimer triangle

Right recurrent laryngeal nerve

Muscular coat, longitudinal layer

Muscular coat, circular layer

Esophageal (submucosal) glands

Esophageal lumen

Adventitia

Venous plexus in submucosa

Muscularis, longitudinal layer

Muscularis, circular layer

Submucosa

Mucosa, muscular layer

Mucosa, lamina propria

Mucosa, epithelial layer

A Esophageal inlet (upper esophageal sphincter)

Posterior view. The muscular posterior wall of the pharynx has been divided and reflected laterally, and the uppermost esophageal segment has been opened posteriorly. At the posterior junction of the longitudinal esophageal musculature with the pharyngeal musculature, the longitudinal muscles are thin and do not span the full circumference of the esophagus. This area of muscular weakness ("Laimer triangle") is a site of vulnerability for the development of diverticula (see p. 73). This diagram shows the esophagus with an expanded, stellate lumen near the esophageal inlet, as it would appear during swallowing. While in the resting state, the esophageal inlet usually has the form of a transverse slit. The musculature of the upper esophagus is a continuation of the (skeletal) pharyngeal muscles and consists of striated fibers that give way distally to smooth muscle (not shown here).

B Microscopic structure of the esophageal wall

Transverse section through an esophagus in the contracted (left) and relaxed state (right). The layers of the esophageal wall are typical of a hollow viscus in the digestive tract:

- The *mucosa*, which consists of an epithelial layer, lamina propria, and muscular layer. The epithelial layer is composed of stratified, non-keratinized squamous epithelium (for mechanical resistance to food passage).
- The *submucosa*, a loose layer of connective tissue that contains numerous glands (esophageal glands) whose secretions lubricate the mucosa to facilitate food passage. Particularly in the lower esophagus, the submucosa contains numerous veins that participate in the closure of the esophageal outlet (see **Cc**).
- The *muscularis*, consisting of an inner layer of circular muscle and an outer layer of longitudinal muscle. Smooth-muscle contractions aid in the peristaltic propulsion of food.
- The *adventitia*, a layer of loose connective tissue that tethers the esophagus to the mediastinal connective tissue and is firmly attached to the connective tissue of the posterior tracheal wall.

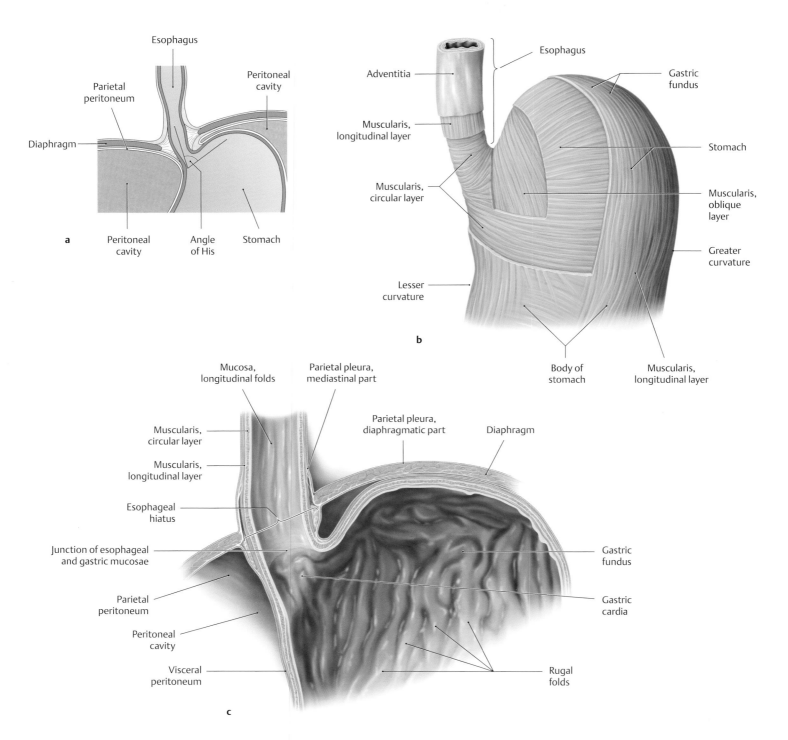

a

- Esophagus
- Parietal peritoneum
- Diaphragm
- Peritoneal cavity
- Peritoneal cavity
- Angle of His
- Stomach

b

- Adventitia
- Esophagus
- Muscularis, longitudinal layer
- Muscularis, circular layer
- Lesser curvature
- Gastric fundus
- Stomach
- Muscularis, oblique layer
- Greater curvature
- Body of stomach
- Muscularis, longitudinal layer

c

- Mucosa, longitudinal folds
- Parietal pleura, mediastinal part
- Parietal pleura, diaphragmatic part
- Diaphragm
- Muscularis, circular layer
- Muscularis, longitudinal layer
- Esophageal hiatus
- Junction of esophageal and gastric mucosae
- Parietal peritoneum
- Peritoneal cavity
- Visceral peritoneum
- Gastric fundus
- Gastric cardia
- Rugal folds

C Esophageal outlet and esophageal closure

Functional closure of the esophageal outlet is an important mechanism for preventing the backflow of gastric contents, especially hydrochloric acid, into the distal esophagus (gastroesophageal reflux). This mechanism is essential because the esophageal mucosa, unlike the gastric mucosa, is vulnerable to corrosive injury by stomach acid. As a result, repeated exposure to hydrochloric acid can cause esophageal inflammation (reflux esophagitis). Early, relatively mild forms of this reflux ("heartburn") are often manifested by a burning retrosternal pain that is most pronounced in the supine position (at night!). Effective closure of the esophagus is based on several factors:

- Narrowing of the esophageal outlet by:
  - the circular muscles of the esophagus (see **b**) and
  - submucous venous plexuses, which raise longitudinal folds in the esophageal mucosa (see **c**). These prominent veins function as portosystemic collaterals in response to an obstruction of portal venous blood flow (see p. 119). Together, the esophageal circular muscles and venous plexuses provide "angiomuscular closure" at the esophagogastric junction.
- The structurally narrow muscular esophageal hiatus in the diaphragm (see **c**)
- Connective tissue and fat surrounding the esophagogastric junction (**c**)
- Continuity of the esophageal and gastric musculature (**b**), and the oblique angle at which the esophagus joins the stomach just below the diaphragm (the angle of His, see **a**).

2.4 Trachea: Thoracic Location and Relations

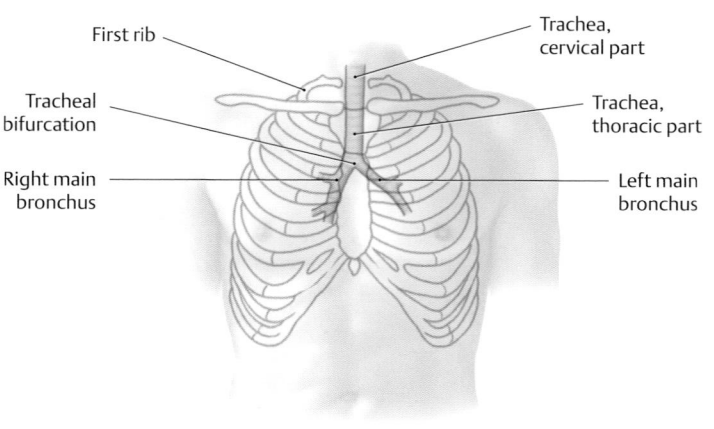

A The trachea projected onto the neck and thorax

The trachea is located in the mediastinum and lies precisely in the median plane. The initial, cervical part of the trachea begins just below the larynx, and its thoracic part ends at the tracheal bifurcation (see **B**). The trachea expands during inspiration and contracts during expiration. The projection in the figure shows the appearance of the trachea at functional residual capacity (relaxed end-expiration).

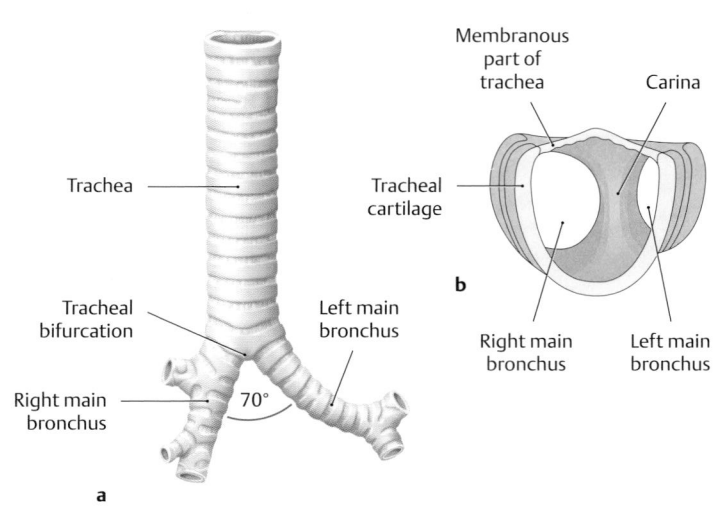

B Shape of the trachea

a Anterior view, **b** superior view of the tracheal bifurcation.

The trachea is a flexible air-conducting tube 10 to 12 cm long. At the approximate level of the T 3–T 4 vertebral bodies, it bifurcates into the left and right main (principal) bronchi, which form an angle of approximately 55–70°. Viewed from the anterior side, the tracheal bifurcation lies just below the junction of the manubrium and body of the sternum.

Note: The right main bronchus is more vertical than the left main bronchus (see p. 82), and therefore it is more common for aspirated foreign bodies to enter the right main bronchus than the left. This also makes it easier to view the interior of the right main bronchus with an endoscope. Owing to the asymmetry of the heart and the associated asymmetrical position of the lungs, the left main bronchus is slightly longer than the right.

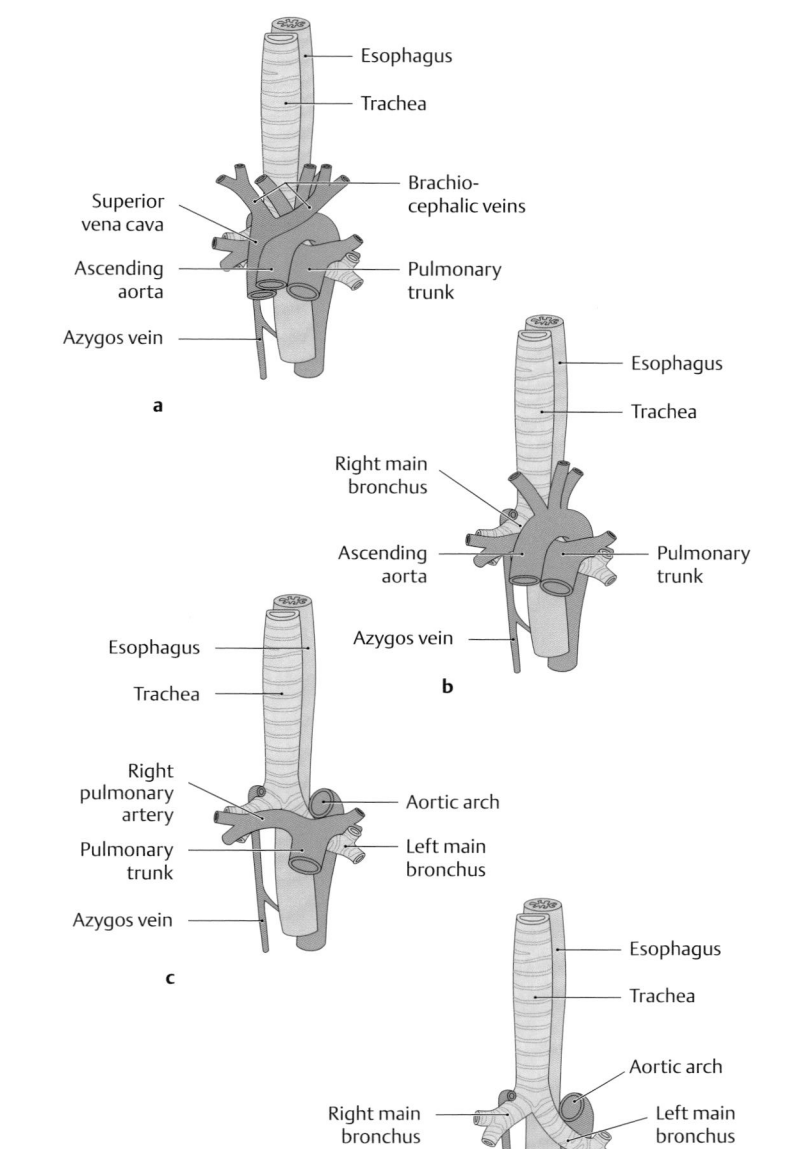

C Topographical relations (after Agur)

Anterior view. With its proximity to the base of the heart and surrounding vessels, the trachea has complex topographical relations with neighboring structures. In the drawings above, structures are progressively removed to obtain greater exposure of the trachea and bronchi.

a With all structures intact, the trachea can be seen anterior to the esophagus. The tracheal bifurcation is covered by the aortic arch and pulmonary artery (see also p. 120).

b With the superior vena cava and brachiocephalic veins removed, the right main bronchus is just visible and the azygos vein is seen "riding" on the right upper lobar bronchus.

c The ascending aorta and much of the aortic arch have been removed, exposing the tracheal bifurcation and pulmonary arteries.

d With the pulmonary trunk removed, the aorta "rides" upon the left main bronchus.

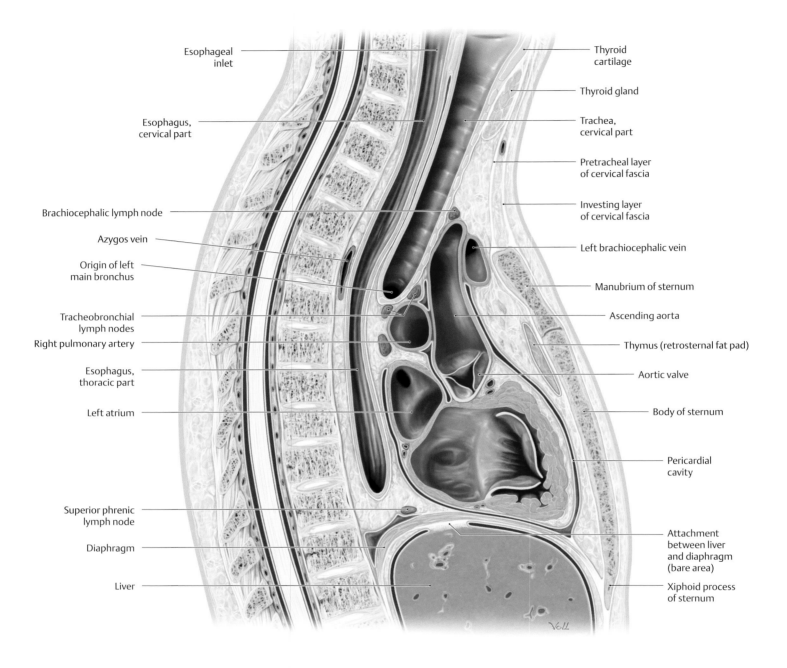

Esophageal inlet

Esophagus, cervical part

Brachiocephalic lymph node

Azygos vein

Origin of left main bronchus

Tracheobronchial lymph nodes

Right pulmonary artery

Esophagus, thoracic part

Left atrium

Superior phrenic lymph node

Diaphragm

Liver

Thyroid cartilage

Thyroid gland

Trachea, cervical part

Pretracheal layer of cervical fascia

Investing layer of cervical fascia

Left brachiocephalic vein

Manubrium of sternum

Ascending aorta

Thymus (retrosternal fat pad)

Aortic valve

Body of sternum

Pericardial cavity

Attachment between liver and diaphragm (bare area)

Xiphoid process of sternum

D The trachea in situ

Midsagittal section viewed from the right side. The pericardium, heart, trachea, and esophagus have been transected. In this simplified lateral view, it can be seen that the trachea, which is just anterior to the esophagus, angles posteriorly as it descends from the neck through the thorax: After entering the chest through the thoracic inlet, it runs *behind* the vessels surrounding the heart. The shape and anatomical relations of the bronchial tree beyond this level are determined by the segmental organization of the lungs (pp. 78–79).

2.5 Lung: Thoracic Location and Relations

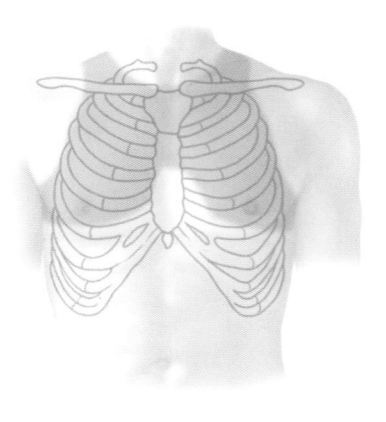

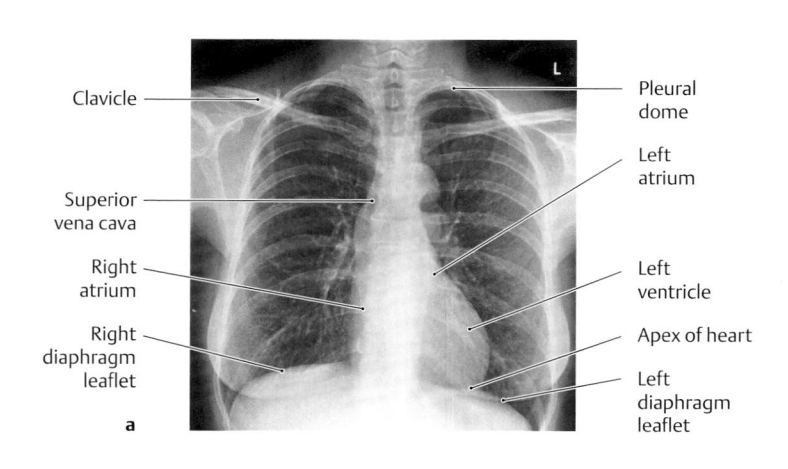

Labels on radiograph (a): Clavicle, Superior vena cava, Right atrium, Right diaphragm leaflet, Pleural dome, Left atrium, Left ventricle, Apex of heart, Left diaphragm leaflet

a

A Percussion field of the lungs

Anterior view. The air-filled lungs constitute a resonant cavity that produces a *sonorous lung sound* on percussion of the chest. The sonorous lung field extends cranially, with attenuation, to the apices of the lungs at the thoracic inlet. It also extends to the front of the chest, again with attenuation, and closely approaches the anterior midline (costomediastinal recess with anterior lung margin on deep inspiration, see p. 91). The fluid-filled heart dampens the lung sounds, producing an area of cardiac dullness (see p. 99). A sharp transition from lung sound to liver sound is clearly audible at the inferior border of the right lung, since the liver is a solid organ with less resonance (medium-pitched, nonsonorous percussion sound).

Note: The lung percussion field does not precisely match the anatomical extent of the lungs because only well-aerated portions of the lung are sonorous to percussion. The anatomical extent of the lungs is greater than the percussion field.

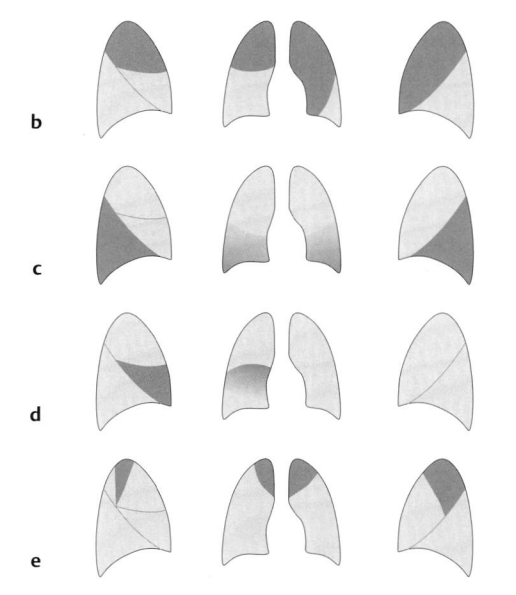

b

c

d

e

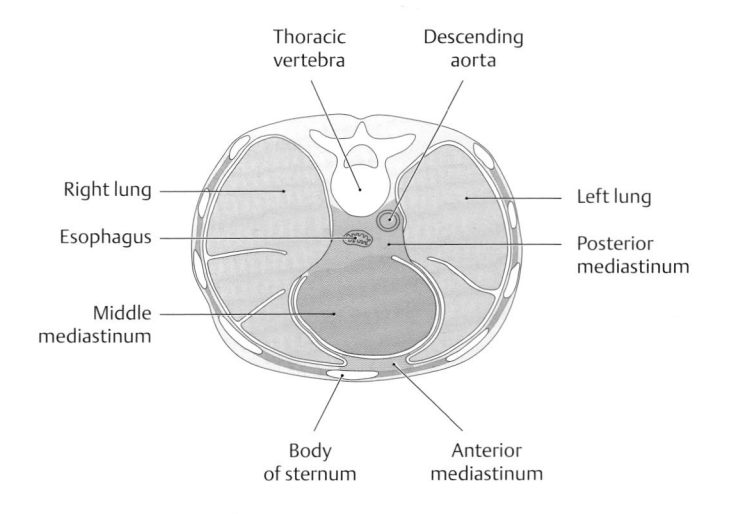

Labels: Thoracic vertebra, Descending aorta, Right lung, Esophagus, Left lung, Posterior mediastinum, Middle mediastinum, Body of sternum, Anterior mediastinum

C Radiographic appearance of the normal lungs and opacities in diseased lung

a Radiographic appearance of the lungs, anterior view. Different regions of the lungs show different degrees of lucency in the chest radiograph. The perihilar region of the lung (where the main bronchi enter the lung and vessels enter and leave the lung) is less radiolucent than the peripheral region, which contains small-caliber vascular branches and segmental bronchi. Additionally, the perihilar lung region is partly covered by the heart. These "shadows" appear as white or bright areas on the radiograph. The same effect is observed in diseased lung areas, which appear more opaque as a result of fluid infiltration (inflammation) or tissue proliferation (neoplasia) (see **b−e**). These opacities are easier to detect in the peripheral part of the lung, which is inherently more radiolucent than the perihilar lung.

b−e Opacity in lung diseases: lateral and anterior views of the right and left lungs.

b Opacity in both lungs. **c** Opacity in both lower lobes. **d** Middle lobe opacity (in the right lung). **e** Opacity in the apical segments of both lungs.

Opacities that follow the lines of segmental lung boundaries are almost invariably due to pulmonary inflammation.

B Position of the lungs in the thorax: topographical relations

Transverse section through the thorax, viewed from above. The lungs completely occupy the left and right pleural cavities flanking the mediastinum. Anteriorly they approach each other in front of the pericardium, and posteriorly they closely approach the vertebral column. The left lung is slightly smaller than the right lung owing to the asymmetrical position of the heart (see **D**).

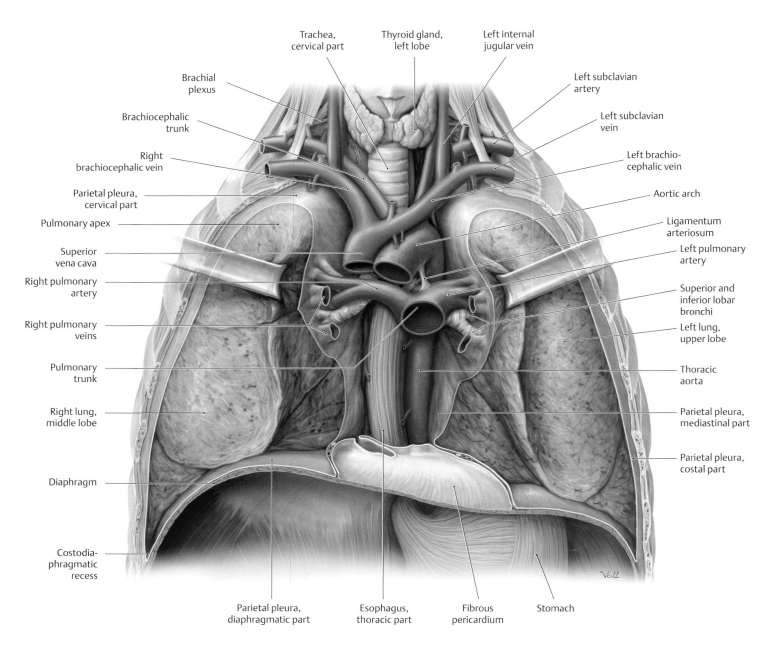

Trachea, cervical part

Thyroid gland, left lobe

Left internal jugular vein

Brachial plexus

Left subclavian artery

Brachiocephalic trunk

Left subclavian vein

Right brachiocephalic vein

Left brachio-cephalic vein

Parietal pleura, cervical part

Aortic arch

Pulmonary apex

Ligamentum arteriosum

Superior vena cava

Left pulmonary artery

Right pulmonary artery

Superior and inferior lobar bronchi

Right pulmonary veins

Left lung, upper lobe

Pulmonary trunk

Thoracic aorta

Right lung, middle lobe

Parietal pleura, mediastinal part

Parietal pleura, costal part

Diaphragm

Costodia-phragmatic recess

Parietal pleura, diaphragmatic part

Esophagus, thoracic part

Fibrous pericardium

Stomach

D The lungs in situ

Anterior view of the opened thorax (depiction simplified). The heart and pericardium have been removed. The vessels surrounding the heart have been transected, and all mediastinal connective tissues have been removed. The lungs have been retracted laterally to stretch and expose the main bronchi. The abdominal cavity has been opened and eviscerated, leaving only the stomach in place. The cervical part of the trachea is still visible below the cricoid cartilage. Shortly below its entry into the chest through the thoracic inlet, the trachea is almost completely obscured by the great vessels (see p. 97). The thoracic part of the esophagus can be seen below the tracheal bifurcation, which lies directly behind the ascending aorta. The lungs in the pleural cavities closely approach the vertebral column *posteriorly,* while *anteriorly* they extend in front of the pericardium and narrow the anterior mediastinum. Percussion of the chest yields a "sonorous" lung sound (see **A**) which is dulled by the heart and pericardium. The extent of the lungs depends on the phase of respiration (see p. 93), but the apices of the lungs always extend into the thoracic inlet, which is closed by a condensation of loose connective tissue—the suprapleural membrane. The apical lung tissue is pictured here as soft and pliant, corresponding to its natural consistency. It should be noted that when the pleural cavities are opened at operation, the lungs tend to collapse toward the hilum owing to their elastic recoil; they do not completely fill the pleural cavity as shown here. (For clarity, the lungs are portrayed in an expanded state.)

2.6 Lung: Shape and Structure

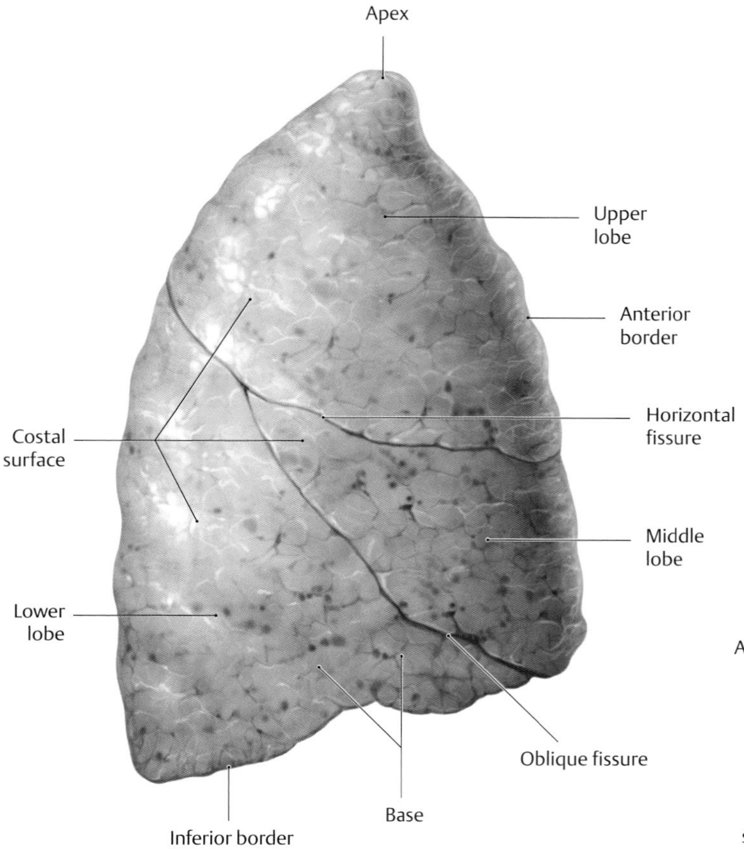

Apex

Upper lobe

Anterior border

Horizontal fissure

Costal surface

Middle lobe

Lower lobe

Oblique fissure

Inferior border

Base

a Right lung, lateral view

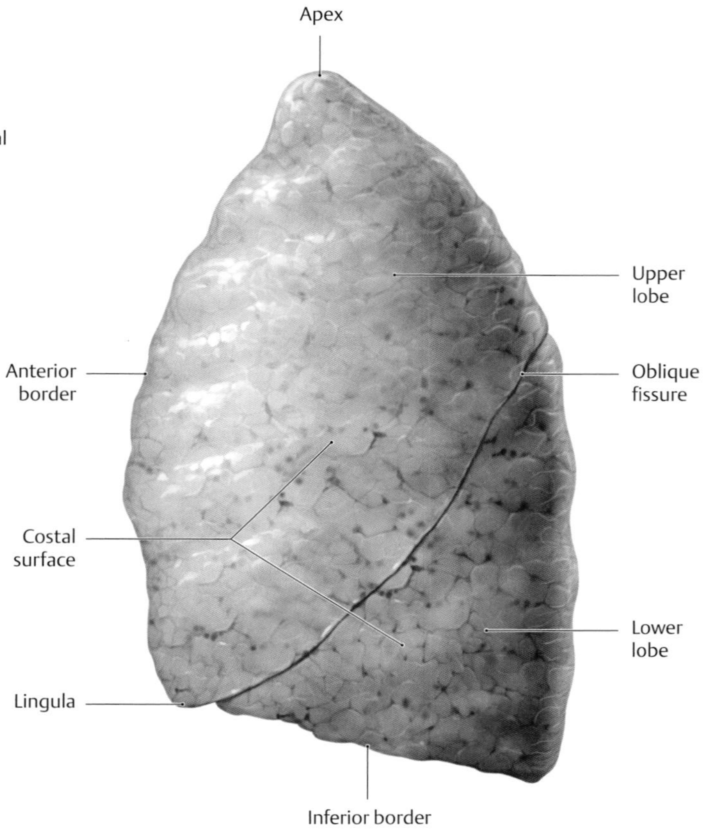

Apex

Upper lobe

Anterior border

Oblique fissure

Costal surface

Lower lobe

Lingula

Inferior border

b Left lung, lateral view

A Gross anatomy of the left and right lungs (for microanatomy see pp. 86–89)

a, b Lateral view. **c, d** Medial view.

The color of the healthy lung ranges from gray to bluish-pink. Grayish-black particles are often visible beneath the pleural surface (as shown here) and are found even in nonsmokers. They do not necessarily have pathological significance, consisting of dust or carbonaceous particles that have been inhaled and deposited in the lung. A lung that has not been chemically fixed has a soft, spongy texture and collapses when taken from the chest. The shape shown above is the in vivo shape of the dynamically expanded lung (see p. 93). The right lung, with a volume of approximately 1500 cm, is slightly larger than the left lung, which has a volume of approximately 1400 cm (due to the inclination of the heart to the left side.) Each of the lungs is divided into *lobes* by one or more interlobar *fissures:*

- The left lung is divided into two lobes (superior and inferior) by one oblique fissure.

- The right lung consists of three lobes (superior, middle, and inferior) separated by one *oblique* fissure and one *horizontal* fissure. The pulmonary fissures are completely lined by visceral pleura.

Note: Owing to the steep angle of the oblique fissure in the left lung, the lingula of the upper lobe forms part of the base of the left lung.

The smallest morphologically distinct and autonomous structural unit of the lung is the *lobule*, which is aerated by a bronchiole. The pulmonary lobules are separated from one another by (often incomplete) fibrous interlobular septa, demarcating numerous polyhedral areas that may be visible on the lung surface.

Aside from the differences noted above, both lungs have the same basic parts:

- The apex, which extends into the thoracic inlet
- The base, which rests on the diaphragm

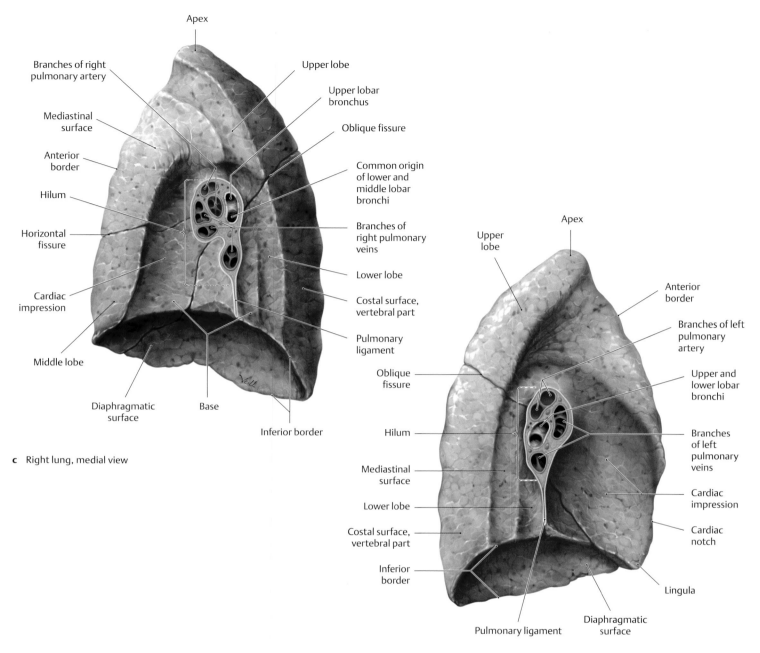

c Right lung, medial view

d Left lung, medial view

- Surfaces of the lung:
  - Costal surface: relates laterally and posteriorly to the ribs. The vertebral part of the costal surface faces the vertebral column (see **c, d**).
  - Mediastinal surface: relates medially to the mediastinum.
  - Diaphragmatic surface (see **c, d**): relates inferiorly to the diaphragm.
  - Interlobar (fissural) surfaces. In the chemically fixed specimen, impressions from the ribs are visible on the costal surface, a cardiac impression on the mediastinal surface, and an impression from the diaphragm leaflet on the diaphragmatic surface. The left lung additionally has a distinct cardiac *notch* in its anterior border.
- Borders of the lung:
  - Anterior border: sharp, thin border located at the junction of the costal and mediastinal surfaces (inserts into the costomediastinal recess).

  - Inferior border: located at the junction of the diaphragmatic and costal or mediastinal surfaces, sharp at the costal surface (inserts into the costodiaphragmatic recess) and blunt at the mediastinal surface.
- Hilum: area where bronchi and neurovascular structures enter and leave the mediastinal surface. The *root* of the lung comprises all of the blood vessels, lymphatics, bronchi, and nerves that enter and emerge at the hilum. Elements of the bronchial tree are generally located in the posterior part of the hilum. Pulmonary venous branches are anterior and inferior, and pulmonary arterial branches are found mainly in the upper part of the hilum.

Both lungs are invested by a serous membrane, the *visceral pleura* (pulmonary pleura), which is reflected at the mediastinal surface to continue as the parietal pleura. This pleural fold is ruptured when the lung is removed, appearing as the *pulmonary ligament*.

2.7 Trachea and Bronchial Tree: Shape and Structure

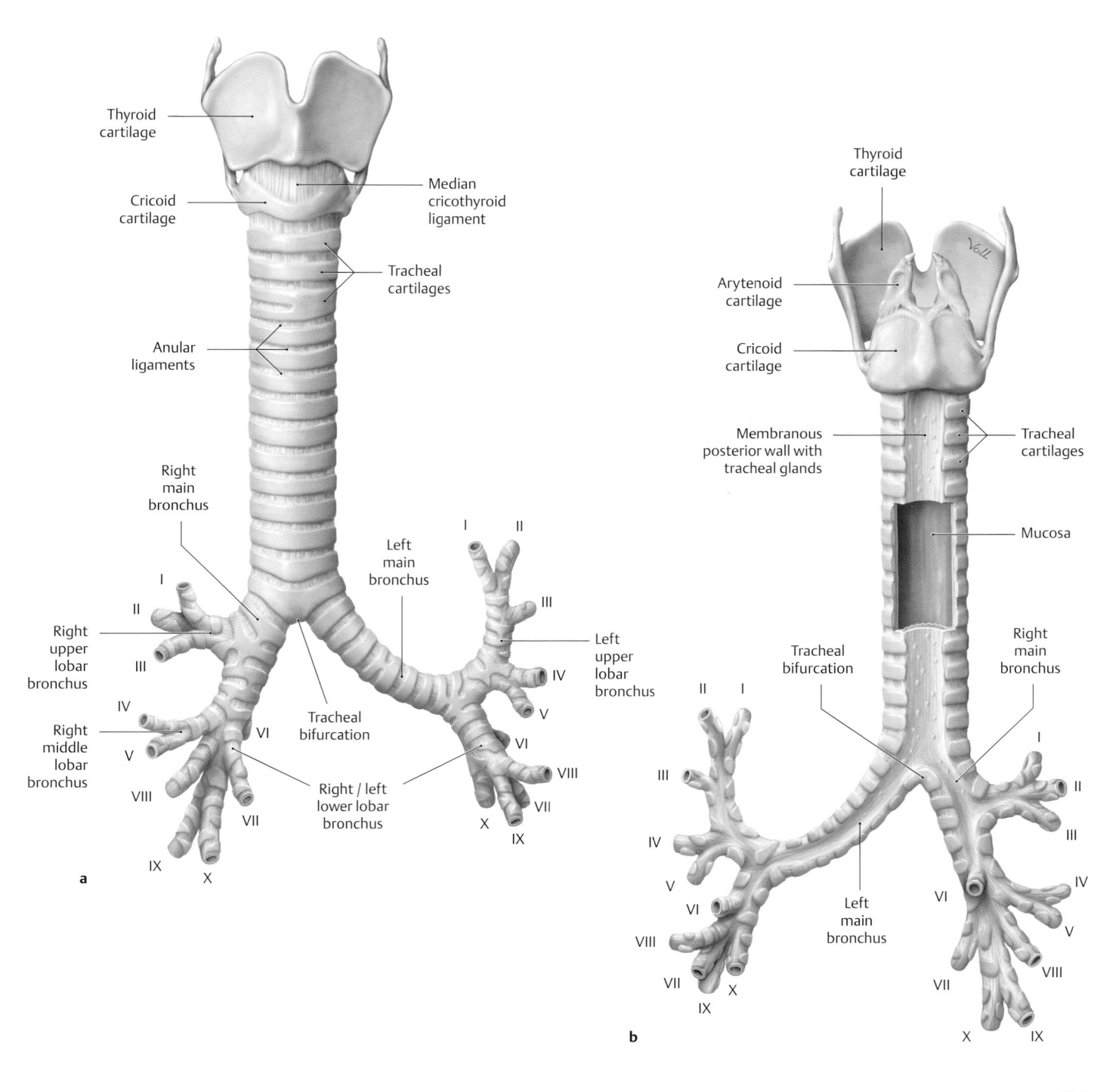

A Structure of the trachea and bronchial tree

a Lateral view, **b** posterior view with opened posterior wall.

The trachea consists of 16–20 horseshoe-shaped rings composed of hyaline cartilage (the tracheal cartilages) and a membranous posterior wall composed of connective tissue and tracheal muscle (not shown here). The tracheal cartilages are interconnected longitudinally by collagenous connective tissue (anular ligaments). The two parts of the trachea are clearly distinguishable:

- Cervical part: extends from the first tracheal cartilage below the cricoid cartilage of the larynx at the level of the C6 / C7 vertebrae to the thoracic inlet (see p. 77).

- Thoracic part: extends from the thoracic inlet to the tracheal bifurcation, where the trachea divides into the right and left main bronchi at the level of the T4 vertebra. A cartilaginous spur at the tracheal bifurcation (the carina, not shown here, see p. 76) projects upward into the tracheal lumen.

The left and right main bronchi divide into two or three *lobar bronchi*, respectively, which subsequently branch into segmental bronchi (see **C**).

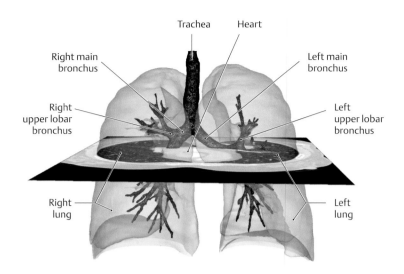

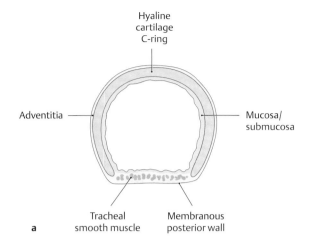

B Reconstruction of the bronchial tree from cross-sectional images

Anterior view. The bronchial tree can be scanned in a series of sectional images and reconstructed in three dimensions from the individual scans. The result is a three-dimensional display with high optical resolution. A CT section displaying the heart and lungs is shown for orientation purposes. This examination is noninvasive, unlike the older technique of bronchography (radiographic contrast examination of the bronchi). Because of the high resolution of the scans, even subtle changes in the bronchial tree can be detected and accurately localized in three dimensions. This is a very precise technique for localizing a malignancy that is particularly common in smokers: bronchial carcinoma.

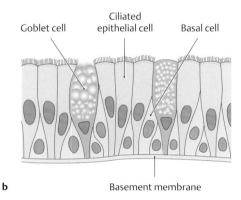

C Divisions of the trachea and bronchial tree

Right main bronchus	Left main bronchus
Right upper lobar bronchus	*Left upper lobar bronchus*
Apical segmental bronchus (I)	Apicoposterior segmental
Posterior segmental bronchus (II)	bronchus (I, II)
Anterior segmental bronchus (III)	Anterior segmental bronchus (III)
Right middle lobar bronchus	
Lateral segmental bronchus (IV)	Superior lingular bronchus (IV)
Medial segmental bronchus (V)	Inferior lingular bronchus (V)
Right lower lobar bronchus	*Left lower lobar bronchus*
Superior segmental bronchus (VI)	Superior segmental bronchus (VI)
Medial basal segmental bronchus (VII)	Medial basal segmental bronchus (VII)
Anterior basal segmental bronchus (VIII)	Anterior basal segmental bronchus (VIII)
Lateral basal segmental bronchus (IX)	Lateral basal segmental bronchus (IX)
Posterior basal segmental bronchus (X)	Posterior basal segmental bronchus (X)

D Wall structure of the trachea and main bronchi

a **Histological organization of the wall of the trachea:** The trachea is a fibroelastic tube supported by spaced C-shaped rings of hyaline cartilage. The open end of each ring is closed by a membranous posterior wall. The entire tube is lined by a *mucosa*, consisting of an epithelial layer (**b**), with an underlying lamina propria of loose connective tissue containing a fibroelastic band at its base. Below the mucosa is a submucosa containing seromucous glands that secrete a protective mucous film. The membranous wall that closes the open end of the tracheal cartilage contains circularly-oriented smooth muscle (trachealis) with additional longitudinal bands. The outermost component is an adventitial layer of connective tissue. Microscopic structure changes substantially at different levels of the bronchial tree (see pp. 86–89).

b **The tracheal epithelium:** Facing the tracheal lumen is a pseudostratified respiratory epithelium with three prominent cell types: columnar *ciliated cells*, which drive mucus and particles along the tracheal surface toward the pharynx, *goblet cells*, which secrete mucus, and *basal cells*, which do not span the full height of the epithelium. Basal cells are mitotic precursors for other cell types in the epithelium. A thick basement membrane underlies this epithelium. The tracheal epithelium contains several other intrinsic cell types, not depicted, as well as lymphocytes and mast cells that have migrated from underlying connective tissue. Prolonged exposure to irritants such as tobacco smoke increases the number of goblet cells and decreases the flow of secretions, compromising airway clearance.

Note: The epithelium of the carina, unlike that of the rest of the trachea, consists of nonkeratinized squamous cells.

2.8 Lung: Segmentation

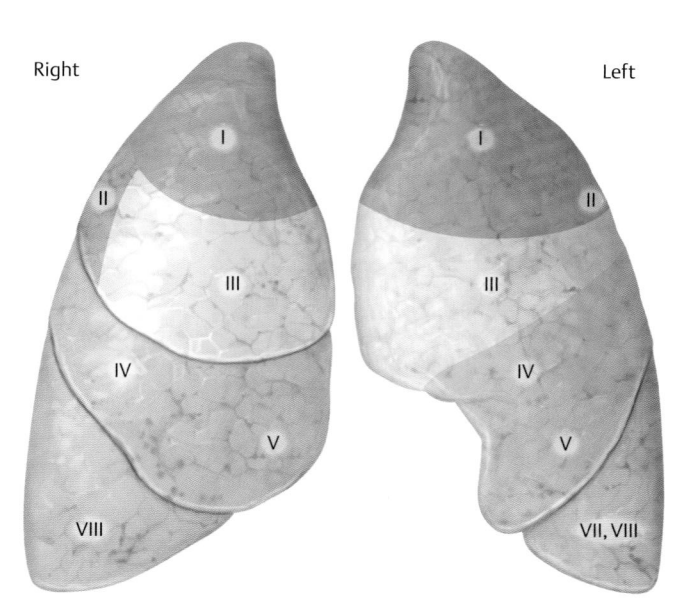

a Lungs, anterior view

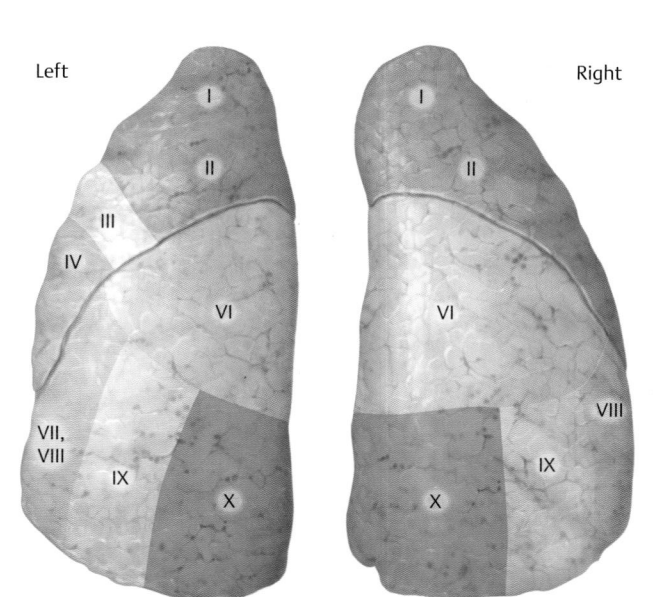

b Lungs, posterior view

A Segmental architecture of the lungs

Anterior view (**a**) and posterior view (**b**) of the right and left lungs (lateral and medial views are shown in **C**).

The segmental architecture of the lung relates directly to the branching pattern of the bronchial tree (see p. 83). The basic structural unit of the lung is the *lobe*, whose boundaries are clearly defined on the surface of the lung by the interlobar fissures. Each lobe is further subdivided into *segments*—wedge-shaped functional units whose apex points toward the pulmonary hilum. The pulmonary segments are incompletely separated from one another by thin connective tissue and are not discernible as separate units on the lung surface. Passing to the center of each segment are a *segmental bronchus* and a *segmental branch of the pulmonary artery* (segmental artery), constituting the "bronchopulmo-nary segment" or "bronchoarterial segment." The segments, in turn, consist of subsegments defined by the further branching pattern of the segmental bronchi. Each lung consists basically of ten segments. Due to the presence of the cardiac notch in the *left* lung, however, segment VII of that lung is often so small that it is not considered a separate segment but part of segment VIII. As noted above, the segmental boundaries are not visible on the surface of the lung. For partial resections of the lung (see **D**), the targeted segments are identified by clamping off the segmental artery. As the devascularized segment blanches, it contrasts sharply with the surrounding tissues that are still perfused. Intrasegmental blood flow can also be demonstrated by ultrasound scanning. The pulmonary segments are named and numbered as shown in table **B**.

B Segmental architecture of the lungs

Right lung	Left lung
Upper lobe	*Upper lobe*
Apical segment (I)	Apicoposterior segment (I + II)
Posterior segment (II)	
Anterior segment (III)	Anterior segment (III)
Middle lobe	
Lateral segment (IV)	Superior lingular segment (IV)
Medial segment (V)	Inferior lingular segment (V)
Lower lobe	*Lower lobe*
Superior segment (VI)	Superior segment (VI)
Medial basal segment (VII)	[Medial basal segment (VII)]
Anterior basal segment (VIII)	Anterior basal segment (VIII)
Lateral basal segment (IX)	Lateral basal segment (IX)
Posterior basal segment (X)	Posterior basal segment (X)

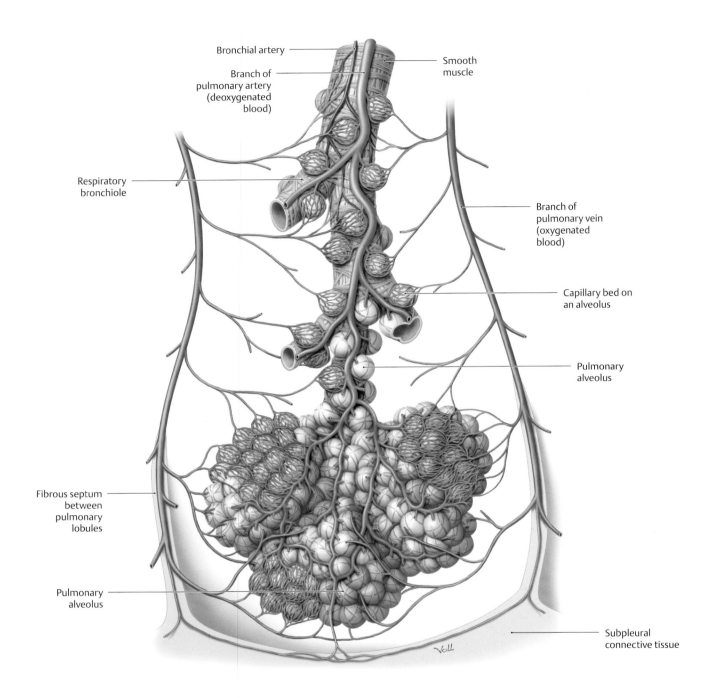

Bronchial artery

Branch of
pulmonary artery
(deoxygenated
blood)

Smooth
muscle

Respiratory
bronchiole

Branch of
pulmonary vein
(oxygenated
blood)

Capillary bed on
an alveolus

Pulmonary
alveolus

Fibrous septum
between
pulmonary
lobules

Pulmonary
alveolus

Subpleural
connective tissue

Voll

C Vascular circuit of a respiratory bronchiole
A respiratory bronchiole and associated alveolar sacs of one of its terminal branches, as illustrated on p. 87, is reproduced here with the local vascular tree superimposed. Note that, as in **B**, the pulmonary arterial branch is depicted in blue because of its deoxygenated blood, while
the corresponding pulmonary venous branch is shown in red because
its blood has been replenished with oxygen. The lung has two separate
vascular systems—pulmonary arteries and veins for gas exchange (vasa
publica), and much smaller-diameter bronchial arteries and veins (vasa
privata) for supplying the metabolic needs of the parts of the lung itself
—bronchi and larger-diameter bronchioles—that do not have direct access to oxygen (see p. 122).

Numerous anastomoses between the vasa publica (pulmonary artery
and vein) and the vasa privata (bronchial artery and vein) help to ensure
that a pulmonary embolism (occlusion of a pulmonary arterial branch
by a blood clot) will not inevitably destroy the dependent lung tissue
and cause pulmonary infarction. The pulmonary system is selectively
vulnerable to such emboli because it is the first capillary bed that all the
blood travels through after being collected from the body into the right
heart; most pulmonary emboli originate in stagnant blood in the veins
of the legs. The collateral circulation cannot compensate for large emboli, which cause massive damage and produce sudden life-threatening
obstructions of pulmonary blood flow.

2.11 **Diaphragm**

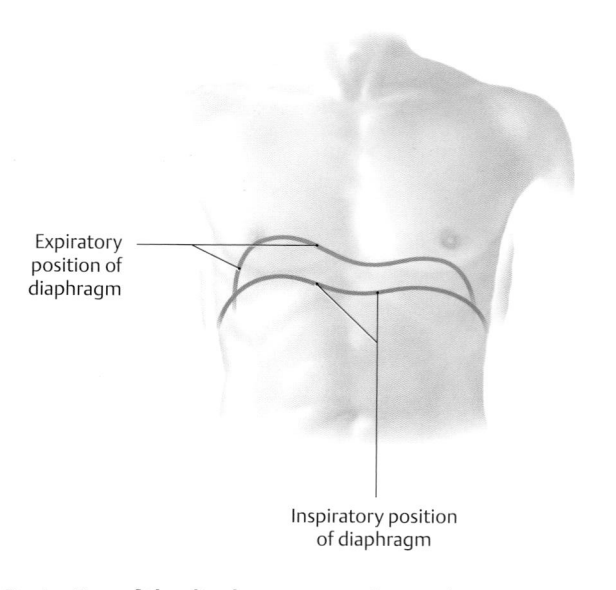

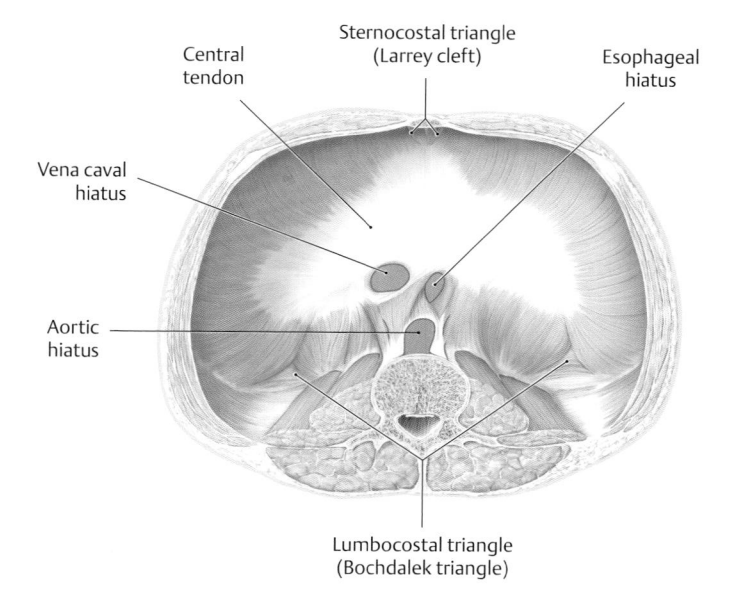

A Projection of the diaphragm onto the trunk

Anterior view. The positions of the diaphragm in expiration (blue) and inspiration (red) are shown. The right hemidiaphragm rises as high as the fourth rib during expiration, and the diaphragm may fall almost to the level of the seventh rib at full inspiration.

Note:

- The exact position of the diaphragm depends on body type, sex, and age.
- The left diaphragm leaflet is lower than the right due to the asymmetrical position of the heart.
- Inspiration is marked by an overall depression of the diaphragm and also by a flattening of the diaphragm leaflets.
- The diaphragm is higher in the supine position (pressure from the intra-abdominal organs) than in the standing position.
- The degree of diaphragmatic movement during inspiration can be assessed by noting the movement of the hepatic border, which is easily palpated.
- The diaphragm in a cadaver occupies a higher level than the expiratory position in vivo due to the loss of muscular tone.

B Openings in the diaphragm

Inferior view. This unit deals only with the openings in the diaphragm and the structures that pass between the thorax and abdomen (see **C**). Details on the shape and structure of the diaphragm may be found in Vol. I, *General Anatomy and Musculoskeletal System*. Topographically, the diaphragm closes the thoracic outlet and forms its inferior boundary. Openings can develop in the diaphragm because the spaces between the different parts of the diaphragm are closed only by connective tissue and because neurovascular structures pierce the muscle tissue or tendinous center of the diaphragm. The larger openings are clinically important because they create potential weak spots through which abdominal organs may herniate into the chest. These hernias are most commonly located at the esophageal hiatus. The openings and transmitted structures are reviewed in Table **C**.

C Openings in the diaphragm and transmitted structures

Openings	Transmitted structures
Vena caval hiatus (at the level of the T 8 vertebra)	Inferior vena cava Phrenico-abdominal branch of right phrenic nerve (the left phrenico-abdominal branch pierces the muscle)
Esophageal hiatus (at the level of the T 10 vertebra)	Esophagus Anterior and posterior vagal trunks (on the esophagus)
Aortic hiatus (at the level of the T 12 / L 1 vertebrae)	Descending aorta Thoracic duct
Apertures in the medial crus	Azygos vein, hemiazygos vein, splanchnic nerves
Apertures between the medial and lateral crura	Sympathetic trunk
Sternocostal triangle	Internal thoracic artery and vein, superior epigastric artery and vein

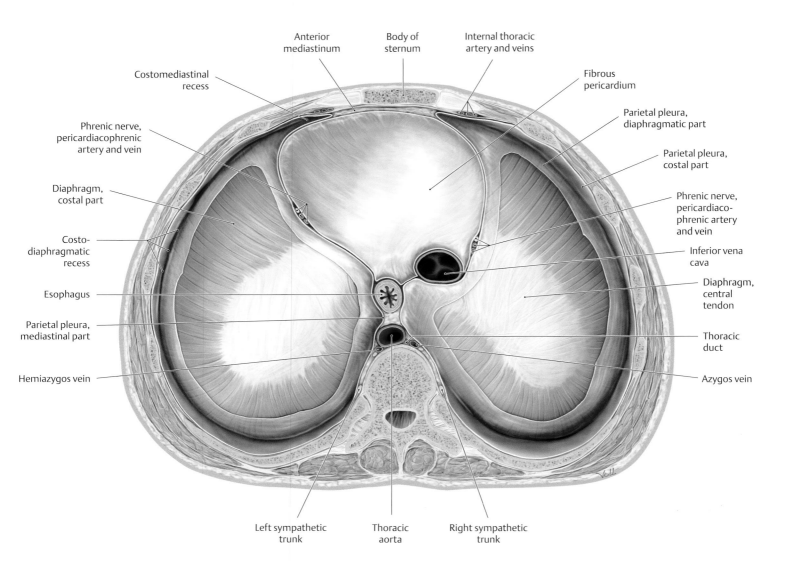

Anterior mediastinum

Body of sternum

Internal thoracic artery and veins

Fibrous pericardium

Costomediastinal recess

Parietal pleura, diaphragmatic part

Phrenic nerve, pericardiacophrenic artery and vein

Parietal pleura, costal part

Diaphragm, costal part

Phrenic nerve, pericardiaco-phrenic artery and vein

Costo-diaphragmatic recess

Inferior vena cava

Diaphragm, central tendon

Esophagus

Thoracic duct

Parietal pleura, mediastinal part

Hemiazygos vein

Azygos vein

Left sympathetic trunk

Thoracic aorta

Right sympathetic trunk

D Closure of the thoracic outlet: diaphragm

Superior view. The heart and lung have been removed, and the parietal pleura has been windowed over a large area of the diaphragm. Owing to the superior convexity of the diaphragm, a recess is formed between the parietal layers of the pleura. This *costodiaphragmatic recess* is lined by the costal and diaphragmatic parts of the parietal pleura. Another recess, the *costomediastinal recess*, is largely independent of the diaphragm convexity. It is lined by the costal and mediastinal parts of the parietal pleura, and it is bounded externally by the ribs and the posterior surface of the sternum and internally by the anterior wall of the pericardium. During inspiration, portions of the lungs expand into the "complementary spaces" formed by these recesses (see p. 93). The anterior mediastinum is a narrow space filled with fat and connective tissue located between the posterior surface of the sternum, the pericardium, and the costomediastinal recess. The phrenic nerve and the pericardiacophrenic artery and vein descend to the diaphragm by passing between the pericardium and the mediastinal part of the parietal pleura. Covered by parietal pleura, the internal thoracic artery and vein descend on the right and left sides of the sternum and pierce the diaphragm through the cleft (not visible here) in the sternocostal triangle. Posteriorly, very close to the vertebral column, the thoracic aorta, azygos and hemiazygos veins, thoracic duct, and portions of the sympathetic trunk pass through the diaphragm as they enter or leave the abdomen.

2.12 **Respiratory Mechanics**

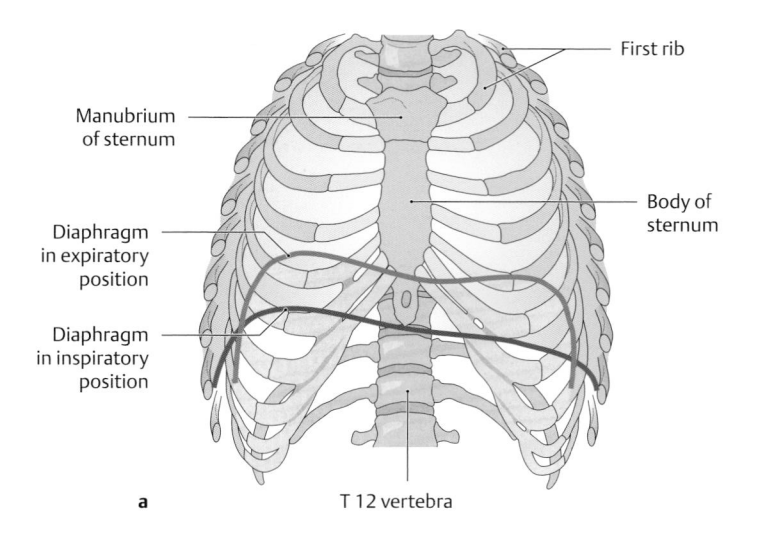

a

First rib

Manubrium
of sternum

Body of
sternum

Diaphragm
in expiratory
position

Diaphragm
in inspiratory
position

T 12 vertebra

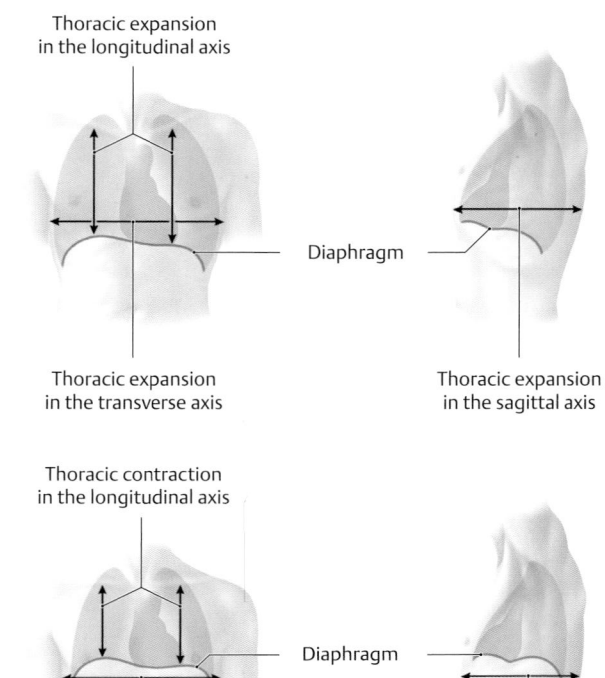

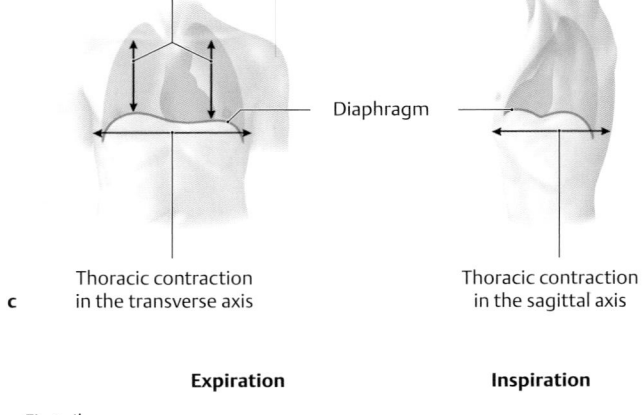

Thoracic expansion
in the longitudinal axis

Diaphragm

b   Thoracic expansion
in the transverse axis

Thoracic expansion
in the sagittal axis

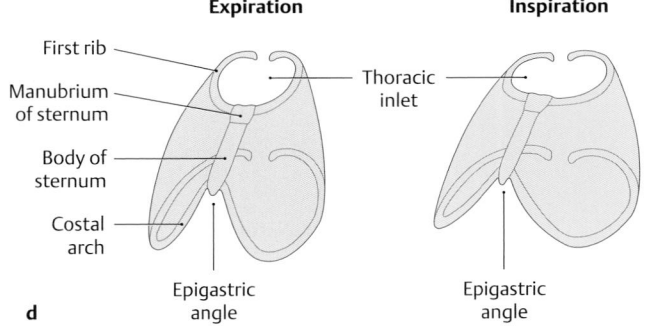

Thoracic contraction
in the longitudinal axis

Diaphragm

c   Thoracic contraction
in the transverse axis

Thoracic contraction
in the sagittal axis

A Basic principles of respiratory mechanics

The mechanics of external respiration (as opposed to the internal respiration of cells and tissues) are based on a rhythmical increase and decrease in the thoracic volume, with an associated expansion and contraction of the lungs. As the lung expands, the pressure within the lung falls and air is drawn into the lung (inspiration). As the lung contracts, the pulmonary pressure rises and air is expelled from the lung (expiration). Thus, contrary to a common misconception, air is not pumped into the lungs during respiration but is sucked into the lungs by the "bellows effect," a negative intrapulmonary pressure. The ribs, the thoracic muscles (especially the intercostal muscles), and the elastic fibers in the lung interact as follows during respiration:

- When the diaphragm moves to the **inspiratory position** (red), the ribs are elevated by the intercostal muscles (chiefly the external intercostals) and the scalene muscles. Because the ribs are curved and are directed obliquely downward, elevation of the ribs expands the chest transversely (toward the flanks) and anteriorly. Meanwhile the diaphragm leaflets are lowered by muscular contraction (red outline in **a**), causing the chest to expand inferiorly. The epigastric angle is also increased (see **d**). These processes result in an overall expansion of the thoracic volume.
- When the diaphragm moves to the **expiratory position** (blue), the chest becomes smaller in all dimensions and the thoracic volume is decreased. This process does not require additional muscular energy. The muscles that are active during inspiration are relaxed, and the lung contracts as the myriad elastic fibers in the lung tissue that were stretched on inspiration release their stored energy, causing an elastic recoil. For forcible expiration, however, the muscles that assist expiration (mainly the internal intercostal muscles) can actively lower the rib cage more rapidly and to a greater extent than is possible by passive elastic recoil alone.

Expiration   **Inspiration**

First rib

Manubrium
of sternum

Body of
sternum

Costal
arch

Thoracic
inlet

Epigastric
angle

Epigastric
angle

d

B Respiratory muscles

Active during inspiration	Active during expiration
Scaleni	Internal intercostal muscles
External intercostal muscles	Transversus thoracis
Intercartilaginous muscles	Subcostal mucosa
Serratus posterior superior and inferior	
Diaphragm	

When the upper limb is fixed (e.g., by bracing the arm on a table), the muscles of the shoulder girdle, whose primary action is to move the shoulder girdle, can elevate and expand the thorax, to which they are attached. They can also function as auxiliary respiratory muscles during forced respiration, when breathing is made difficult (dyspnea) by disease.

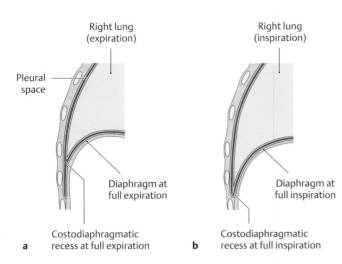

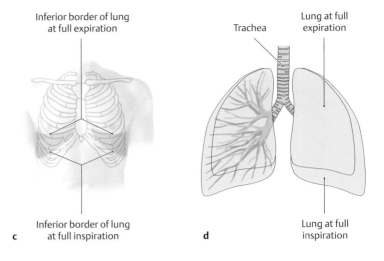

a   Costodiaphragmatic recess at full expiration   b   Costodiaphragmatic recess at full inspiration   c   Inferior border of lung at full inspiration   d   Lung at full inspiration

C Respiratory changes in lung volume

a–c Respiratory contraction and expansion of the lung. Capillary forces in the pleural space cause the lung to "stick" to the wall of the pleural cavity, forcing the lung to follow changes in the thoracic volume. This is particularly evident in the pleural recesses—sites where the lung does not fully occupy the pleural cavity at functional residual capacity (the resting position between inspiration and expiration, see p. 79). As the dome of the diaphragm flattens during inspiration (see p. 90), the costodiaphragmatic recess expands and the lung is "sucked" into the resulting space, though it does not fill it completely.

During expiration, the lung retracts from the recess somewhat. The respiratory changes in the volume of the costodiaphragmatic recess lead to considerable displacement of the inferior lung borders (**c**).

d Respiratory movements of the bronchial tree. As the thoracic volume changes during respiration, the entire bronchial tree moves within the lung. These structural movements are more pronounced in portions of the bronchial tree that are more distant from the pulmonary hilum.

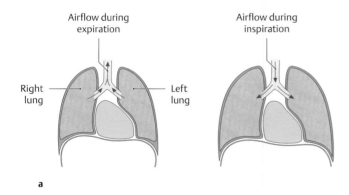

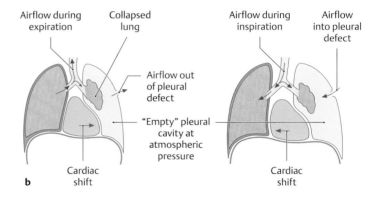

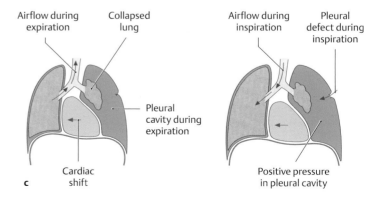

D Change in respiratory mechanics due to pneumothorax

a Normal respiratory mechanics: The pleural space is hermetically sealed on all sides.

b Pneumothorax: With injury to the left parietal pleura, outside air can enter the pleural space. The mechanical effect of the capillary pleural space (see **C**) is lost, and the left lung collapses from the inherent elasticity of its connective tissue. It no longer participates in respiration. The right pleural cavity is intact and can function independently. Air is sucked into the opened pleural cavity during inspiration and is expelled during expiration. Because normal respiratory pressure variations still prevail in the right pleural cavity but are absent on the left side due to the pleural defect, the mediastinum shifts toward the normal side during expiration and returns toward the midline during inspiration ("mediastinal flutter").

c Tension pneumothorax (valve pneumothorax): Tissue that has been traumatically detached and displaced covers the defect in the pleural cavity from the inside like a mobile flap, preventing the expulsion of air. Air passes through the defect in one direction only: from outside to inside. Because of this check-valve mechanism, a small amount of air enters the pleural cavity with each breath but cannot escape,

similar to air being pumped into a bicycle tire. The mediastinum is gradually shifted toward the normal side (mediastinal shift), which may cause kinking of the vessels around the heart. Without treatment, tension pneumothorax is invariably fatal.

2.13 Prenatal and Postnatal Circulation

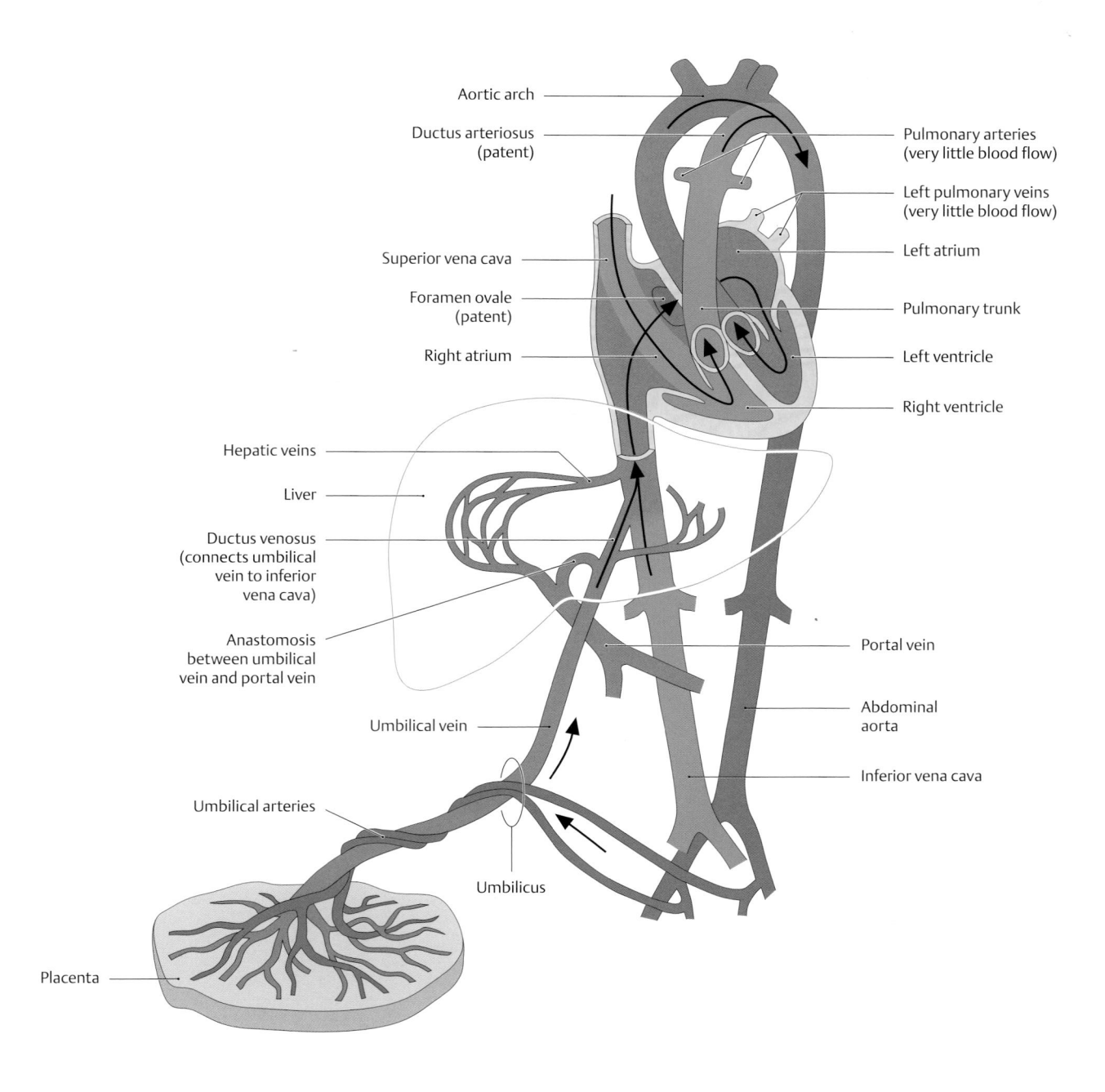

Aortic arch
Ductus arteriosus (patent)
Pulmonary arteries (very little blood flow)
Left pulmonary veins (very little blood flow)
Superior vena cava
Left atrium
Foramen ovale (patent)
Pulmonary trunk
Right atrium
Left ventricle
Right ventricle
Hepatic veins
Liver
Ductus venosus (connects umbilical vein to inferior vena cava)
Anastomosis between umbilical vein and portal vein
Portal vein
Abdominal aorta
Umbilical vein
Inferior vena cava
Umbilical arteries
Umbilicus
Placenta

A Prenatal circulation (after Fritsch and Kühnel)
The prenatal circulation is characterized by:

- very little pulmonary blood flow
- gas exchange in the placenta
- nutrient delivery to the fetus through the placenta
- a right-to-left shunt in the heart

The fetal **lungs** have not yet expanded, are not aerated, and have minimal blood flow. Consequently, the exchange of O_2 and CO_2 takes place outside the fetus in the placenta. Oxygen- and nutrient-rich blood from the fetal part of the placenta is delivered to the fetus by the unpaired umbilical vein. Near the liver, the umbilical vein empties into the inferior vena cava through a venovenous anastomosis, the ductus venosus. Oxygen-poor blood in the inferior vena cava mixes with oxygen-rich blood (from the umbilical vein). The umbilical vein has another venovenous anastomosis with the portal vein, which carries nutrient-rich blood into the liver for metabolic processing. Blood flow in the **heart** is characterized by a right-to-left shunt. Blood from both venae cavae flows into the right atrium. Blood from the inferior vena cava is channeled past an endocardial flap (the valve of the inferior vena cava) and through the patent foramen ovale into the left atrium. Blood from the superior vena cava passes through the right ventricle into the pulmonary trunk, but it does not enter the unexpanded fetal lungs. Instead it passes directly into the aorta through an arterioarterial anastomosis, the ductus arteriosus, and is distributed to the peripheral fetal vessels. Blood returns to the placenta through the paired umbilical arteries (branch of the internal iliac artery). Since very little blood perfuses the lungs, blood is not delivered to the left atrium by the pulmonary veins.

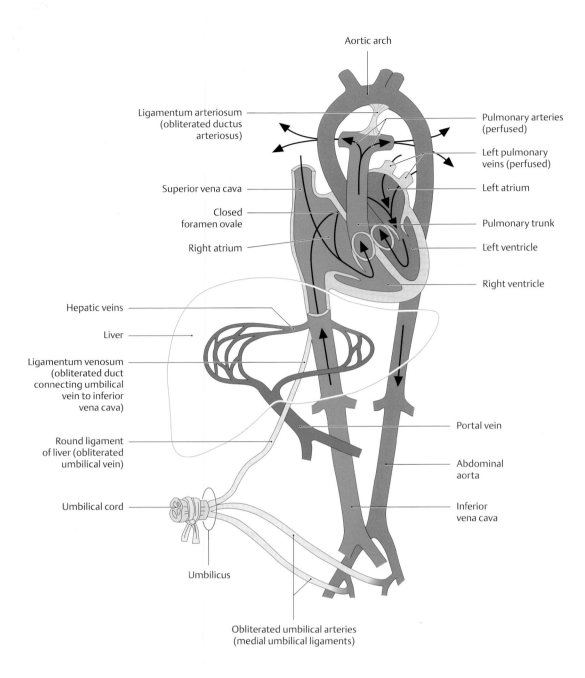

Aortic arch

Ligamentum arteriosum
(obliterated ductus
arteriosus)

Pulmonary arteries
(perfused)

Left pulmonary
veins (perfused)

Superior vena cava

Left atrium

Closed
foramen ovale

Pulmonary trunk

Right atrium

Left ventricle

Right ventricle

Hepatic veins

Liver

Ligamentum venosum
(obliterated duct
connecting umbilical
vein to inferior
vena cava)

Round ligament
of liver (obliterated
umbilical vein)

Portal vein

Abdominal
aorta

Umbilical cord

Inferior
vena cava

Umbilicus

Obliterated umbilical arteries
(medial umbilical ligaments)

B Postnatal circulation (after Fritsch and Kühnel)
At birth, the circulatory system undergoes a radical alteration in terms of gas exchange and hemodynamics. The postnatal circulation is characterized by:

- pulmonary respiration and pulmonary gas exchange
- loss of the placental circulation
- functional occlusion of the right-to-left shunt and fetal anastomoses

When respiration begins, the lungs are expanded and aerated, becoming the essential organs of gas exchange. Vascular resistance falls dramatically in the vessels of the expanded lungs. The pressure in the right atrium plummets, causing an endocardial flap valve in the left atrium to close over the foramen ovale and occlude it (the pressure in the left atrium is now higher than in the right atrium). The contraction of smooth muscle in the ductus arteriosus also functionally occludes that opening. This functional constriction is mediated by oxygen tension and by bradykinin produced by the lungs. The duct eventually involutes to leave a fibrous ligamentum arteriosum. The right ventricle pumps

blood through the pulmonary arteries into the expanded lungs. Blood from the left ventricle is pumped through the aorta and distributed to all body regions before returning through the venae cavae to the right atrium. The right and left sides of the postnatal heart are hemodynamically separate. The umbilical vein is no longer perfused, and the ductus venosus connecting it to the inferior vena cava is occluded (eventually scarring to form the ligamentum venosum). The duct connecting the umbilical vein to the liver is also obliterated, and the umbilical vein usually becomes fibrous over its entire length, forming the round ligament of the liver (ligamentum teres hepatis). Only the proximal portions of the umbilical arteries remain patent while the distal parts are obliterated, forming a medial umbilical ligament on each side.
Note: The persistence of a patent ductus arteriosus causes the lung to be "flooded" with blood from the aorta, which is at high pressure, resulting in secondary damage to the pulmonary arteries. Treatment consists of surgical closure of the patent ductus. If the umbilical vein remains patent, a rise of intrahepatic pressure can cause a reversal of blood flow from the liver to the umbilicus (see portosystemic collaterals, p. 293).

2.14 Heart: Anterior View

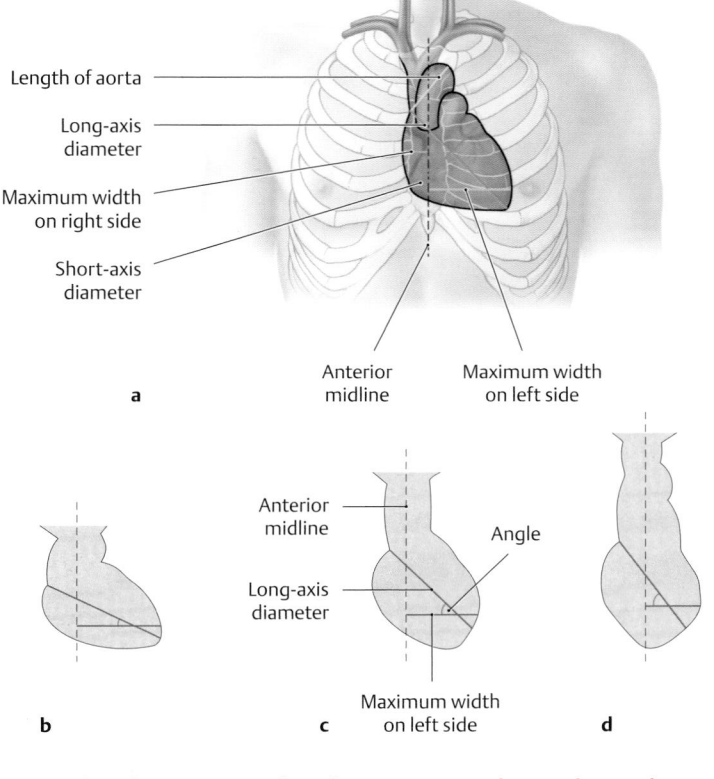

Length of aorta

Long-axis diameter

Maximum width on right side

Short-axis diameter

Anterior midline

Maximum width on left side

a

Anterior midline

Angle

Long-axis diameter

Maximum width on left side

b   c   d

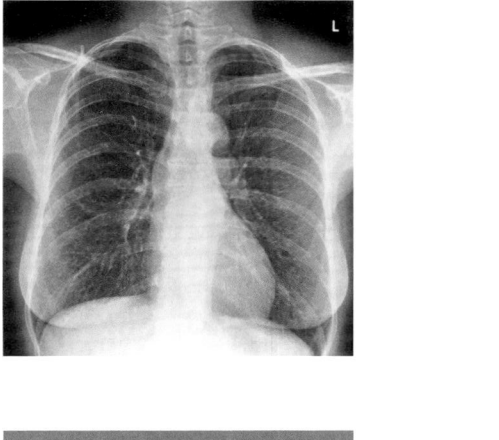

a

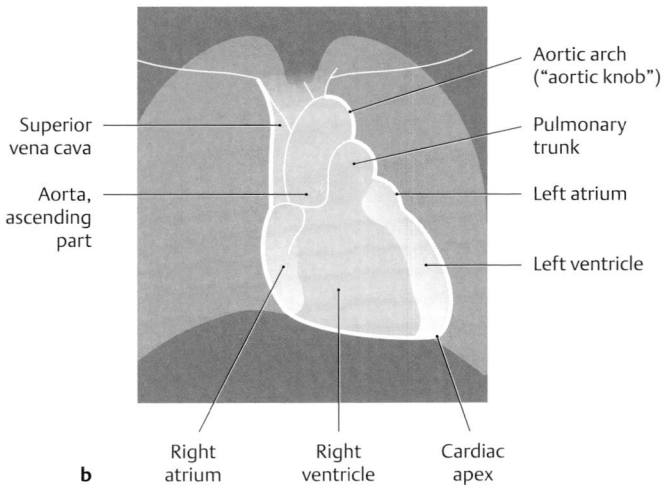

Superior vena cava

Aorta, ascending part

Aortic arch ("aortic knob")

Pulmonary trunk

Left atrium

Left ventricle

Right atrium   Right ventricle   Cardiac apex

b

A Cardiac dimensions and configurations in a chest radiograph
(after Rauber and Kopsch)

The heart is located behind the sternum in the middle portion of the inferior mediastinum. Because of its asymmetrical position, more of the heart is to the left of the sternum than to the right (the structures that form the cardiac borders are shown in **B**). Virtual lines can be drawn over the cardiac silhouette on radiographs (**a**) and can be used to evaluate the size and configuration of the heart. The critical cardiac dimensions are the long-axis diameter, transverse diameter, and short-axis diameter. The long-axis and short-axis diameters can be directly measured on the radiograph, while the transverse diameter is calculated as the sum of the maximum cardiac widths to the right and left of the midline (measured at different levels). The angle between the long-axis diameter and the maximum width to the left of the anterior midline can be measured to assess the cardiac configuration (**b–d**), which may be classified (left to right) as transverse, oblique, or vertical. The exact configuration of the heart is dependent upon both the patient's body type and the point of the respiratory cycle at the moment the image is created.

B Radiographic appearance of the heart: anterior view

The right atrium and superior vena cava form the **right cardiac border** while the aortic arch (called the "aortic knob" on radiographs), pulmonary trunk, left atrium, and left ventricle form the **left cardiac border**. The short intrathoracic segment of the inferior vena cava can be seen directly above the diaphragm when the latter is completely depressed at full inspiration. The right ventricle lies behind the sternum and is "lost" in the cardiac silhouette, but for clarity it has been outlined in the diagram. The schematic diagram is illustrative only and may vary considerably with individual body type, respiratory phase, and degree of cardiac training (cardiac chamber enlargement) (see **A**).

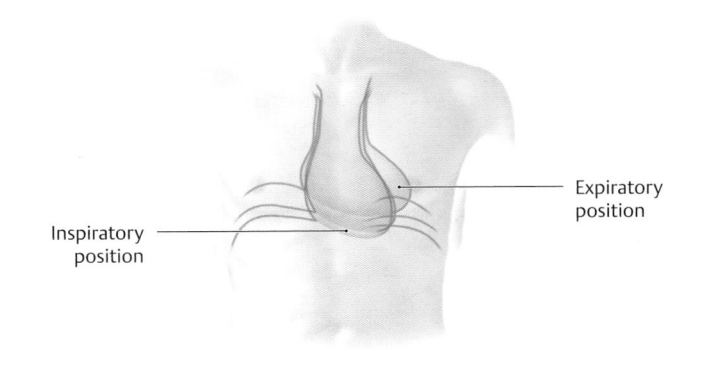

Expiratory position

Inspiratory position

C Respiratory changes in the cardiac borders

Owing to the strong fibrous attachment of the pericardium to the diaphragm, the heart must follow the respiratory movements of the diaphragm. When the diaphragm falls during inspiration, the heart descends as well (red). Since the heart has an oblique orientation in the chest, it appears to assume a more upright position and the cardiac silhouette becomes narrower. The heart also rotates slightly clockwise when viewed from above, displaying a greater portion of the left atrium (which, like the left ventricle, helps to form the cardiac border). During expiration (purple), the cardiac apex moves upward while the heart assumes a more horizontal orientation, broadening the cardiac borders.

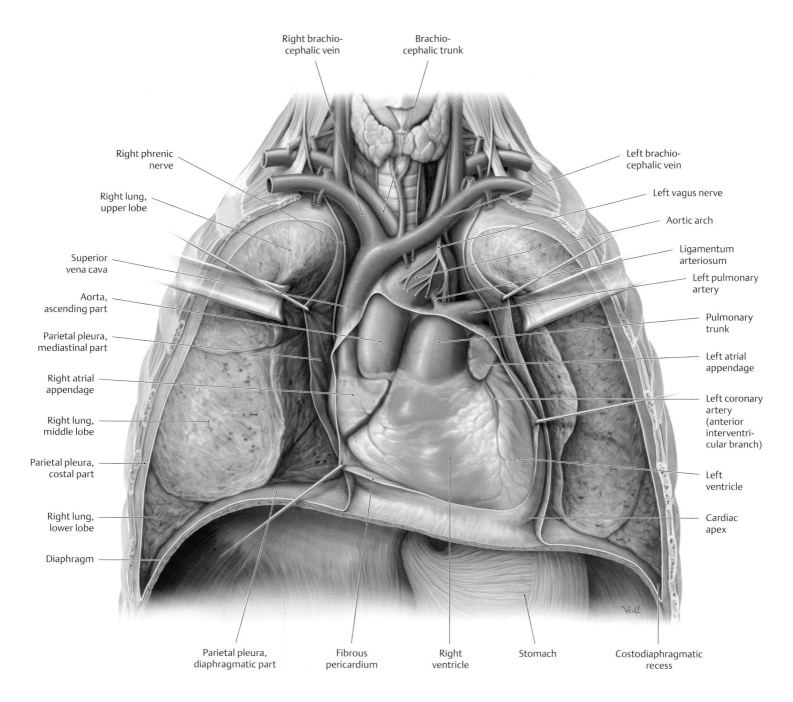

Right brachio-cephalic vein

Brachio-cephalic trunk

Right phrenic nerve

Right lung, upper lobe

Superior vena cava

Aorta, ascending part

Parietal pleura, mediastinal part

Right atrial appendage

Right lung, middle lobe

Parietal pleura, costal part

Right lung, lower lobe

Diaphragm

Left brachio-cephalic vein

Left vagus nerve

Aortic arch

Ligamentum arteriosum

Left pulmonary artery

Pulmonary trunk

Left atrial appendage

Left coronary artery (anterior interventricular branch)

Left ventricle

Cardiac apex

Parietal pleura, diaphragmatic part

Fibrous pericardium

Right ventricle

Stomach

Costodiaphragmatic recess

D The heart in situ, anterior view

Simplified illustration. The chest has been widely opened, and the pleural cavities and fibrous pericardium have been cut open. The connective tissue has been removed from the anterior mediastinum to display the heart. Although the pleural cavities have been opened, the lungs are not shown in a collapsed state. The heart lies within the pericardium, which is firmly attached to the diaphragm (see **C**) but is mobile in relation to the parietal pleura. A longitudinal axis drawn from the base to the apex of the heart demonstrates that this "long axis" is directed forward and downward from right to left. Thus the heart, when viewed from the front, has an oblique orientation and is tilted counterclockwise within the chest. Along this axis it appears slightly "rolled" in a posterior direction. Thus the right ventricle faces forward, as pictured here,

while the left ventricle is only partly visible. As a result, all of the great vessels cannot be seen even when the base of the heart is viewed from the front. The short pulmonary veins are covered by the cardiac silhouette because they terminate at the left atrium, which is directed posteriorly. It is easy to identify the right and left atrial appendages, which partially define the right and left cardiac borders on radiographs. The cardiac apex points downward and to the left. Most of it is still covered by pericardium in this dissection. Its movement, called the apical beat, is palpable as a fine motion in the fifth intercostal space on the left midclavicular line (see p. 109). The thin serous membrane of the epicardium (see p. 67) gives the surface of the heart a shiny appearance. Under this membrane are clusters of fatty tissue in which the coronary vessels are embedded.

2.15 Heart: Lateral and Superior Views

A Topographical relations

Left lateral view (stomach not to scale). The heart, enclosed in its pericardium, rests broadly on the diaphragm in the middle mediastinum and extends almost to the posterior surface of the sternum. The base of the heart, which is occupied by the roots of the great vessels, is directed superiorly, posteriorly, and slightly to the right due to the orientation of the cardiac axis (see p. 96). The left atrium in particular is very closely related to the esophagus. As a result, atrial enlargement due to heart disease (e.g., a congenital defect of the left atrioventricular valve, see p. 106) may cause extrinsic narrowing of the esophagus.

The close proximity of the heart and esophagus forms the basis for esophageal electrocardiography, in which the electrical activity of the heart is recorded with a probe passed down the esophagus (a sensitive procedure that can detect even very subtle abnormalities of electrical heart activity). The esophagus also provides access for transesophageal echocardiography.

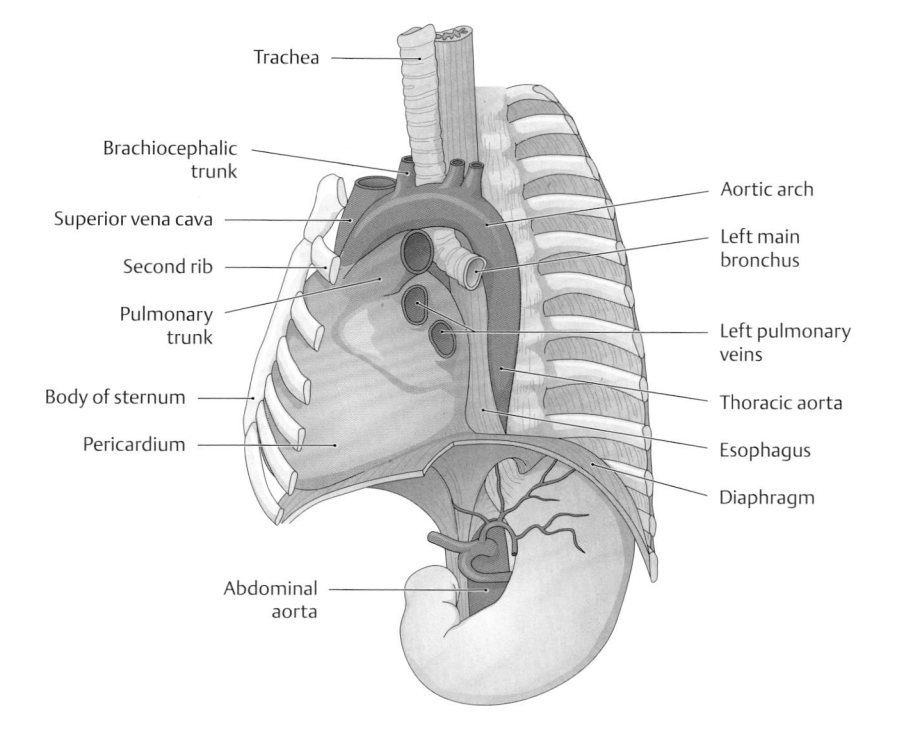

B Radiographic appearance of the heart: lateral view

The diaphragm leaflets and lungs are faintly visible in this left lateral view. The radiograph and correlative drawing clearly show how narrow the anterior mediastinum is when compared with the relatively broad

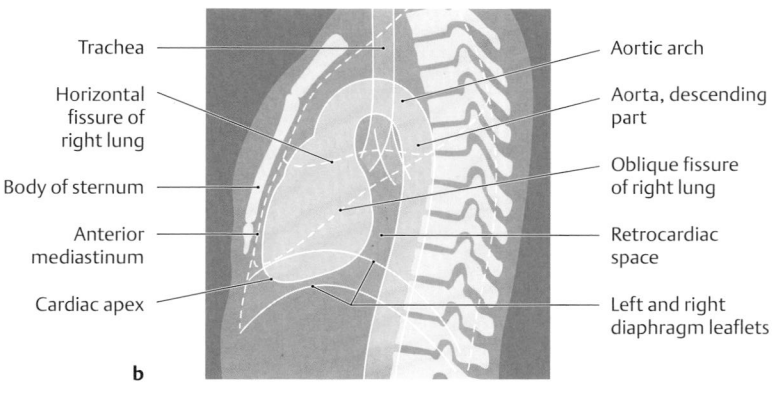

retrocardiac (Holzknecht) space, which is traversed by the esophagus (not shown here) and several neurovascular structures (see **D**). The aortic arch forms a sling over the left main bronchus.

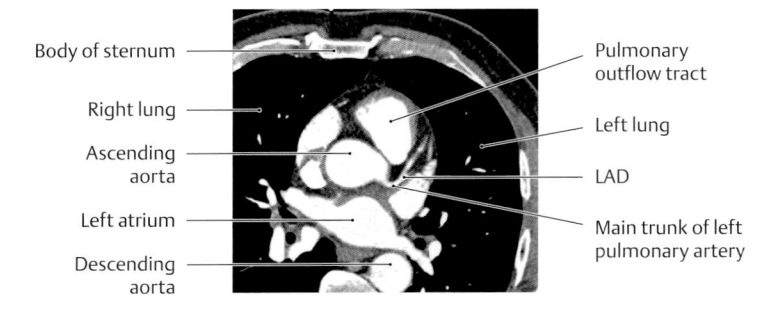

C Appearance of the heart on MRI

Magnetic resonance image of the normal thorax. The cardiac chambers are clearly displayed because of their fluid content, while the lungs are not visualized. The axial MRI slice is viewed from below, so the right side of the image corresponds to the anatomical left side. Blood-filled cardiac chambers and adjacent vascular segments appear white in the image. LAD = left anterior descending coronary artery.

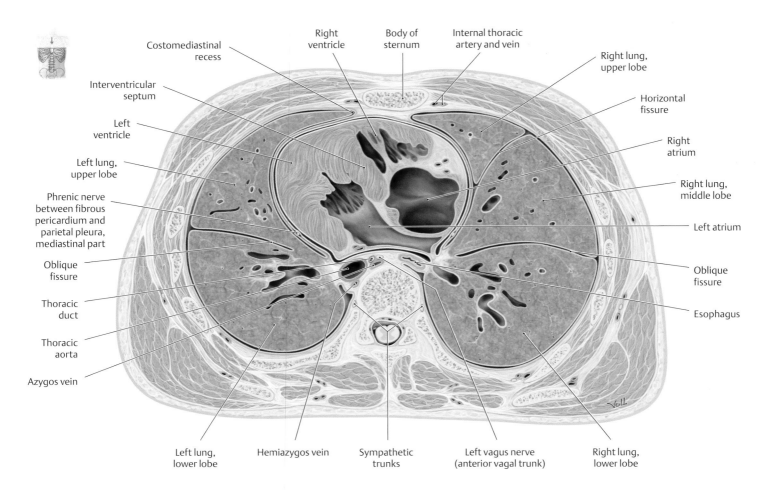

Costomediastinal recess — Right ventricle — Body of sternum — Internal thoracic artery and vein — Right lung, upper lobe

Interventricular septum — Horizontal fissure

Left ventricle — Right atrium

Left lung, upper lobe — Right lung, middle lobe

Phrenic nerve between fibrous pericardium and parietal pleura, mediastinal part — Left atrium

Oblique fissure — Oblique fissure

Thoracic duct — Esophagus

Thoracic aorta

Azygos vein

Left lung, lower lobe — Hemiazygos vein — Sympathetic trunks — Left vagus nerve (anterior vagal trunk) — Right lung, lower lobe

D The heart in situ, superior view

Transverse section through the thorax at the level of T 8 vertebra. Viewing the transverse section from above demonstrates the asymmetrical position of the heart in the middle mediastinum and its slight degree of physiologic counterclockwise rotation: the left ventricle faces downward and to the left, while the right ventricle faces forward and to the right. The right ventricle thus lies almost directly behind the posterior wall of the sternum (with only the narrow anterior mediastinum intervening, see **B**). The left atrium is in very close relationship to the esophagus. The costomediastinal recess is interposed between the

heart and *sternum* on the right and left sides (see **E**). A relatively small space is available between the heart and *vertebral column* for the passage of neurovascular structures and organs: thoracic aorta, esophagus, thoracic duct, azygos and hemiazygos veins, and portions of the autonomic nervous system. Each lung bears an indentation from the heart called the cardiac impression. This impression is larger in the left lung than in the right lung because of the heart's asymmetric position. The potential spaces between the pleural layers and the serous portions of the pericardium are considerably smaller than pictured here.

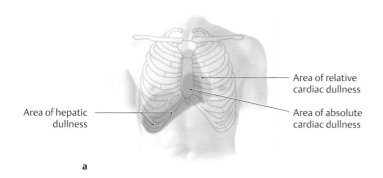

Area of hepatic dullness — Area of relative cardiac dullness — Area of absolute cardiac dullness

a

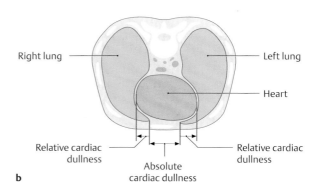

Right lung — Left lung

Heart

Relative cardiac dullness — Relative cardiac dullness

Absolute cardiac dullness

b

E Cardiac dullness on percussion of the chest

Anterior view (**a**) and transverse section viewed from above (**b**). In contrast to the sonorous sound that is produced by the percussion of *air-filled* lung (see p. 78), the *fluid-filled* heart produces a flat sound on percussion known as *cardiac dullness*. The dullness may be *absolute* (at sites where there is no lung tissue to moderate cardiac dullness) or *relative* (at sites where lung tissue overlies the heart and adds resonance to the percussion sound). Accordingly, the area of absolute cardiac dullness

is located between the chest wall and heart while the area of relative cardiac dullness is located over the right and left costomediastinal recesses, which contain small expansions of lung tissue (see **b**).

Note: Cardiac dullness gives way to hepatic dullness in the epigastrium and right hypochondriac region due to the anatomical extent of the liver (see **a**). The boundaries of the heart can be roughly estimated from the area of cardiac dullness because the sound characteristics at the cardiac borders contrast with the more resonant lung sounds.

2.16 Heart: Shape and Structure

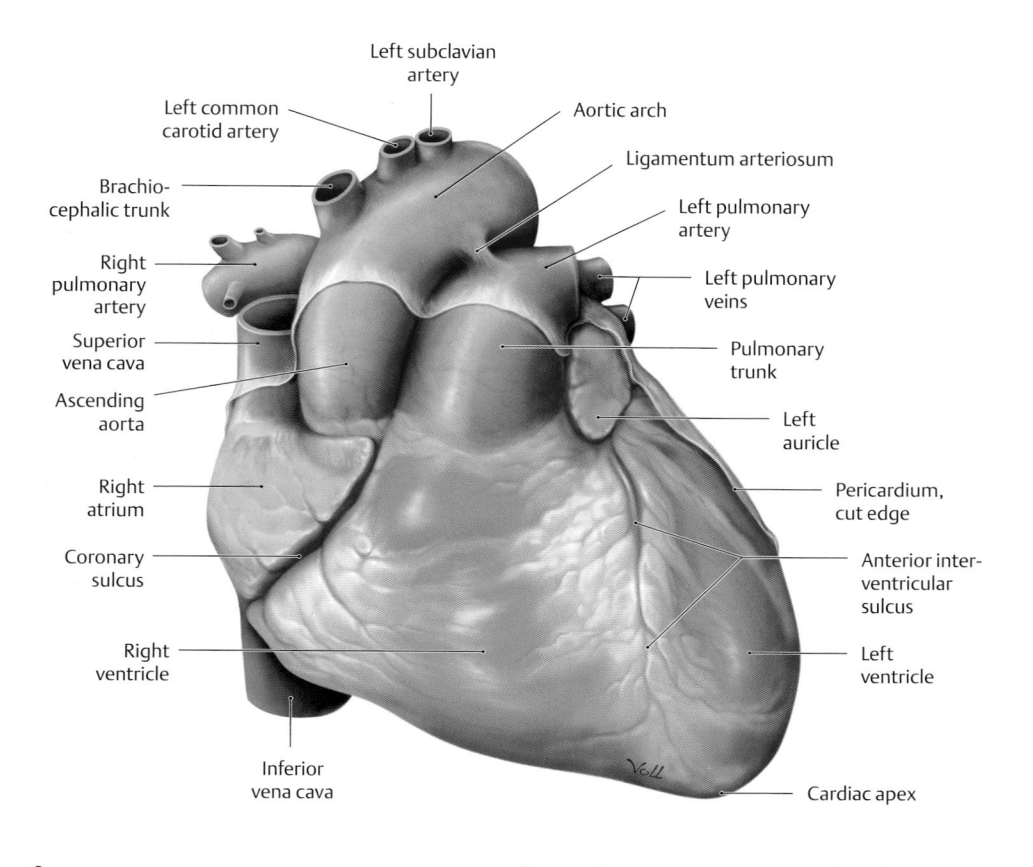

Left subclavian artery

Left common carotid artery

Aortic arch

Brachio-cephalic trunk

Ligamentum arteriosum

Right pulmonary artery

Left pulmonary artery

Superior vena cava

Left pulmonary veins

Ascending aorta

Pulmonary trunk

Right atrium

Left auricle

Coronary sulcus

Pericardium, cut edge

Right ventricle

Anterior inter-ventricular sulcus

Inferior vena cava

Left ventricle

Cardiac apex

A Heart, sternocostal surface
Anterior view. The heart is a muscular hollow organ shaped approximately like a flattened cone. It consists topographically of a base, apex, and three surfaces:

- The base of the heart, which is occupied by entering and emerging vessels, is directed superiorly, posteriorly, and to the right.
- The apex is directed inferiorly, anteriorly, and to the left.
- The surfaces are described as anterior (sternocostal), posterior, and inferior (diaphragmatic) (see **B**).

The sternocostal surface of the heart is formed chiefly by the right ventricle, whose boundary with the left ventricle is marked by the anterior interventricular sulcus. The left ventricle (occupying the inferior and posterior cardiac surfaces) forms the left border and apex of the

heart. The *anterior interventricular sulcus* contains the anterior interventricular branch of the left coronary artery (see p. 124) and the anterior interventricular (great cardiac) vein. Both vessels are embedded in fat and almost completely occupy the groove, so that the anterior surface of the heart appears nearly smooth. The left and right atria are separated from the ventricles by the *coronary sulcus*, which also transmits coronary vessels (the intrinsic vessels of the heart, see pp. 124–127). The right atrial appendage lies at the root of the ascending aorta, the left atrial appendage at the root of the pulmonary trunk. The origin of the right pulmonary artery from the pulmonary trunk is hidden by the ascending aorta. For clarity, all three illustrations in this series (**A, C, D**) show sites where the visceral layer of the pericardium is reflected to form the parietal layer. The pericardium extends onto the roots of the great arteries.

B Surfaces of the heart

Surface	Orientation	Cardiac chambers that form the surface (with vessels)
Anterior (sternocostal) surface	Directed anteriorly toward the posterior surface of the sternum and the ribs	• Right atrium with right atrial appendage • Right ventricle • Small part of left ventricle with cardiac apex • Left atrial appendage • Ascending aorta, superior vena cava, pulmonary trunk
Posterior surface	Directed posteriorly toward the posterior mediastinum	• Left atrium with termination of four pulmonary veins • Left ventricle • Part of right atrium with termination of superior and inferior venae cavae
Inferior (diaphragmatic) surface (clinically: the posterior wall)	Directed inferiorly toward the diaphragm	• Left ventricle with cardiac apex • Right ventricle • Part of right atrium with termination of inferior vena cava

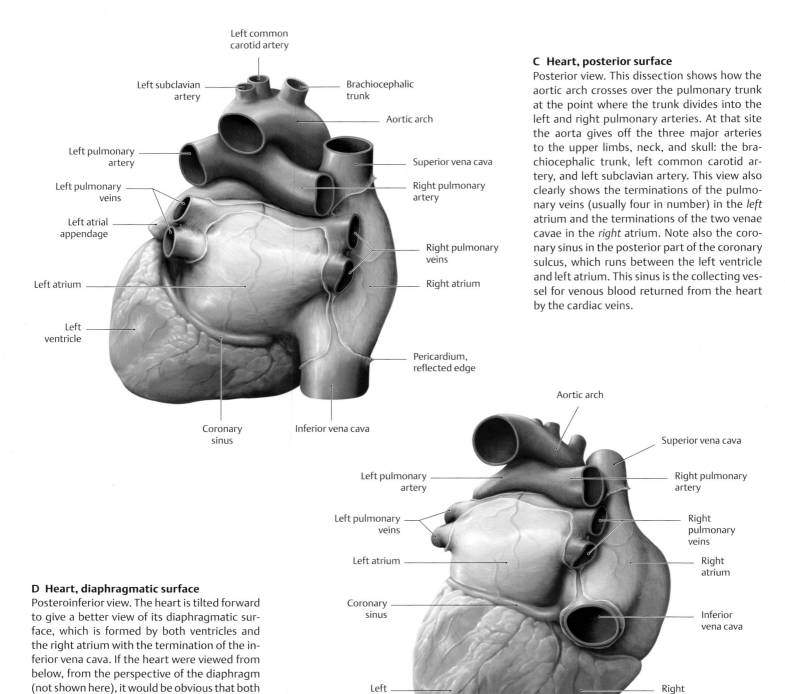

Left common carotid artery

Left subclavian artery

Brachiocephalic trunk

Aortic arch

Left pulmonary artery

Superior vena cava

Left pulmonary veins

Right pulmonary artery

Left atrial appendage

Right pulmonary veins

Left atrium

Right atrium

Left ventricle

Pericardium, reflected edge

Coronary sinus

Inferior vena cava

Aortic arch

Superior vena cava

Left pulmonary artery

Right pulmonary artery

Left pulmonary veins

Right pulmonary veins

Left atrium

Right atrium

Coronary sinus

Inferior vena cava

Left ventricle

Right ventricle

Posterior interventricular sulcus

Cardiac apex

C Heart, posterior surface

Posterior view. This dissection shows how the aortic arch crosses over the pulmonary trunk at the point where the trunk divides into the left and right pulmonary arteries. At that site the aorta gives off the three major arteries to the upper limbs, neck, and skull: the brachiocephalic trunk, left common carotid artery, and left subclavian artery. This view also clearly shows the terminations of the pulmonary veins (usually four in number) in the *left* atrium and the terminations of the two venae cavae in the *right* atrium. Note also the coronary sinus in the posterior part of the coronary sulcus, which runs between the left ventricle and left atrium. This sinus is the collecting vessel for venous blood returned from the heart by the cardiac veins.

D Heart, diaphragmatic surface

Posteroinferior view. The heart is tilted forward to give a better view of its diaphragmatic surface, which is formed by both ventricles and the right atrium with the termination of the inferior vena cava. If the heart were viewed from below, from the perspective of the diaphragm (not shown here), it would be obvious that both venae cavae are in alignment: Looking into the inferior vena cava, one can see through the terminal part of the superior vena cava.

E Structure of the cardiac wall

Term	Location	Composition
Endocardium	Innermost layer, lines the cavities of the heart	Single layer of flat epithelium, continuous with vascular endothelium in blood vessels
Myocardium	Middle layer and thickest part of the heart wall; motor for the pumping action of the heart (see pp. 102, 103)	Complex arrangement of muscle fibers
Epicardium	Outermost layer of the heart wall; part of the pericardium (see p. 67), forming its visceral layer	Serous membrane

2.17 Heart:
Muscular Structure (Myocardium)

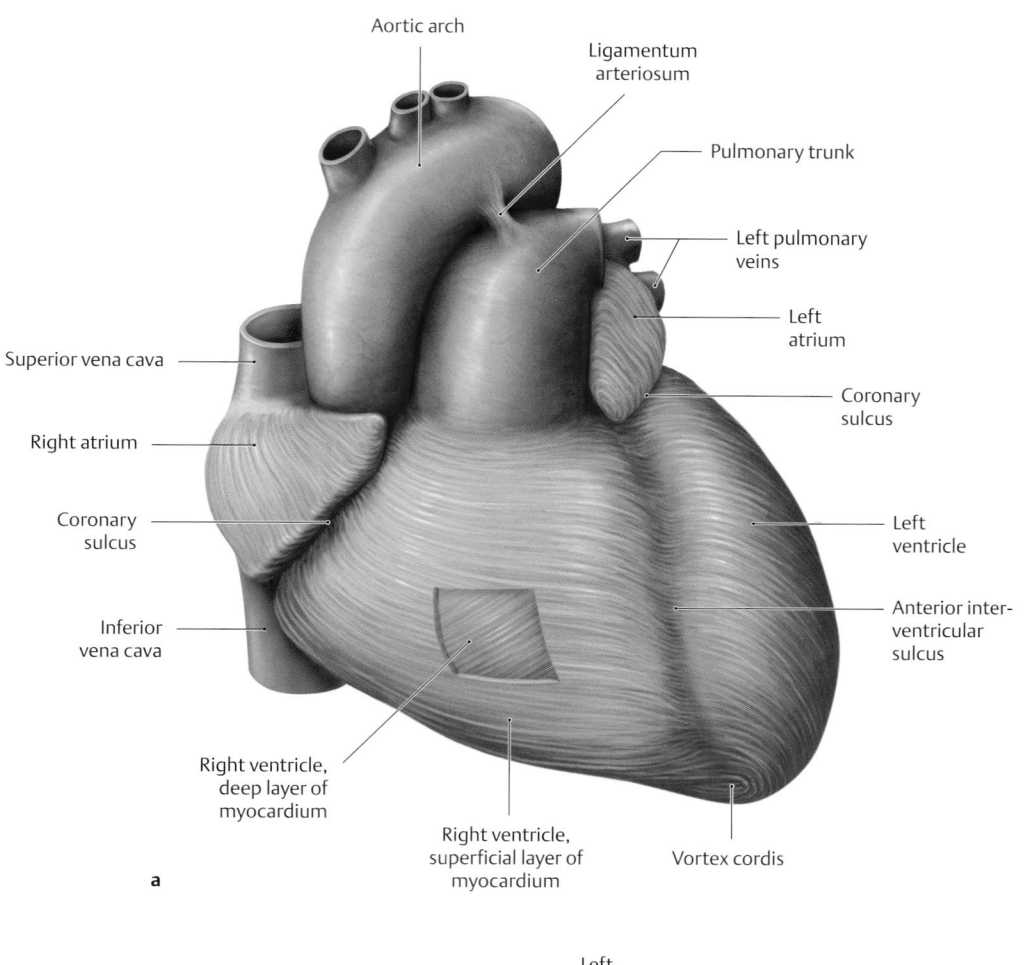

Aortic arch

Ligamentum arteriosum

Pulmonary trunk

Left pulmonary veins

Left atrium

Superior vena cava

Coronary sulcus

Right atrium

Coronary sulcus

Left ventricle

Inferior vena cava

Anterior interventricular sulcus

Right ventricle, deep layer of myocardium

Right ventricle, superficial layer of myocardium

Vortex cordis

a

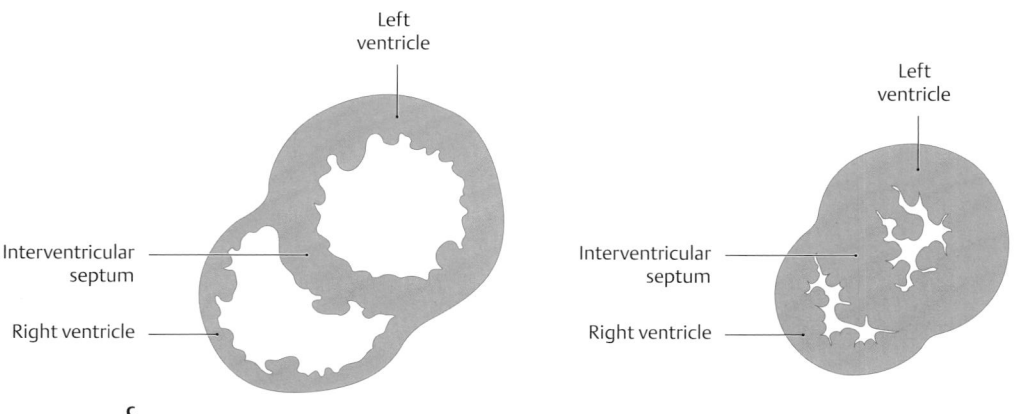

Left ventricle

Left ventricle

Interventricular septum

Interventricular septum

Right ventricle

Right ventricle

c

A Myocardial architecture

a, **b** External musculature of the heart, simplified anteroinferior view. The muscular walls of the right and left ventricles have been windowed to display the deeper fibers.

Note: The epicardium has been removed in **a** and **b** along with the subepicardial fat. The coronary vessels are not shown in order to display more clearly the cardiac surface grooves (anterior and posterior interventricular sulci).

The **musculature of the atria** is arranged in two layers, superficial and deep. The superficial layer (shown here) extends over the atria and is common to both, whereas each atrium has its own deep layer. Looped and annular muscle fibers extend down to the atrioventricular boundary and also encircle the venous orifices. The **ventricular musculature** has a complex arrangement, consisting basically of a superficial (subepicardial), middle, and deep (subendocardial) layer. The superficial layer joins apically with the deeper layers to form a whorled arrangement of muscle fibers around the cardiac apex (vortex cordis). The right ventricle, which is a lowpressure system (see **c**), is less muscular than the left and almost completely lacks a middle layer. The subendocardial layer forms the trabeculae carneae and papillary muscles (see **d** and p. 107).

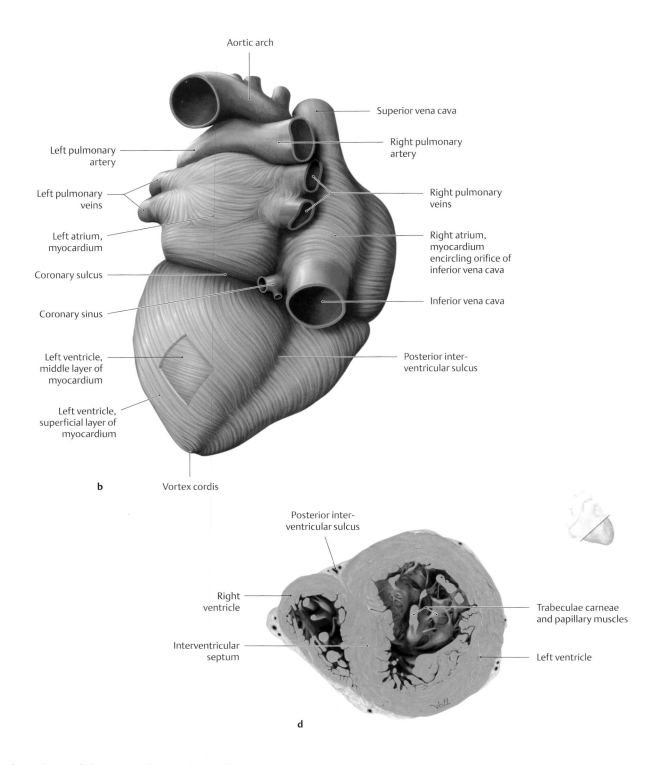

Aortic arch

Superior vena cava

Left pulmonary
artery

Right pulmonary
artery

Left pulmonary
veins

Right pulmonary
veins

Left atrium,
myocardium

Right atrium,
myocardium
encircling orifice of
inferior vena cava

Coronary sulcus

Coronary sinus

Inferior vena cava

Left ventricle,
middle layer of
myocardium

Posterior inter-
ventricular sulcus

Left ventricle,
superficial layer of
myocardium

b Vortex cordis

Posterior inter-
ventricular sulcus

Right
ventricle

Trabeculae carneae
and papillary muscles

Interventricular
septum

Left ventricle

d

The histological unit of the myocardium is the cardiac myocyte, a specialized form of cardiac muscle cell. Unlike their electronically isolated counterparts in skeletal muscle, cardiac myocytes form a *syncytium* in which membrane depolarization and contraction spread in a wave.

c, d Myocardial cross-sections perpendicular to the long axis of the heart, viewed from above. **c** Schematic representation: The left heart is in an expanded state (diastole), the right heart in a contracted state (systole). **d** Transverse section through a specimen during diastole.

All the sections clearly demonstrate the difference in thickness between the left and right ventricular myocardia: The left ventricle is part of the high-pressure system, and therefore its myocardium must generate a significantly higher pressure (120–140 mmHg during ventricular contraction) than the right ventricle (approximately 25–30 mmHg). The difference in thickness is most pronounced during ventricular contraction (see **c**). Section **d** shows how the coronary vessels and subepicardial fat fill the sulci in the heart.

2.18 Heart: Atria and Ventricles

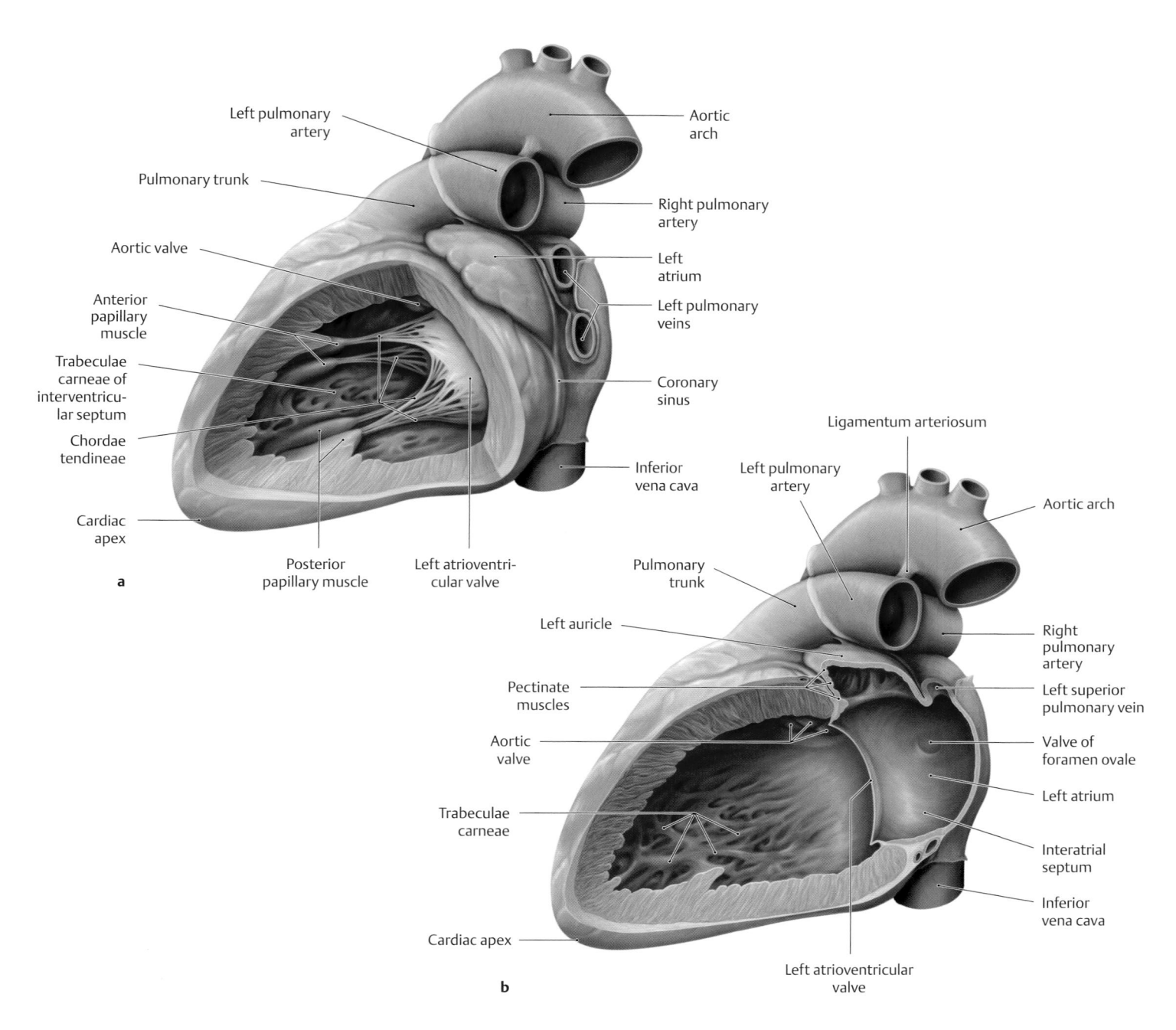

Left pulmonary artery

Pulmonary trunk

Aortic valve

Anterior papillary muscle

Trabeculae carneae of interventricular septum

Chordae tendineae

Cardiac apex

Posterior papillary muscle

Left atrioventricular valve

a

Aortic arch

Right pulmonary artery

Left atrium

Left pulmonary veins

Coronary sinus

Inferior vena cava

Ligamentum arteriosum

Left pulmonary artery

Aortic arch

Pulmonary trunk

Left auricle

Pectinate muscles

Aortic valve

Trabeculae carneae

Cardiac apex

Left atrioventricular valve

b

Right pulmonary artery

Left superior pulmonary vein

Valve of foramen ovale

Left atrium

Interatrial septum

Inferior vena cava

A Chambers of the left heart

Left lateral view. **a** Ventricle, **b** ventricle and atrium. The ventricular and atrial walls have been opened.

The **left atrium** is smaller than the right (see **Ba**). Its muscular wall is thin (low-pressure system) and is smooth in areas derived embryologically from the orifices of the pulmonary veins. The rest of the atrium is lined by pectinate muscles. The pulmonary veins, usually four in number, terminate in the left atrium. Occasionally a narrow tissue fold (valve of the foramen ovale) is found on the interatrial septum, formed by a protrusion of the fossa ovalis into the left atrium. It marks the site of fusion between the embryonic septum primum and septum secundum.

The **left ventricle** has an inflow tract and outflow tract. The *inflow tract* begins at the left atrioventricular orifice, which is guarded by the left atrioventricular valve (see p. 106). The muscular ridges of the trabec-

ulae carneae project into the lumen of the ventricular inflow tract. Specialized extensions of the trabeculae, the papillary muscles, are attached to the cusps of the left atrioventricular valve by collagenous cords, the chordae tendineae (see p. 106). The *outflow tract* of the left ventricle has smooth inner walls and lies close to the interventricular septum. It leads to the aorta and is capped by the aortic valve at the root of the ascending aorta (see p. 108). The interventricular septum consists largely of muscle tissue (muscular part), and only a small portion near the aorta consists entirely of connective tissue (membranous part). The placement of the interventricular septum between the cardiac chambers is marked externally by the anterior and posterior interventricular sulci on the cardiac surface. The muscular wall of the left ventricle is thick (high-pressure system), having approximately three times the thickness of the right ventricular wall (see **Bb**). The chambers of the left (and right) heart are lined by endocardium.

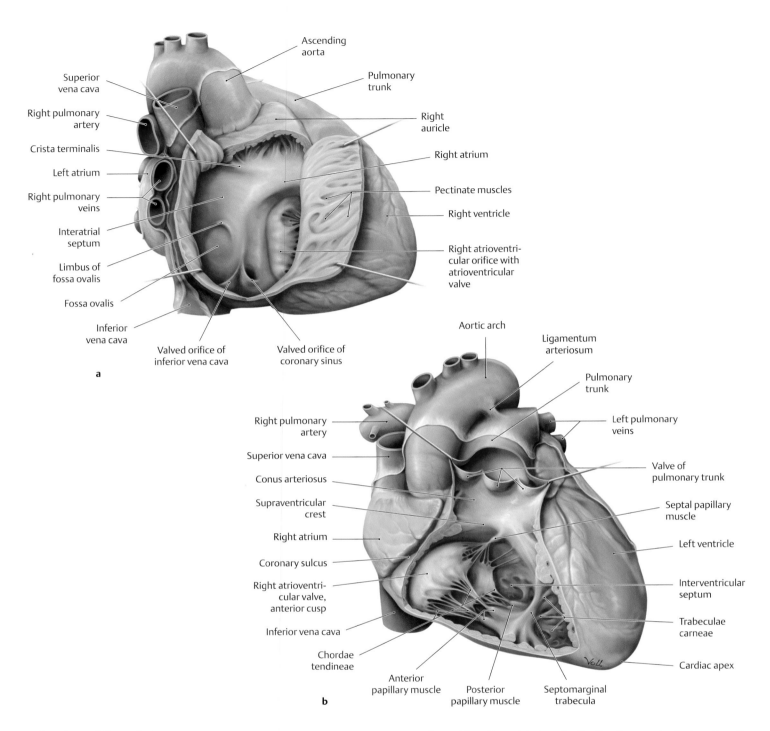

B Chambers of the right heart
a Right lateral view of the atrium. **b** Anterior view of the ventricle. The ventricular and atrial walls have been broadly opened, and the heart wall has been cut open to display the internal chambers.

The **right atrium** (see **a**) consists of a posterior and anterior segment. The *posterior* segment with the smooth-walled sinus venarum (not visible here) bears the orifices of the superior and inferior venae cavae. A small valve at the orifice of the inferior vena cava (valve of the inferior vena cava) directs blood in the *prenatal* circulation through the foramen ovale in the interatrial septum. Because the foramen ovale is sealed shut postnatally, becoming the fossa ovalis (surrounded by a rounded margin, the limbus), this valve atrophies after birth. The orifice of the coronary sinus also bears a small crescent-shaped valve (valve of the coronary sinus). The *anterior* segment, which comprises the actual atrium with the atrial appendage (auricle), is separated from the posterior segment by a ridge, the crista terminalis. Small muscular trabeculae, the pectinate muscles, arise from the crista terminalis, giving this segment an irregular wall texture. The wall of the right atrium is thin (low-pressure system).

The **right ventricle** is divided into two segments by two muscular ridges, the supraventricular crest and septomarginal trabecula: the inflow tract posteroinferiorly (with the heart positioned in situ) and the outflow tract anterosuperiorly (see also p. 113). As in the left ventricle, the wall of the right ventricular *inflow tract* is studded with trabeculae carneae, and papillary muscles are attached by chordae tendineae to the right atrioventricular valve. The *outflow tract* is cone-shaped and consists mainly of the conus arteriosus, which has a smooth wall. The right ventricular outflow tract expels blood into the pulmonary trunk, whose orifice is guarded by the pulmonary valve. The wall of the right ventricle is relatively thin (low-pressure system).

2.19 Heart: Overview of the Cardiac Valves; the Atrioventricular Valves

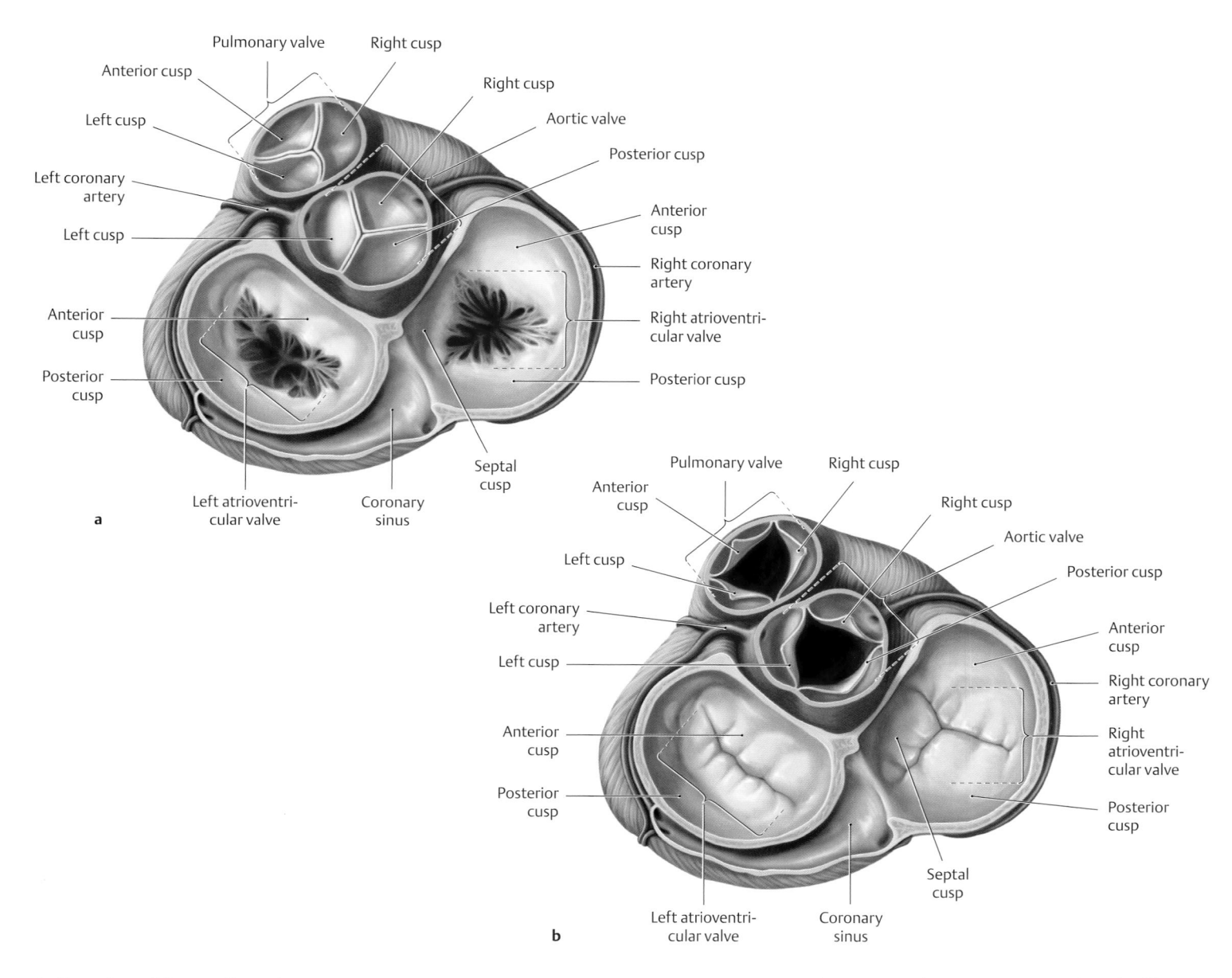

A Overview of the cardiac valves

Plane of the cardiac valves viewed from above. The atria have been removed, and the great arteries have been transected at their roots. The cardiac valves are classified into two types—atrioventricular and semilunar.

Atrioventricular valves. Located between the atria and ventricles, the left and right atrioventricular valves are composed of thin, avascular connective tissue covered by endocardium. They are classified mechanically as *sail valves* (see **B**) because the chordae tendoneae (see **B**) constrain the movement of each cusp like the teathering ropes on a sail. The function of these valves is to prevent the reflux of blood from the ventricles into the atria.

- The *left atrioventricular valve* has two cusps *(bicuspid valve):* an anterior cusp (anteromedial) and a posterior cusp (posterolateral). The anterior cusp is continuous with the wall of the aorta. The alternate term *mitral valve* is derived from the two major cusps, which are similar in shape to a bishop's miter. Subdivisions in the lateral margins of the otherwise smooth valve have led some anatomists to describe small accessory cusps called the commissural cusps (usually two). These

are not true cusps, however, and are not connected to the fibrous anulus of the cardiac skeleton (see **C**). The cusps are tethered by papillary muscles (see **B**).

- The *right atrioventricular valve* has three cusps *(tricuspid valve):* anterior, posterior, and septal. One or two small accessory cusps may also be found; they do not extend to the fibrous anulus.

Semilunar valves. These valves have three crescent-shaped cusps of approximately equal size placed at the orifices of the pulmonary trunk (pulmonary valve) and aorta (aortic valve). Like the atrioventricular valves, they are composed of thin connective tissue covered by endocardium. The semilunar valves are classified mechanically as *pocket valves* because their cusps pouch into the ventricle like bulging pockets. The wall of the aorta and pulmonary trunk show slight dilations just above the valve (the pulmonary and aortic sinuses). The aortic sinuses expand the cross-section of the aorta, forming the aortic bulb. The right and left coronary arteries branch off the base of the aorta just past the aortic valve (see pp. 124–127 for details). The drawings illustrate the function of the valves during ventricular diastole (relaxation) (**a**) and ventricular systole (contraction) (**b**).

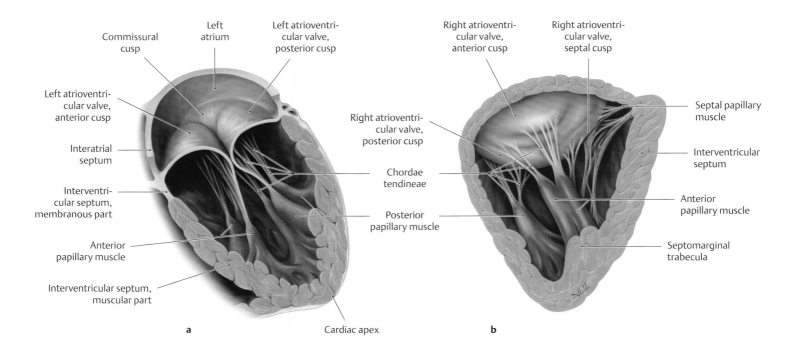

a   Cardiac apex   b

B Atrioventricular valves and papillary muscles

Anterior view of the left (**a**) and right (**b**) atrioventricular valves. The drawings represent a very early phase of ventricular contraction in which the atrioventricular valves have just closed. The papillary muscles are clearly displayed. There are *three* papillary muscles for the *three* cusps of the right atrioventricular valve (anterior, posterior, and septal papillary muscles) and *two* papillary muscles for the *two* cusps of the left atrioventricular valve (anterior and posterior papillary muscles). The papillary muscles (specialized extensions of the trabeculae carneae) are attached to the free margins of the valve cusps by tendinous cords (the chordae tendineae). When the papillary muscles contract (valve clo-

sure), the chordae tendineae are shortened to restrict the motion of the valve cusps. This keep the cusps from opening into the atria during ventricular contraction (systole), thereby preventing the regurgitation of blood back into the atria.

Note: Like other myocardial regions, the myocardium of the papillary muscles may suffer necrosis due to a myocardial infarction, leaving the corresponding cusp prone to prolapse into the atrium. Conversely, pathological shortening of the chordae may also prevent the valve from closing completely. This also would allow blood to regurgitate into the atrium during ventricular systole, producing an audible heart murmur (see p. 113).

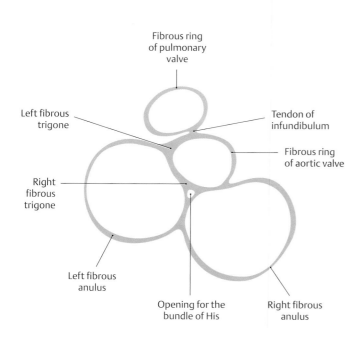

C Skeleton of the heart

Valve plane viewed from above. The skeleton of the heart is a layer of connective tissue (often with considerable fat) that completely separates the myocardium from the cardiac ventricles and atria. The components of the cardiac skeleton in a *narrow sense* are as follows:

- The right and left fibrous anuli and intervening fibrous trigones
- The fibrous ring of the aortic valve, which is connected to both fibrous anuli
- The membranous part of the interventricular septum (not shown here)

In a *broad sense*, the fibrous ring of the pulmonary valve also contributes to the cardiac skeleton. It is connected by a collagenous band (tendon of infundibulum) to the fibrous ring of the aortic valve. The atrioventricular valves are anchored to the fibrous anuli, while the semilunar valves are each attached by connective tissue to their valvular fibrous rings. Thus, the cardiac skeleton in the broad sense provides a mechanical framework for all the cardiac valves. Besides *mechanically stabilizing* the heart, the fibrous skeleton also functions as an *electrical insulator* between the atria and ventricles. The electrical impulses that stimulate cardiac contractions (see pp. 110 and 111) can pass from the atrium to the ventricles only through the bundle of His, and there is only one opening in the fibrous skeleton (in the right fibrous trigone) which transmits that bundle.

107

2.20 Heart: Semilunar Valves and Sites for Auscultating the Cardiac Valves

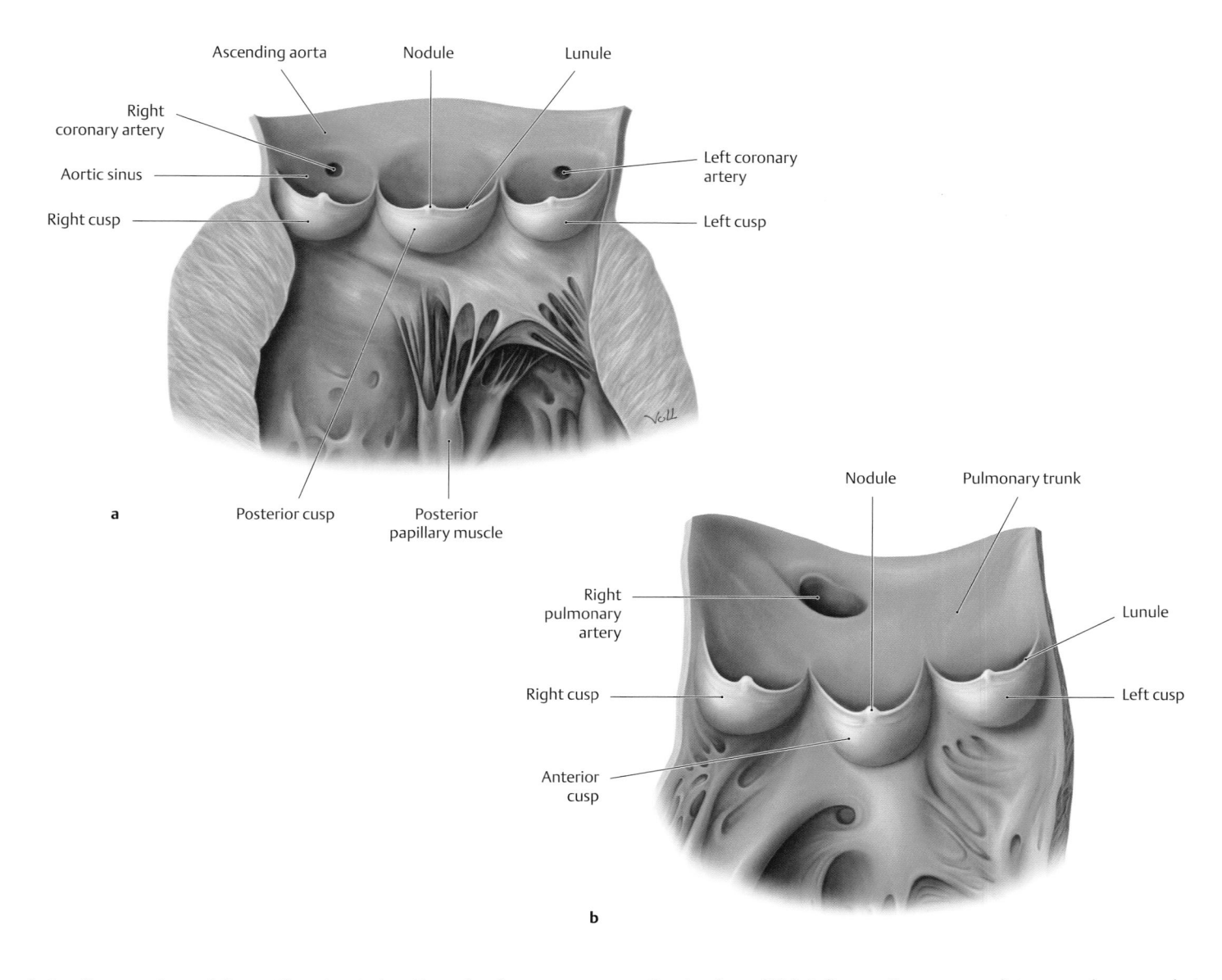

A Semilunar valves of the outflow tracts (aortic and pulmonary valve)

The aortic valve (**a**) and pulmonary valve (**b**) have been displayed by cutting open the ascending aorta and pulmonary trunk and opening them up like a book. The aortic valve and pulmonary valve close the ventricular outflow tracts during diastole:

- The aortic valve closes the left ventricular outflow tract.
- The pulmonary valve closes the right ventricular outflow tract.

These valves almost completely prevent the regurgitation of blood expelled by the ventricles. The origins of the left and right coronary arteries can be clearly identified in the aortic sinuses past the semilunar cusps (**a**), and the origin of the right pulmonary artery can be identified in the pulmonary trunk (**b**). The free margin of each semilunar cusp is thickened centrally to form a valvular nodule, and on each side of the nodule is a fine rim called the lunule. The nodule and lunule ensure that the margins of the cusps appose tightly and completely during valve closure. Both the atrioventricular valves (see p. 106) and the semilunar valves may undergo pathological changes, usually due to inflamma-

tion (endocarditis). Inflammation may result in secondary vascularization of the initially avascular valves, causing them to undergo fibrotic changes that stiffen the valves and compromise their function. There are two main abnormalities of valvular mechanics, which may coexist in the same valve:

- Valvular stenosis: *Opening* of the valve is impaired, causing a reduction of blood flow across the valve. Usually this creates a pressure overload on the chamber proximal to the obstruction.
- Valvular insufficiency: *Closure* of the valve is impaired, allowing blood to regurgitate into the chamber proximal to the valve. Such a pathological reflux creates a volume overload on the affected cardiac segments. When the load exceeds a certain magnitude, surgical replacement of the valve may be necessary to prevent further damage to the heart.
- Stenosis and insufficiency may coexist: A valve may become stuck in an intermediate position, unable to open or close completely.

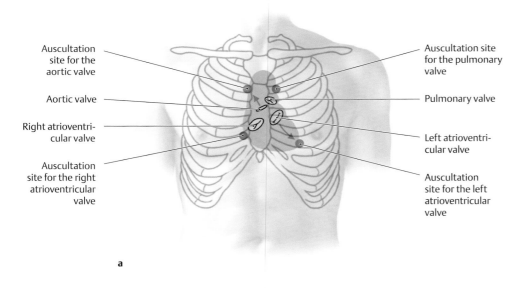

a

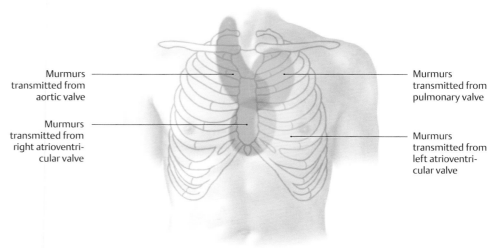

b

B Auscultation of the cardiac valves

In the healthy heart, blood does not generate a perceptible sound as it flows across the cardiac valves. But if the valves are functionally impaired as a result of disease (stenosis, insufficiency), the blood flow at the cardiac valves becomes turbulent. This type of flow produces audible sounds that are transmitted via the bloodstream. In most cases these sounds (murmurs) are not heard best over the anatomical projections of the valves on the chest wall (due to sound muffling by the thick cardiac wall), but are heard more clearly at sites located downstream from the valves (see **C**).

Diagram **a** shows the anatomical projections of the valves on the chest wall in relation to the sites where the valves are auscultated, and **b** shows the areas over which transmitted valvular murmurs can be auscultated on physical examination. The auscultation sites are located approximately at the center of the areas for auscultating transmitted valvular murmurs. Table **C** compares the anatomical projections of the valves with their auscultation sites.

Note: As a result of sound transmission, the aortic valve, while part of the *left* heart, is auscultated on the *right* side of the chest. The pulmonary valve, while part of the right heart, is auscultated on the *left* side. Normal heart sounds are described on p. 112.

C Anatomical projections and auscultation sites of the cardiac valves

Valve	Anatomical projection	Auscultation site
Left atrioventricular valve	Fourth / fifth costal cartilage on the left side	Fifth intercostal space on the midclavicular line
Right atrioventricular valve	Sternum at the level of the fifth costal cartilage	Right fifth intercostal space close to the sternum
Aortic valve	Left sternal border at the level of the third rib	Right second intercostal space close to the sternum
Pulmonary valve	Left sternal border at the level of the third costal cartilage	Left second intercostal space close to the sternum

2.21 Heart: Impulse Formation and Conduction System

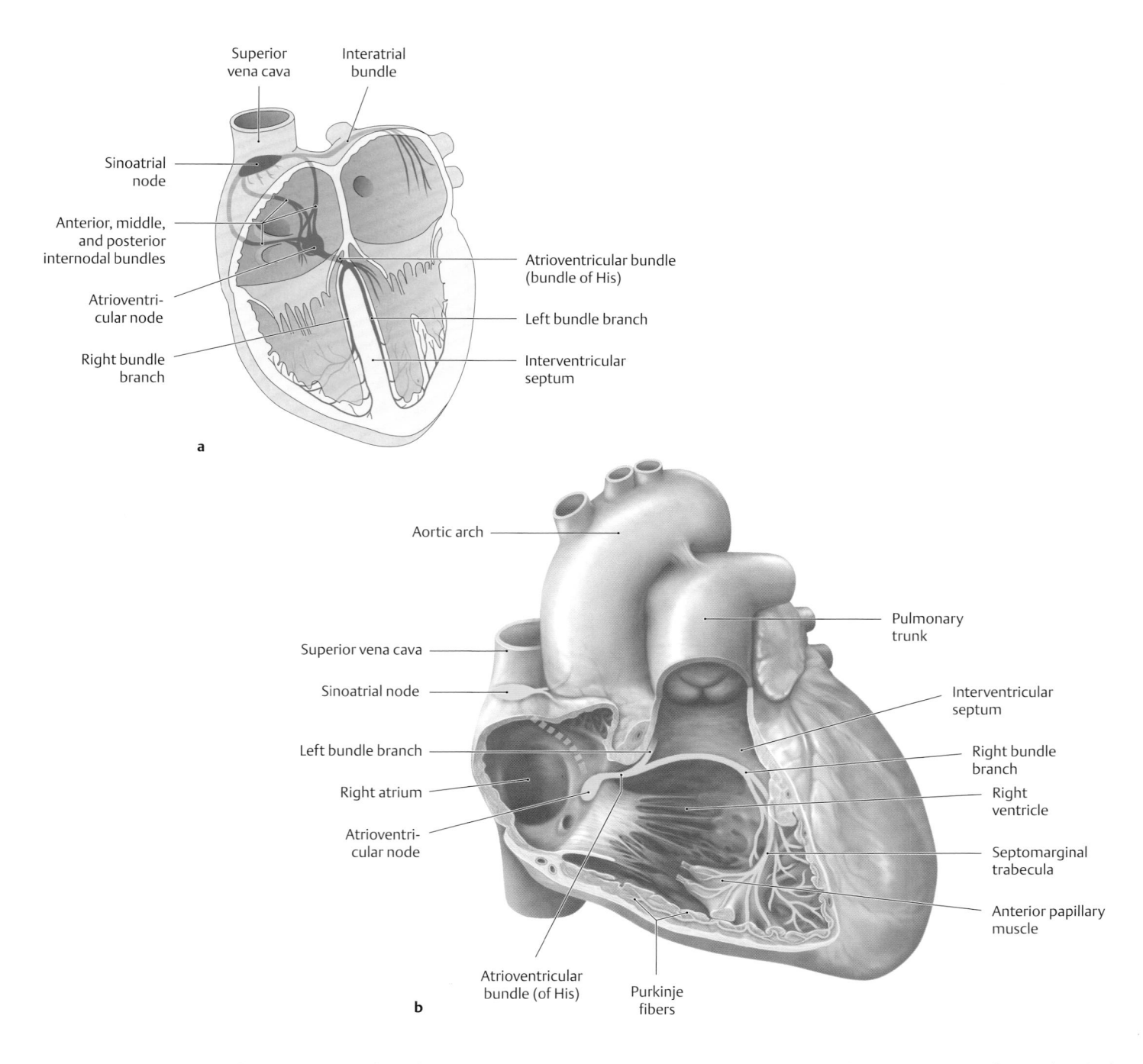

a

b

A Overview of cardiac impulse formation and conduction

Anterior view (**a**), right lateral view (**b**), left lateral view (**c**).

Even when the extrinsic nervous control of the heart is completely disrupted, it continues to beat. When supplied with oxygen and nutrients, it can even keep beating after it has been removed from the chest. This is made possible by an intrinsic, independent system that generates and conducts excitatory impulses in the heart. This system consists of specialized myocardial cells and has four main parts:

- Sinoatrial node (SA node, sinus node)
- Atrioventricular node (AV node)
- Atrioventricular bundle (AV bundle, bundle of His)
- Right and left bundle branches

SA node (the "pacemaker" of the heart, approximately 1 cm long). The cardiac impulse begins in the SA node, a subepicardial node located on the posterior side of the right atrium near the orifice of the superior vena cava. The SA node generates salvos of impulses which stimulate the atrial myocardium at a resting rate of 60–70 beats / min. The atrial impulses spread rapidly toward the ventricles (particularly in the crista terminalis and internodal bundles between the SA and AV nodes, as shown by electrophysiologic studies). The impulses travel from the AV node to the bundle of His, which distributes branches to the ventricular myocardium. (Direct impulse conduction from the atrium to the ventricles is normally prevented by the insulating effect of the fibrous skeleton.)

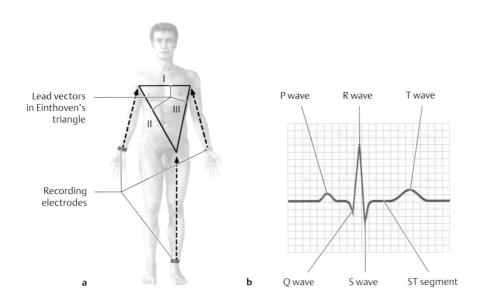

B Recording the electrical activity of the heart

The cardiac impulse that travels across the heart can be detected with electrodes and recorded over time as an electrocardiogram (ECG).

a ECG using three electrodes that separately record electrical heart activity along three axes or "vectors" (Einthoven limb leads).

b Tracing illustrates the ECG components of one cardiac cycle (one "heartbeat"). The cycle consists of a definite sequence of waves, segments, and intervals. The shape of the tracing is useful in determining whether the conduction of the cardiac impulse is normal or abnormal (e.g., due to myocardial infarction).

A standard ECG examination includes additional leads (Goldberger, Wilson).

Lead vectors in Einthoven's triangle

Recording electrodes

a

P wave   R wave   T wave

Q wave   S wave   ST segment

b

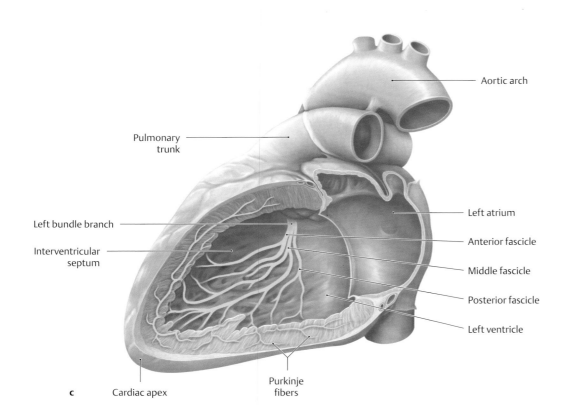

Aortic arch

Pulmonary trunk

Left atrium

Left bundle branch

Anterior fascicle

Interventricular septum

Middle fascicle

Posterior fascicle

Left ventricle

Purkinje fibers

c   Cardiac apex

AV node (approximately 5 mm long): located in the interatrial septum near the orifice of the coronary sinus. This node delays impulse conduction to the ventricles, allowing both atria to depolarize before ventricular contraction begins. It can also generate impulses spontaneously, but at a considerably lower rate than the SA node (approximately 40–50 depolarizations / min). Because of its slower rate, the AV node cannot act as a pacemaker for the heart when the SA node is intact.

Atrioventricular bundle (of His) (approximately 2 cm long). The atrioventricular bundle (of His) is subendocardial while still in the atrium. It then passes through the right fibrous trigone (see p. 107) to enter the ventricular septum, where it divides (in the membranous part of the septum) into the right and left bundle branches. The AV bundle conducts impulses from the AV node to the ventricles.

Left bundle branch: branches to the left from the bundle of His and divides into three main fascicles (anterior, middle, and posterior).

Right bundle branch: initially continues in the ventricular septum toward the cardiac apex and is then distributed to the ventricular wall. The main trunk of the right bundle branch enters the septomarginal trabecula, known also as the "moderator band." Finally the impulse is distributed throughout the ventricular myocardium by the Purkinje fibers.

Note: The Purkinje fibers stimulate the ventricular walls in a retrograde direction, proceeding from the cardiac apex toward the atria. Thus the apical myocardium contracts first, pulling the apex of the heart toward the plane of the valves. The papillary muscles, which are stimulated by direct fibers from the bundle branches, contract before the ventricular walls to ensure that the AV valves remain closed during ventricular systole.

111

2.22 Mechanical Action of the Heart

Phases of the heartbeat

The heartbeat consists of two main phases: contraction (systole) and relaxation (diastole). A total of four phases are distinguished in the contraction and expansion of the ventricles:

Ventricular systole:

- Isovolumetric contraction phase: The ventricular myocardium contracts and tightens around the blood column within the ventricle. All valves are closed, i.e., the AV valves are *already* closed (ventricular pressure exceeds the atrial pressure), and the aortic and pulmonary valves are *still* closed (ventricular pressure is still lower than the intra-arterial pressure). Isovolumetric contraction of the myocardium around the blood column produces a mechanical vibration that is audible as the first heart sound.
- Ejection phase: The AV valves remain closed and prevent the reflux of ventricular blood into the atria. As the intraventricular pressure exceeds the pressure in the arteries, the aortic and pulmonary valves open, and blood flows into the aorta and pulmonary trunk.

Ventricular diastole:

- Relaxation phase: The ventricular myocardium relaxes. All valves are closed during this phase: The AV valves are *still* closed, and the aortic and pulmonary valves are *already* closed (to prevent the reflux of ejected blood back into the ventricles). Closure of the aortic and pulmonary valves ("slamming doors") is audible as the second heart sound. Occasionally the arterial valves close at slightly different times, producing a divided second heart sound.
- Filling phase: The intraventricular pressure is very low, and the arterial valves remain closed. The AV valves open, and blood flows into the ventricles. Ventricular filling results more from the movement of the valve plane than from atrial contraction: The valve plane moves toward the cardiac apex during systole, and it returns very quickly to its initial position during diastole, "throwing itself" over the blood column.

Note: During both the isovolumetric contraction phase and the relaxation phase, there are periods in which all the valves are closed. By contrast, there is no point in the cardiac cycle when all valves are open!

Heart sounds are normal acoustical phenomena produced by the heart. Abnormal valvular heart sounds (murmurs) are described on p. 109. Although the first heart sound is generated by ventricular contraction itself, that first sound is clinically associated with closure of the atrioventricular valves.

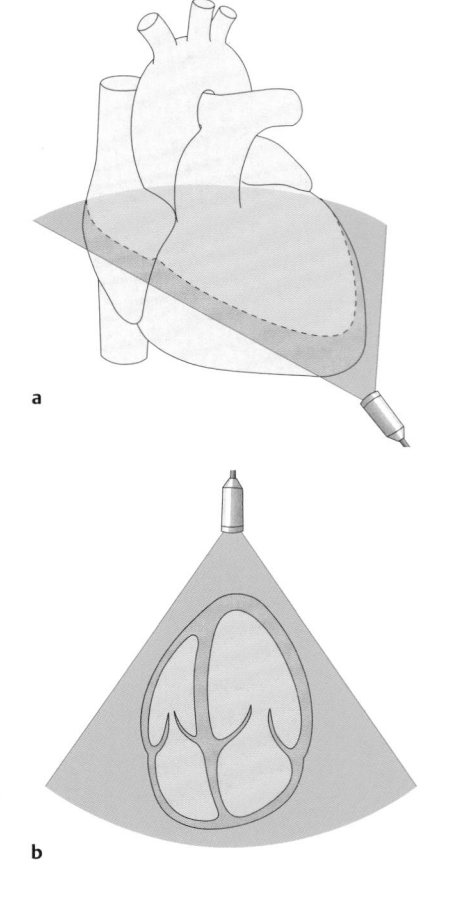

a

b

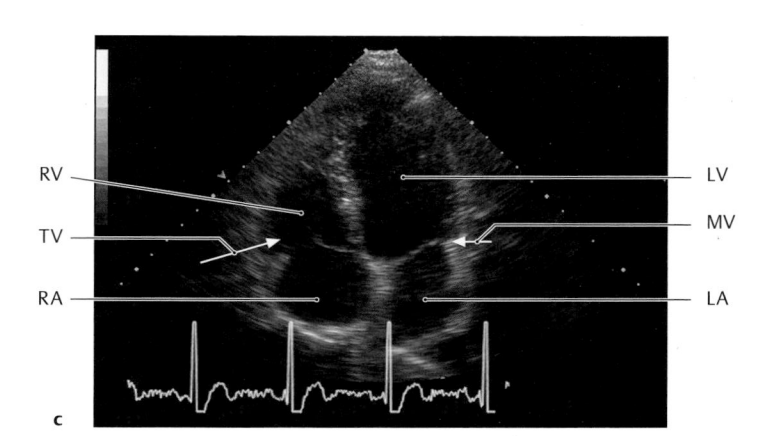

RV — LV
TV — MV
RA — LA

c

A Ultrasound imaging of the heart (after Flachskampf)

The "four-chamber view."

a Placement of the ultrasound probe relative to the heart. **b** Position of the heart in the ultrasound beam. **c** Ultrasound image of the heart. The probe is angled from the cardiac apex to the right ventricle, directing the main beam along the approximate anatomical axis of the heart. Scanning in this plane demonstrates all four chambers of the heart (the ventricles are displayed above the atria). The left cardiac chambers appear on the right side of the image, the right chambers on the left side. The left and right atrioventricular valves, the interventricular septum, and the interatrial septum are clearly visualized. The size of the heart, the shape of the individual chambers, and the shape and function of the valves can be accurately evaluated with ultrasound.

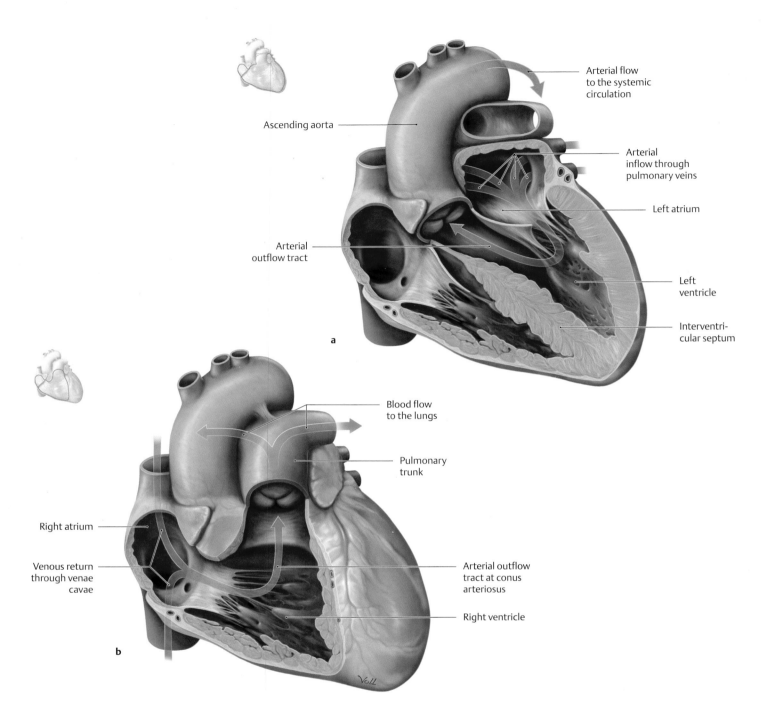

Ascending aorta

Arterial flow to the systemic circulation

Arterial inflow through pulmonary veins

Left atrium

Arterial outflow tract

Left ventricle

Interventricular septum

a

Blood flow to the lungs

Pulmonary trunk

Right atrium

Venous return through venae cavae

Arterial outflow tract at conus arteriosus

Right ventricle

b

B Blood flow in the heart

The septa between the atria and ventricles functionally divide the heart into two main parts: the right heart and left heart. The cardiac valves define the direction of blood flow through both sides of the heart, enabling the right and left heart to function as finely coordinated tandem pumps.

Blood flow in the right heart (b): Anterior view with the right atrium and right ventricle cut open. Venous blood from the superior and inferior venae cavae flows into the sinus venarum and enters the right atrium. From there it flows across the open right atrioventricular valve and passes through the right atrioventricular orifice along the inflow tract into the right ventricle. Inside the ventricle it is redirected into the outflow tract and pumped through the open pulmonary valve (shown closed here) and conus arteriosus into the pulmonary trunk. From there it flows through the pulmonary arteries into the lungs, where it is oxygenated. The right heart pumps blood with a low oxygen tension.

Blood flow in the left heart (a): Left anterior view. All of the cardiac chambers have been cut open anteriorly. Oxygenated blood from the lungs flows across the open left atrioventricular valve and through the left atrioventricular orifice along the inflow tract into the left ventricle. There it is rerouted into the outflow tract and flows across the open aortic valve (shown closed here) through the aortic orifice into the ascending aorta for distribution throughout the systemic circulation (after first perfusing the coronary arteries). The left heart pumps blood with a high oxygen tension.

3.1 Thoracic Aorta

Right common carotid
artery and right
internal jugular vein

Left common carotid
artery and left
internal jugular vein

Right subclavian
artery and vein

Left subclavian
artery and vein

Superior
vena cava

Ascending
aorta

Right
pulmonary veins

Pulmonary
trunk

Diaphragm

Cardiac apex

A Projection of the heart and vessels onto the chest wall

Anterior view. The two great arterial vessels in the thorax are the *aorta* and the *pulmonary trunk*. Because the pulmonary arteries run a very short distance before entering the lungs, they are discussed under the heading of the pulmonary vessels (see pp. 120 and 121).

The *ascending* aorta is "in the shadow" of the sternum on the PA chest radiograph, while the aortic arch ("aortic knob") forms the superior left portion of the left heart border. The descenting aorta is hiddeen by the heart itself.

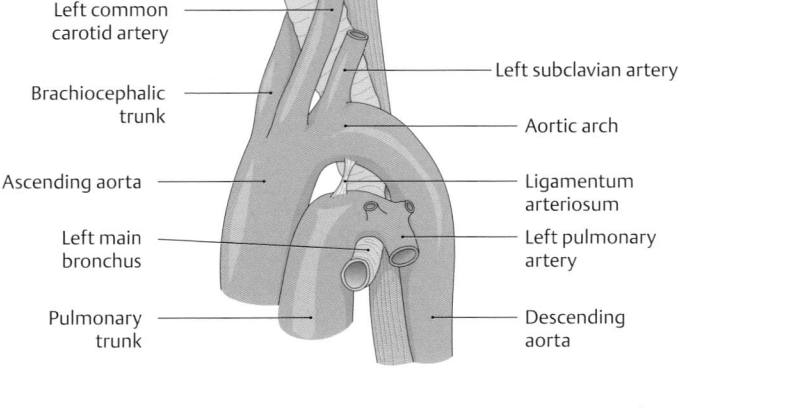

Trachea

Esophagus

Left common
carotid artery

Brachiocephalic
trunk

Left subclavian artery

Ascending aorta

Aortic arch

Ligamentum
arteriosum

Left main
bronchus

Left pulmonary
artery

Pulmonary
trunk

Descending
aorta

B Parts of the aorta and their relationship to the trachea and esophagus

Left lateral view. The aorta consists of three main parts:

• Ascending aorta: arises from the left ventricle, is dilated near the heart to form the aortic bulb (not visible here).
• Aortic arch: the arched portion of the aorta between the ascending and descending

parts, runs posteriorly and to the left. A constriction may persist as an embryonic remnant in this part of the aorta (the aortic isthmus, not shown here).
• Descending aorta: consists of the thoracic and abdominal portions of the aorta (see **D**).

C Functional groups of arteries that supply the thoracic organs

These are mainly vessels that supply the *organs and internal structures* of the thorax. The intrathoracic branches of the aorta can be divided into four main functional groups:

Arteries to the head and neck
(see pp. 10, 11) **or to the upper limb:**
• Brachiocephalic trunk with:
  – Right common carotid artery
  – Right subclavian artery
• Thyroid ima artery (present in only 10 % of the population)
• Left common carotid artery
• Left subclavian artery

Direct aortic branches that supply intrathoracic structures:
• Visceral branches to thoracic organs (heart, trachea, bronchi, and esophagus):
  – Right and left coronary arteries
  – Tracheal branches
  – Pericardial branches
  – Bronchial branches
  – Esophageal branches
• Parietal branches to the internal (mainly posterolateral) chest wall and diaphragm:
  – Posterior intercostal arteries
  – Right and left superior phrenic arteries

Indirect paired branches (not arising directly from the aorta) that are distributed primarily to the head and neck but give off branches, usually small, that enter the chest and supply intrathoracic organs:
• Inferior thyroid artery (from the thyrocervical trunk = branch of subclavian artery) with:
  – Esophageal branches
  – Tracheal branches

Indirect paired branches which supply the chest wall (mostly anterior, some inferior), usually in the form of parietal branches, and may give off other branches to intrathoracic organs (visceral sub-branches):
• Internal thoracic artery (from the subclavian artery) with:
  – Thymic branches
  – Mediastinal branches
  – Anterior intercostal branches
  – Pericardiacophrenic artery (with branches to the pericardium and diaphragm)
  – Musculophrenic artery (with a branch to the diaphragm)

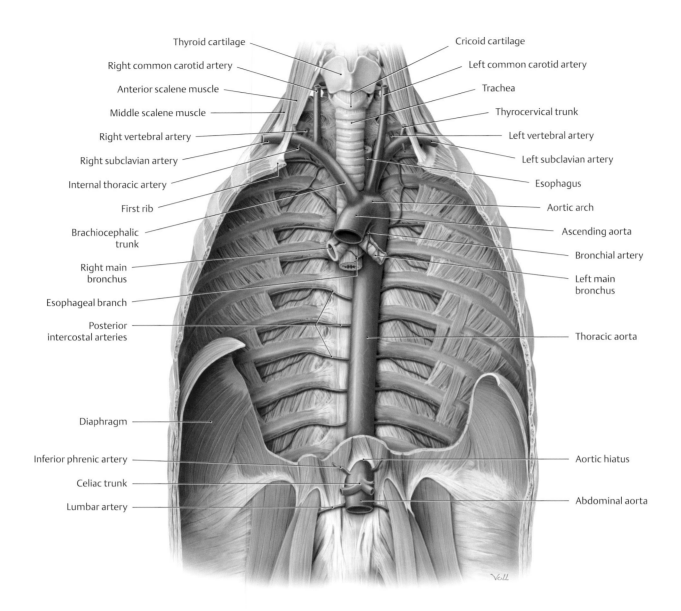

Thyroid cartilage
Cricoid cartilage
Right common carotid artery
Left common carotid artery
Anterior scalene muscle
Trachea
Middle scalene muscle
Thyrocervical trunk
Right vertebral artery
Left vertebral artery
Right subclavian artery
Left subclavian artery
Internal thoracic artery
Esophagus
First rib
Aortic arch
Brachiocephalic trunk
Ascending aorta
Right main bronchus
Bronchial artery
Esophageal branch
Left main bronchus
Posterior intercostal arteries
Thoracic aorta
Diaphragm
Inferior phrenic artery
Aortic hiatus
Celiac trunk
Abdominal aorta
Lumbar artery

D Position of the aorta in the thorax

Anterior view. The pleura, internal fasciae, and most thoracic organs have been removed, and the diaphragm has been windowed to display more of the thoracic cavity. The branches of the aorta (see **C** and p. 263) supply blood to all the organs, delivering almost 5 liters of blood per minute throughout the body. The thoracic aorta is thick-walled, particularly in its ascending segment and arch, but these walls are also elastic. During the systolic wave of pressure as the left ventricle contracts, these segments of the aorta dilate rapidly and then recoil. This serves to absorb and dissipate the pressure wave to produce a steadier, more even flow of blood in the arteries farther away from the heart. Because the aortic arch runs posteriorly and to the left, the relationship of the aorta to the trachea and esophagus changes as the vessel passes inferiorly through the chest (see also **B** and p. 118). The most anterior part of the aorta is the *ascending aorta*. The *aortic arch* then passes to the left side

of the trachea, arching over the left main bronchus. It passes initially to the left of the esophagus but then descends *posterior* to the esophagus and anterior to the vertebral column. Because of this relationship, an abnormal outpouching of the aortic wall (aneurysm) may narrow the esophagus and cause swallowing difficulties (dysphagia). The thoracic aorta pierces the diaphragm at the aortic hiatus (junction of the T 11/ T 12 vertebrae), becoming the abdominal aorta (see p. 263).

Note: In rare cases the aortic arch is constricted behind the ligamentum arteriosum (see **B**). This constriction is normal in the embryonic circulation, but its persistence after birth may produce the clinical manifestations of a *coarctation of the aorta*. This includes hypertension in the head, neck, and upper limbs, insufficient blood flow in the lower extremities, and left ventricular hypertrophy (due to chronic excessive workload and pressure).

3.2 Vena Cava and Azygos System

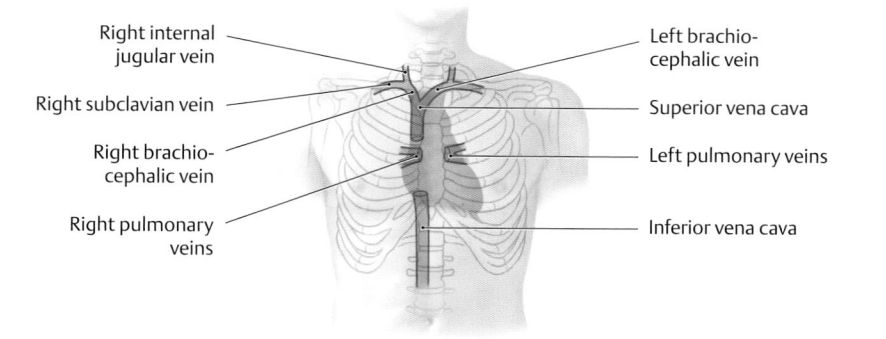

Right internal jugular vein
Right subclavian vein
Right brachio-cephalic vein
Right pulmonary veins

Left brachio-cephalic vein
Superior vena cava
Left pulmonary veins
Inferior vena cava

A Projection of the venae cavae onto the skeleton

Anterior view. The *superior* vena cava lies to the right of the midline and appears at the right sternal border on radiographs. Formed by the confluence of the two brachiocephalic veins, the superior vena cava enters the right atrium of the heart from above, forming its border in the

PA chest radiograph (see p. 96). The *inferior vena cava* runs a very short distance within the thorax (approximately 1 cm, not shown here). Immediately after piercing the diaphragm (at the vena caval hiatus), it passes through the pericardium and ends by opening into the right atrium of the heart from below. It has no tributaries within the chest (the pulmonary veins are described on pp. 120 and 121).

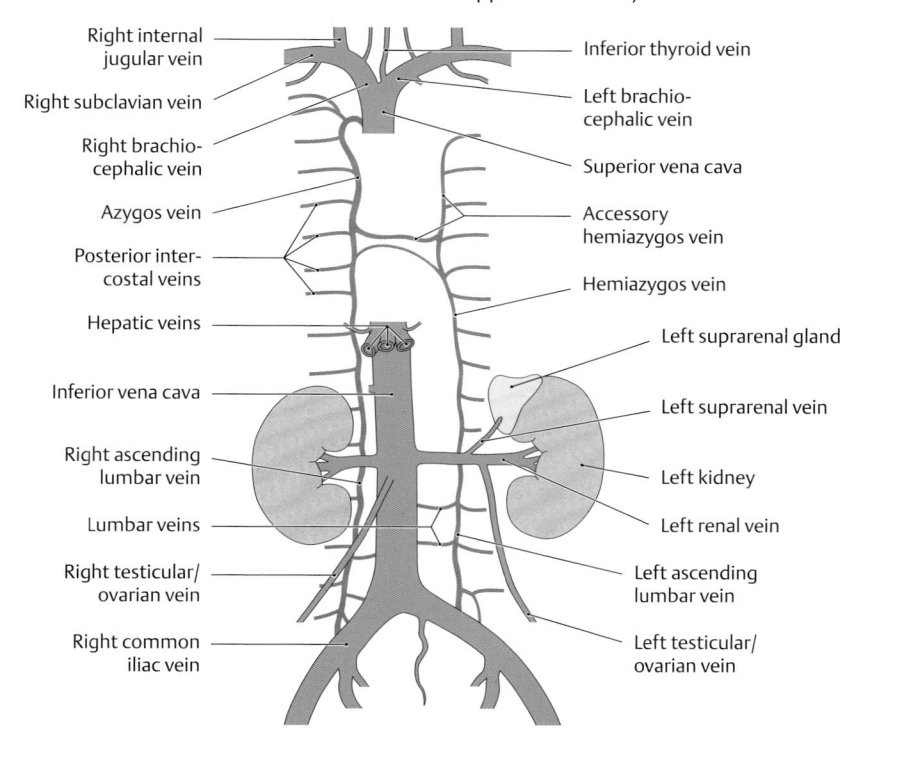

Right internal jugular vein
Right subclavian vein
Right brachio-cephalic vein
Azygos vein
Posterior inter-costal veins
Hepatic veins
Inferior vena cava
Right ascending lumbar vein
Lumbar veins
Right testicular/ovarian vein
Right common iliac vein

Inferior thyroid vein
Left brachio-cephalic vein
Superior vena cava
Accessory hemiazygos vein
Hemiazygos vein
Left suprarenal gland
Left suprarenal vein
Left kidney
Left renal vein
Left ascending lumbar vein
Left testicular/ovarian vein

B The azygos system

Anterior view. The venous drainage of the thorax is handled mainly by the long azygos system, which runs vertically through the chest. The *azygos vein* runs to the right of the vertebral column, the *hemiazygos vein* to the left. The hemiazygos vein empties into the azygos vein, which in turn empties into the superior vena cava. An *accessory hemiazygos vein* is frequently present in the upper left thorax; it may open independently into the azygos vein or by way of the hemiazygos vein. The azygos system receives tributaries from the mediastinum

and from portions of the chest wall, predominantly in the central and lower thorax.
Note: The azygos vein empties into the superior vena cava, while the ascending lumbar veins on both sides open into the inferior vena cava via the lumbar veins and the common iliac veins. In this way the azygos system creates a shunt between the superior and inferior venae cavae, called the "cavocaval anastomosis." If drainage from the inferior vena cava is obstructed, venous blood can still reach the superior vena cava and enter the right heart by passing through the azygos system (see **D** and p. 292).

C Functional groups of veins that drain the thoracic organs

These are mainly vessels that drain the *organs and internal structures* of the thorax. All of them drain ultimately to the superior vena cava, whose tributaries in the chest can be divided into four main functional groups:

Veins that drain the head and neck (see pp. 12 and 13) **or the upper limb:**

- Left and right brachiocephalic vein with:
  – Right and left subclavian veins
  – Right and left internal jugular veins
  – Right and left external jugular veins
  – Supreme intercostal veins
  – Pericardial veins
  – Left superior intercostal vein

Veins that drain intrathoracic structures (open into the accessory hemiazygos vein or hemiazygos vein on the left side, into the azygos vein on the right side). Blood from both territories is collected in the azygos vein, which empties into the superior vena cava. The tributaries can be grouped as follows:

- Visceral branches that drain the trachea, bronchi, and esophagus:
  – Tracheal veins
  – Bronchial veins
  – Esophageal veins
- Parietal branches that drain the inner chest wall and diaphragm:
  – Posterior intercostal veins
  – Right and left superior phrenic vein
  – Right superior intercostal vein

Indirect paired tributaries of the superior vena cava that descend from the head and neck but receive smaller veins that drain thoracic organs:

- Inferior thyroid vein (= tributaries of the brachiocephalic vein) with:
  – Esophageal veins
  – Tracheal veins

Indirect paired tributaries of the superior vena cava that mainly drain the anterior chest wall as parietal branches but may also receive tributaries (visceral sub-branches) from organs:

- Internal thoracic vein (opens into the brachiocephalic vein) with:
  – Thymic veins
  – Mediastinal tributaries
  – Anterior intercostal veins
  – Pericardiacophrenic vein (with tributaries from the pericardium and diaphragm)
  – Musculophrenic vein (with a tributary from the diaphragm)

Note: Structures of the superior mediastinum may also drain directly to the brachiocephalic veins (e.g., via the tracheal veins, esophageal veins, and mediastinal veins).

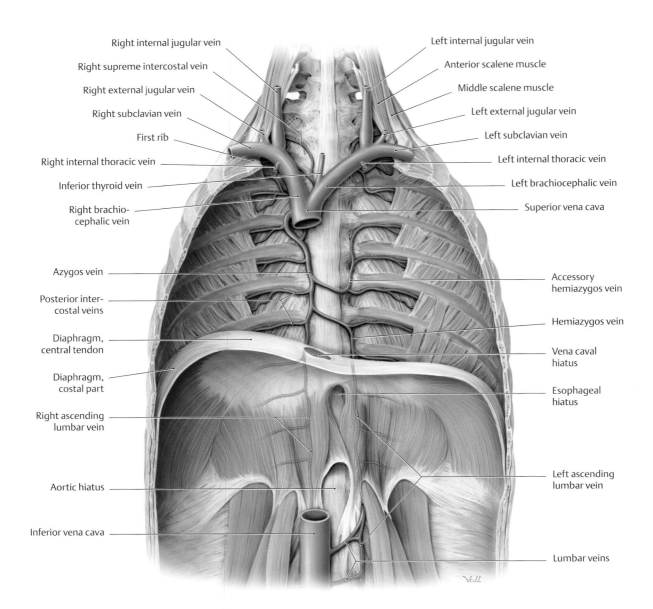

Right internal jugular vein
Right supreme intercostal vein
Right external jugular vein
Right subclavian vein
First rib
Right internal thoracic vein
Inferior thyroid vein
Right brachio-cephalic vein
Azygos vein
Posterior inter-costal veins
Diaphragm, central tendon
Diaphragm, costal part
Right ascending lumbar vein
Aortic hiatus
Inferior vena cava

Left internal jugular vein
Anterior scalene muscle
Middle scalene muscle
Left external jugular vein
Left subclavian vein
Left internal thoracic vein
Left brachiocephalic vein
Superior vena cava
Accessory hemiazygos vein
Hemiazygos vein
Vena caval hiatus
Esophageal hiatus
Left ascending lumbar vein
Lumbar veins

D Superior vena cava and azygos system in the thorax
Anterior view. The thorax has been cut open and the organs, internal fasciae, and serous membranes have been removed. The inferior vena cava has been removed at the level of the L 1/ L 2 vertebrae to display the right ascending lumbar vein. The **superior vena cava** is formed by the confluence of the two brachiocephalic veins at the approximate level of the T 2 / T 3 junction, to the right of the median plane. Each brachio-cephalic vein is formed in turn by the union of the internal jugular vein and subclavian vein. The azygos vein ascends on the right side of the ver-tebral column and opens into the posterior right aspect of the superior vena cava just below the union of the brachiocephalic veins. The right and left ascending lumbar veins pass upward through the diaphragm to form the **azygos vein** on the right side and the **hemiazygos vein** on the left side. At the level of the T 7 vertebra, the hemiazygos vein crosses over the vertebral column from the left side and opens into the azygos vein. In this dissection the accessory hemiazygos vein drains separately into the azygos vein after crossing over the vertebral column from left to right. Not infrequently, however, the hemiazygos vein and accessory hemiazygos vein are interconnected by anastomoses.

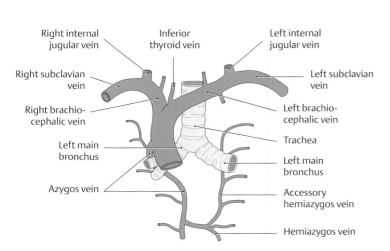

Right internal jugular vein
Inferior thyroid vein
Left internal jugular vein
Right subclavian vein
Left subclavian vein
Right brachio-cephalic vein
Left brachio-cephalic vein
Trachea
Left main bronchus
Left main bronchus
Azygos vein
Accessory hemiazygos vein
Hemiazygos vein

E Relations of the trachea, superior vena cava, and azygos system
The superior vena cava lies to the right of the trachea. The left brachio-cephalic vein passes anterior to the trachea from the left side to unite with the right brachiocephalic vein. The azygos vein ascends posterior to the right main bronchus and turns anteriorly to enter the superior vena cava from behind (the azygos vein "rides" upon the right main bronchus). The accessory hemiazygos vein ascends behind the left main bronchus and may open independently into the azygos vein or may join the hemiazy-gos vein to form a common trunk that opens into the azygos vein.

3.3   Arteries and Veins of the Esophagus

A Blood vessels of the esophagus
a Arteries, **b** veins.

Posterior wall of the thorax and upper abdomen, viewed from the anterior aspect. All of the thoracic organs have been removed except for the esophagus and part of the trachea. The proximal portion of the stomach has been left in the abdomen.

Note: The esophagus is supplied by three groups of arteries, consistent with its division into three parts (see p. 70), and it is likewise drained by three venous groups.

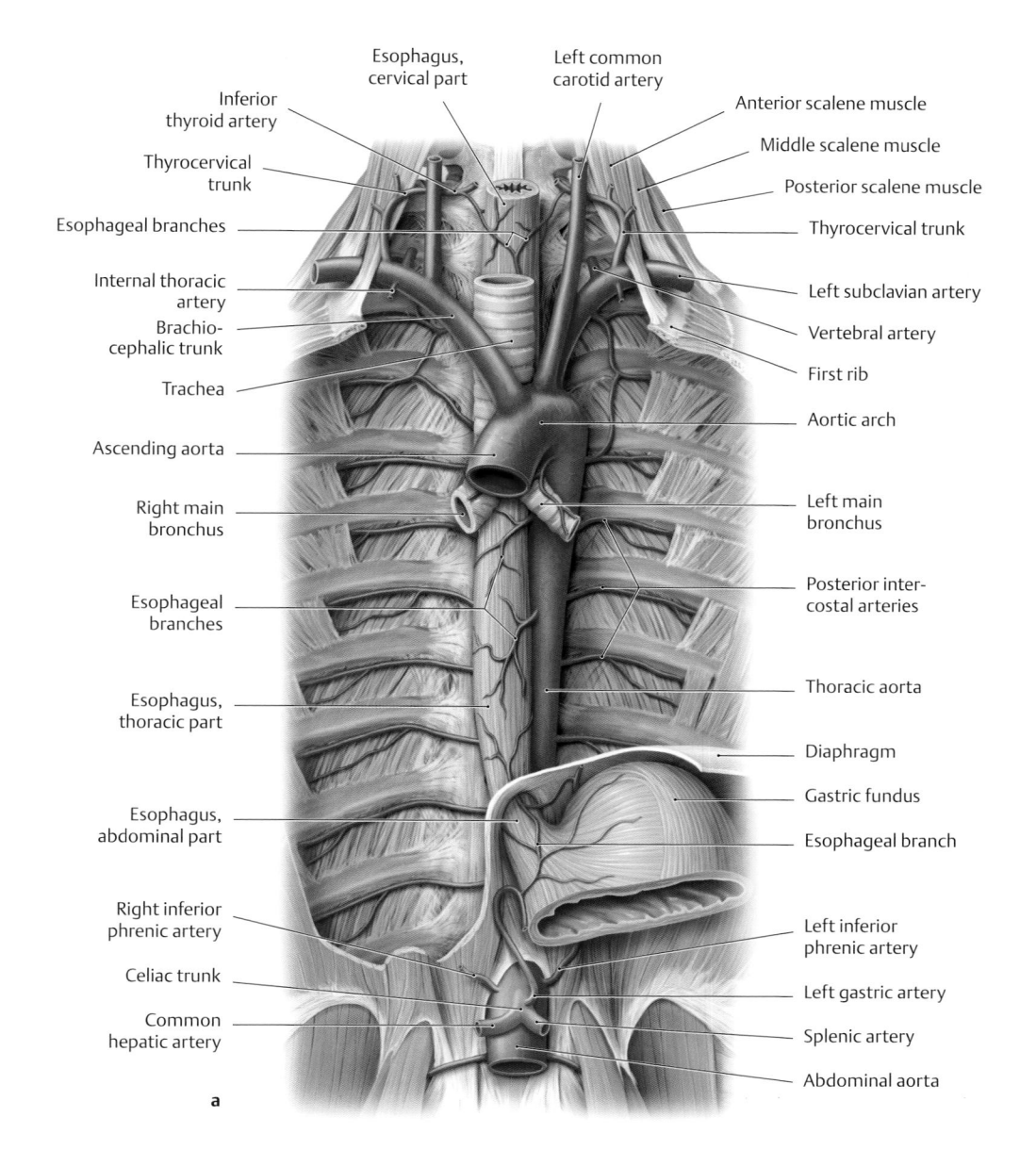

a

Labels (left, top to bottom): Inferior thyroid artery; Thyrocervical trunk; Esophageal branches; Internal thoracic artery; Brachio-cephalic trunk; Trachea; Ascending aorta; Right main bronchus; Esophageal branches; Esophagus, thoracic part; Esophagus, abdominal part; Right inferior phrenic artery; Celiac trunk; Common hepatic artery

Labels (top center): Esophagus, cervical part; Left common carotid artery

Labels (right, top to bottom): Anterior scalene muscle; Middle scalene muscle; Posterior scalene muscle; Thyrocervical trunk; Left subclavian artery; Vertebral artery; First rib; Aortic arch; Left main bronchus; Posterior inter-costal arteries; Thoracic aorta; Diaphragm; Gastric fundus; Esophageal branch; Left inferior phrenic artery; Left gastric artery; Splenic artery; Abdominal aorta

B Arterial supply and venous drainage of the esophagus

Part of esophagus	Arterial supply	Venous drainage (see Ab)

• Cervical part	• Esophageal branches
	  – Usually from the inferior thyroid artery or
	  – Direct branches (rare, not shown here) from the thyrocervical trunk or common carotid artery
		• Esophageal veins
		  – Drain to inferior thyroid vein or
		  – Left brachiocephalic vein

• Thoracic part	• Esophageal branches from the thoracic aorta, distributed to the anterior and posterior sides of the esophagus	• Esophageal veins
		  – Drain at upper left into the accessory hemiazygos vein or left brachiocephalic vein
		  – Drain at lower left into the hemiazygos vein
		  – Drain into the azygos vein on the right side

• Abdominal part (smallest arteries and veins serving the esophagus)	• Esophageal branch of the left gastric artery	• Esophageal veins draining into the left gastric vein

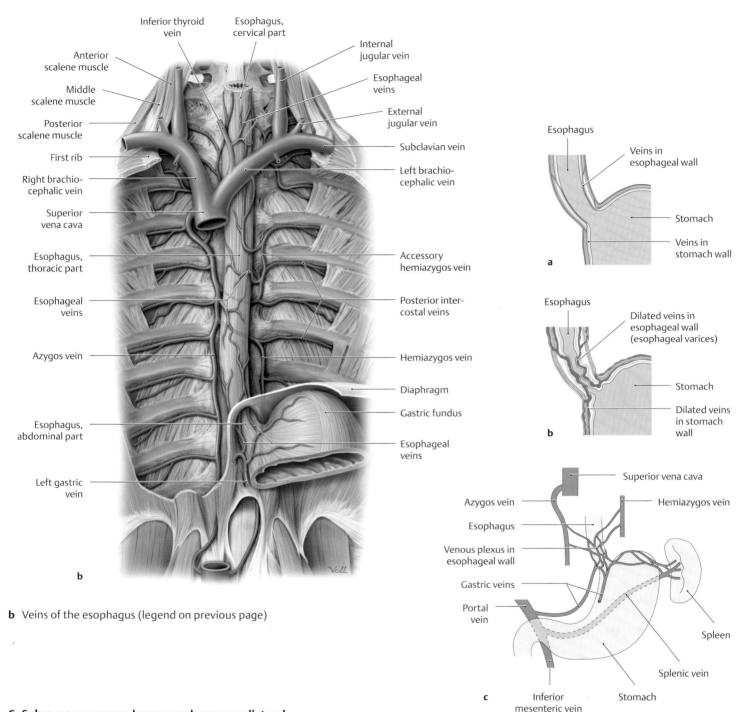

Inferior thyroid vein

Esophagus, cervical part

Anterior scalene muscle

Middle scalene muscle

Posterior scalene muscle

First rib

Right brachio-cephalic vein

Superior vena cava

Esophagus, thoracic part

Esophageal veins

Azygos vein

Esophagus, abdominal part

Left gastric vein

Internal jugular vein

Esophageal veins

External jugular vein

Subclavian vein

Left brachio-cephalic vein

Accessory hemiazygos vein

Posterior inter-costal veins

Hemiazygos vein

Diaphragm

Gastric fundus

Esophageal veins

Esophagus

Veins in esophageal wall

Stomach

Veins in stomach wall

a

Esophagus

Dilated veins in esophageal wall (esophageal varices)

Stomach

Dilated veins in stomach wall

b

Superior vena cava

Azygos vein

Hemiazygos vein

Esophagus

Venous plexus in esophageal wall

Gastric veins

Portal vein

Spleen

Splenic vein

Stomach

c   Inferior mesenteric vein

b

b Veins of the esophagus (legend on previous page)

C Submucous venous plexuses and venous collaterals

a, b Submucous venous plexuses and varices in the esophagus (after Stelzner): The smallest tributaries of the esophageal veins pass through all layers of the esophageal wall, accompanied by arterial branches, to the lamina propria of the mucosa. In the adjacent, thicker submucosa they form an extensive plexus that contributes to functional closure of the esophagus at the junction of its thoracic and abdominal parts (see p. 75). This venous plexus is continuous with an analogous plexus at the gastric inlet. With any obstruction of portal venous flow to the liver (as in cirrhosis associated with chronic alcoholism), these anastomoses provide a collateral pathway by which the venous blood flow may be diverted into the submucous venous plexuses of the esophagus, causing them to undergo varicose dilation (esophageal varices, see **b**). There may be associated abnormal dilation of the gastric veins.

c Esophageal venous collaterals (after Strohmeyer and Dölle). Venous anastomoses provide two routes for draining the veins at the junction of the thoracic and abdominal parts of the esophagus:

1. Via the azygos or hemiazygos vein to the superior vena cava (thoracic route)
2. Via the left gastric vein to the portal vein (abdominal route)

Thus, when portal venous flow becomes obstructed in the liver (cirrhosis), blood may be diverted through the esophageal veins to the superior vena cava (portosystemic collaterals, see p. 293).

3.4 Pulmonary Arteries and Veins

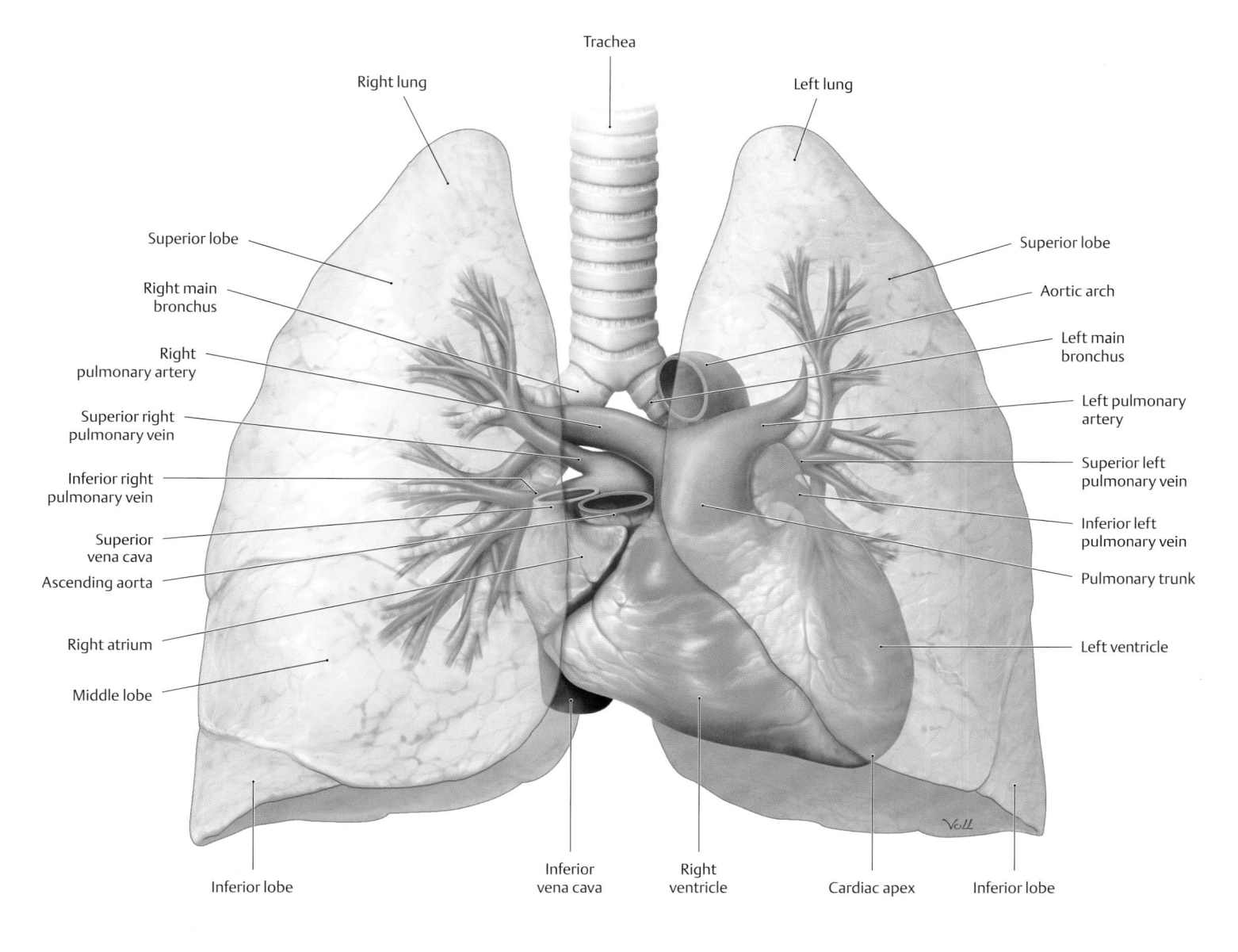

A Topographical anatomy of the pulmonary vessels
Anterior view of a "heart-lung preparation." The venae cavae have been cut close to the heart, and a segment has been removed from the ascending aorta and arch to display the division of the pulmonary trunk, which is inferior to the aortic arch, and the origin of the right pulmonary artery. The lungs and heart are shown partially transparent. The arteries and veins that pass to the lung are divided into two groups:

- *Pulmonary arteries and veins*, which carry blood to the lungs and back for *gas exchange* (O_2, CO_2)
- *Bronchial arteries and veins* (not shown here), which *supply blood* to parts of the lungs themselves (see p. 122).

The **divisions of the pulmonary arteries** basically follow the branching pattern of the bronchial tree (see p. 82). Two or three arterial branches,

called lobar arteries, accompany the two (left) or three (right) lobar bronchi into the lung. (The lobar arteries are larger than the lobar bronchi.) As the bronchial tree branches into *segmental bronchi*, the arteries similarly divide into *segmental arteries*. The artery and its associated bronchus are always placed at the center of the structural lung unit, first occupying the *center of a lobe*, then the *center of a bronchopulmonary segment* (see p. 84).

The **divisions of the pulmonary veins** do not follow the branching pattern of the bronchial tree, instead coursing between pulmonary segments to collect blood from within (intrasegmental veins) and among (intersegmental veins) adjacent segments. Thus pulmonary veins are named differently than pulmonary arteries (see **C** and **D**).

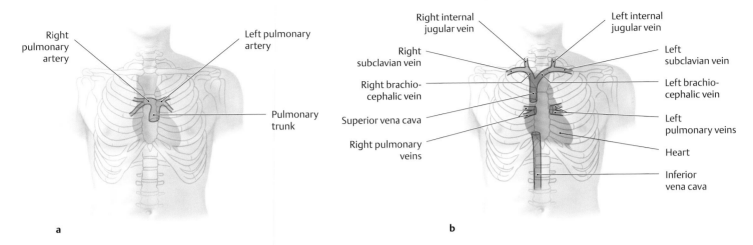

B Projection of the pulmonary arteries and veins onto the chest wall
Anterior view.

a Projection of the pulmonary arteries onto the chest wall. The pulmonary trunk arises from the right ventricle, which is anterior owing to the slightly rotated position of the heart, and divides into a left and right pulmonary artery for each lung. The pulmonary trunk appears on chest radiographs as a knob-like shadow on the left cardiac border (see p. 96) above the ventricles.

Note: The pulmonary trunk lies to the left of the midline in the chest. As a result, the right pulmonary artery (length approximately 2–3 cm) is longer than the left pulmonary artery.

b Projection of the pulmonary veins onto the chest wall. Normally, a pair of pulmonary veins open into the left atrium on each side. Taken together, the right and left pulmonary veins and both venae cavae form an asymmetrical cruciform pattern on the chest radiograph.

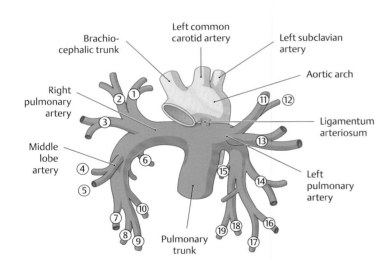

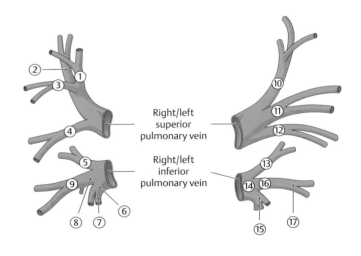

C The pulmonary arteries and their branches

Right lung Right pulmonary artery	Left lung Left pulmonary artery
Superior lobe arteries ① Apical segmental artery ② Posterior segmental artery ③ Anterior segmental artery	*Superior lobe arteries* ⑪ Apical segmental artery ⑫ Posterior segmental artery ⑬ Anterior segmental artery
Middle lobe artery ④ Lateral segmental artery ⑤ Medial segmental artery	⑭ Lingular artery
Inferior lobe arteries ⑥ Superior segmental artery ⑦ Anterior basal segmental artery ⑧ Lateral basal segmental artery ⑨ Posterior basal segmental artery ⑩ Medial basal segmental artery	*Inferior lobe arteries* ⑮ Superior segmental artery ⑯ Anterior basal segmental artery ⑰ Lateral basal segmental artery ⑱ Posterior basal segmental artery ⑲ Medial basal segmental artery

D The pulmonary veins and their tributaries

Right lung Right pulmonary veins	Left lung Left pulmonary veins
Right superior pulmonary vein ① Apical vein ② Posterior vein ③ Anterior vein ④ Middle lobe vein	*Left superior pulmonary vein* ⑩ Apicoposterior vein ⑪ Anterior vein ⑫ Lingular vein
Right inferior pulmonary vein ⑤ Superior vein ⑥ Common basal vein ⑦ Inferior basal vein ⑧ Superior basal vein ⑨ Anterior basal vein	*Left inferior pulmonary vein* ⑬ Superior vein ⑭ Common basal vein ⑮ Inferior basal vein ⑯ Superior basal vein ⑰ Anterior basal vein

121

3.5 Bronchial and Diaphragmatic Arteries and Veins

A Bronchial arteries and veins

Anterior view. The trachea and bronchi are shown partially transparent.

a Arterial supply of the bronchi: The bronchi derive their blood supply from the thoracic aorta via bronchial arterial branches that follow the divisions of the main bronchi. It is not uncommon for one of the bronchial arteries to arise from a posterior intercostal artery (usually on the right side), rather than directly from the aorta. Given the relationship of the bronchi to the thoracic aorta, the bronchial arteries usually enter the bronchi from the posterior side.
Note: The trachea is supplied with arterial blood by small tracheal branches (not shown here) that may arise from the thoracic aorta, the internal thoracic artery, or the thyrocervical trunk, depending on the level of the trachea that is supplied.

b Venous drainage of the bronchi: The bronchi are drained by bronchial veins, which usually open into the accessory hemiazygos vein on the left side. On the right side, the veins may drain via collaterals into the azygos vein, but may also empty into the pulmonary veins, causing a small amount of deoxygenated bronchial blood to be mixed with the much larger outflow of pulmonary blood on its way to the left atrium. Small tracheal veins (not shown here) empty into the superior vena cava, left brachiocephalic vein, or internal thoracic vein at different levels of the trachea.

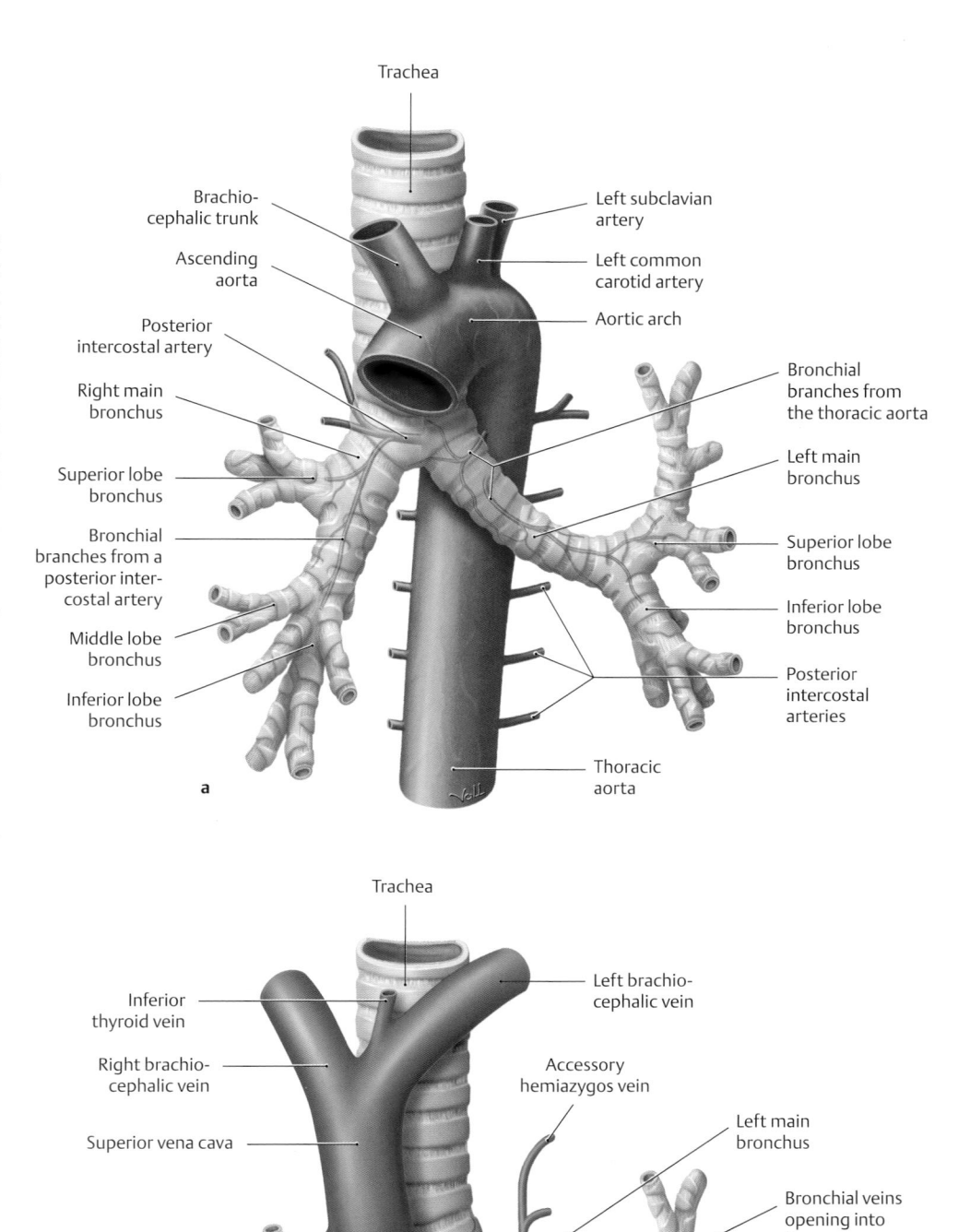

a

b

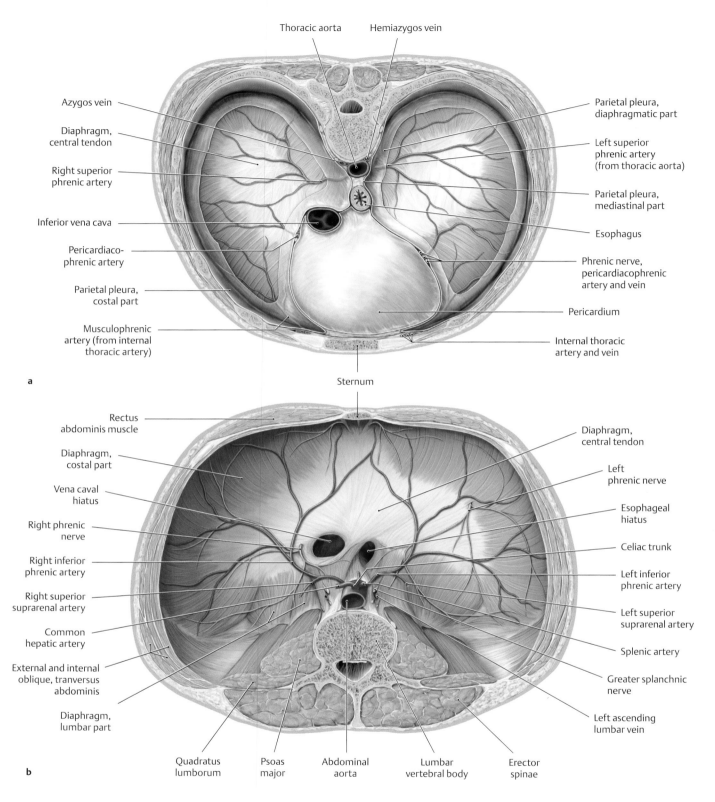

Thoracic aorta

Hemiazygos vein

Azygos vein

Diaphragm, central tendon

Right superior phrenic artery

Inferior vena cava

Pericardiaco-phrenic artery

Parietal pleura, costal part

Musculophrenic artery (from internal thoracic artery)

Parietal pleura, diaphragmatic part

Left superior phrenic artery (from thoracic aorta)

Parietal pleura, mediastinal part

Esophagus

Phrenic nerve, pericardiacophrenic artery and vein

Pericardium

Internal thoracic artery and vein

a

Sternum

Rectus abdominis muscle

Diaphragm, costal part

Vena caval hiatus

Right phrenic nerve

Right inferior phrenic artery

Right superior suprarenal artery

Common hepatic artery

External and internal oblique, tranversus abdominis

Diaphragm, lumbar part

Diaphragm, central tendon

Left phrenic nerve

Esophageal hiatus

Celiac trunk

Left inferior phrenic artery

Left superior suprarenal artery

Splenic artery

Greater splanchnic nerve

Left ascending lumbar vein

Quadratus lumborum

Psoas major

Abdominal aorta

Lumbar vertebral body

Erector spinae

b

B Arteries of the diaphragm

a Superior surface of the diaphragm viewed from above. The parietal pleura (diaphragmatic part) has been removed over a broad area, leaving the pericardium in place. Three (pairs of) arteries supply the superior surface of the diaphragm:

- Superior phrenic artery: arises from the thoracic aorta just above the diaphragm and supplies the largest area of the diaphragm.
- Pericardiacophrenic artery: runs close to the pericardium and gives off branches to the diaphragm.
- Internal thoracic artery: supplies the diaphragm by direct branches or via the musculophrenic artery.

b Inferior surface of the diaphragm viewed from below. The parietal peritoneum has been completely removed. The inferior surface of the diaphragm is supplied by the paired inferior phrenic arteries, the highest branches of the abdominal aorta.

The **diaphragmatic veins** (not shown here) mainly accompany the arteries:

- Inferior phrenic veins: open into the inferior vena cava.
- Superior phrenic veins: usually open into the azygos vein on the right side and into the hemiazygos vein on the left side.

123

3.6 Coronary Vessels (Coronary Arteries and Cardiac Veins): Anatomy and Relations

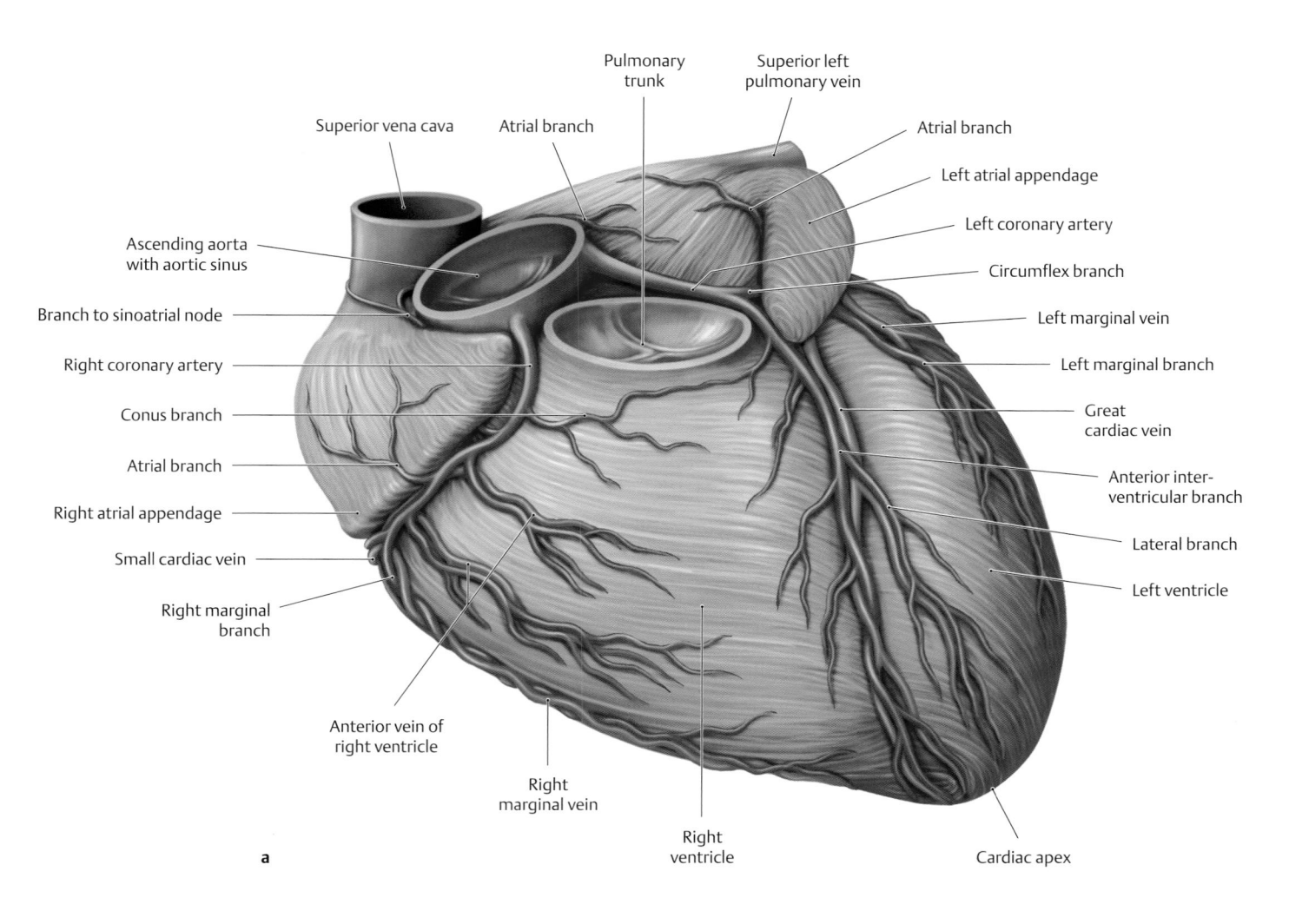

a

A Coronary arteries and cardiac veins
a Anterior view of the sternocostal surface of the heart.
b Posteroinferior view of the diaphragmatic surface of the heart.

Because the heart functions continuously to pump blood, it has a high oxygen demand. This demand is met by the right and left coronary arteries—intrinsic cardiac vessels that have an extensive capillary network. The coronary arteries spring from small dilations in the aorta (the aortic sinuses) located just above the aortic valve. The **left coronary artery** is usually slightly larger than the right and divides into two main branches:

- Circumflex branch: runs in the coronary sulcus (boundary between the atrium and ventricle) around the *left* side of the heart to the posterior heart wall.
- Anterior interventricular branch: runs in the anterior interventricular sulcus (boundary between the ventricles) to the cardiac apex. Each of these vessels gives off smaller branches (see p. 126).

The **right coronary artery,** usually smaller than the left, runs in the coronary sulcus around the *right* side of the heart to the posterior wall, where it forms the posterior interventricular branch. It also gives off numerous branches (see p. 126).

Note: The coronary arteries are functional end-arteries because they form anastomoses that are not adequate for reciprocal blood flow (see also p. 127). The coronary arteries must efficiently deliver blood to an organ with constant high metabolic demand that is itself at elevated pressure, especially during systole. This difficult requirement is achieved in part by the anatomical relation between the aortic valve and the origin of the coronary arteries, just superior to the valve leaflets. As the left ventricle completes its contraction and the distended aorta begins to recoil, the aortic valve is forced closed by the backflow and a local surge in pressure (a pressure *hammer*) develops. This pressure hammer drives blood into the coronary arteries. The heart is thus efficiently perfused at the maximum pressure that the cardiovascular system can reach.

The **cardiac veins** usually course with the coronary arteries and consist of the great, middle and small cardiac veins. These veins open on the posterior heart wall into the *coronary sinus*, which empties into the right atrium. Additional smaller veins (smallest cardiac veins, not shown here, thebesian veins) open directly into the cardiac chambers, mainly the right atrium.

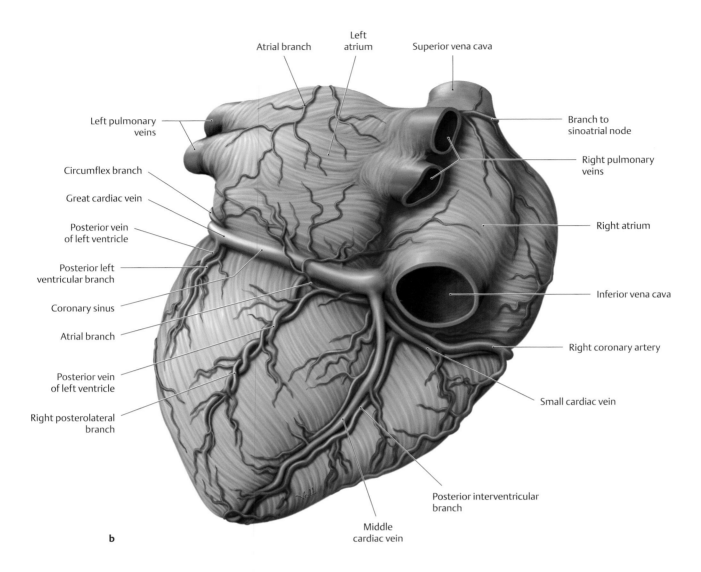

b Posteroinferior view of the diaphragmatic surface of the heart (legend on previous page).

B Branches of the coronary arteries

Left coronary artery	Right coronary artery
• Circumflex branch	• Branch to sinoatrial node
• Atrial branch	• Atrial branch
• Left marginal branch	• Right marginal branch
• Anterior interventricular branch	• Posterior interventricular branch
• Conus branch	• Conus branch
• Lateral branch	• Right posterolateral branch
• Posterior left ventricular branch	• Branch to atrioventricular node
• Interventricular septal branches	• Interventricular septal branches

Note: The left and right coronary arteries arise from the aortic sinus just superior to the aortic valve cusps.

C Divisions of the cardiac veins

Great cardiac vein
- Left marginal vein
- Anterior interventricular vein
- Posterior vein of left ventricle

Middle cardiac vein

Small cardiac vein
- Anterior vein of right ventricle
- Right marginal vein

Posterior vein of left ventricle

Note: Blood from the cardiac veins passes through the coronary sinus into the right atrium.

3.7 Coronary Vessels: Distribution of the Coronary Arteries

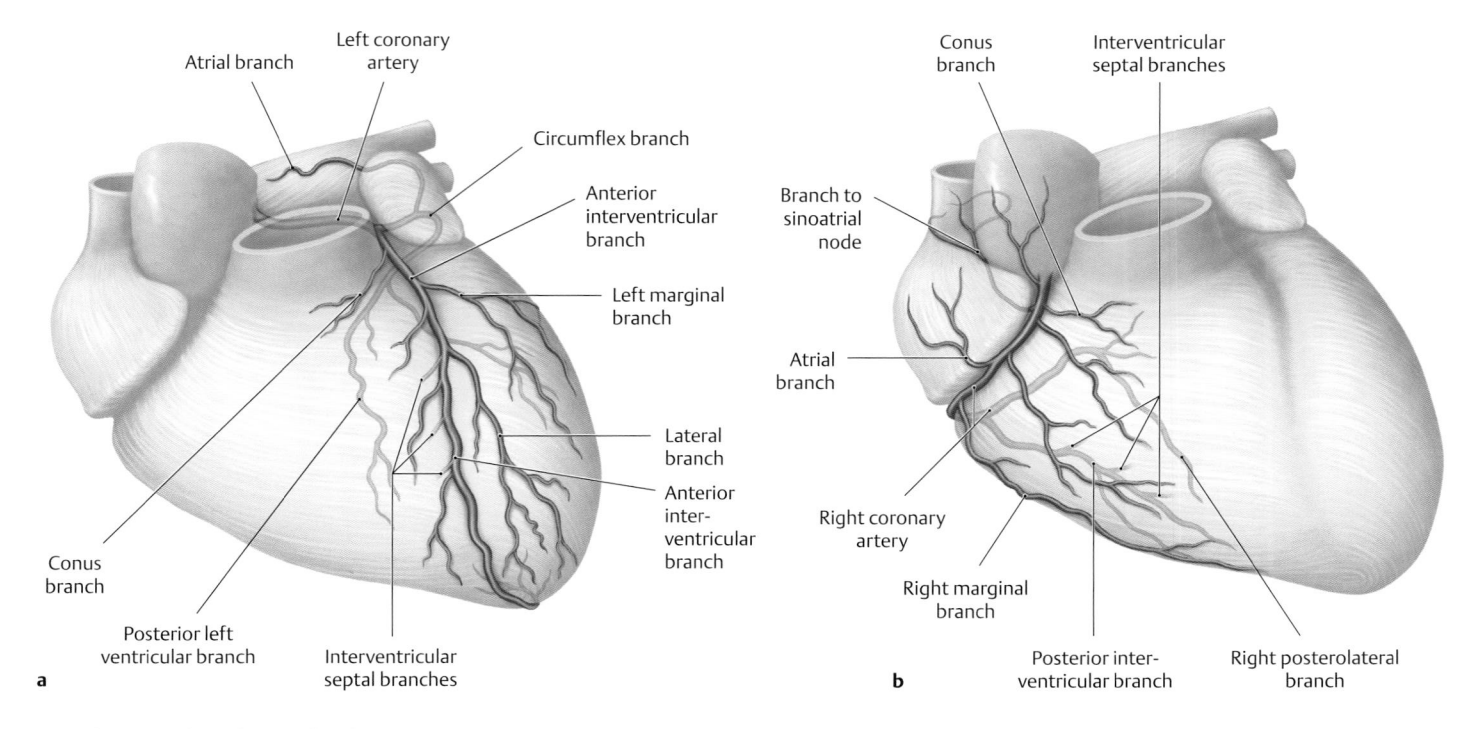

A Distribution of the left and right coronary arteries
The drawings illustrate a "balanced" type of coronary circulation (see **C**). See **B** for details.

B Distribution of the left and right coronary arteries

Distribution	Left coronary artery	Right coronary artery
Left atrium	Atrial branches and an intermediate atrial branch of the circumflex branch	
Right atrium		Atrial branches and an intermediate atrial branch
Left ventricle • Anterior wall • Lateral wall • Posterior wall	 • Anterior interventricular branch and its lateral branch • Left marginal branch of the circumflex branch * • Partly by the posterior left ventricular branch of the circumflex branch	 • Partly by the right posterolateral branch
Right ventricle • Anterior wall • Lateral wall • Posterior wall	 • Strip near the septum by the conus branch and small twigs from the anterior interventricular branch	 • Conus branch with smaller twigs and the right marginal branch • Right marginal branch • Posterior interventricular branch
Interventricular septum	Interventricular septal branches (supply the larger anterior part of the septum)	Interventricular septal branches (supply the smaller posterior part of the septum)
Sinoatrial node (sinus node)		Branch to the sinoatrial node
Atrioventricular node (AV node)		Branch to the atrioventricular node

* The left marginal branch has a variable origin. It typically arises from the circumflex branch, but often it springs from the anterior interventricular branch (as shown in **A**).

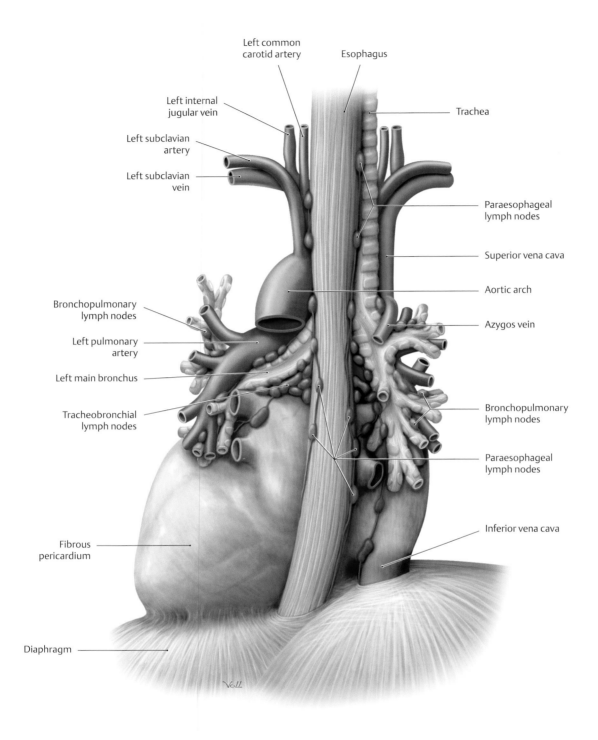

Left common
carotid artery

Esophagus

Left internal
jugular vein

Trachea

Left subclavian
artery

Left subclavian
vein

Paraesophageal
lymph nodes

Superior vena cava

Bronchopulmonary
lymph nodes

Aortic arch

Left pulmonary
artery

Azygos vein

Left main bronchus

Tracheobronchial
lymph nodes

Bronchopulmonary
lymph nodes

Paraesophageal
lymph nodes

Inferior vena cava

Fibrous
pericardium

Diaphragm

C Thoracic lymph nodes, posterior view
The numerous lymph nodes located at the divisions of the main bronchi into lobar bronchi are often called the "hilar" lymph nodes because
they are located in the region of the pulmonary hilum (not shown here).
Frequently they are the first group of lymph nodes to be affected by pulmonary disease (tuberculosis, malignant tumors).

4.3 The Thymus

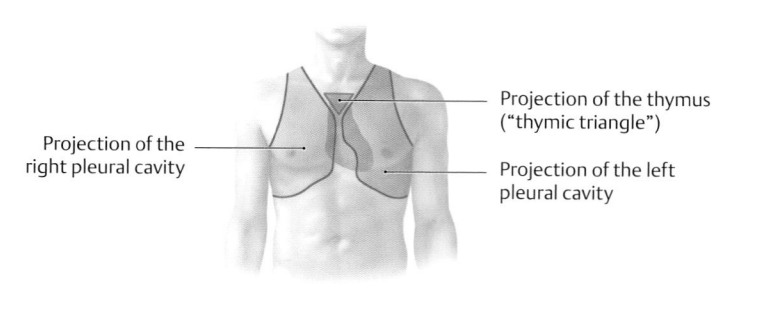

A Projection of the thymus onto the chest wall

For clarity, the pleural cavities have also been projected onto the chest wall. The thymus lies in the superior mediastinum and extends down into the anterior mediastinum, where it is anterior to the heart and great vessels and posterior to the sternum. The area in which the thymus projects onto the chest wall is sometimes called the "thymic triangle." On the chest radiograph of a very small child, the large thymus may appear to broaden the silhouette of the cardiac base.

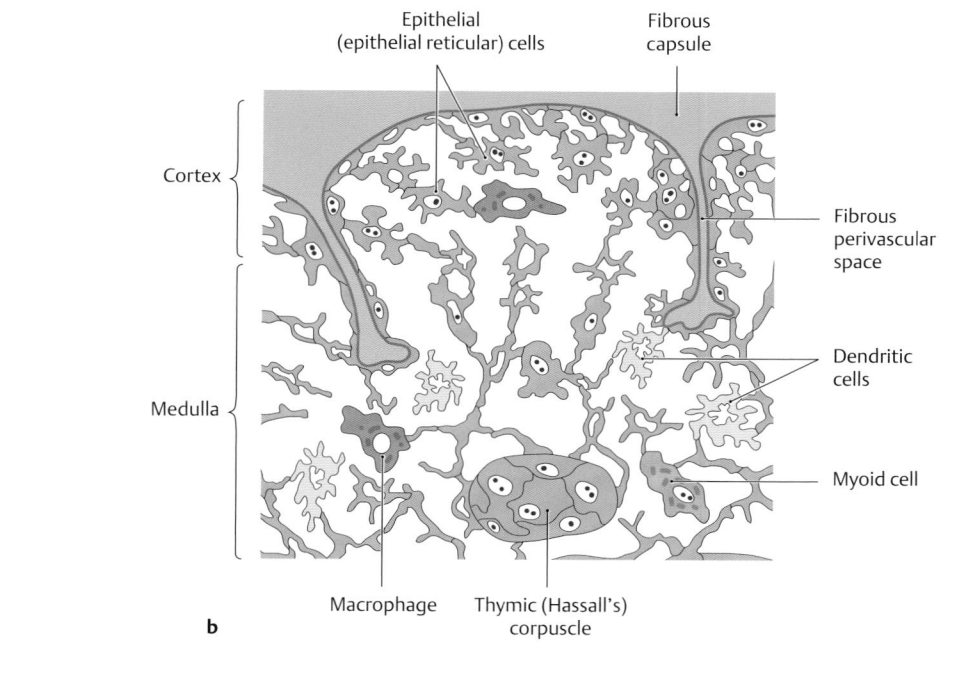

B Histological structure of the thymus

a **Structure of the thymus in adolescence (above) and old age (below).** The thymus is a primary lymphatic (lymphoepithelial) organ that has a predominantly endodermal origin (third pharyngeal pouch) but also contains ectodermal elements. It plays a central role in the maturation of T (thymus) lymphocytes and their differentiation into immunologically competent cells. Additionally, immune-modulating hormones (thymosin, thymopoietin, thymulin) are produced in the thymus. Congenital absence of the thymus results in severe immunodeficiency. The thymus consists of a cortex and medulla. The cortex appears much darker-staining due to the predominance of thymocytes (precursors to T-lymphocytes). The inner medullary region appears lighter-staining as a result of fewer thymocytes and an increase in the number of epithelial cells. Fine, vascularized trabeculae extend from the delicate fibrous capsule of the thymus into the parenchyma, subdividing the organ into numerous lobules.

b **Functional architecture** (as described by Lüllmann-Rauch). The thymus consists of a basic epithelial framework (= lymphoepithelial organ). During embryonic development, the precursors of T-lymphocytes migrate into the thymus and mature (under the control of the epithelial cells) into immunocompetent T-lymphocytes. The epi-

thelial cells form a densely packed, subcapsular layer that creates a boundary between the interior of the thymus and the cortical capillaries in the fibrous trabeculae (the "blood-thymus barrier," not shown here). Epithelial (epithelial reticular) cells with long processes join together in the cortex and medulla to form a three-dimensional network that encloses the thymocytes. (Thymocytes are not shown here in order to display other cell types clearly.) Epithelial cells in the medulla aggregate to form the thymic (Hassall's) corpuscles. The innermost cells in large thymic corpuscles often degenerate into a homogeneous mass. The function of the thymic corpuscles is not yet fully understood. The thymus contains several other cell types as well:

- Macrophages (phagocytosis of thymocytes)
- Dendritic cells (antigen presentation)
- Myoid cells (function unclear)

Maturation of the thymocytes occurs during their migration from the cortex to the medulla. A mature T-lymphocyte can recognize foreign antigens and differentiate them from endogenous cells ("autotolerance").

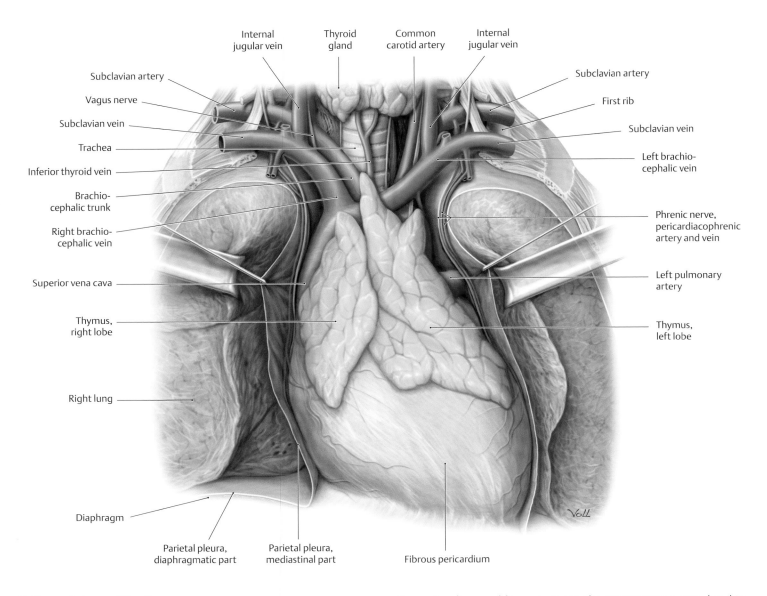

Internal jugular vein

Thyroid gland

Common carotid artery

Internal jugular vein

Subclavian artery

Vagus nerve

Subclavian vein

Trachea

Inferior thyroid vein

Brachio-cephalic trunk

Right brachio-cephalic vein

Superior vena cava

Thymus, right lobe

Right lung

Diaphragm

Parietal pleura, diaphragmatic part

Parietal pleura, mediastinal part

Fibrous pericardium

Subclavian artery

First rib

Subclavian vein

Left brachio-cephalic vein

Phrenic nerve, pericardiacophrenic artery and vein

Left pulmonary artery

Thymus, left lobe

C Size and shape of the thymus

Anterior view into the superior mediastinum of a 2-year-old child. The thymus is still well developed at this age, consisting of two prominent lobes (right and left) that are subdivided by fibrous septa into numerous lobules. Usually the thymus is apposed to the anterior surface of the pericardium and lies anterior to the superior vena cava, brachiocephalic veins, and aorta. In a small child, the thymus may extend up into the neck almost to the level of the thyroid gland, lying posterior to the pretracheal lamina of the cervical fascia. When the thymus reaches its greatest size during puberty, it has a maximum weight of 20–50 g.

4.4 Lymphatic Drainage of the Esophagus

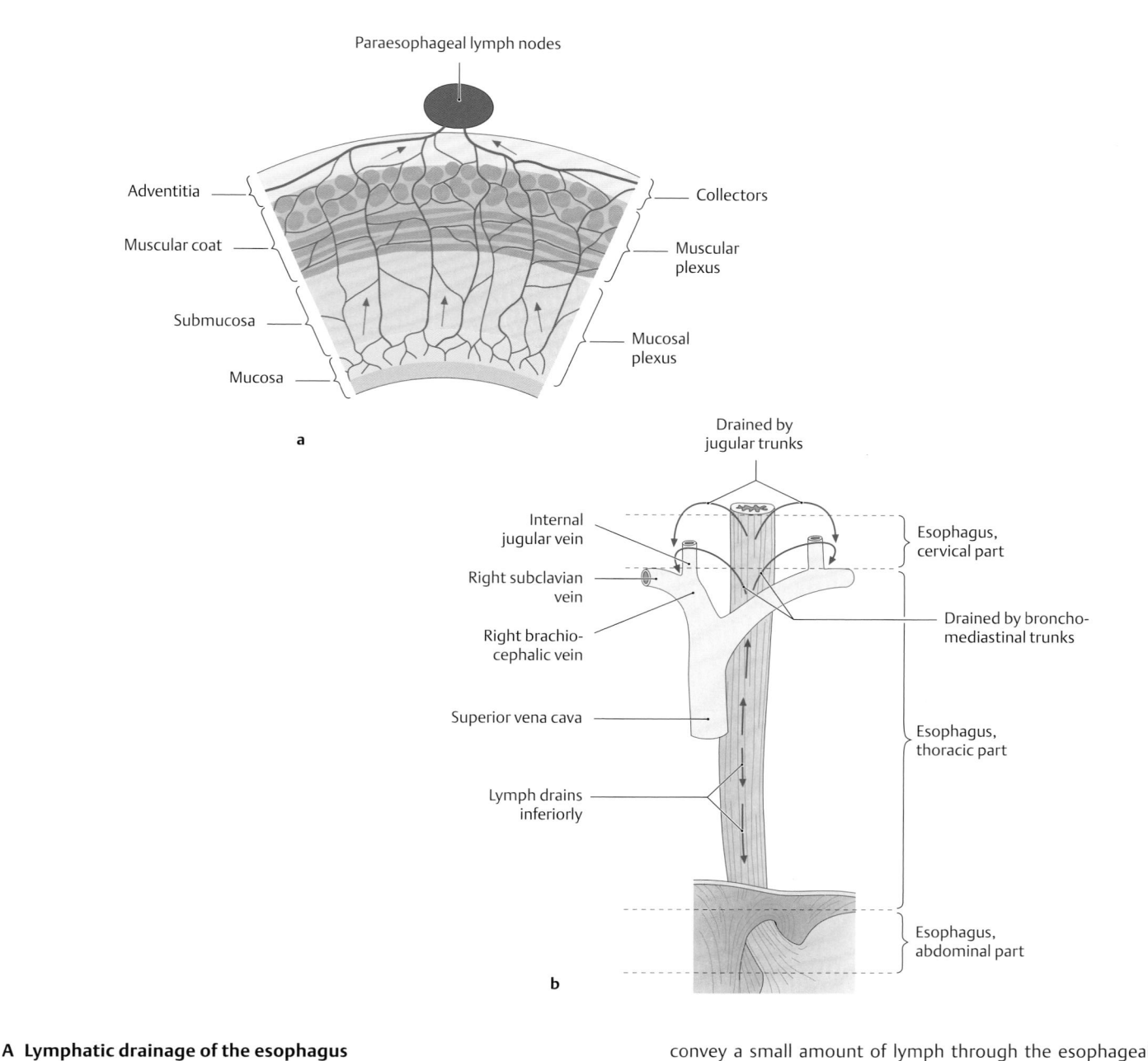

A Lymphatic drainage of the esophagus

a Lymphatic drainage of the esophageal wall, **b** lymphatic drainage at different levels of the esophagus.

Lymph from the esophagus flows from inside to outside through the various wall layers (**a**), draining initially to the lymph nodes that are distributed along the esophageal wall (paraesophageal lymph nodes, see **B**). There are three principal directions of lymphatic drainage, which correspond roughly to the three divisions of the esophagus (**b**):

- The *cervical part* of the esophagus drains cranially, mainly to the deep cervical lymph nodes and then to the jugular trunk.
- The *thoracic part* of the esophagus drains in two principal directions:
  - Cranially to the bronchomediastinal trunks (upper half).
  - Inferiorly (partly *via* the *superior* phrenic lymph nodes) to the bronchomediastinal trunks (lower half). Fine lymphatic vessels may

convey a small amount of lymph through the esophageal hiatus into the upper abdomen to the abdominal part of the esophagus (lymph may drain to the *inferior* phrenic lymph nodes as well as the celiac nodes). The "watershed" area for these two flow directions lies at the approximate midpoint of the thoracic esophagus, whose upper part may also drain to tracheal lymph nodes.

- The *abdominal part* of the esophagus, like the stomach, drains to the celiac lymph nodes (not shown here). Thus, when the flow direction in these lowest esophageal lymph nodes is reversed (a simple change of body posture or intracavitary pressure change due to breathing or bearing down can alter the direction of lymph flow), lymph from the stomach (which may bear malignant cells from gastric carcinoma) can reflux across the diaphragm and enter the thoracic nodes.

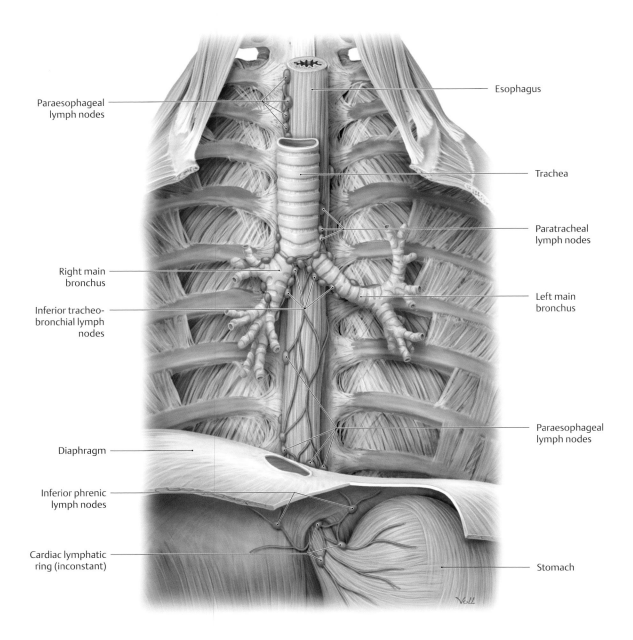

Paraesophageal lymph nodes

Esophagus

Trachea

Paratracheal lymph nodes

Right main bronchus

Inferior tracheo-bronchial lymph nodes

Left main bronchus

Paraesophageal lymph nodes

Diaphragm

Inferior phrenic lymph nodes

Cardiac lymphatic ring (inconstant)

Stomach

B Lymph nodes of the esophagus

Anterior view of the opened thorax. All thoracic organs, with the exception of a portion of the trachea, the main bronchi, and the esophagus have been removed. Part of the abdomen is shown, and the stomach has been retracted slightly downward. A portion of the diaphragm has been excised to display the esophageal hiatus. The esophagus is covered by a network of fine lymphatic vessels that carry lymph to the paraesophageal lymph nodes. Lymph from the paraesophageal nodes drains to collecting nodes or directly into the jugular trunk or the right and left bronchomediastinal trunks (see **A**). Esophageal lymphatics near the tracheal bifurcation also communicate with the (inferior) tracheobronchial lymph nodes. Lymphatic vessels descend with the esophagus through the esophageal hiatus, and they may connect at the abdominal level with the inconstant cardiac lymphatic ring that surrounds the cardiac orifice of the stomach (drains to the celiac lymph nodes). The esophageal lymph nodes at this level may also connect with the lymph nodes on the inferior surface of the diaphragm (*inferior* phrenic lymph nodes). *Note:* The paraesophageal lymph nodes are classified as a subgroup of the mediastinal lymph nodes (see also p. 129).

4.5 Lymphatic Drainage of the Trachea, Bronchial Tree, and Lungs

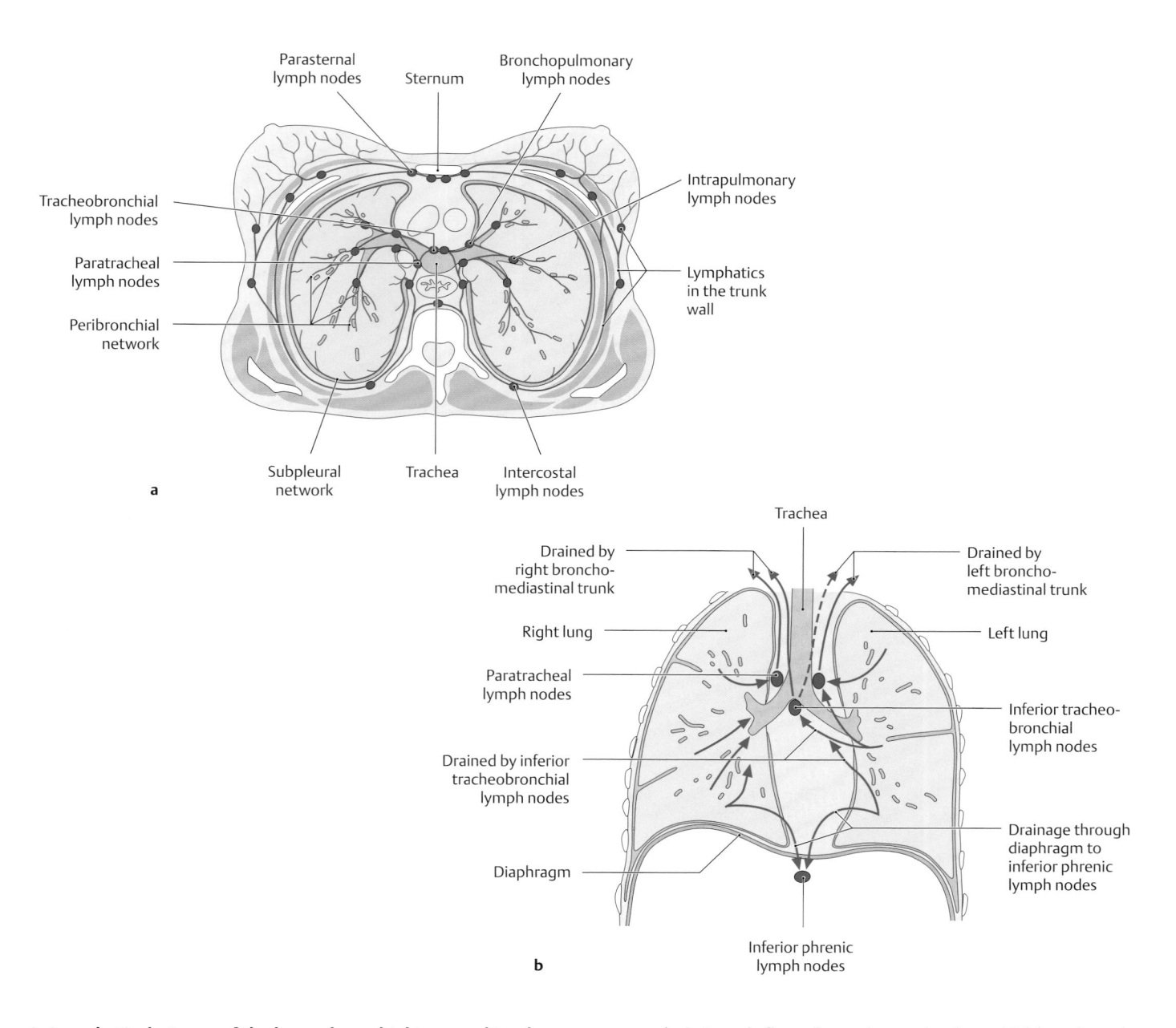

A Lymphatic drainage of the lungs, bronchial tree, and trachea

a, b Transverse and coronal sections viewed from above (**a**) and from the front (**b**). The lymphatic drainage of the lungs and bronchi is handled by two separate networks of delicate lymphatic vessels (see **b**):

- The *peribronchial network* follows the branching pattern of the bronchial tree (see p. 82) and collects lymph from the bronchi and most of the lungs.
- The *subpleural network* (smaller) bordering the lungs collects lymph from peripheral lung areas and from the *visceral* pleura. The parietal pleura (part of the chest wall!) is drained by the intercostal and parasternal lymph nodes of the chest wall.

These two networks communicate at the pulmonary hilum and convey lymph *cranially*, ultimately to the tracheobronchial lymph nodes (deep tissue areas may drain to the intrapulmonary or bronchopulmonary nodes, but the lung as a whole is drained by the tracheobronchial

nodes). Lymph flows from the tracheobronchial lymph nodes to the paratracheal nodes and bronchomediastinal trunks, which terminate at the junction of the subclavian and internal jugular veins independently or after joining the thoracic duct or right lymphatic duct.

Note: Lymph from the *left* lower lobe may also drain to the right bronchomediastinal trunk via (inferior) tracheobronchial lymph nodes. The lower lobes of *both* lungs may drain cranially, but they may also drain inferiorly to the superior phrenic lymph nodes or may drain through the diaphragm to the inferior phrenic nodes.

The **trachea** drains to the paratracheal lymph nodes, which may empty directly into the jugular trunk or indirectly via the bronchomediastinal lymph nodes.

Note: Tracheobronchial lymph nodes that lie very close to the pulmonary hilum are known in clinical parlance as the "hilar lymph nodes." Their enlargement in response to pathological processes may be detectable by imaging studies.

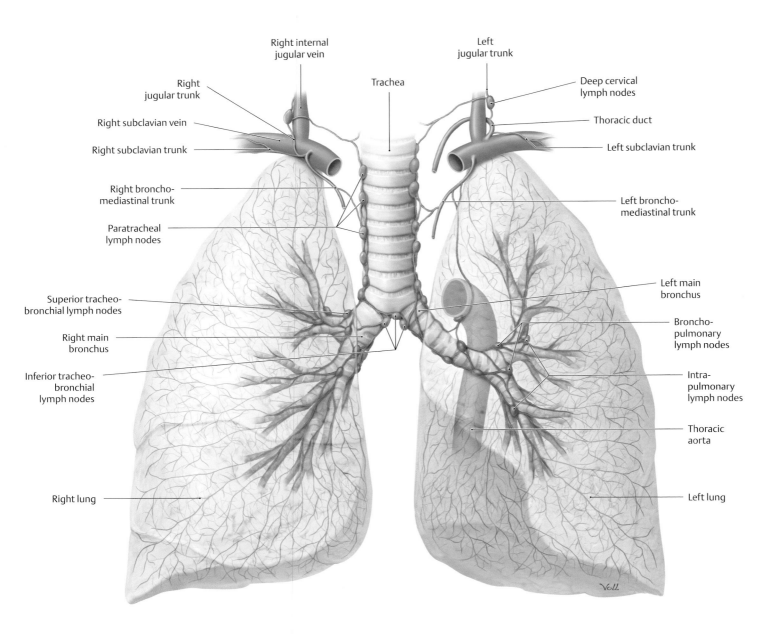

Right internal
jugular vein

Left
jugular trunk

Trachea

Right
jugular trunk

Deep cervical
lymph nodes

Right subclavian vein

Thoracic duct

Right subclavian trunk

Left subclavian trunk

Right broncho-
mediastinal trunk

Left broncho-
mediastinal trunk

Paratracheal
lymph nodes

Left main
bronchus

Superior tracheo-
bronchial lymph nodes

Broncho-
pulmonary
lymph nodes

Right main
bronchus

Intra-
pulmonary
lymph nodes

Inferior tracheo-
bronchial
lymph nodes

Thoracic
aorta

Right lung

Left lung

B Lymph nodes of the trachea, bronchi, and lungs
Anterior view. The following lymph nodes can be distinguished inside
and outside the lungs, listed in order from deep to superficial (see **A**):

- Inside the lung: intrapulmonary lymph nodes in the lung tissue and
  at the divisions of the segmental bronchi; bronchopulmonary lymph
  nodes at the division of the lobar bronchi.

- Outside the lung: inferior and superior tracheobronchial lymph nodes
  at the tracheal bifurcation and on both main bronchi; paratracheal
  lymph nodes along both sides of the trachea.

4.6 Lymphatic Drainage of the Diaphragm, Heart, and Pericardium

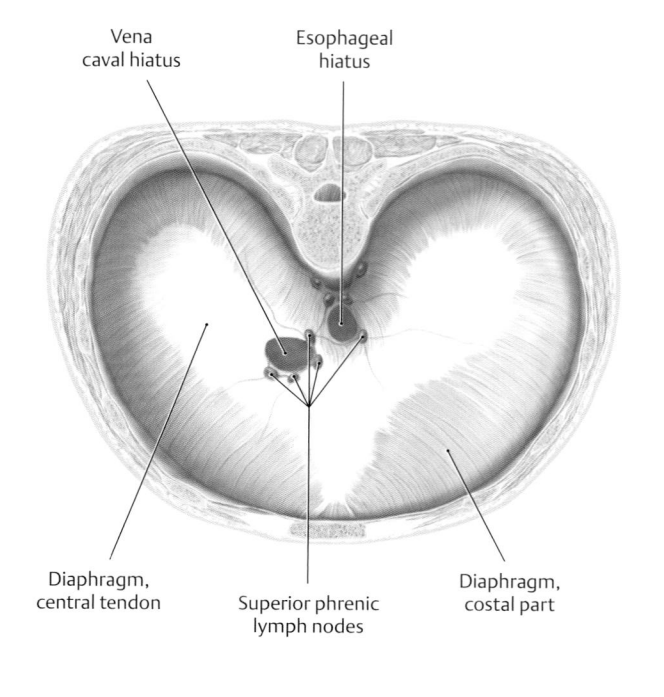

Vena caval hiatus

Esophageal hiatus

Diaphragm, central tendon

Superior phrenic lymph nodes

Diaphragm, costal part

A Lymph nodes and lymphatic drainage of the diaphragm
Superior view. The lymph nodes of the diaphragm are divided into two groups based on their location:

- Superior phrenic lymph nodes on the superior surface of the diaphragm
- Inferior phrenic lymph nodes on the inferior surface of the diaphragm (not shown here, see pp. 297 and 302)

The **superior phrenic lymph nodes**, then, are *thoracic* lymph nodes that collect lymph from the diaphragm, lower esophagus (see p. 134), lung, and also from the liver (by a transdiaphragmatic route, see p. 129). The superior lymph nodes on the right side are involved in hepatic drainage. The superior lymph nodes drain to the bronchomediastinal trunk. The **inferior phrenic lymph nodes** are *abdominal* lymph nodes; they collect lymph from the diaphragm and usually convey it to a lumbar trunk (see p. 297). They may also collect lymph from the lower lobes of the lungs (see p. 136).

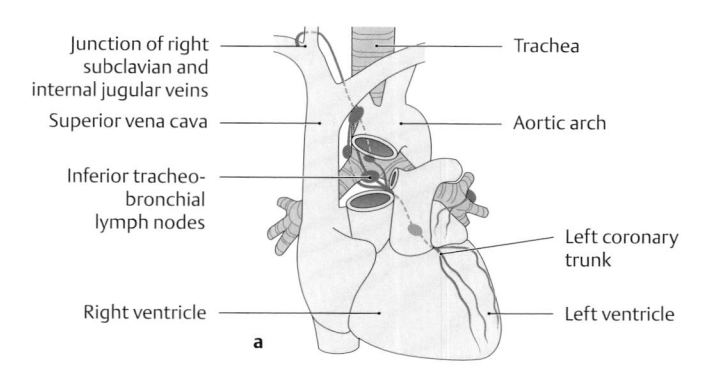

Junction of right subclavian and internal jugular veins

Superior vena cava

Inferior tracheo-bronchial lymph nodes

Right ventricle

Trachea

Aortic arch

Left coronary trunk

Left ventricle

a

B Lymphatic drainage of the heart (after Földi and Kubik)
The heart viewed from the anterior aspect (**a**, **b**) and posterior aspect (**c**).
The **lymphatic drainage of the ventricles (and part of the atria)** can be roughly divided into two regions (see **a** and **b**):

- The *left region* (**a**) encompasses the left ventricle, a small strip of the right ventricle, and portions of the left atrium. It conveys its lymph through a "left coronary trunk" to the inferior tracheobronchial lymph nodes, which drain to the junction of the right subclavian and internal jugular veins (directly or via the right bronchomediastinal trunk).
- The *right region* (**b**) mainly encompasses the right ventricle and portions of the right atrium. It conveys its lymph through a "right coronary trunk" along the ascending aorta and then to the junction of the left subclavian and internal jugular veins.

This arrangement creates two "crossed" pathways for lymphatic drainage:

- Right region → "right coronary trunk" → junction of the left subclavian and internal jugular veins
- Left region → "left coronary trunk" → junction of the right subclavian and internal jugular veins

Lymphatic drainage of the rest of the atria: Portions of the atria that are outside the above region drain to the inferior tracheobronchial lymph nodes or to the ipsilateral bronchopulmonary lymph nodes and thence to the bronchomediastinal trunks.

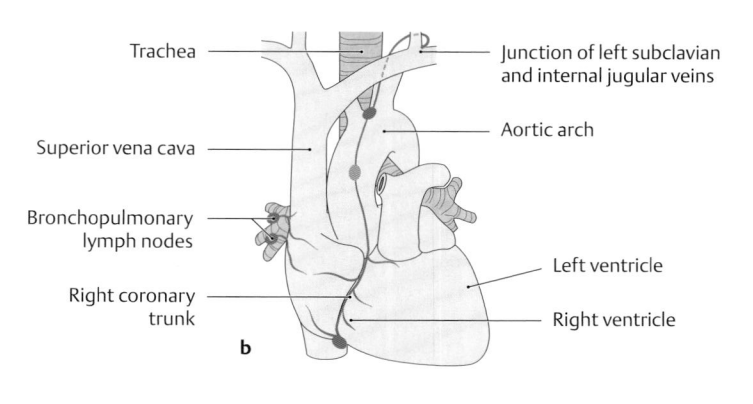

Trachea

Junction of left subclavian and internal jugular veins

Aortic arch

Superior vena cava

Bronchopulmonary lymph nodes

Right coronary trunk

Left ventricle

Right ventricle

b

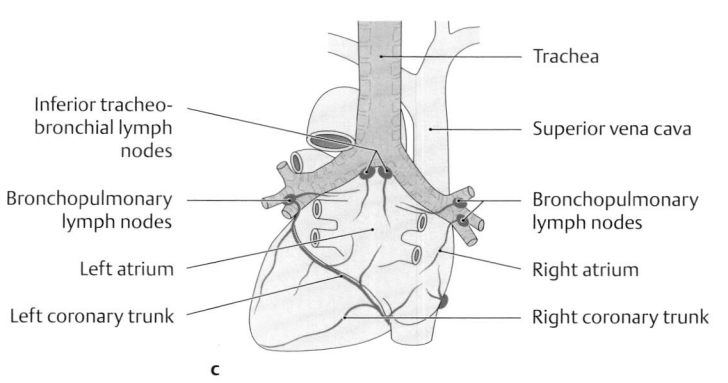

Inferior tracheo-bronchial lymph nodes

Bronchopulmonary lymph nodes

Left atrium

Left coronary trunk

Trachea

Superior vena cava

Bronchopulmonary lymph nodes

Right atrium

Right coronary trunk

c

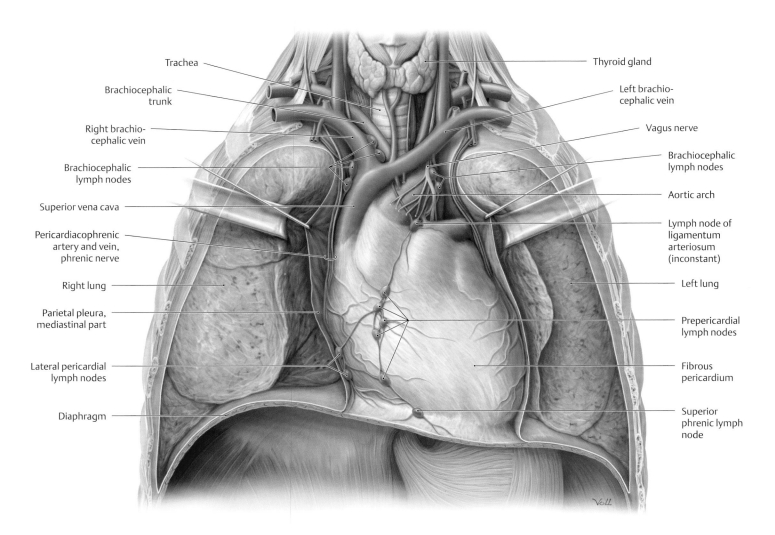

Trachea

Brachiocephalic trunk

Right brachio-cephalic vein

Brachiocephalic lymph nodes

Superior vena cava

Pericardiacophrenic artery and vein, phrenic nerve

Right lung

Parietal pleura, mediastinal part

Lateral pericardial lymph nodes

Diaphragm

Thyroid gland

Left brachio-cephalic vein

Vagus nerve

Brachiocephalic lymph nodes

Aortic arch

Lymph node of ligamentum arteriosum (inconstant)

Left lung

Prepericardial lymph nodes

Fibrous pericardium

Superior phrenic lymph node

C Lymph nodes and lymphatic drainage of the pericardium
Anterior view of the opened thorax. The pleural cavities have been opened, and the lungs and pleura have been retracted laterally. Lymph node groups of varying size (prepericardial and lateral pericardial lymph nodes) lie anterior and adjacent to the pericardium and are interconnected by a network of fine lymphatic vessels. These pericardial lymph nodes may drain inferiorly (to the superior phrenic lymph nodes) or cranially (usually to the brachiocephalic lymph nodes). Lymph from the pericardial lymph nodes is ultimately conveyed to the bronchomediastinal trunks (see p. 129), which open at the junction of the right or left subclavian and internal jugular veins.

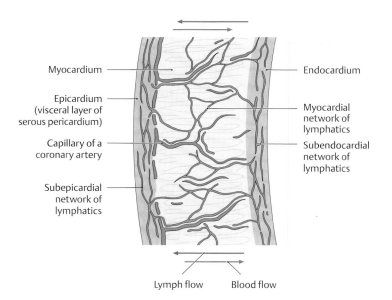

Myocardium

Epicardium (visceral layer of serous pericardium)

Capillary of a coronary artery

Subepicardial network of lymphatics

Endocardium

Myocardial network of lymphatics

Subendocardial network of lymphatics

Lymph flow   Blood flow

D Lymphatic drainage of the heart wall (after Földi and Kubik)
Section through the heart wall. There are three networks of densely interconnected lymphatic vessels, corresponding to the three layers of the heart wall:

• Epicardium (= visceral layer of the serous pericardium): A subepicardial network collects lymph from the epicardium and from the other two networks. The subepicardial network conveys the lymph to the collecting vessels and lymph nodes of the heart.
• Myocardium: The very extensive myocardial network collects lymph from the myocardium and also from the subendocardial network. Lymphatic vessels of the myocardial network often follow the distribution of the blood capillaries that arise from the coronary arteries. Thus the blood (red arrows) and lymph (green arrows) flow in opposite directions.
• Endocardium: A subepicardial network collects lymph from the endocardium and conveys it to the subendocardial network, either directly or via the myocardial network.

139

5.1　Overview of Thoracic Innervation

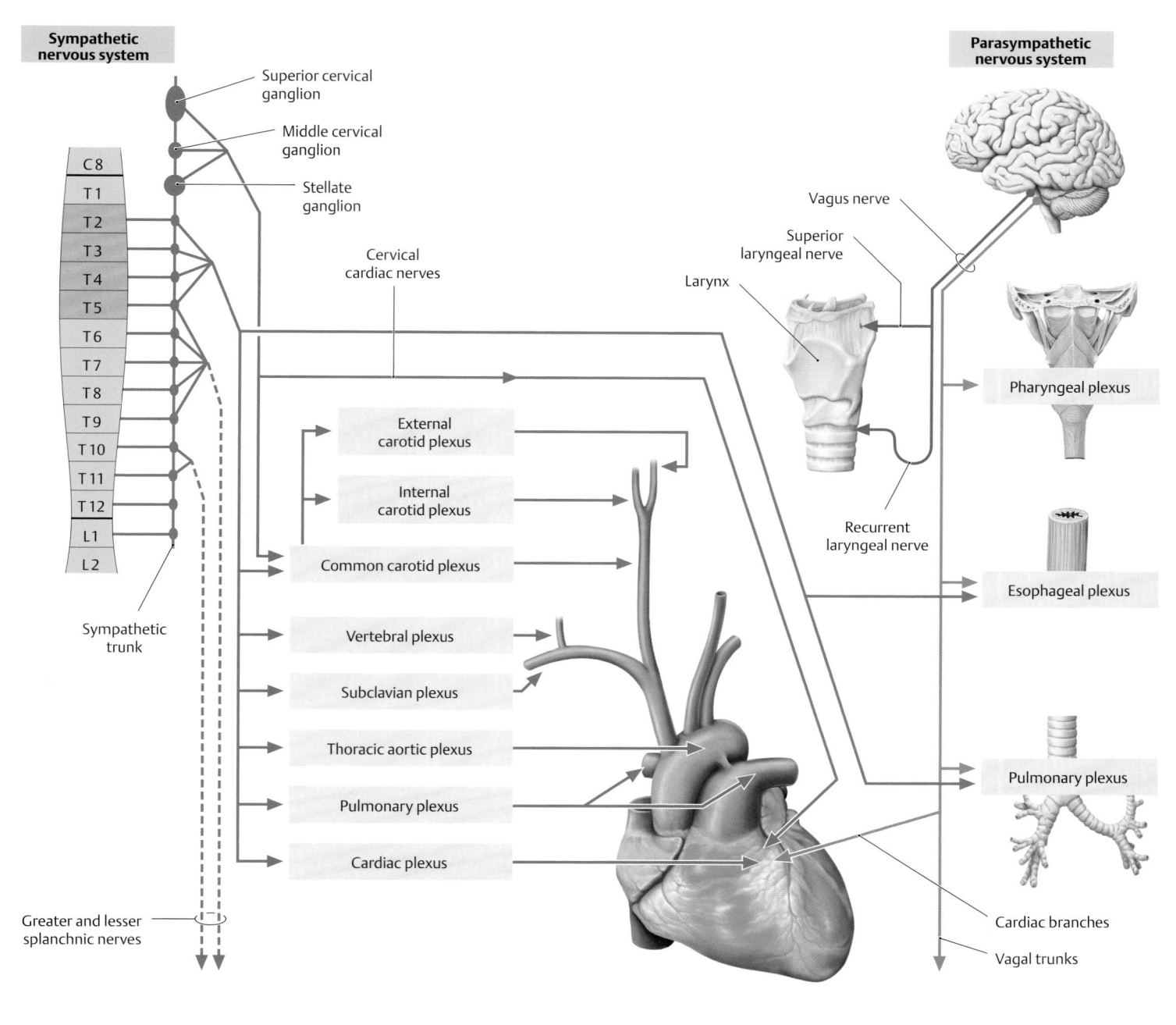

A　Organization of the sympathetic and parasympathetic nervous systems in the thorax

With the prominent exceptions of the phrenic nerve (pp. 146–147) and intercostal nerves (**B**), thoracic innervation is largely autonomic, arising from either the paravertebral sympathetic trunks or the parasympathetic vagus nerves.

Sympathetic organization: The peripheral sympathetic system consists of a two-neuron relay, with presynaptic (preganglionic) fibers arising from neurons in the spinal cord. These axons synapse onto neurons in the paired paravertebral sympathetic ganglia, which send axons to innervate the thoracic viscera and blood vessels.

The cell bodies of the presynaptic motor neurons are located in the lateral horns of the thoracolumbar spinal cord (T 1 to L 2); the neurons involved in sympathetic innervation of the thorax are concentrated in upper thoracic levels. Axons from the paravertebral ganglion cells (postsynaptic [postganglionic] fibers) follow several courses: some fibers follow intercostal nerves to innervate blood vessels and glands in the chest wall; others accompany arteries to visceral targets; other groups of postganglionic axons gather in the greater and lesser splanchnic nerves

and enter the abdomen (see p. 306).

Parasympathetic organization: The peripheral parasympathetic nervous system has a similar two-neuron relay, but its presynaptic neurons are in the brainstem and the ganglion cells are scattered in microscopic groups in their target organs. The vagus nerve (CN X) carries presynaptic parasympathetic motor axons from brainstem neurons into the thorax and gives off the following branches:

- Cardiac branches to the cardiac plexus (heart, see pp. 144 and 145)
- Esophageal branches to the esophageal plexus (esophagus, see p. 143)
- Tracheal branches (trachea, see p. 142); bronchial branches to the pulmonary plexus (bronchi, pulmonary vessels see p. 142)

The vagus nerves continue beyond these branches, following the esophagus into the abdomen (see p. 307).

Note: The vagus nerve also carries visceral sensory axons (mostly pressure sensation) for thoracic organs. The sensory neuron cell bodies are in the inferior vagal ganglion (nodose) (see p. 19); the first synapse in this sensory pathway is in the brainstem.

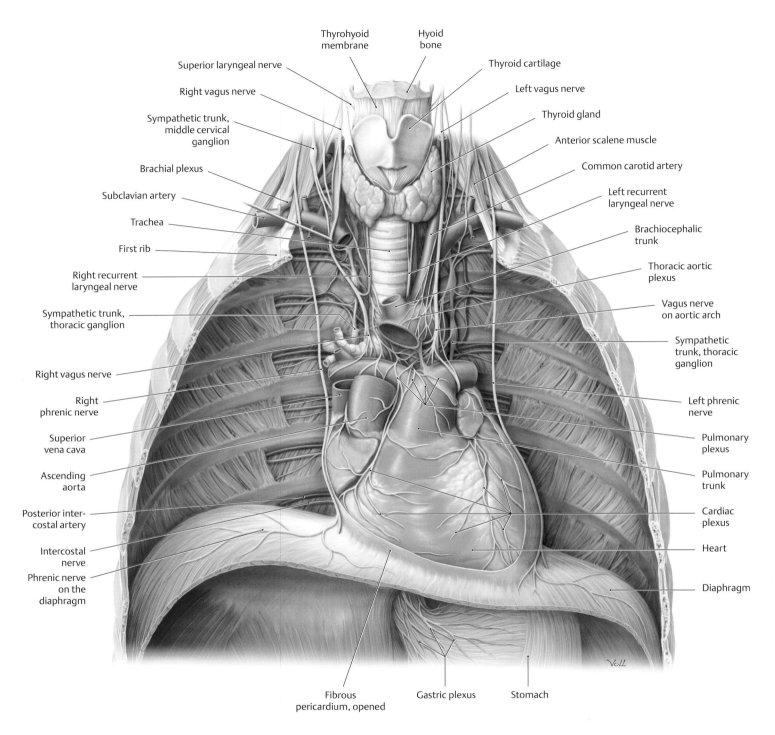

Thyrohyoid membrane

Hyoid bone

Superior laryngeal nerve

Thyroid cartilage

Right vagus nerve

Left vagus nerve

Sympathetic trunk, middle cervical ganglion

Thyroid gland

Anterior scalene muscle

Brachial plexus

Common carotid artery

Subclavian artery

Left recurrent laryngeal nerve

Trachea

Brachiocephalic trunk

First rib

Right recurrent laryngeal nerve

Thoracic aortic plexus

Sympathetic trunk, thoracic ganglion

Vagus nerve on aortic arch

Right vagus nerve

Sympathetic trunk, thoracic ganglion

Right phrenic nerve

Left phrenic nerve

Superior vena cava

Pulmonary plexus

Ascending aorta

Pulmonary trunk

Posterior inter-costal artery

Cardiac plexus

Intercostal nerve

Heart

Phrenic nerve on the diaphragm

Diaphragm

Fibrous pericardium, opened

Gastric plexus

Stomach

D Autonomic nerves of the heart

Anterior view of the opened thorax with the lungs, pleura, and internal fasciae removed. The pericardium has been broadly opened anteriorly. The vessels surrounding the heart are intact except for a portion of the ascending aorta, which has been removed to display the right pulmonary artery. Part of the upper abdomen is also shown. The cardiac plexus, pulmonary plexus, and thoracic aortic plexus can be clearly identified on the heart and surrounding vessels. These plexuses receive fibers from the vagus nerves and sympathetic trunk. The **right and left vagus nerves** initially run in the anterior part of the superior mediasti-

num. After giving off branches to the plexuses, they enter the posterior mediastinum (see **A**). **Sympathetic fibers** pass to the cardiac plexus in the form of the cervical cardiac nerves (from the three cervical ganglia) and thoracic cardiac branches (from the thoracic ganglia) (see **A**).
Note: Most of the autonomic fibers in the plexuses are extremely fine, but in this dissection they are shown larger for clarity. The phrenic nerve does not innervate the heart but does give off somatosensory branches to the pericardium (pericardial branches, not shown here) in the middle mediastinum on its way to the diaphragm (see p. 146).

5.4 Innervation of the Pericardium and Diaphragm

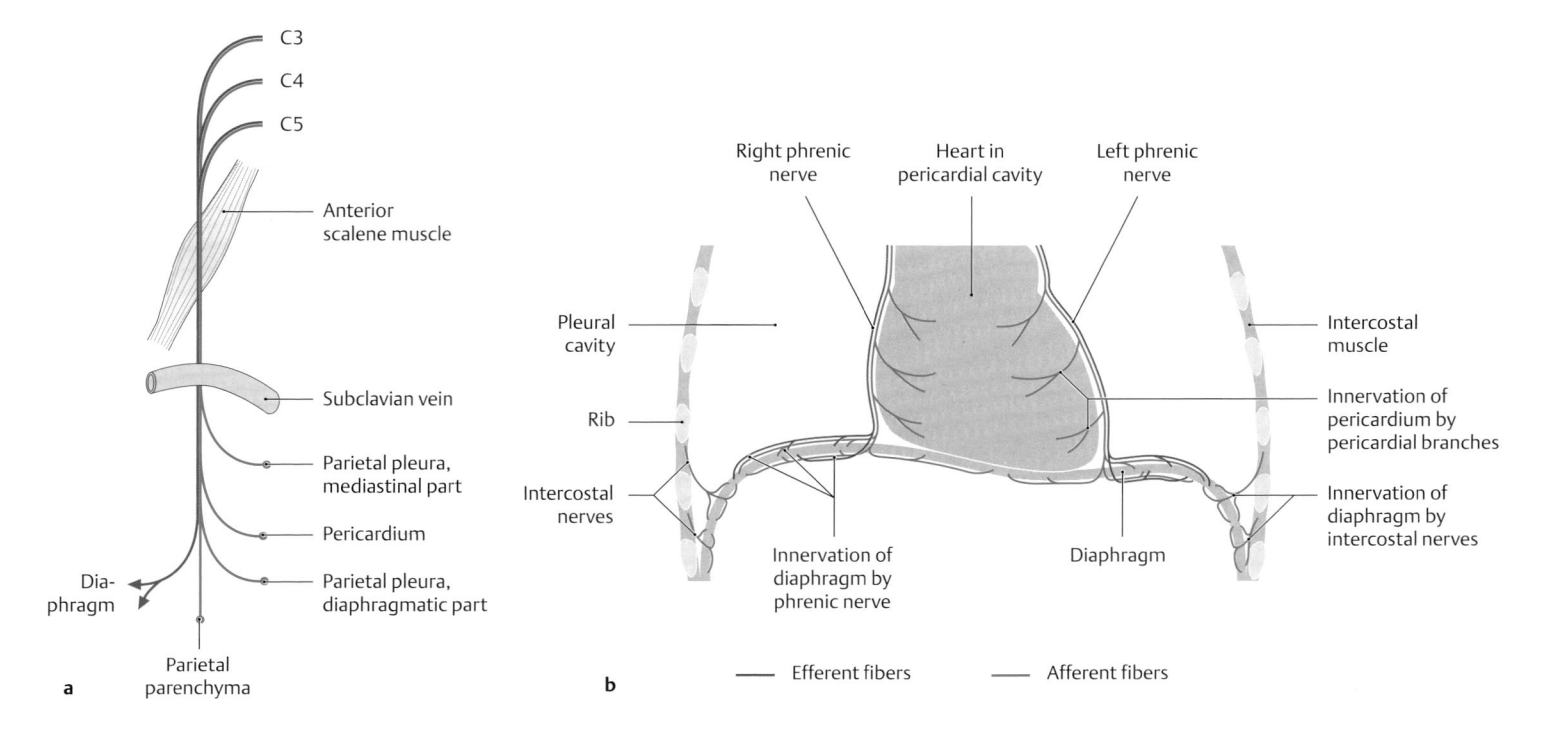

a

C3
C4
C5

Anterior scalene muscle

Subclavian vein

Parietal pleura, mediastinal part

Pericardium

Dia-phragm

Parietal pleura, diaphragmatic part

Parietal parenchyma

b

Right phrenic nerve

Heart in pericardial cavity

Left phrenic nerve

Pleural cavity

Rib

Intercostal nerves

Innervation of diaphragm by phrenic nerve

Diaphragm

Intercostal muscle

Innervation of pericardium by pericardial branches

Innervation of diaphragm by intercostal nerves

—— Efferent fibers   —— Afferent fibers

A Innervation of the diaphragm and pericardium

The diaphragm and pericardium are supplied by the phrenic nerve, a somatomotor and somatosensory spinal nerve that arises from the cervical plexus, specifically from the C1–C4 spinal cord segments (mainly C4, see **a**). The phrenic nerve descends to the diaphragm while giving off branches to the mediastinal pleura and pericardium (pericardial branches). It contains both efferent (motor) and afferent (sensory) fibers, the latter being responsible for pain conduction from the serous membranes that cover the diaphragm. A phrenicoabdominal branch passes through the diaphragm to the peritoneum on its inferior surface.

Sensory distribution:
- Fibrous pericardium and the parietal layer of the serous pericardium
- Large portions of the diaphragmatic part of the parietal pleura
- Portions of the mediastinal part of the parietal pleura

- The parietal peritoneum on the inferior surface of the diaphragm
- The peritoneum covering the inferior diaphragmatic surface.

Motor distribution: diaphragm.

Areas of the diaphragm near the ribs also receive somatosensory innervation from the tenth and eleventh intercostal nerves (see **b**) and from the subcostal nerve (T12, not visible). An accessory phrenic nerve (not shown here) is occasionally observed as fibers from C5 (C6) join with the phrenic nerve via the subclavian nerve. The *blood vessels* of the diaphragm and pericardium receive autonomic innervation like other vessels.

Note: Bilateral disruption of the phrenic nerve (e.g., due to a high transection of the cervical spinal cord) leads to bilateral paralysis of the diaphragm. Because the diaphragm is the dominant muscle of respiration, bilateral diaphragmatic paralysis is usually fatal.

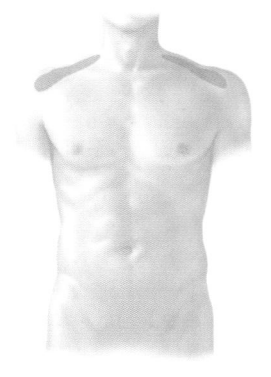

B Referred pain from the diaphragm

As with other thoracic viscera, pain caused by trauma or pathology of the diaphragm may not be localized to the site of injury but may seem to be originating at different locations, a phenomenon called "referred pain." This is easily understood for the diaphragm, whose sensory innervation from the phrenic nerve is associated with mid-cervical levels of the spinal cord, where the phrenic nerve originates from branches of the cervical plexus. Diaphragmatic pain is thus referred to cutaneous areas at those cervical levels, specifically to the anterior aspect of the shoulder girdles. These areas, and others associated with referred pain from different visceral organs, are known as *Head zones* or lines (from Henry Head (1860–1941), British neurologist). Because the phrenic nerve provides sensory innervation to the parietal peritoneum under the diaphragm, and because of the proximity of the gallbladder to the diaphragm on the right side, gallbladder inflammation may thus cause pain that seems to come from the right shoulder girdle.

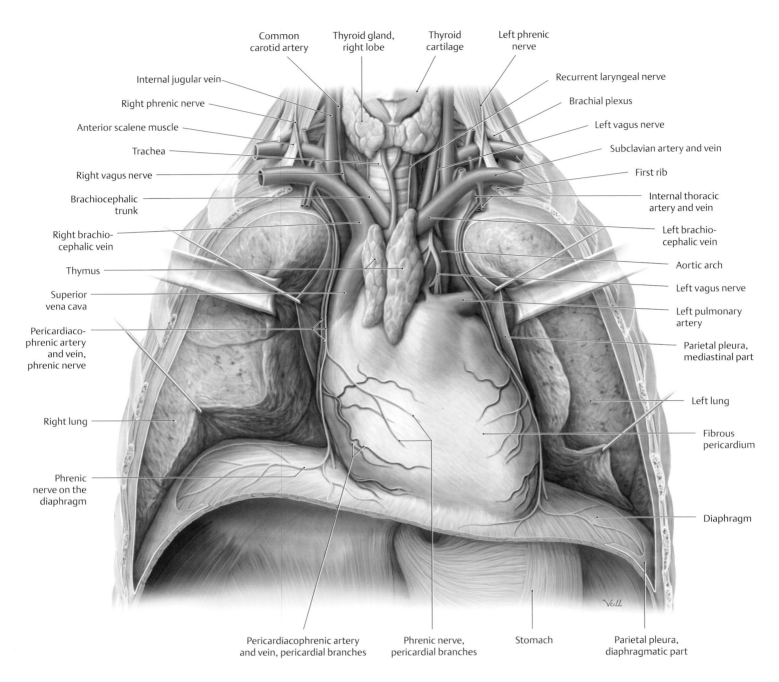

Common carotid artery
Thyroid gland, right lobe
Thyroid cartilage
Left phrenic nerve
Internal jugular vein
Right phrenic nerve
Anterior scalene muscle
Trachea
Right vagus nerve
Brachiocephalic trunk
Right brachio-cephalic vein
Thymus
Superior vena cava
Pericardiaco-phrenic artery and vein, phrenic nerve
Right lung
Phrenic nerve on the diaphragm

Recurrent laryngeal nerve
Brachial plexus
Left vagus nerve
Subclavian artery and vein
First rib
Internal thoracic artery and vein
Left brachio-cephalic vein
Aortic arch
Left vagus nerve
Left pulmonary artery
Parietal pleura, mediastinal part
Left lung
Fibrous pericardium
Diaphragm

Pericardiacophrenic artery and vein, pericardial branches
Phrenic nerve, pericardial branches
Stomach
Parietal pleura, diaphragmatic part

C Course of the phrenic nerve in the thorax

Anterior view. The pleural cavities have been opened and the lungs have been retracted laterally. When the chest is opened from the front, the right and left phrenic nerves can be seen at once in the superior and middle mediastinum because of their anterior location. The paired phrenic nerves initially course on the anterior scalene muscle. The nerve then passes anterior to the subclavian artery and posterior to the subclavian vein to the thoracic inlet on each side. The phrenic nerve is joined in the chest by the pericardiacophrenic artery and vein from the internal thoracic artery and vein. This neurovascular bundle runs close to the superior vena cava on the right side and close to the aortic arch on the left side before passing directly to the surface of the fibrous pericardium, where it gives off pericardial branches. It thus descends in the potential space between the pericardium and mediastinal pleura. As a spinal nerve, the phrenic nerve contains both sensory and motor fibers.

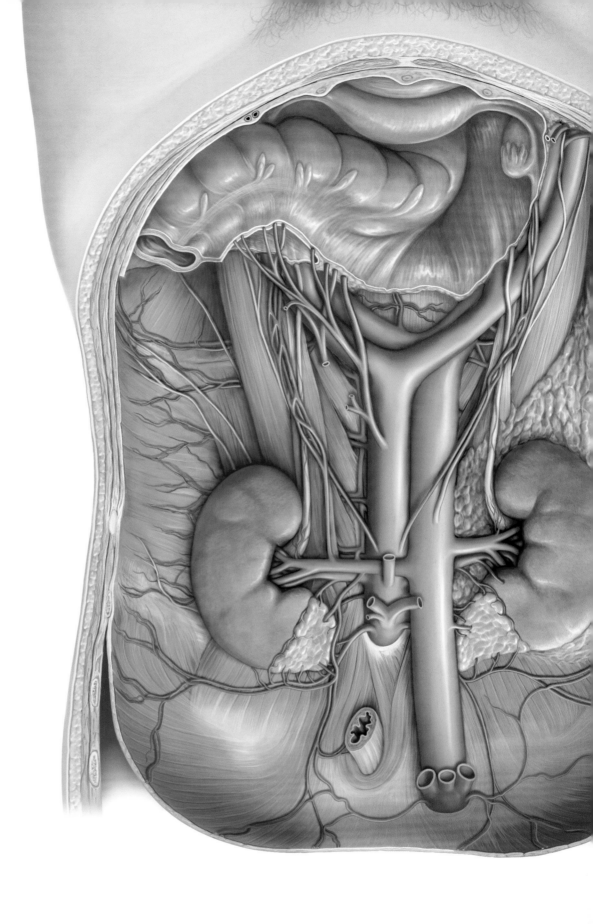

Abdomen and Pelvis

1.1 Location of the Abdominal and Pelvic Organs and their Projection onto the Trunk Wall

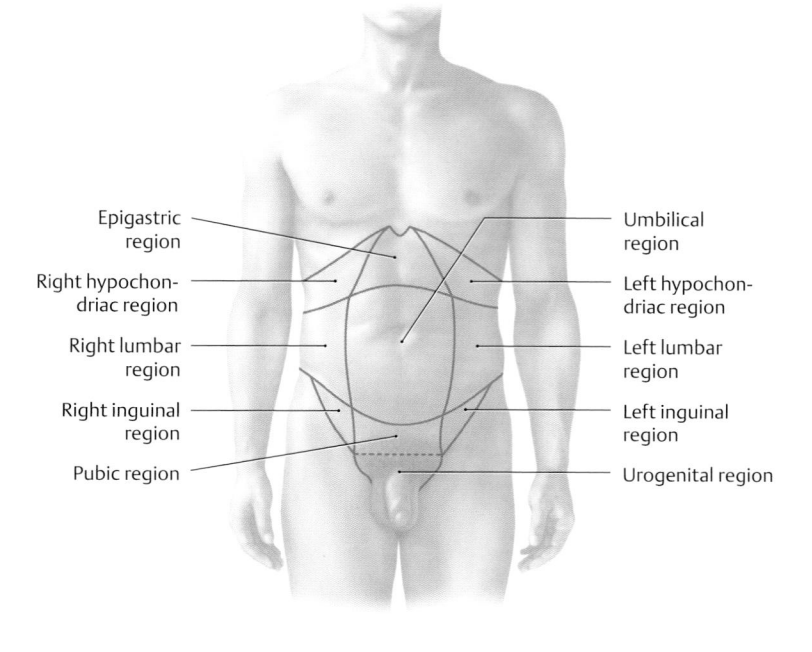

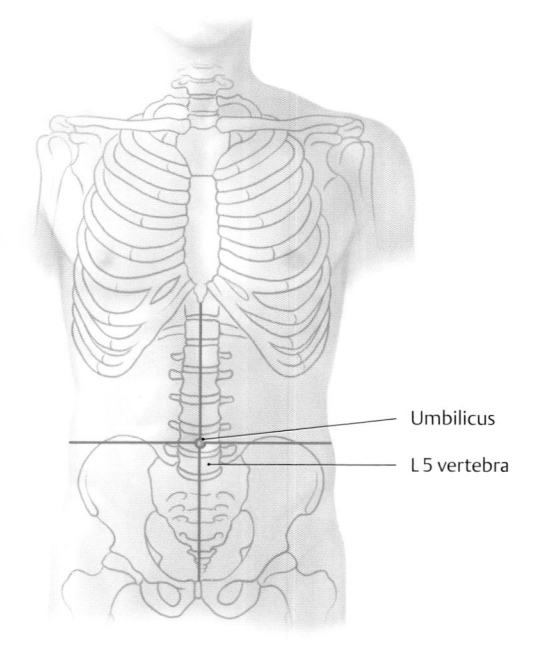

A Regions of the anterior trunk wall

Three levels can be identified on the abdominal wall from above downward: the epigastrium, mesogastrium, and hypogastrium. Each level consists of three regions:

- The median region of the epigastrium is the *epigastric region*. It is flanked laterally by the right and left hypochondriac regions.
- The median region of the mesogastrium is the *umbilical region*, which is bounded laterally by the right and left lumbar regions.
- The median region of the hypogastrium is the *pubic region*, which is flanked by the right and left inguinal regions. The pubic region is bounded inferiorly by the *urogenital region*.

The levels of the abdomen are defined by horizontal planes that are determined by palpable bony landmarks (see **C**).

B Quadrants of the anterior trunk wall

The quadrants of the anterior trunk wall are centered on the umbilicus, which lies at the level of the L 3–4 vertebral body and are named right and left upper and lower quadrant (RUQ, LUQ, RLQ, LLQ).

C Horizontal (transverse) planes in the anterior trunk wall

The anterior trunk wall is divided transversely by the following imaginary planes of section:

- **Xiphosternal plane:** passes through the synchondrosis between the *xiphoid* process and body of the *sternum*.
- **Transpyloric plane:** plane midway between the jugular notch of the sternum and the superior border of the pubic symphysis. Located at the level of the L 1 vertebra, it divides the anterior trunk wall into upper and lower halves. The pylorus of the stomach is generally located slightly *below* this plane.
- **Subcostal plane:** passes through the *lowest points of the costal arch* of the tenth rib at the level of the L 3 vertebral body. It marks the boundary between the epigastrium and mesogastrium (see **A**).
- **Supracristal plane:** passes through the junction of the L 4 vertebra, connecting the *highest points on the iliac crests*.
- **Intertubercular plane:** connects the *iliac tubercles* and passes through the L 5 vertebral body. The intertubercular plane marks the boundary between the mesogastrium and hypogastrium.
- **Interspinal plane:** connects the two *anterior superior iliac spines*.

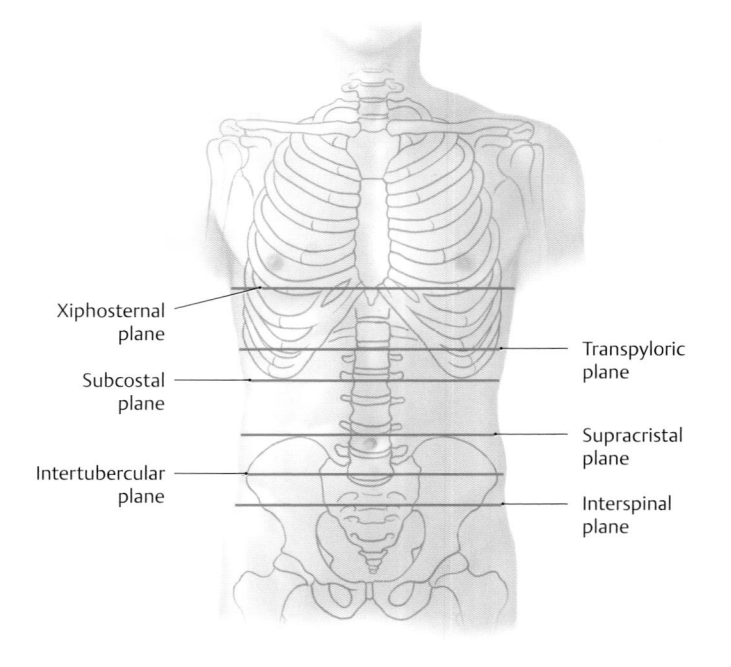

Note: The three upper planes are variable in their location, which depends on the position and shape of the thoracic cage. The key variables are respiratory position, age, sex, and constitutional type.

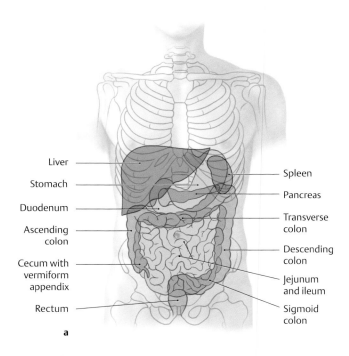

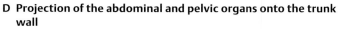

a

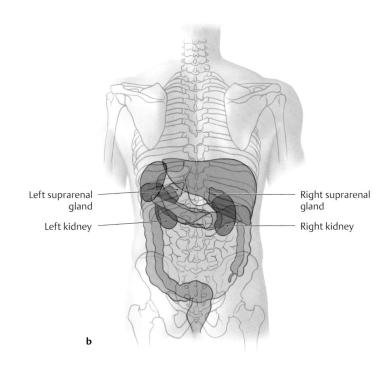

b

D Projection of the abdominal and pelvic organs onto the trunk wall

a Anterior trunk wall, **b** posterior trunk wall.

The surface projection of organs on the trunk wall depends on body posture, age, constitutional type, sex, nutritional state, and respiratory position. *Note* the overlap of the abdominal and thoracic cavities: Perforating injuries of the abdominal cavity that involve the liver, for example, may also involve the pleural cavity ("multicavity injury"). The projections of individual organs are shown in **E**.

E Projection of anatomical structures in the abdomen and pelvis onto the vertebral column

The spinal notation refers to vertebral bodies.

T 7	Superior border of the liver
T 12	Aortic hiatus
L 1	• Transpyloric plane (generally the pylorus is at or below this plane) • Gallbladder fundus • Renal hilum • Superior part of the duodenum • Pancreas (neck) • Origin of the celiac trunk • Origin of the superior mesenteric artery • Attachment of the transverse mesocolon • Spleen (hilum)
L 1 / L 2	Origin of the renal arteries
L 2	Duodenojejunal flexure
L 3	Origin of the inferior mesenteric artery
L 3 / L 4	Umbilicus
L 4	Aortic bifurcation
L 5	Origin of the inferior vena cava from the common iliac veins
S 3	Upper (cranial) border of the rectum

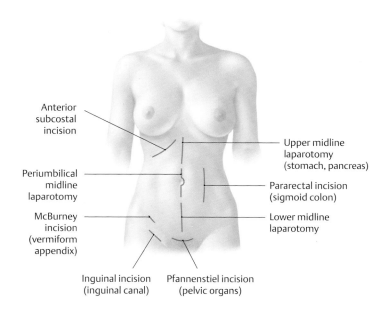

F Placement of surgical skin incisions in the anterior abdominal wall

Note: The periumbilical midline incision passes around the *left* side of the umbilicus to avoid cutting the remnant of the umbilical vein on the *right* side (the ligamentum teres of the liver, see p. 155). This umbilical vein remnant is generally but not always obliterated, and injury to the vessel, if it is still patent, may cause significant bleeding.

The McBurney incision is also called the *gridiron incision* because it changes direction in different planes of the trunk wall. The muscles of the trunk wall can be divided less traumatically by tailoring the direction of the cut to the prevailing fiber direction of the various muscle layers.

1.2   Divisions of the Abdominal and Pelvic Cavities

The organs of the abdomen and pelvis can be classified according to various topographical criteria:

- By layers in the anteroposterior direction (**A**)
- By levels in the craniocaudal direction (**B**)
- As intra- or extraperitoneal based on their peritoneal investment (**C, D**)

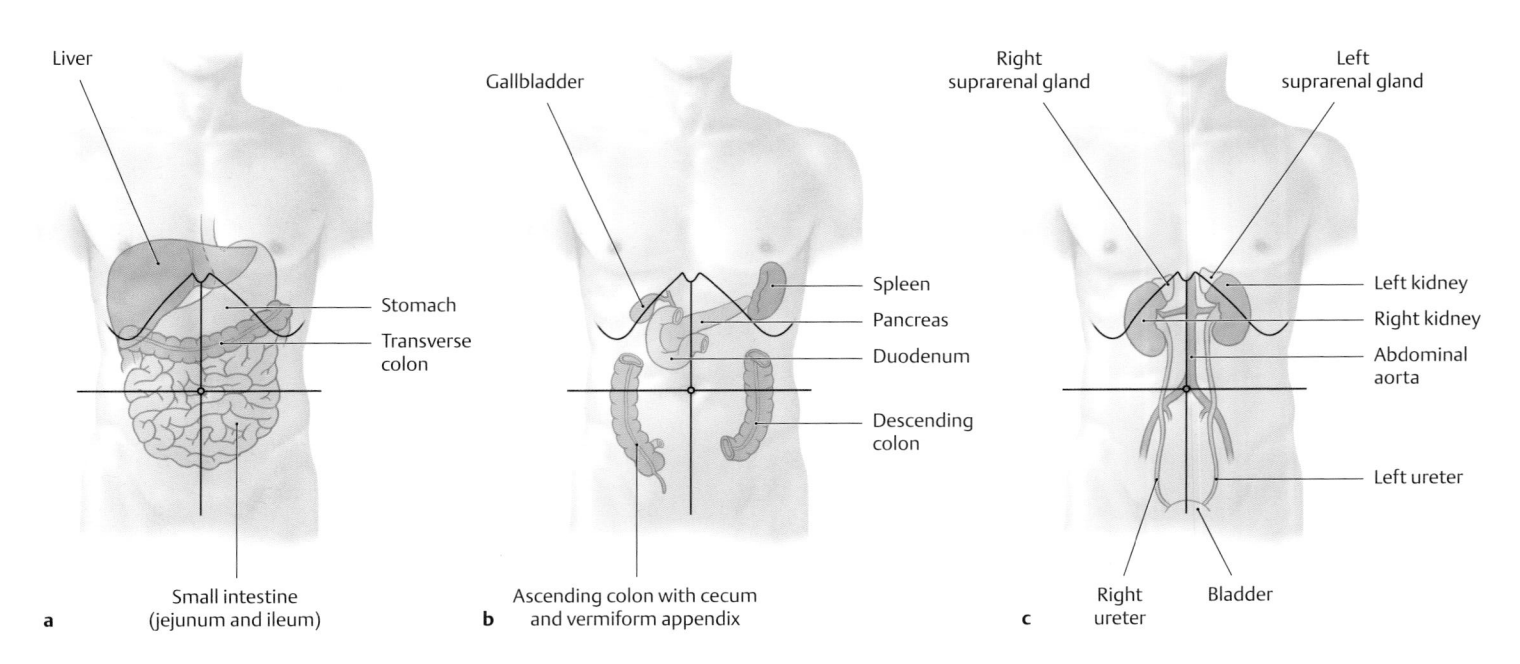

a Liver — Stomach — Transverse colon — Small intestine (jejunum and ileum)

b Gallbladder — Spleen — Pancreas — Duodenum — Descending colon — Ascending colon with cecum and vermiform appendix

c Right suprarenal gland — Left suprarenal gland — Left kidney — Right kidney — Abdominal aorta — Left ureter — Right ureter — Bladder

A Classification of the abdominal and pelvic organs by layers
The abdominal and pelvic organs can be roughly divided into three layers in the anteroposterior direction. This classification is particularly useful from a surgical standpoint.
Note: Larger organs may occupy more than one layer (see p. 154).

a Anterior layer: liver, transverse colon, jejunum, ileum, and bladder (for clarity not shown here, but shown with the other urinary organs in **c**)
b Middle layer: liver, duodenum, pancreas, spleen, ascending and descending colon, and uterus (not shown for clarity, extends into the anterior layer)
c Posterior layer: great vessels, kidneys, ureters, and suprarenal glands (for clarity, the bladder is shown in its relationship to the other urinary organs).

B Classification of the abdominal and pelvic organs by levels
In this classification the organs are roughly assigned to craniocaudal levels based on their relationship to the transverse mesocolon (upper and lower abdominal organs, see p. 159) and lesser pelvis (pelvic organs). Because the kidneys and adrenal glands are retroperitoneal, they are not listed in the table. When the kidney is projected onto the abdominal wall, its inferior pole extends into the lower abdomen.

Level	Organs located there
Upper abdomen (above the transverse mesocolon)	• Stomach • Duodenum • Liver • Gallbladder and biliary tract • Spleen • Pancreas
Lower abdomen (between the transverse mesocolon and pelvic inlet plane)	• Small intestine (excluding the duodenum) • Large intestine (excluding the rectum) *Note:* The transverse colon, while located in the upper abdomen, is classified functionally as part of the lower abdomen.
Lesser pelvis	• Bladder • Rectum • Uterus, fallopian tube, ovary, and vagina • Portions of the vas deferens, prostate, and seminal gland (the testis and epididymis are outside the pelvic cavity)

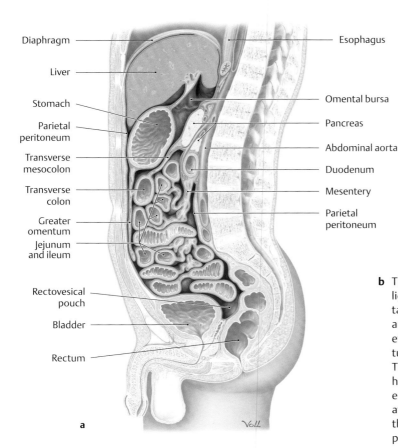

Diaphragm — Esophagus

Liver —

Stomach —

Parietal peritoneum —

Transverse mesocolon —

Transverse colon —

Greater omentum —

Jejunum and ileum —

Rectovesical pouch —

Bladder —

Rectum —

— Omental bursa

— Pancreas

— Abdominal aorta

— Duodenum

— Mesentery

— Parietal peritoneum

a

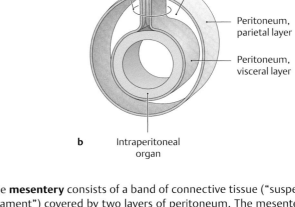

Mesentery Peritoneal cavity

— Peritoneum, parietal layer

— Peritoneum, visceral layer

b   Intraperitoneal organ

C Classification of the abdominal and pelvic organs by their relationship to the peritoneum and mesentery

a Midsagittal section (kidneys outside the sectional plane) viewed from the left side. The **peritoneum** (shown in red) divides the abdomen and pelvis into a serous cavity, the peritoneal cavity, and a connective-tissue space, the extraperitoneal space (for further subdivisions, see below; the anterolateral portions of the extraperitoneal space between the parietal and visceral peritoneum contain *no organs* and are disregarded here).

Note: Clinically, the *rectum* is sometimes subdivided into an extraperitoneal fixed rectum and an intraperitoneal mobile rectum (which may have a small mesentery). Surgical procedures on the fixed rectum are less hazardous, as they can be performed without opening the peritoneal cavity.

b The **mesentery** consists of a band of connective tissue ("suspensory ligament") covered by two layers of peritoneum. The mesentery attachment to the organ is continuous with the visceral peritoneum, and the attachment to the body wall is continuous with the parietal peritoneum. The mesentery transmits the neurovascular structures that supply the intraperitoneal organs "suspended" from it. The presence of the mesentery causes the *intraperitoneal* organs to have greater mobility than extraperitoneal organs without a mesentery. Nevertheless, the intraperitoneal organs still maintain a relatively constant position because they are attached to the wall of the peritoneal cavity. *Extraperitoneal* organs* are either embedded primarily in the connective tissue of the extraperitoneal space (primarily retroperitoneal) or they become attached secondarily to the wall of the peritoneal cavity by peritoneal fusion (secondarily retroperitoneal). It is only the flexibility of the extraperitoneal connective tissue that allows these organs (e.g., the rectum and bladder) to undergo necessary changes in size and shape.

Note: Although the intraperitoneal liver possesses a mesentery in the form of anterior and posterior peritoneal folds (ventral and dorsal mesenteries), the part of the liver that is attached to the diaphragm lacks a peritoneal covering (the "bare area"). Thus the liver is not freely mobile, but it does move with the respiratory excursions of the diaphragm.

* "Extraperitoneal" occasionally refers to an organ that is not in contact with the peritoneum when formed.

D Extra- and intraperitoneal organs

Extra- and intraperitoneal organs	Organs
Intraperitoneal	These organs are completely covered by peritoneum and are attached by a mesentery to the posterior wall of the peritoneal cavity (the liver and stomach are also attached to the anterior wall).
• In the abdominal peritoneal cavity	• Stomach, small intestine (some of the superior part of the duodenum plus the jejunum and ileum), spleen, liver, and gallbladder; cecum with the vermiform appendix (the cecum has a variable peritoneal covering, and portions of variable size may be retroperitoneal); and the large intestine (transverse colon and sigmoid colon)
• In the pelvic peritoneal cavity	• Fundus and body of the uterus, the ovaries, and the fallopian tubes
Extraperitoneal	These organs either lack a peritoneal covering (e.g., the kidneys) or are partially covered by peritoneum (e.g., the duodenum, pancreas, and bladder), usually on their anterior or superior surface; they do not have a mesentery.
• Retroperitoneal (behind the peritoneal cavity) – Primarily retroperitoneal (already retroperitoneal when formed)	• Kidneys, suprarenal glands (not visible here, lateral to this midsagittal plane), and ureters
– Secondarily retroperitoneal (enter the retroperitoneum during embryonic development)	• Duodenum (descending, horizontal and ascending [partial]); pancreas; ascending and descending colon; rectum *up to* the sacral flexure
• Infraperitoneal / subperitoneal (below the peritoneal cavity / below the pelvic peritoneal cavity)	• Bladder and distal ureters, prostate, seminal vesicle, uterine cervix, vagina, and rectum *past* the sacral flexure

1.3 Peritoneal Relationships in the Abdomen and Pelvis: Overview and Anterior Abdominal Wall

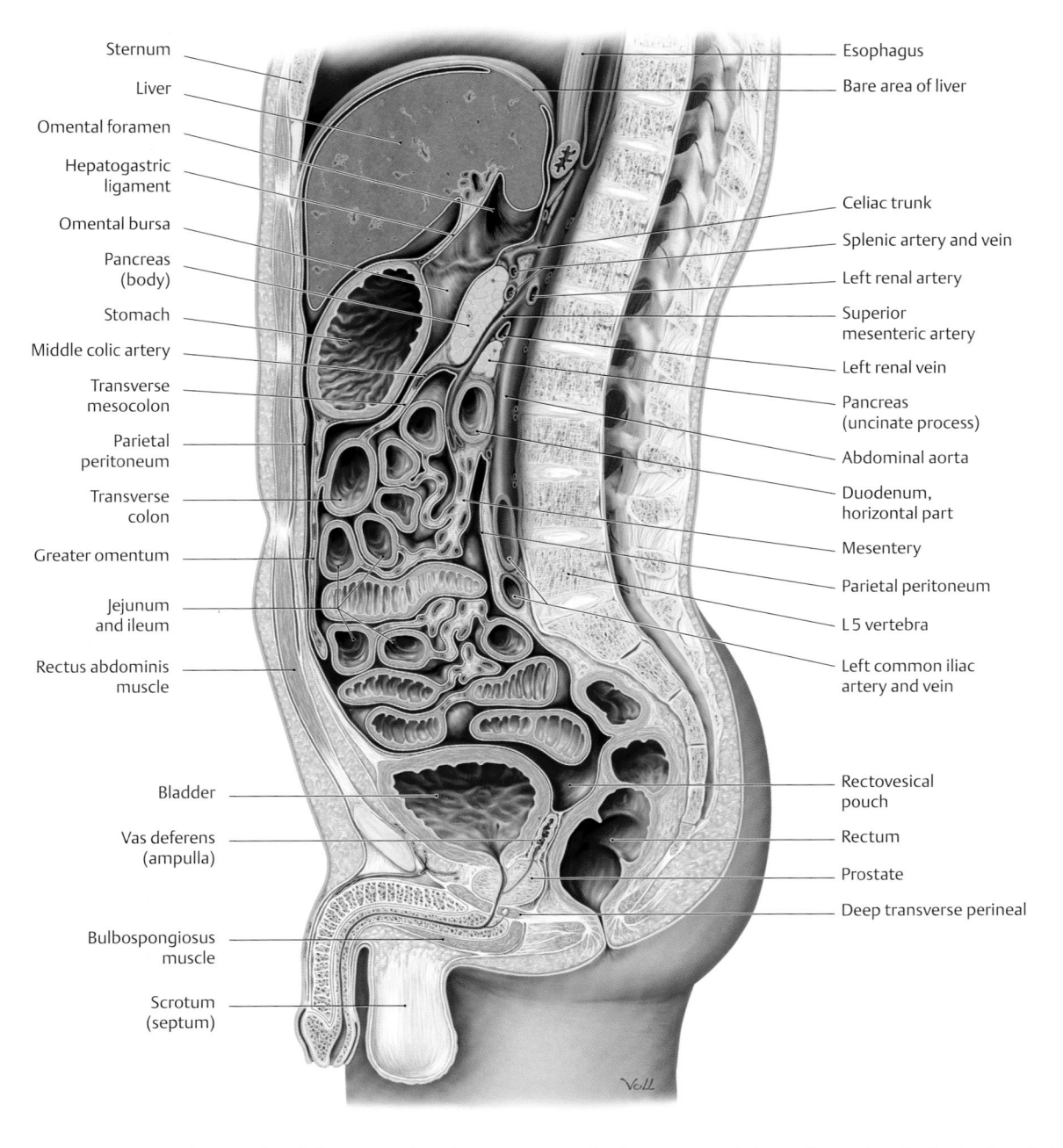

A Overview of peritoneal relationships in the abdomen and male pelvis*

Midsagittal section (kidneys outside the plane of section), viewed from the left side. The peritoneal cavity is basically a closed cavity that is lined by *parietal* peritoneum and surrounded on all sides by the *extra*peritoneal cavity. The extraperitoneal cavity is slit-like laterally, anteriorly, and superiorly. Only its posterior portion (retroperitoneum) and inferior portion (extraperitoneal space of the pelvis) are true *spaces* that contain organs (see **D**, p. 153). Since the organs and walls of the peritoneal cavity are covered by peritoneum, the intraperitoneal organs can easily glide upon one another. The *extra*peritoneal organs, such as the bladder and rectum, are only partially covered by peritoneum or do not have a peritoneal covering. The bladder, for example, is covered by peritoneum only on its superior surface, enabling it to expand upward as it fills with urine (important in percutaneous bladder aspiration, see p. 234).

Note: The lowest part of the peritoneal cavity in the female is the *recto-uterine pouch* (known clinically as the *cul-de-sac*). The lowest part of the peritoneal cavity in the male is the *rectovesical pouch*. Blood, pus, or tumor cells may collect at that site as a result of intra-abdominal inflammation or neoplasia. In females, a fluid sample can be obtained for diagnostic analysis by passing a needle into the cul-de-sac through the posterior vaginal fornix. The female pelvis contains an additional peritoneal fossa located between the bladder and uterus: the narrow vesicouterine pouch (see p. 174).

---

* The following illustrations present a series of dissections that progressively trace the peritoneal relationships through the peritoneal cavity to its posterior wall and into the retroperitoneum.

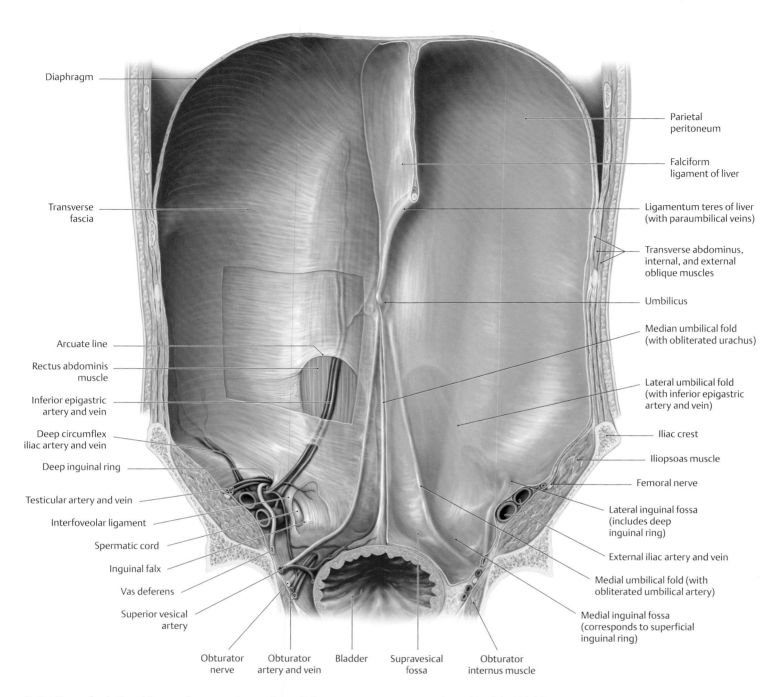

Diaphragm

Transverse fascia

Arcuate line

Rectus abdominis muscle

Inferior epigastric artery and vein

Deep circumflex iliac artery and vein

Deep inguinal ring

Testicular artery and vein

Interfoveolar ligament

Spermatic cord

Inguinal falx

Vas deferens

Superior vesical artery

Obturator nerve

Obturator artery and vein

Bladder

Supravesical fossa

Obturator internus muscle

Parietal peritoneum

Falciform ligament of liver

Ligamentum teres of liver (with paraumbilical veins)

Transverse abdominus, internal, and external oblique muscles

Umbilicus

Median umbilical fold (with obliterated urachus)

Lateral umbilical fold (with inferior epigastric artery and vein)

Iliac crest

Iliopsoas muscle

Femoral nerve

Lateral inguinal fossa (includes deep inguinal ring)

External iliac artery and vein

Medial umbilical fold (with obliterated umbilical artery)

Medial inguinal fossa (corresponds to superficial inguinal ring)

B Peritoneal relationships on the posterior surface of the abdominal wall

Posterior surface of the anterior abdominal wall, viewed from the posterior aspect. The peritoneum on the left side has been removed to display the contents of the peritoneal folds (umbilical folds). They are formed by the peritoneum that covers structures on the posterior surface of the anterior trunk wall. The parietal peritoneum lying between the folds raised by these structures forms shallow depressions called fossae.

Peritoneal folds (umbilical folds):

- One median umbilical fold: This is where the parietal peritoneum covers the median umbilical ligament, which is the obliterated urachus (remnant of the allentois that is obliterated during embryonic development).
- *Note:* Incomplete obliteration of the urachus may lead to umbilical fistulae in postnatal life.
- Two medial umbilical folds: sites where the parietal peritoneum covers the umbilical artery (the portion of the artery that becomes occluded at birth).

- Two lateral umbilical folds: sites where the parietal peritoneum covers the inferior epigastric artery and vein.

Each of the *paired umbilical arteries* consists of a proximal patent part (which gives rise to the superior vesical artery and, in males, the branch to the vas deferens) and a distal occluded part. The *unpaired umbilical vein* is usually obliterated to form the ligamentum teres of the liver.

Peritoneal fossae:

- Two supravesical fossae
- Two medial inguinal fossae (posterior to the superficial inguinal ring)
- Two lateral inguinal fossae (in which the deep inguinal ring is located)

Note: The *deep inguinal ring* (internal inguinal ring) is a structural weak point in the abdominal wall which forms the entrance to the inguinal canal. This canal provides a path for a path for the descent of the testis during normal development, but also creates a potential route for the herniation of abdominal viscera (indirect inguinal hernia).

1.4 Peritoneal Cavity: Dissections to Display the Abdominal Viscera

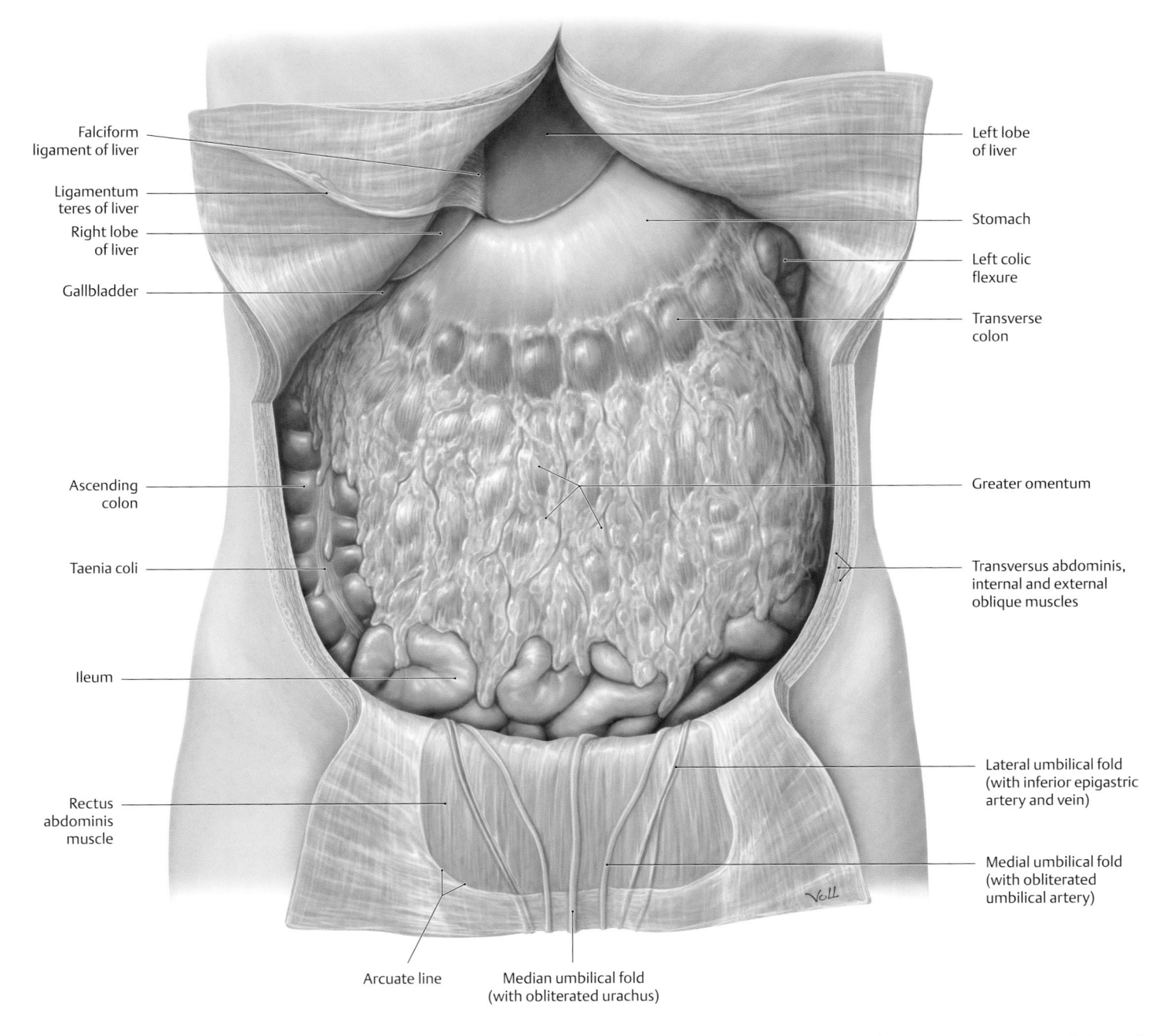

Falciform ligament of liver

Ligamentum teres of liver

Right lobe of liver

Gallbladder

Ascending colon

Taenia coli

Ileum

Rectus abdominis muscle

Left lobe of liver

Stomach

Left colic flexure

Transverse colon

Greater omentum

Transversus abdominis, internal and external oblique muscles

Lateral umbilical fold (with inferior epigastric artery and vein)

Medial umbilical fold (with obliterated umbilical artery)

Arcuate line

Median umbilical fold (with obliterated urachus)

A The greater omentum in situ

Anterior view. The layers of the abdominal wall have been opened and retracted to display the greater omentum in its normal anatomical position. The greater omentum is draped over the loops of small intestine, which are visible only at the inferior border of the omentum. The greater omentum is an apron-like fold of peritoneum suspended from the greater curvature of the stomach and covering the anterior surface of the transverse colon. It develops from the embryonic dorsal mesogastrum, which becomes greatly enlarged to form a peritoneal sac suspended from the greater curvature (see p. 165). The greater omentum is relatively mibile, and is subject to considerable variation. Not infre-

quently, adhesions form between the greater omentum and the peritoneal covering of organs, especially as a result of local inflammation. While these adhesions help contain the spread of inflammation, they also limit the mobility of the organ to which the omentum is adherent. Peritoneal adhesions may undergo fibrotic changes over time, forming tough bands of scar tissue that may cause extrinsic narrowing and obstruction of organs such as the small intestine. In many cases the greater omentum also assumes importance as a lymphoid organ through the secondary acquisition of lymph nodes. The lesser omentum is described on p. 164.

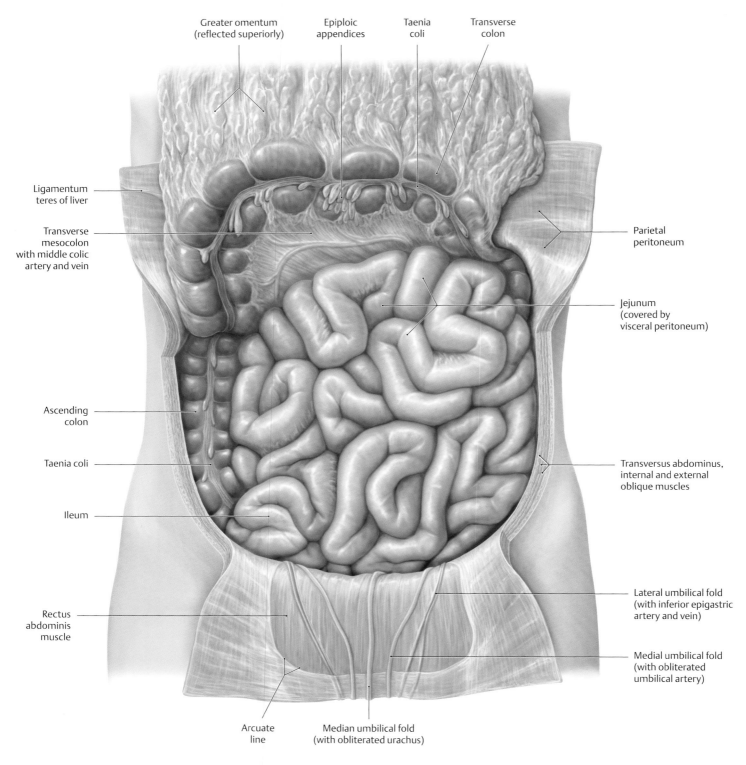

Greater omentum (reflected superiorly)

Epiploic appendices

Taenia coli

Transverse colon

Ligamentum teres of liver

Transverse mesocolon with middle colic artery and vein

Parietal peritoneum

Jejunum (covered by visceral peritoneum)

Ascending colon

Taenia coli

Transversus abdominus, internal and external oblique muscles

Ileum

Rectus abdominis muscle

Lateral umbilical fold (with inferior epigastric artery and vein)

Medial umbilical fold (with obliterated umbilical artery)

Arcuate line

Median umbilical fold (with obliterated urachus)

B Dissection with the greater omentum reflected superiorly and the small intestine in situ

Anterior view. The greater omentum has been reflected superiorly, carrying with it the transverse colon, to demonstrate how the intraperitoneal part of the small intestine is framed by the colon segments. The *transverse mesocolon* divides the peritoneal cavity into a supracolic part and an infracolic part (see **B**, p.152).

The large epithelial surface area of the peritoneum is important clinically:

- With bacterial infection (caused by external trauma or the seepage of septic material from an inflamed appendix), pathogenic micro-organisms can easily spread within the peritoneal cavity, where bacterial toxins are readily absorbed and carried into the bloodstream. As a result, bacterial peritonitis (inflammation of the peritoneum) generally constitutes a very serious and life-threatening condition.
- Localized inflammations may result in peritoneal adhesions and scar-tissue bands (see **A**).
- The large surface area can be utilized for *peritoneal dialysis* in patients with renal failure: A dialysis solution instilled into the peritoneal cavity can absorb waste products from the blood through the peritoneum, allowing them to be removed from the body.

1.5 Peritoneal Cavity: Mesenteries and Drainage Spaces

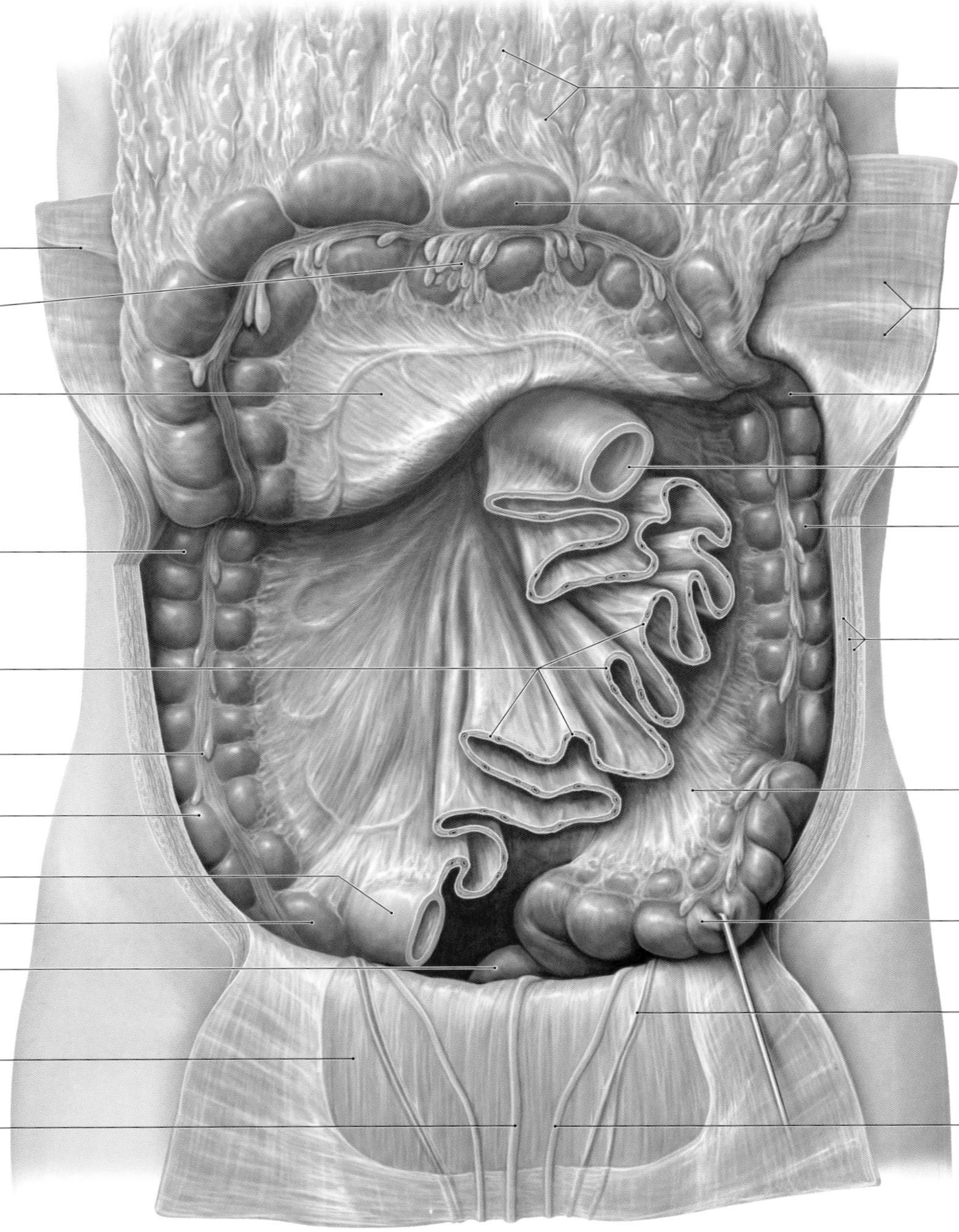

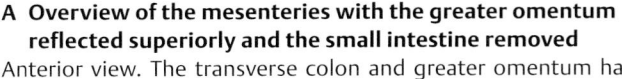

Greater omentum (reflected superiorly)

Transverse colon

Ligamentum teres of liver

Epiploic appendices

Transverse mesocolon

Parietal peritoneum

Left colic flexure

Jejunum

Descending colon

Right colic flexure

Transversus abdominus, internal and external oblique muscles

Mesentery (cut edge)

Taenia coli

Sigmoid mesocolon

Ascending colon

Ileum

Cecum

Rectum

Sigmoid colon

Lateral umbilical fold (with inferior epigastric artery and vein)

Rectus abdominis muscle

Median umbilical fold (with obliterated urachus)

Medial umbilical fold (with obliterated umbilical artery)

A Overview of the mesenteries with the greater omentum reflected superiorly and the small intestine removed

Anterior view. The transverse colon and greater omentum have been reflected superiorly and the intraperitoneal small intestine has been removed, leaving short stumps of jejunum and ileum. Three principal mesenteries are distinguishable in relation to the small and large intestine (the structure of the mesentery is described on p.153):

- The mesentery of the small intestine (the mesentery proper)
- The transverse mesocolon
- The sigmoid mesocolon (called also the mesosigmoid, see **D**, p. 163)

The origins of the mesenteries are shown in **B**. *Smaller mesenteries* are found on the vermiform appendix (*mesoappendix*) and rarely the upper part of the rectum (*mesorectum*, see **C**).

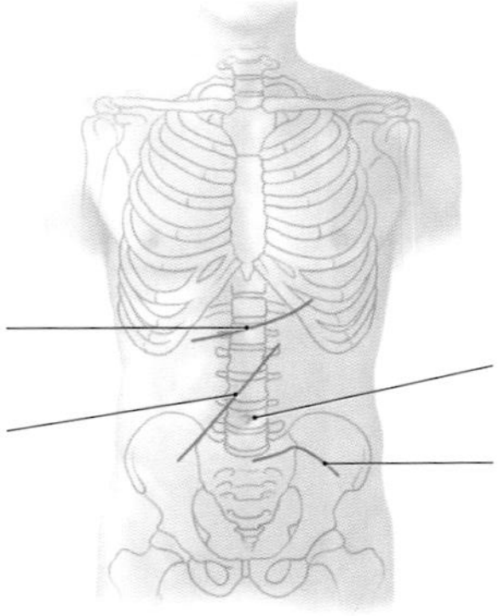

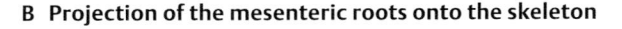

Transverse mesocolon

L 4 vertebra

Mesentery

Sigmoid mesocolon

B Projection of the mesenteric roots onto the skeleton

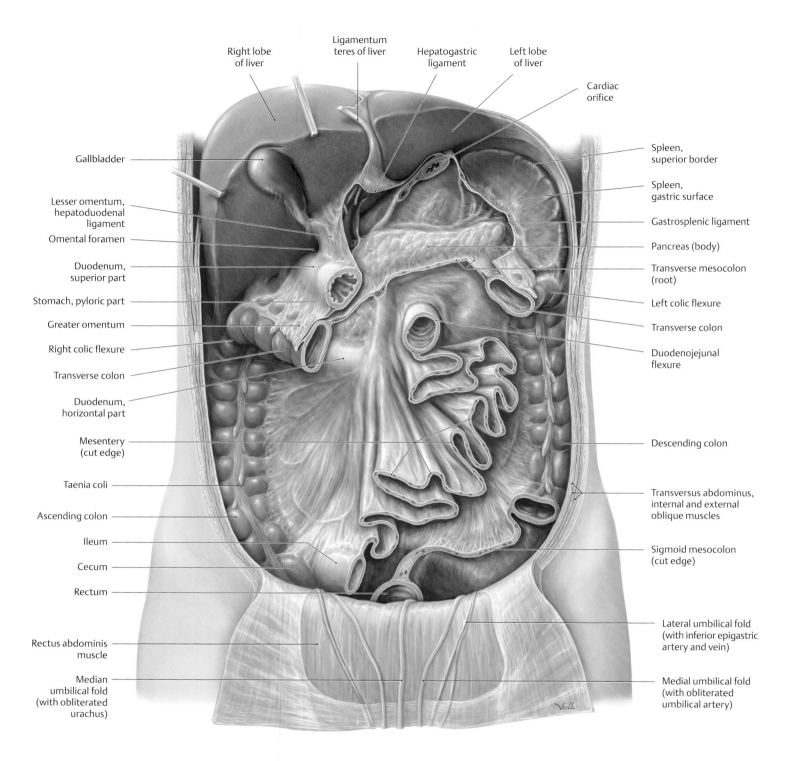

Right lobe of liver

Ligamentum teres of liver

Hepatogastric ligament

Left lobe of liver

Cardiac orifice

Gallbladder

Lesser omentum, hepatoduodenal ligament

Omental foramen

Duodenum, superior part

Stomach, pyloric part

Greater omentum

Right colic flexure

Transverse colon

Duodenum, horizontal part

Mesentery (cut edge)

Taenia coli

Ascending colon

Ileum

Cecum

Rectum

Rectus abdominis muscle

Median umbilical fold (with obliterated urachus)

Spleen, superior border

Spleen, gastric surface

Gastrosplenic ligament

Pancreas (body)

Transverse mesocolon (root)

Left colic flexure

Transverse colon

Duodenojejunal flexure

Descending colon

Transversus abdominus, internal and external oblique muscles

Sigmoid mesocolon (cut edge)

Lateral umbilical fold (with inferior epigastric artery and vein)

Medial umbilical fold (with obliterated umbilical artery)

C Overview of the mesenteries* with the greater omentum removed

Anterior view. The mesenteries have been exposed by removing the stomach, jejunum, and ileum, leaving short stumps of small intestine. The liver has been reflected superiorly to display one part of the lesser omentum: the hepatoduodenal ligament, which connects the liver to the pylorus and duodenum. The other part of the lesser omentum, the hepatogastric ligament (peritoneal fold between the liver and lesser curvature of the stomach), has been removed with the stomach, opening the anterior wall of the omental bursa. Most of the transverse colon and sigmoid colon have been removed to display the roots of the transverse mesocolon and sigmoid mesocolon.

Note: The ascending and descending *colon* become attached to the posterior wall of the peritoneal cavity during the fourth month of embryonic development. The mesentaries of the ascending and descending *colon* become fused to the posterior wall of the peritoneal cavity. The *transverse* mesocolon crosses over the duodenum, whose mesentery also fuses to the posterior wall of the peritoneal cavity during embryonic development (see p. 179). The transverse mesocolon necessarily passes over this "retroperitoneal portion" of the duodenum because of its attachment to the posterior wall of the peritoneal cavity (see also **B**, p. 161). Developmentally, almost all of the mesenteries are *dorsal* mesenteries. Only upper abdominal organs like the stomach and liver have *ventral* mesenteries.

* "Mesentery" in the broad sense refers to any of the peritoneal folds attached to the small and large intestine. "Mesentery" in the strict sense refers specifically to the mesentery of the jejunum and ileum, and consequently the terms "mesojejunum" and "mesoileum" are not used.

1.6 Peritoneal Cavity: Peritoneal Relationships and Recesses on the Posterior Abdominal Wall

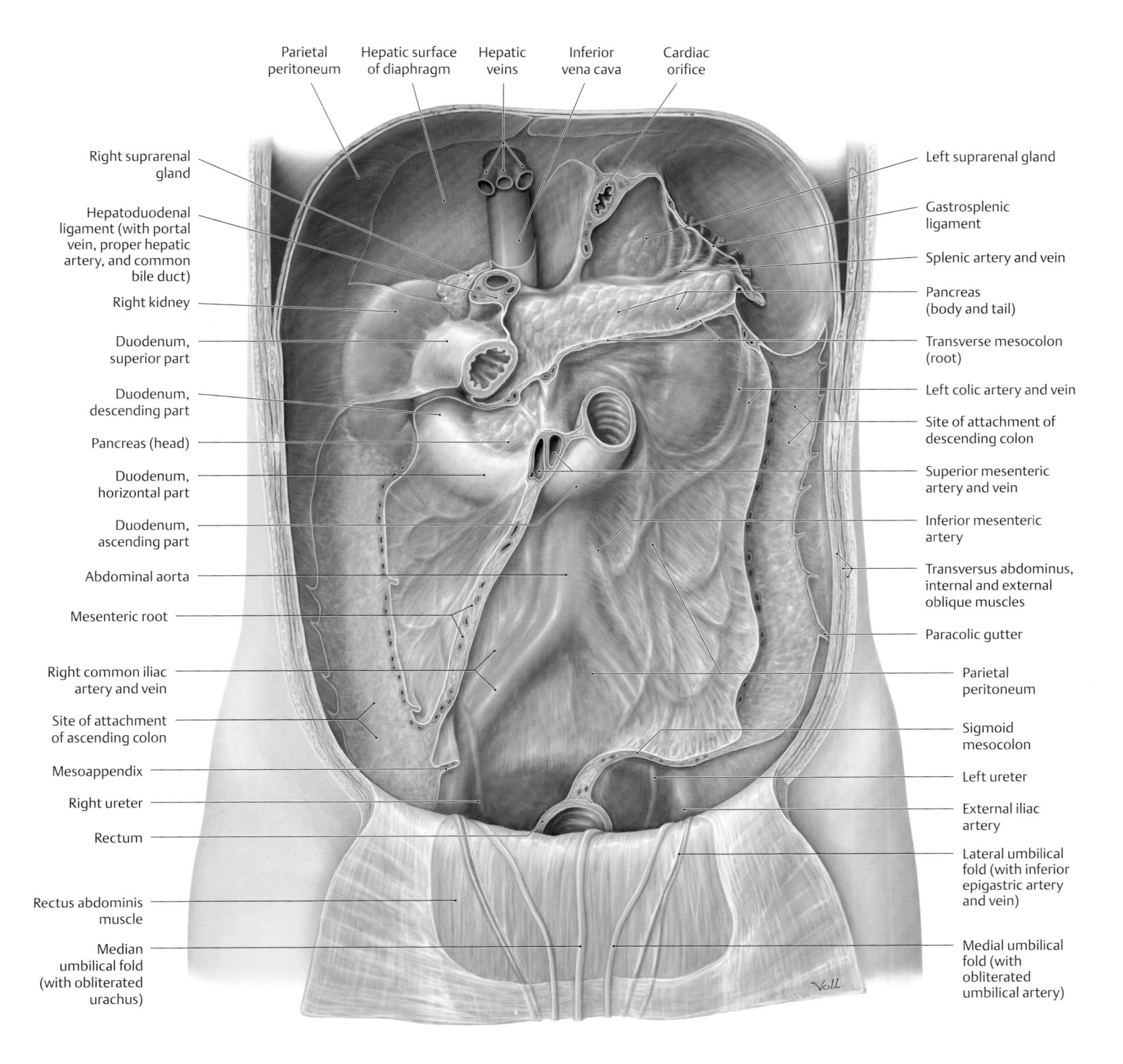

Parietal peritoneum
Hepatic surface of diaphragm
Hepatic veins
Inferior vena cava
Cardiac orifice

Right suprarenal gland

Hepatoduodenal ligament (with portal vein, proper hepatic artery, and common bile duct)

Right kidney

Duodenum, superior part

Duodenum, descending part

Pancreas (head)

Duodenum, horizontal part

Duodenum, ascending part

Abdominal aorta

Mesenteric root

Right common iliac artery and vein

Site of attachment of ascending colon

Mesoappendix

Right ureter

Rectum

Rectus abdominis muscle

Median umbilical fold (with obliterated urachus)

Left suprarenal gland

Gastrosplenic ligament

Splenic artery and vein

Pancreas (body and tail)

Transverse mesocolon (root)

Left colic artery and vein

Site of attachment of descending colon

Superior mesenteric artery and vein

Inferior mesenteric artery

Transversus abdominus, internal and external oblique muscles

Paracolic gutter

Parietal peritoneum

Sigmoid mesocolon

Left ureter

External iliac artery

Lateral umbilical fold (with inferior epigastric artery and vein)

Medial umbilical fold (with obliterated umbilical artery)

A Peritoneal relationships on the posterior wall of the peritoneal cavity

Anterior view of the opened thorax and abdomen. All of the intraperitoneal organs have been removed to display the retroperitoneum (retroperitoneal space). The posterior wall of the peritoneal cavity also forms the anterior wall of the retroperitoneum. Unlike the anterior wall of the peritoneal cavity, which consists largely of muscles and fasciae, much of the posterior wall is formed by the organs in the retroperitoneum, which are visible through the parietal peritoneum in this dissection. For clarity, the retroperitoneal connective tissue and fat have been thinned out to display the course of the retroperitoneal vessels and the ureter (where it crosses in front of the iliac vessels; see **A**, p. 162). The hepatic surface

of the diaphragm is devoid of peritoneum and corresponds to the bare area of the liver. The ascending and descending colon (removed here for clarity) are attached by connective tissue to the posterior wall of the peritoneal cavity, so they are also located in the retroperitoneum (see **C**, p. 159). In this speciman, the area of attachment of the ascending colon extends further inferiorly to the pelvis than usual. The transverse mesocolon, like the transverse colon, is located anterior to the duodenum (i.e., is intraperitoneal). The migration of these organs during embryonic development is described on p. 181. The sigmoid mesocolon crosses anterior to the left iliac vessels and left ureter.

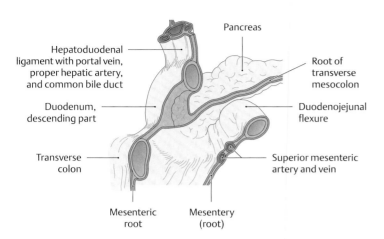

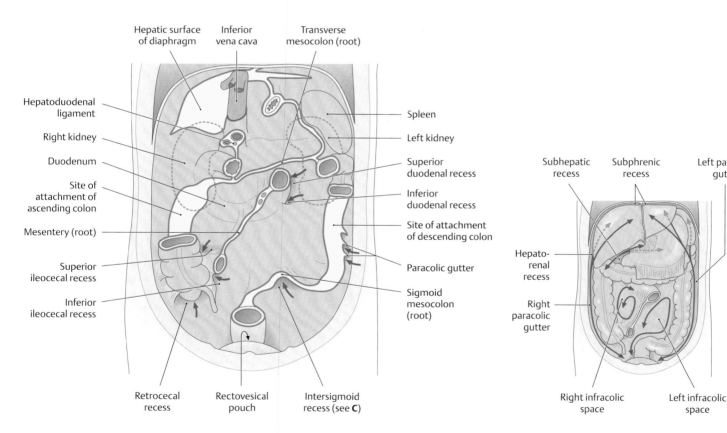

B Peritoneal coverings of the duodenum and pancreas

Anterior view. This diagram shows how the root of the transverse mesocolon crosses over the descending part of the duodenum and the pancreas (both of which are secondarily retroperitoneal).

C Position of the sigmoid mesocolon and intersigmoid recess

The sigmoid colon has been partially removed (left) or reflected superiorly with the sigmoid mesocolon (right). The left ureter descends through the intersigmoid recess in the retroperitoneum.

D Recesses in the posterior wall of the peritoneal cavity

Anterior view of a male abdomen and pelvis. The peritoneum forms recesses or sulci at some sites between the organs (see also **B** and **C**). In a sense, the omental bursa may be considered the largest recess in the peritoneal cavity (see p. 164).

Note: The individual recesses are located between organs or between an organ and the wall of the peritoneal cavity. Freely mobile bowel loops may become entrapped in these recesses ("internal hernia"), hampering the passage of material through the small intestine and potentially causing a life-threatening bowel obstruction ("mechanical ileus").

E Drainage spaces within the peritoneal cavity

Anterior view. The arrangement of the mesenteric roots and sites of organ attachment create partially bounded spaces (recesses or sulci) within the peritoneal cavity. Peritoneal fluid released by the peritoneal epithelium (transudate) can flow freely within these spaces.

1.7 The Retroperitoneum and Its Contents

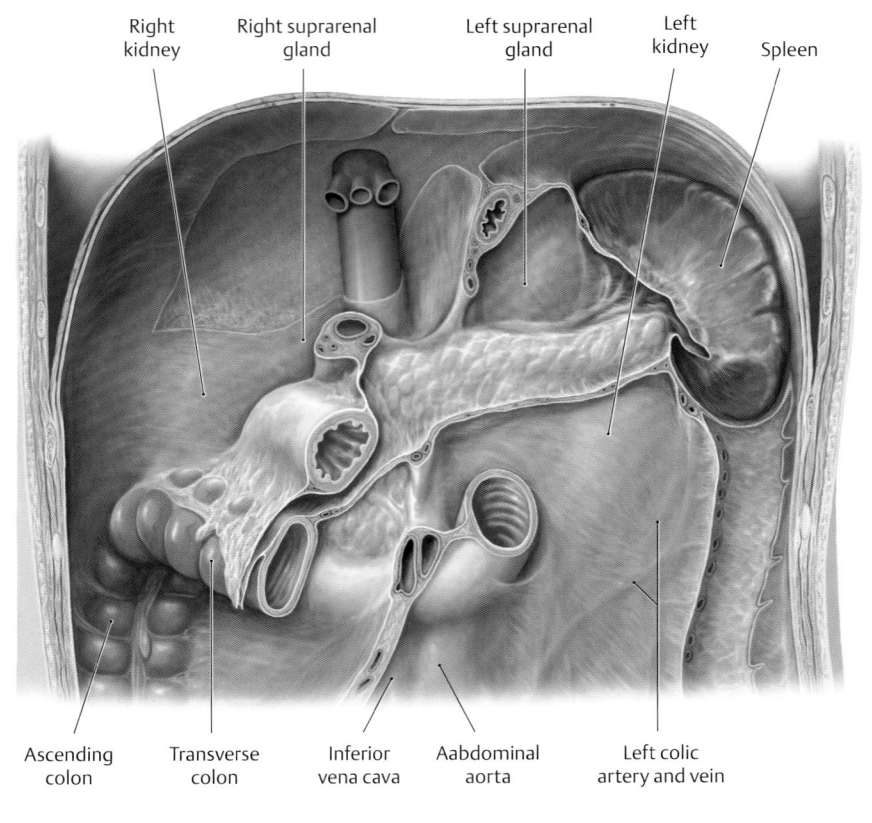

Right kidney — Right suprarenal gland — Left suprarenal gland — Left kidney — Spleen

Ascending colon — Transverse colon — Inferior vena cava — Aabdominal aorta — Left colic artery and vein

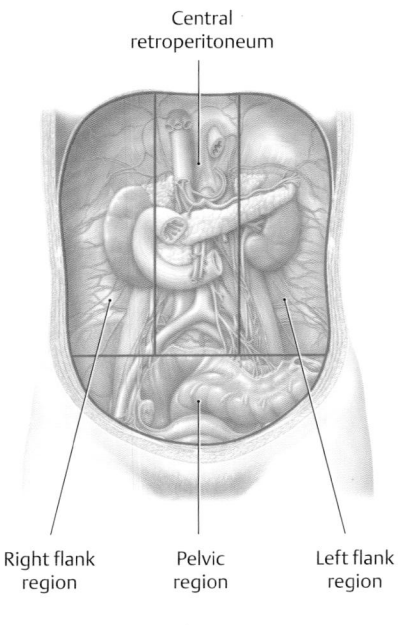

Central retroperitoneum

Right flank region — Pelvic region — Left flank region

A Transperitoneal view of the retroperitoneum

Anterior view. The intraperitoneal organs have been removed except for the spleen and a small part of the transverse colon. The retroperitoneal descending colon has also been removed. The connective tissue and fat in the retroperitoneum are of normal volume in this dissection. The kidneys form in the retroperitoneum during embryonic development and are embedded in the retroperitoneal fat and connective tissue. Thus the kidneys, like the great vessels, are obscured by the anterior wall of the retroperitoneum and are visible only as

bulges behind the parietal peritoneum. Additionally, the prerenal layer of the renal fascia is interposed between the kidneys and the parietal peritoneum (see p. 226). Because the pancreas is secondarily retroperitoneal, it is not fully integrated into the retroperitoneal fat and connective tissue. Being attached to the posterior wall of the peritoneal cavity "only" by fusion of the peritoneal layers, the pancreas can be seen with much greater clarity. Although its anterior surface is covered by peritoneum, that layer is more translucent than the retroperitoneal connective tissue and fat.

C Zones of the retroperitoneum (after von Lanz and Wachsmuth)

The retroperitoneum, like other body cavities, can be divided into zones based on clinical criteria. This type of classification is useful for evaluating what organs may be jointly affected by disease or injury due to their proximity to each other, even if they belong to entirely different functional systems. The retroperitoneum is divided into three zones:

Zone 1: central retroperitoneum with the duodenum and great vessels
Zone 2: left and right flank regions with the kidneys, ureters, ascending colon, and descending colon (omitted here to give a clearer view of the other organs)
Zone 3: pelvic region (corresponding to the hypogastrium) with the bladder, distal ureters, rectum, and internal genitalia

B Organs and neurovascular structures in the retroperitoneum

Organs	Vessels	Nerves
Primarily retroperitoneal (or extraperitoneal): • Right and left kidneys • Right and left suprarenal glands • Right and left ureters *Secondarily retroperitoneal:* • Pancreas • Duodenum: descending and horizontal parts, some of the ascending part • Ascending and descending colon • Variable: portions of the cecum • Rectum to the sacral flexure	• Aorta (abdominal part) and its branches • Inferior vena cava and its tributaries • Ascending lumbar veins • Portal vein (before coursing in the hepatoduodenal ligament) and its tributaries • Lumbar, sacral, and iliac lymph nodes, lumbar trunks, cisterna chyli	• Branches of the lumbar plexus (iliohypogastric, ilioinguinal, genitofemoral, lateral femoral cutaneous, femoral, and obturator nerves) • Sympathetic trunk • Autonomic ganglia and plexuses

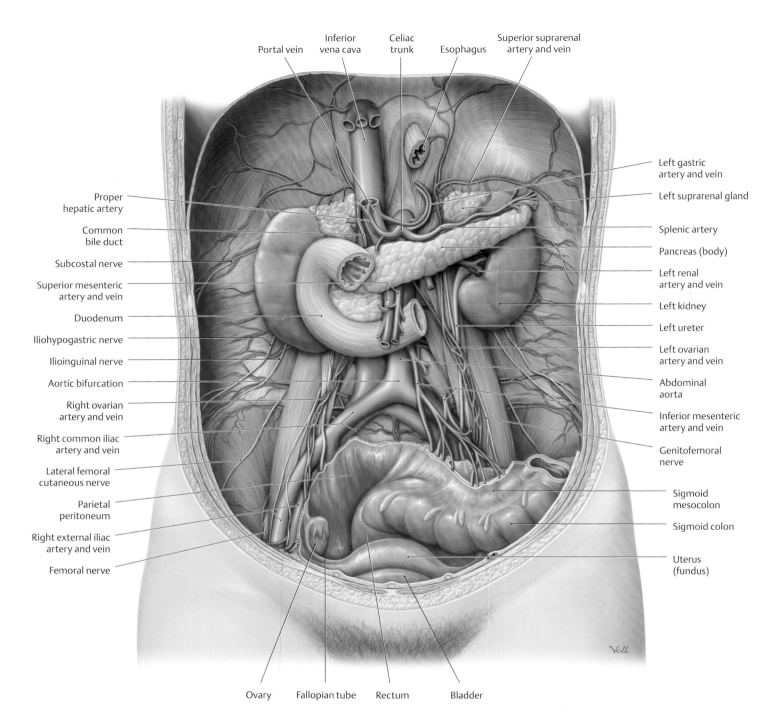

Portal vein
Inferior vena cava
Celiac trunk
Esophagus
Superior suprarenal artery and vein

Proper hepatic artery
Common bile duct
Subcostal nerve
Superior mesenteric artery and vein
Duodenum
Iliohypogastric nerve
Ilioinguinal nerve
Aortic bifurcation
Right ovarian artery and vein
Right common iliac artery and vein
Lateral femoral cutaneous nerve
Parietal peritoneum
Right external iliac artery and vein
Femoral nerve

Left gastric artery and vein
Left suprarenal gland
Splenic artery
Pancreas (body)
Left renal artery and vein
Left kidney
Left ureter
Left ovarian artery and vein
Abdominal aorta
Inferior mesenteric artery and vein
Genitofemoral nerve
Sigmoid mesocolon
Sigmoid colon
Uterus (fundus)

Ovary   Fallopian tube   Rectum   Bladder

D Overview of the retroperitoneum

Anterior view of a female abdomen and pelvis. The mesenteries and intraperitoneal organs have been removed except for the sigmoid colon and internal genitalia. Most of the parietal peritoneum has been removed, and the retroperitoneal fat and connective tissue have been almost completely removed. The stump of the esophagus has been drawn slightly inferiorly to provide an anatomical landmark.

Note: Some of the retroperitoneal organs are fully integrated in that space, having formed in the retroperitoneum: the kidneys, suprarenal glands, great vessels, and nerves. Other structures form in the peritoneal cavity and migrate to the retroperitoneum secondarily (the pancreas and duodenum, see **B**). Their visceral peritoneum becomes fused to the parietal peritoneum of the posterior wall, and they retain a peritoneal covering on their anterior surface. The primary retroperitoneal organs do not have a peritoneal covering because they are fully integrated into the retroperitoneal connective tissue.

1.8 Omental Bursa

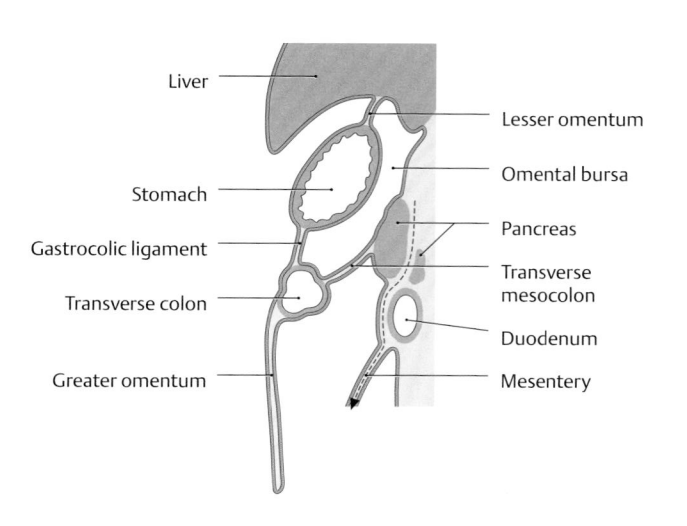

A Shape and location of the omental bursa in sagittal section

Left lateral view. The omental bursa is the largest potential space in the peritoneal cavity. It is located behind the lesser omentum and stomach.

Note: As the stomach rotates during embryonic development, the omental bursa comes to lie posterior to the stomach. The pancreas, which migrates into the retroperitoneum secondarily, thus forms part of the posterior wall of the bursa, which provides a route for gaining surgical access to that organ. As the stomach rotates in the clockwise direction (viewed from the front), its lesser curvature points to the right and also superiorly, simultaneously displacing the liver superiorly and to the right. As a result of this, the omental bursa comes to lie partially posterior to the liver.

B Boundaries of the omental bursa

Anterior	Lesser omentum, gastrocolic ligament
Posterior	Pancreas, aorta (abdominal part), celiac trunk, splenic artery and vein, gastropancreatic fold, left suprarenal gland, superior pole of left kidney
Superior	Liver (with caudate lobe), superior recess of omental bursa
Inferior	Transverse mesocolon, inferior recess of omental bursa
Left	Spleen, gastrosplenic ligament, splenic recess of omental bursa
Right	Liver, duodenal bulb

C Surgical approaches to the omental bursa (see **A**)

- Through the omental foramen (natural opening, see **E**)
- Between the greater curvature of the stomach and the transverse colon through the gastrocolic ligament
- Through the transverse mesocolon after elevating the transverse colon (inferior approach)
- Between the lesser curvature of the stomach and the liver (through the lesser omentum)
- From the greater curvature of the stomach after division of the greater omentum

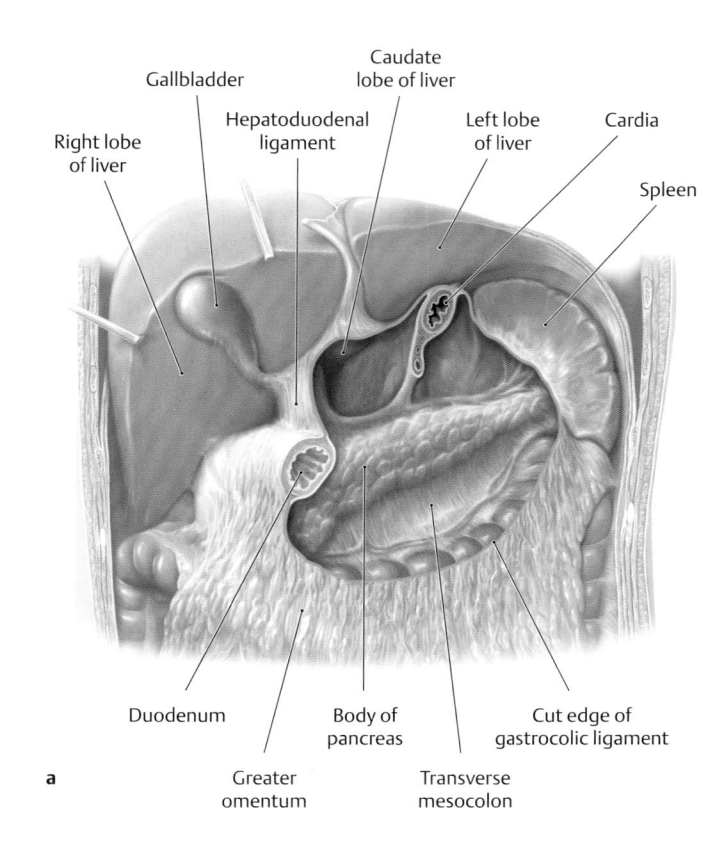

a

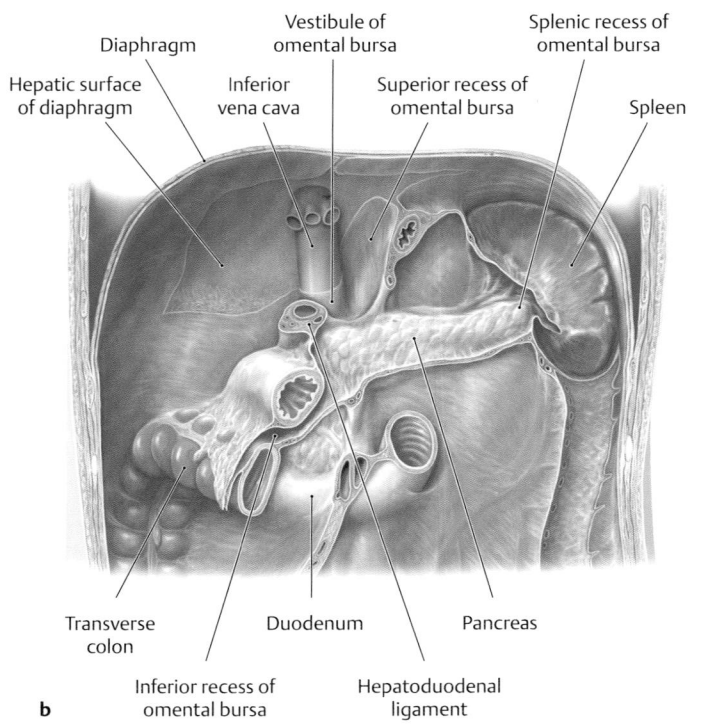

b

D Omental bursa, anterior view

a Boundaries of the omental bursa, also the shape and location of the gastric bed.

b Structure of the posterior wall of the omental bursa.

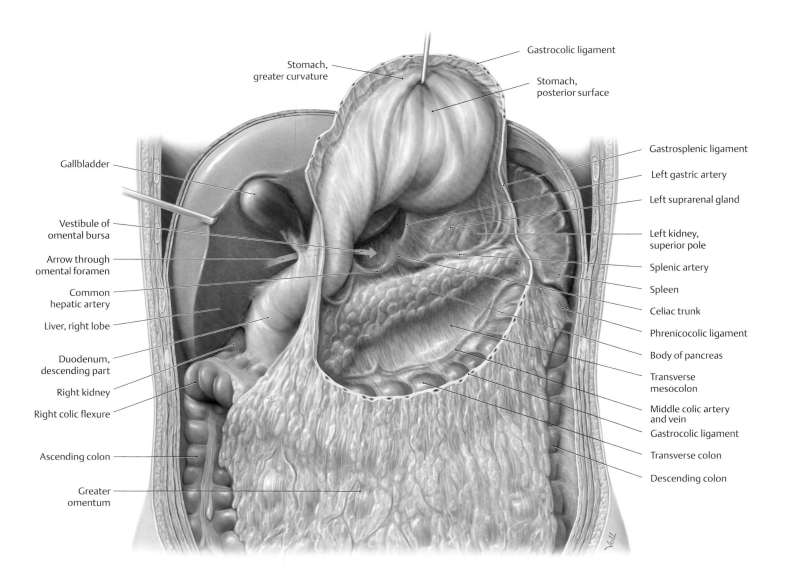

Stomach, greater curvature

Gastrocolic ligament

Stomach, posterior surface

Gallbladder

Gastrosplenic ligament

Left gastric artery

Left suprarenal gland

Vestibule of omental bursa

Left kidney, superior pole

Arrow through omental foramen

Splenic artery

Common hepatic artery

Spleen

Celiac trunk

Liver, right lobe

Phrenicocolic ligament

Duodenum, descending part

Body of pancreas

Right kidney

Transverse mesocolon

Right colic flexure

Middle colic artery and vein

Gastrocolic ligament

Ascending colon

Transverse colon

Descending colon

Greater omentum

E Omental bursa in the upper abdomen
Anterior view. The gastrocolic ligament has been divided, the stomach has been reflected superiorly (surgical approach), and the liver has been retracted superolaterally. The *omental foramen* (arrow) is the only natural orifice of the omental bursa (opens posterior to the hepatoduodenal ligament). The *vestibule* of the omental bursa lies just past the foramen and forms the initial portion of the bursa cavity.

F Transverse section through the omental bursa
Schematic section through the abdomen at the T 12 / L 1 level, viewed from above.
Note the walls and recesses that result from the formation of the bursa during the embryonic rotation of the stomach. Because the initial upper right portion of the embryonic body cavity moves posteriorly as part of the 90° rotation of the stomach, structures that were formerly posterior (spleen) move to the left side while structures that were formerly anterior (liver) move to the right side. Recesses in the omental bursa extend close to these organs (see **B**).

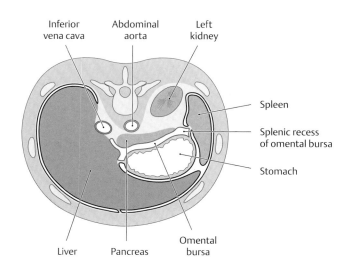

Inferior vena cava

Abdominal aorta

Left kidney

Spleen

Splenic recess of omental bursa

Stomach

Liver

Pancreas

Omental bursa

165

1.9 Transverse Sections through the Abdomen

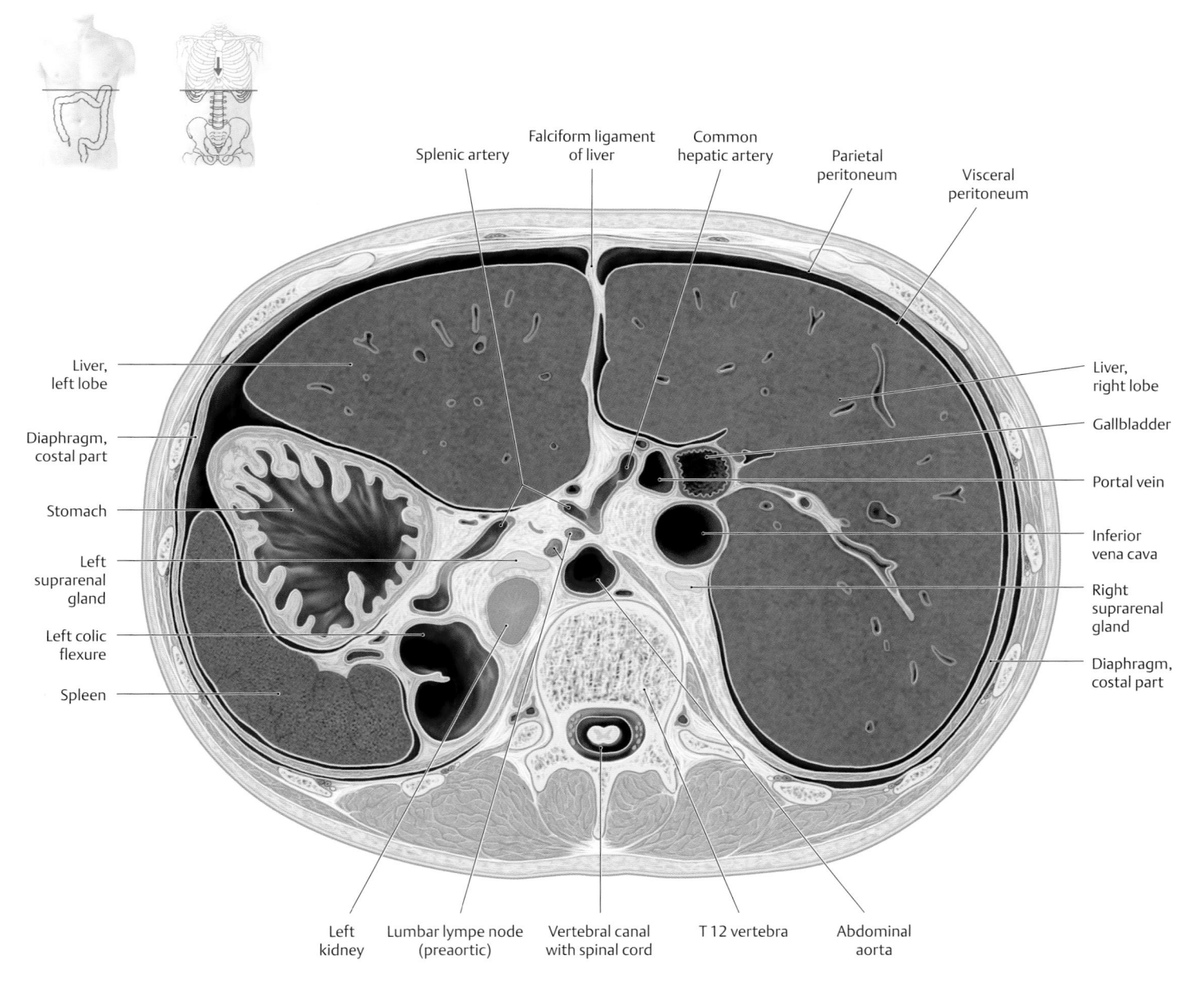

Splenic artery — Falciform ligament of liver — Common hepatic artery — Parietal peritoneum — Visceral peritoneum

Liver, left lobe

Diaphragm, costal part

Stomach

Left suprarenal gland

Left colic flexure

Spleen

Liver, right lobe

Gallbladder

Portal vein

Inferior vena cava

Right suprarenal gland

Diaphragm, costal part

Left kidney — Lumbar lympe node (preaortic) — Vertebral canal with spinal cord — T 12 vertebra — Abdominal aorta

A Transverse section through the abdomen at the level of the T 12 vertebral body

Viewed from above.

Note the anatomical extent of the liver. The single heaviest organ in the body, the liver occupies most of the right upper abdomen and also extends into the left upper abdomen at this level. The hepatoduodenal ligament contains the portal vein, bile ducts, and hepatic arteries. The hepatic veins (not visible in the section) leave the liver in the "bare area," which is *outside* the surface covered by peritoneum. The close proximity of the stomach and spleen results from the development of the liver and stomach: Embryologically, the spleen forms posterior to the stomach in the dorsal mesogastrium. As the stomach rotates, the spleen moves into the left upper abdomen, the quadrant toward which the fundus and greater curvature of the rotated stomach are directed. In the sec-

tion shown above, the left colic flexure occupies an unusually posterior location (normal anatomical variation). Because the section through the flexure is slightly oblique, the ascending part (from the transverse colon) and the descending part (to the descending colon) are incompletely separated, creating the appearance of a uniform tube. The falciform ligament of the liver is derived from the ventral mesentery. The level that most organs occupy in the body is dependent on age, posture, constitutional type, nutritional state, and position of the diaphragm in the breathing cycle. Thus, a transverse section at a certain level is apt to show *considerable variation*, especially in the organs that just border the sectional plane. The section above passes through the left kidney (and left suprarenal gland). The right kidney, which is lower because of the liver, lies below the plane of section. Its position can be inferred, however, from the location of the right suprarenal gland, which is cut by the section.

166

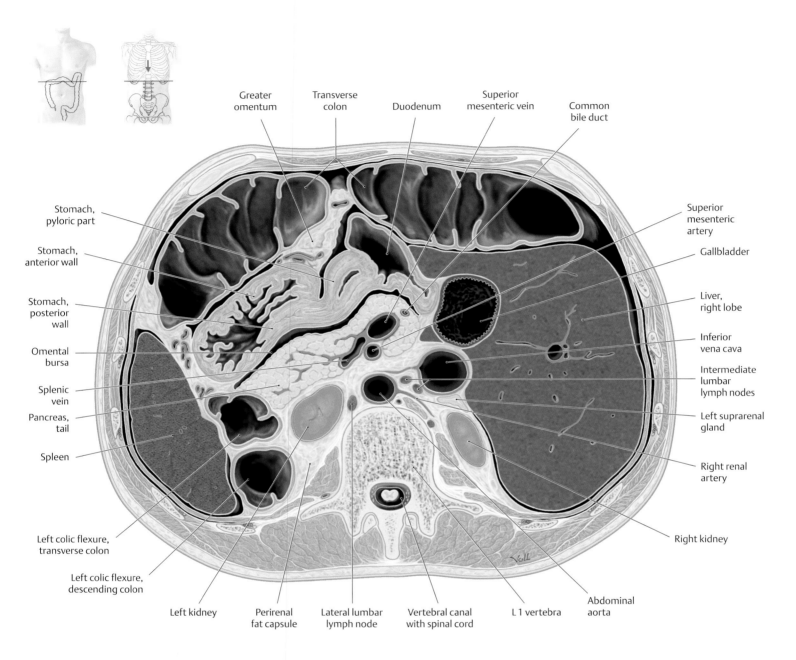

Greater omentum

Transverse colon

Duodenum

Superior mesenteric vein

Common bile duct

Stomach, pyloric part

Stomach, anterior wall

Stomach, posterior wall

Omental bursa

Splenic vein

Pancreas, tail

Spleen

Left colic flexure, transverse colon

Left colic flexure, descending colon

Superior mesenteric artery

Gallbladder

Liver, right lobe

Inferior vena cava

Intermediate lumbar lymph nodes

Left suprarenal gland

Right renal artery

Right kidney

Left kidney

Perirenal fat capsule

Lateral lumbar lymph node

Vertebral canal with spinal cord

L 1 vertebra

Abdominal aorta

B Transverse section through the abdomen at the level of the L 1 vertebral body

Viewed from above.

Note the position of the omental bursa. It extends to the left to the gastrosplenic ligament, which forms the left boundary of the omental bursa. During embryonic rotation of the stomach, the intraperitoneal spleen swings into the left upper abdomen and the bursa moves posteriorly, maintaining its relationship to the spleen in the form of the splenic recess. The omental bursa runs along the full length of the posterior stomach wall. The superior mesenteric artery and vein pass through the substance of the pancreas, and consequently a tumor in the head of the pancreas may cause obstruction of these vessels. The discontinuity in the transverse colon results from the level of the section: the connecting part lies outside the sectional plane. Both kidneys are transected at this level.

1.10 Peritoneal Relationships and Pelvic Spaces: Comparison of Coronal and Parasagittal Sections in the Male and Female

Subdivision of the lesser pelvis by spaces and fasciae

Spaces: The lesser pelvis consists of two spaces: the *pelvic peritoneal cavity* and the *pelvic extraperitoneal space.* The extraperitoneal space is further divided by the levator ani muscle into an upper and lower part (defining the three levels of the lesser pelvis, see **B**). It is occupied by connective tissue of variable density and can be subdivided topographically (based on its relationship to the peritoneum and pelvic wall) into three smaller spaces:

- Retroinguinal space: below the peritoneum and behind the inguinal region
- Retropubic space: between the bladder and pubic symphysis
- Retroperitoneal space: between the peritoneum and sacrum (continuation of the retroperitoneum of the abdomen)

Fasciae: The *pelvic fascia* consists of parietal fascia (covering the structures of the pelvic wall) and visceral fascia (covering the pelvic organs).

The *connective tissue of the visceral fascia* is thickened at sites between and around the organs and is continuous with the adventitia or capsule of the pelvic organs:

- Rectoprostatic fascia: rectovesical septum (male pelvis, located between the rectum and bladder)
- Rectovaginal fascia: rectovaginal septum (female pelvis, located between the rectum and vagina)

The *connective tissue around the organs* is also thickened and generally transmits the neurovascular bundles that supply the organs.

- Lateral rectal ligament
- Lateral ligament of the bladder
- Pubovesicular ligament
- Transverse cervical ligament

A   Peritoneal relationships, fasciae, and spaces in the pelvis
a Male pelvis, anterior view of a coronal section tilted slightly forward. This section displays the peritoneum, fasciae, and connective-tissue spaces around the bladder and prostate.
b Female pelvis, anterior view of a coronal section tilted slightly backward. This section displays the peritoneum, fasciae, and connective-tissue spaces around the uterus and vagina.

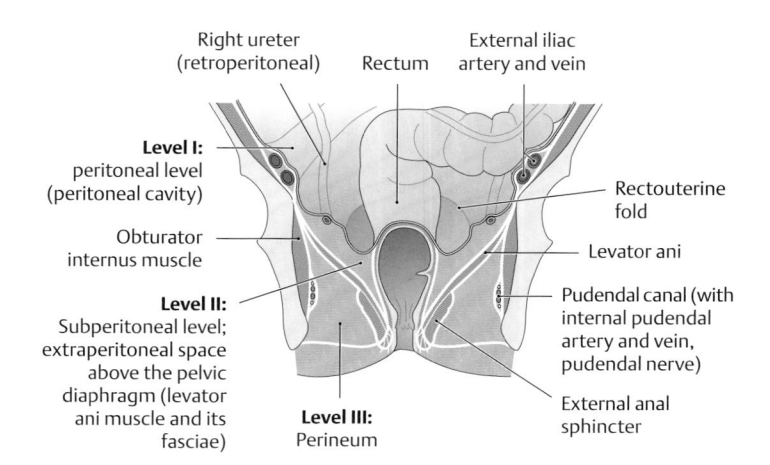

B   The three levels of the pelvis
Anterior view of a posterior coronal section that passes through the lower part of the rectum.
Note: The peritoneum and levator ani muscle divide the pelvis into three levels (see **C**). The rectum subdivides levels II and III into left and right halves. The ureters are retroperitoneal.

C   Organs and structures of the three pelvic levels (see **B**)

Pelvic level	Relationship to peritoneum	Structures at that level
I Peritoneal level	Intraperitoneal	<ul><li>Coils of ileum</li><li>Vermiform appendix</li><li>Sigmoid colon</li></ul>
II Subperito-neal level	Extraperitoneal, *above* the levator ani muscle	<ul><li>Distal ureters</li><li>Internal iliac artery and vein with visceral and parietal branches</li><li>Obturator artery and vein</li><li>Obturator nerve</li><li>Sacral plexus</li><li>Inferior hypogastric plexus</li></ul>
III Perineum	Extraperitoneal, *below* the levator ani muscle	<ul><li>Internal pudendal artery and vein</li><li>Pudendal nerve and its branches</li></ul>

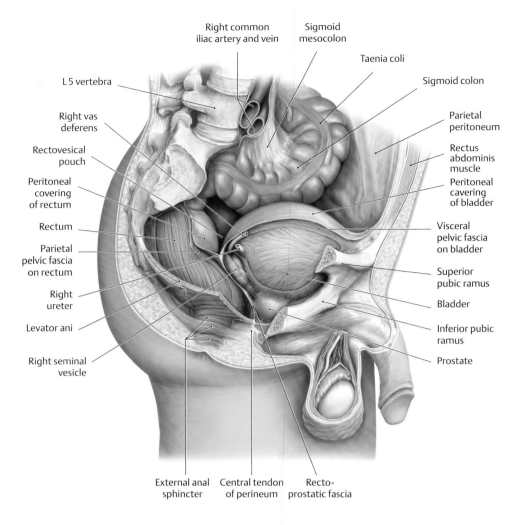

Right common iliac artery and vein
Sigmoid mesocolon
Taenia coli
L 5 vertebra
Right vas deferens
Sigmoid colon
Rectovesical pouch
Parietal peritoneum
Peritoneal covering of rectum
Rectus abdominis muscle
Rectum
Peritoneal covering of bladder
Parietal pelvic fascia on rectum
Visceral pelvic fascia on bladder
Right ureter
Superior pubic ramus
Levator ani
Bladder
Right seminal vesicle
Inferior pubic ramus
Prostate
External anal sphincter
Central tendon of perineum
Recto-prostatic fascia

D Peritoneal relationships in the male pelvis

Parasagittal section, viewed from the right side. The plane of section is slightly lateral to the median plane so that midline structures are also displayed. For clarity, most of the connective tissue in the pelvic extraperitoneal space has been removed. This accounts for the apparently "empty" spaces between the organs.

Note the relationship of the rectum to the pelvic floor and bladder: Between the bladder and rectum is the generally shallow rectovesical pouch, whose specific shape and depth depend on the degree of distention of the bladder and rectum. The lower portions of the rectum and the connective tissue around the rectum (not shown here) are supported by the pelvic diaphragm (chiefly the levator ani muscle). The bladder is shown here in a distended state so that the suprasymphyseal part of the bladder not covered by peritoneum can be seen (this part of the bladder is targeted in a suprapubic bladder aspiration, which is performed with a full bladder to avoid peritoneal injury; see also p. 234).

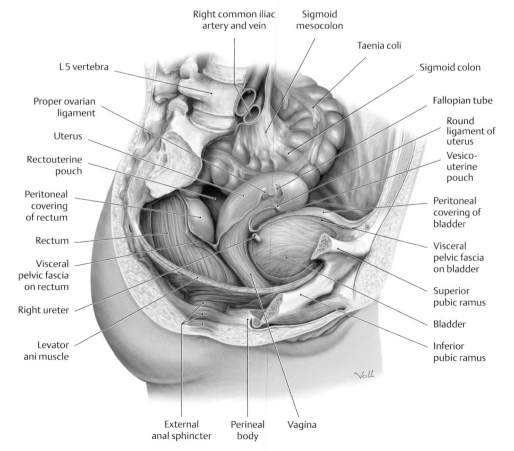

Right common iliac artery and vein
Sigmoid mesocolon
Taenia coli
L 5 vertebra
Sigmoid colon
Proper ovarian ligament
Fallopian tube
Uterus
Round ligament of uterus
Rectouterine pouch
Vesico-uterine pouch
Peritoneal covering of rectum
Peritoneal covering of bladder
Rectum
Visceral pelvic fascia on bladder
Visceral pelvic fascia on rectum
Superior pubic ramus
Right ureter
Bladder
Levator ani muscle
Inferior pubic ramus
External anal sphincter
Perineal body
Vagina

E Peritoneal relationships in the female pelvis

Parasagittal section, viewed from the right side. For clarity, most of the connective tissue has again been removed from the pelvic extraperitoneal space. The extraperitoneal spaces between the bladder, cervix (vagina), and rectum appear empty. Between the uterus and rectum is the generally deep rectouterine pouch, whose specific shape and depth depend on the degree of rectal distention. The vesicouterine pouch lies between the bladder and uterus. The bladder is relatively well distended here, raising the uterus to a slightly more upright position.

1.11 Peritoneal Relationships and Pelvic Spaces: Comparison of Midsagittal Sections in the Male and Female

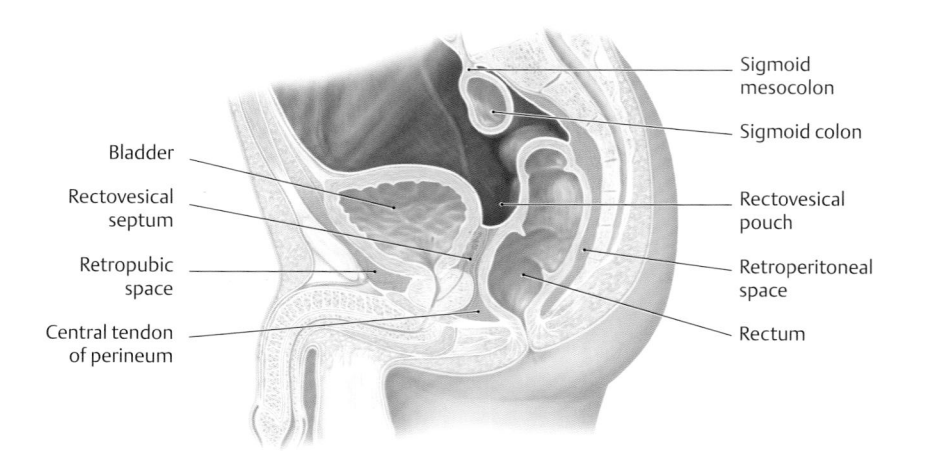

A Visceral fasciae in the male pelvis

Midsagittal section, viewed from the left side. The pelvic space outside the peritoneum, called the pelvic extraperitoneal space, is subdivided by variable bands of connective tissue (fasciae or septa) into fascial spaces that are located between the pelvic wall and an organ or between individual organs. These spaces provide the pelvic organs with some degree of mobility (expansion of the bladder and rectum). They also provide routes for the spread of inflammation or post-traumatic hemorrhage.

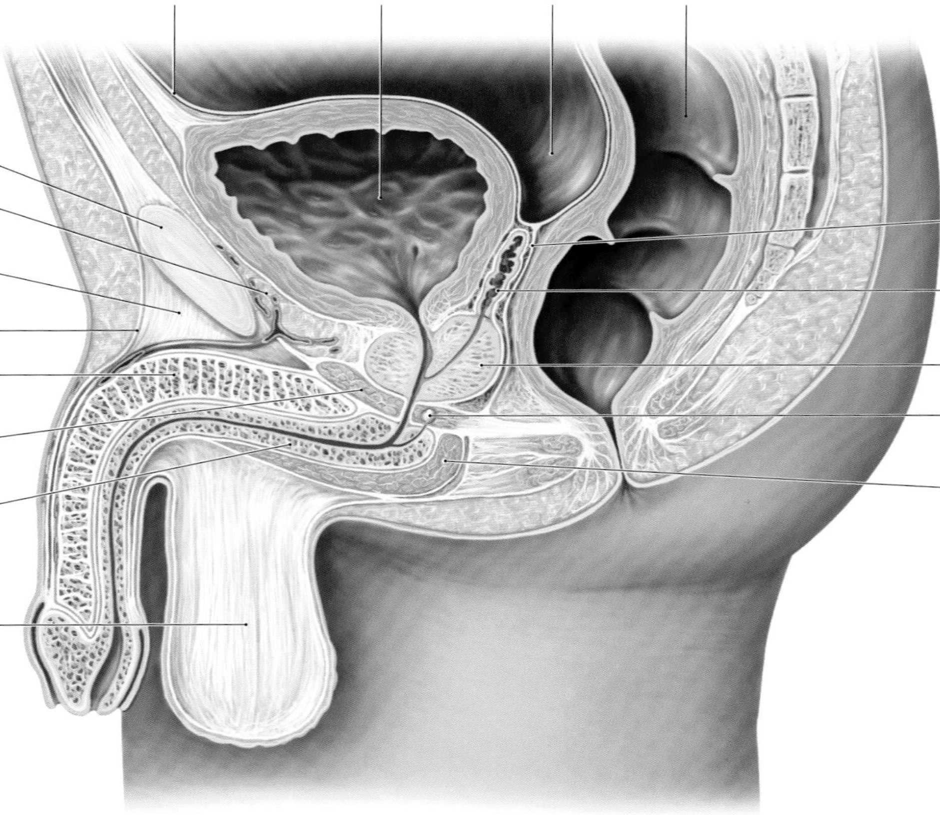

Labels for figure A:
- Sigmoid mesocolon
- Sigmoid colon
- Bladder
- Rectovesical septum
- Rectovesical pouch
- Retropubic space
- Retroperitoneal space
- Central tendon of perineum
- Rectum

Labels for figure B:
- Parietal peritoneum
- Bladder
- Rectovesical pouch
- Rectum
- Pubic symphysis
- Retropubic space
- Suspensory ligament of penis
- Penile fascia
- Corpus cavernosum of penis
- Sphincter urethrae
- Corpus spongiosum of penis
- Scrotal septum
- Rectovesical septum
- Ampulla of vas deferens
- Prostate
- Bulbourethral gland
- Bulbospongiosus muscle

B Peritoneal relationships in the male pelvis

Midsagittal section, viewed from the left side. The bulbourethral gland has been displaced slightly medially to show its position in the sphincter urethrae muscle. The peritoneum is reflected from the anterior wall of the peritoneal cavity onto the upper surface of the bladder. The bladder in this section is shown in a distended state. When the bladder is empty, it is considerably smaller and lies behind the pubic symphysis.

The surface of the empty bladder also bears a transverse crease, the transverse vesical fold. Posteriorly, the peritoneum is reflected from the bladder surface onto the anterior wall of the rectum, forming a small recess termed the rectovesical pouch. The peritoneum does not extend to the prostate. The rectovesical pouch is the lowest part of the male peritoneal cavity.

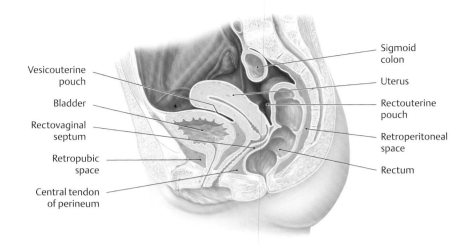

C Visceral fasciae in the female pelvis
Midsagittal section, viewed from the left side. As in the male pelvis, the pelvic extraperitoneal space contains fasciae and septa that determine the boundaries of fascial spaces. The specific spatial relationships are altered relative to the male, however by the presence of the uterus, which is interposed between the bladder and rectum (see **D**). The fascial spaces are greatly distorted during labor and delivery as the connective tissues surrounding the organs are compressed by the passage of the fetus through the birth canal.

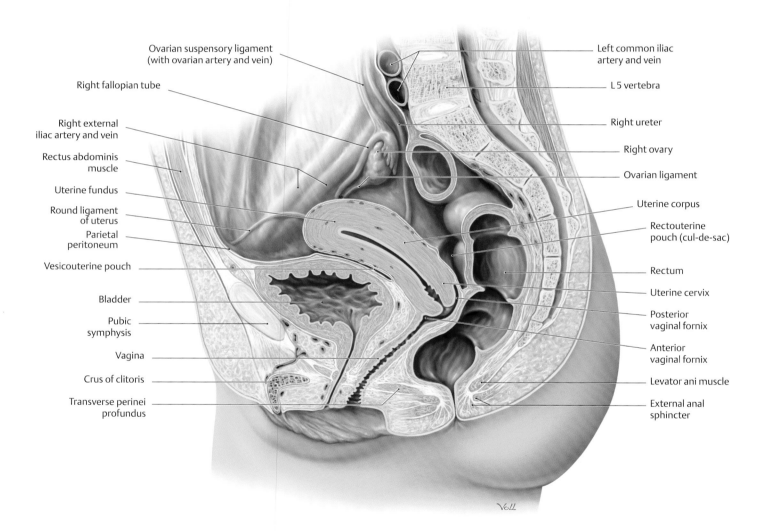

D Peritoneal relationships in the female pelvis
Midsagittal section, viewed from the left side. The small and large intestine have been removed except for the sigmoid colon and rectum.
Note: In the female, the uterus and its ligaments are interposed between the bladder and rectum. This alters the peritoneal relationships in a characteristic way compared with the male pelvis. The peritoneum is reflected from the anterior wall of the peritoneal cavity onto the bladder surface as in the male, but from there it is reflected onto the anterior wall of the uterus. Because the uterus typically occupies an anteflexed and anteverted position on the bladder (see p. 251), the peritoneum be-

tween the bladder and uterus forms a deep but narrow recess, the *vesicouterine pouch*. The reflection of the peritoneum from the posterior wall of the uterus onto the anterior wall of the rectum forms a second recess, the *rectouterine pouch* (known clinically as the *cul-de-sac*). This pouch is the lowest part of the female peritoneal cavity. It is clinically important because it is accessible to transvaginal diagnostic procedures (needle aspiration, endovaginal ultrasound). The bladder in this section is shown in a distended state. As the bladder fills with urine, it raises the uterus to a more upright position.

1.12 Peritoneal Relationships and Spaces in the Male Pelvis

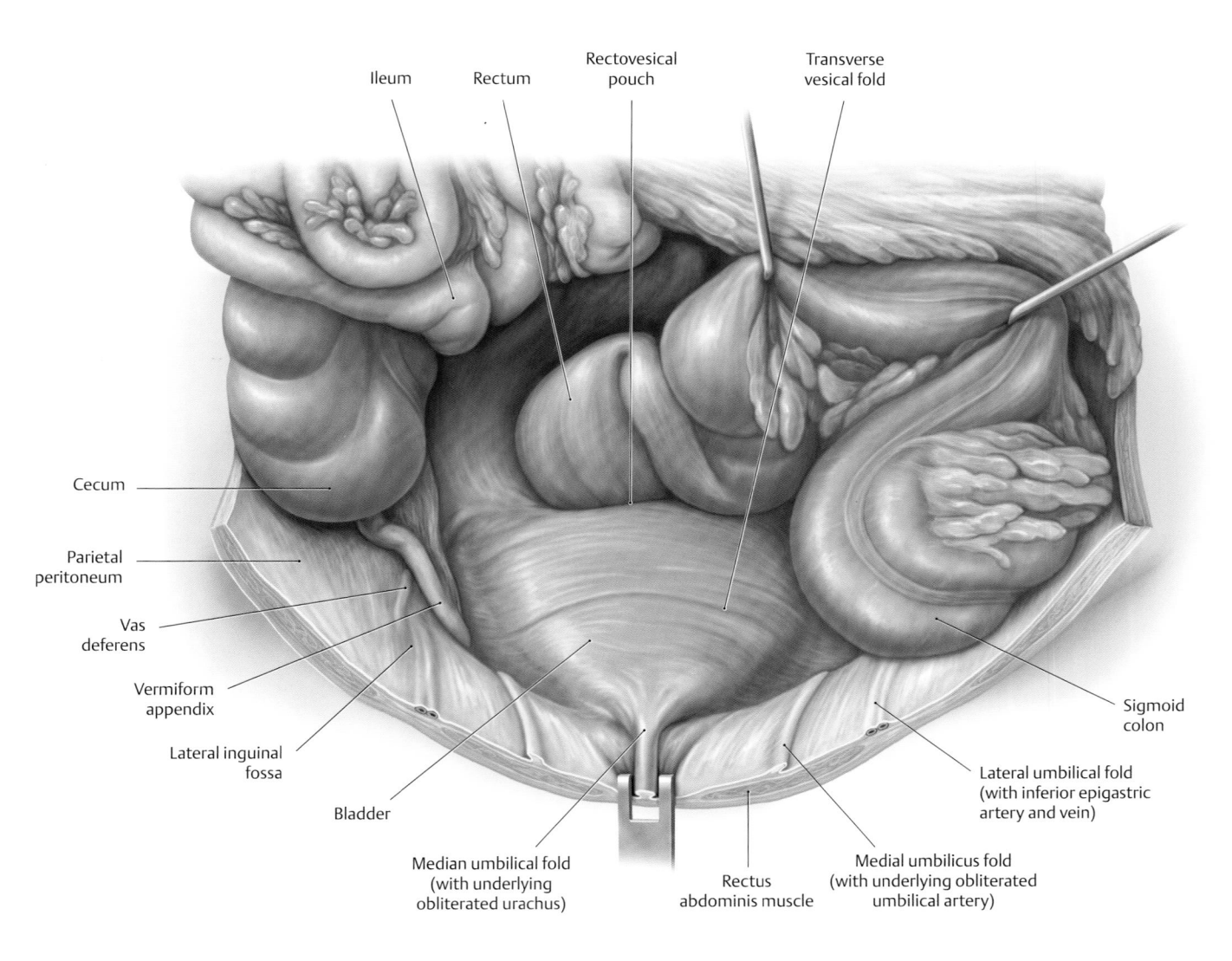

Ileum   Rectum   Rectovesical pouch   Transverse vesical fold

Cecum

Parietal peritoneum

Vas deferens

Vermiform appendix

Lateral inguinal fossa

Bladder

Median umbilical fold (with underlying obliterated urachus)

Rectus abdominis muscle

Medial umbilicus fold (with underlying obliterated umbilical artery)

Lateral umbilical fold (with inferior epigastric artery and vein)

Sigmoid colon

A Peritoneal relationships in the male lesser pelvis

Anterosuperior view. Loops of small intestine and portions of the colon have been retracted laterally and posteriorly to demonstrate the bladder and rectum.

Note: The parietal peritoneum on the anterior abdominal wall is reflected onto the surface of the bladder. It forms a transverse crease in the empty bladder, the transverse vesical fold, which is effaced when the bladder is full. The vas deferens, which passes through the anterior wall via the inguinal canal, is also covered by parietal peritoneum in this area. The peritoneum between the bladder and rectum is deepened into a cavity, the rectovesical pouch.

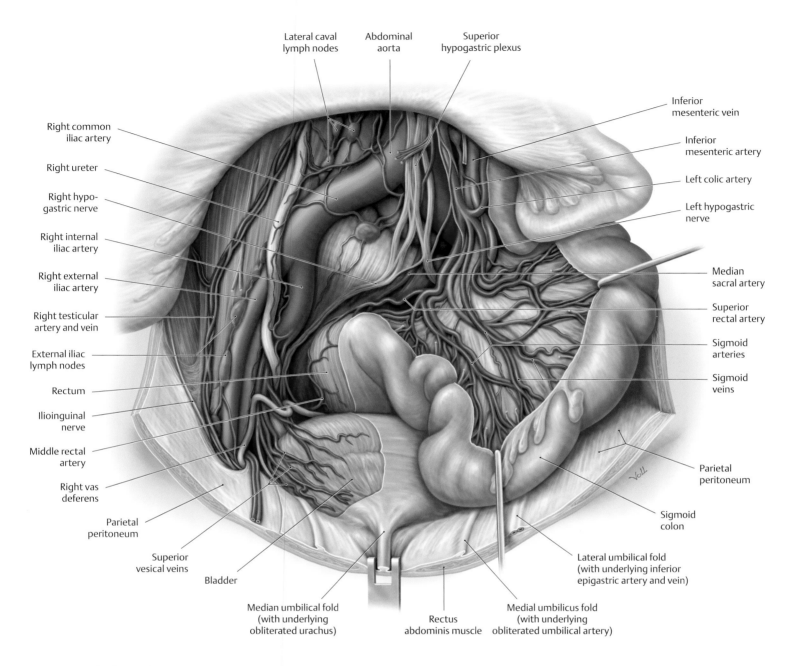

Lateral caval lymph nodes

Abdominal aorta

Superior hypogastric plexus

Inferior mesenteric vein

Inferior mesenteric artery

Left colic artery

Left hypogastric nerve

Right common iliac artery

Right ureter

Right hypogastric nerve

Right internal iliac artery

Right external iliac artery

Right testicular artery and vein

External iliac lymph nodes

Rectum

Ilioinguinal nerve

Middle rectal artery

Right vas deferens

Parietal peritoneum

Superior vesical veins

Bladder

Median umbilical fold (with underlying obliterated urachus)

Rectus abdominis muscle

Medial umbilicus fold (with underlying obliterated umbilical artery)

Median sacral artery

Superior rectal artery

Sigmoid arteries

Sigmoid veins

Parietal peritoneum

Sigmoid colon

Lateral umbilical fold (with underlying inferior epigastric artery and vein)

B Peritoneal relationships in the male lesser pelvis
Anterosuperior view. The sigmoid colon has been retracted laterally. In contrast to **A**, the peritoneum over the sigmoid mesocolon, rectum, bladder, and the posterior and lateral pelvic walls has been partially removed to expose the underlying structures. Lymph nodes and autonomic nerve plexuses are shown schematically for clarity.

Note the site where the ureters pass in front of the iliac vessels. This creates a constricted area in which renal stones may become lodged while passing down the ureter. This crossing site is one of three anatomical constrictions of the ureter (see p. 233).

1.13 Peritoneal Relationships and Spaces in the Female Pelvis

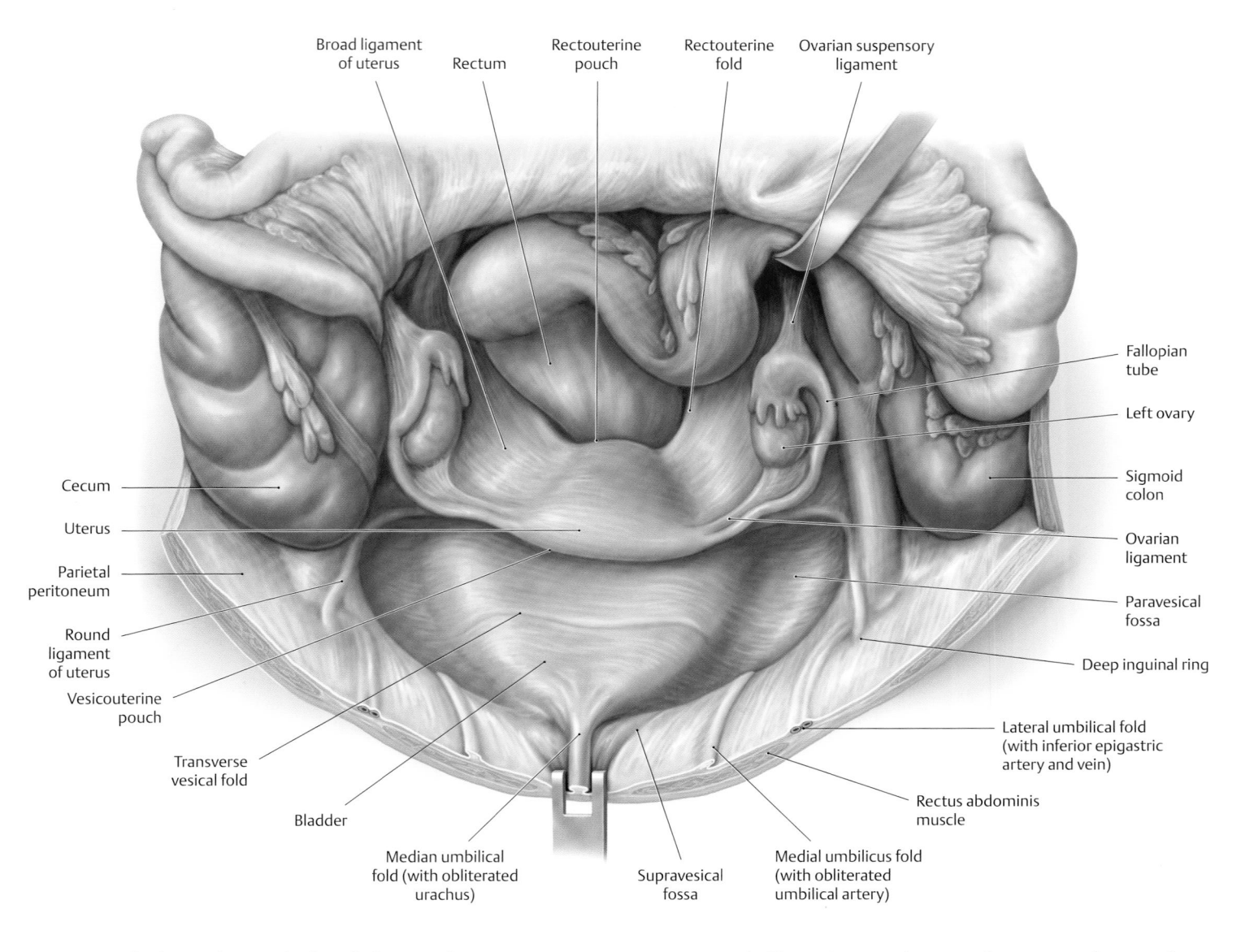

A Peritoneal relationships in the female lesser pelvis
Anterosuperior view. The parietal peritoneum of the anterior abdominal wall is reflected onto the bladder and then is continued onto the uterus and the anterior wall of the rectum. The peritoneum on the bladder covers the bladder apex. The peritoneum covers all of the uterus except for part of the cervix (not visible here), and it covers most of the parametrial connective tissue (parametrium). The peritoneum on the rectum covers the anterior and lateral wall of the upper rectum. The peritoneum is recessed between the bladder and uterus to form the narrow vesico- uterine pouch. The peritoneum between the uterus and rectum forms the broad rectouterine pouch (cul-de-sac), which is the lowest part of the female peritoneal cavity. The ovaries and fallopian tubes are intra- peritoneal organs, and so they are completely covered by peritoneum. The peritoneal cavity in the male is a completely closed cavity. In the female, however, the abdominal end of the patent fallopian tube creates a "potential opening to the outside." The cervical mucus plug of pregnancy creates a germ-proof seal on the uterus that protects the peritoneal cav- ity from ascending infections.

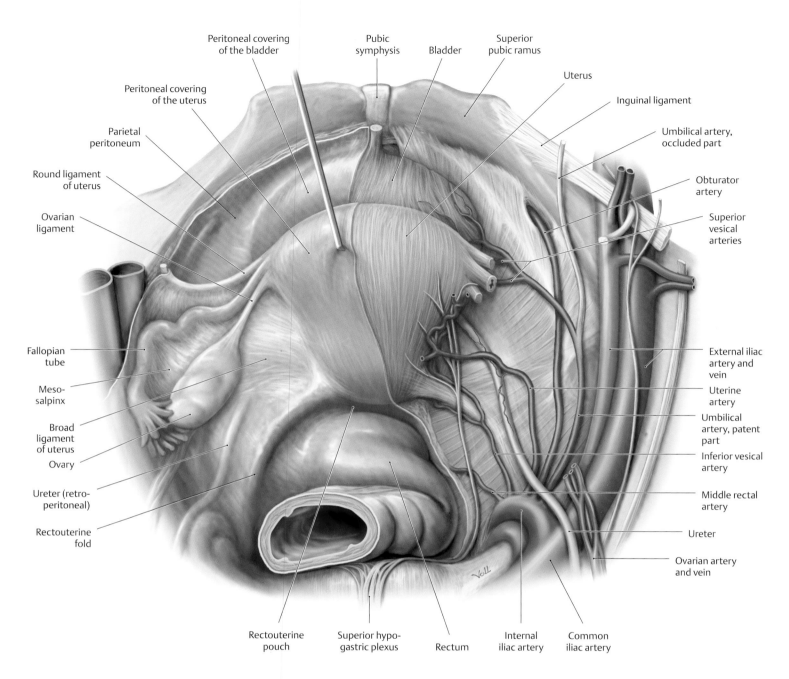

Peritoneal covering of the bladder
Pubic symphysis
Bladder
Superior pubic ramus
Uterus
Peritoneal covering of the uterus
Inguinal ligament
Parietal peritoneum
Umbilical artery, occluded part
Round ligament of uterus
Obturator artery
Ovarian ligament
Superior vesical arteries
Fallopian tube
External iliac artery and vein
Meso-salpinx
Uterine artery
Broad ligament of uterus
Umbilical artery, patent part
Ovary
Inferior vesical artery
Ureter (retro-peritoneal)
Middle rectal artery
Rectouterine fold
Ureter
Ovarian artery and vein
Rectouterine pouch
Superior hypo-gastric plexus
Rectum
Internal iliac artery
Common iliac artery

B Peritoneal relationships in the female lesser pelvis

Posterosuperior view. The peritoneum over the uterus, bladder, and lateral and posterior pelvic walls has been partially removed. The uterus has been retracted forward, and the uterine broad ligament, a part of the parametrium, has been removed on the right side (along with the right ovary and fallopian tube). The uterus normally occupies an ante-verted and anteflexed position (see p. 251) and it overrides the bladder, which pushes the uterus upward as it fills with urine.

As the ureter descends toward the bladder, it passes through the parametrium (removed here on the right side) and inferior to the uterine artery. This proximity of the ureter to the artery should be taken into account during operations on the uterus and parametrium.

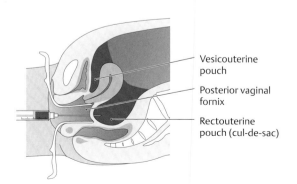

Vesicouterine pouch
Posterior vaginal fornix
Rectouterine pouch (cul-de-sac)

C Needle aspiration of the rectouterine pouch

Midsagittal section of the pelvis, viewed from the left side. A needle can be passed through the posterior vaginal fornix into the rectouterine pouch (known clinically as the cul-de-sac) to obtain a fluid sample for diagnostic analysis. The fluid may consist of blood or pus, for example, that has gravitated to this deepest point in the female peritoneal cavity. In the case illustrated, the cul-de-sac has been markedly expanded by blood, effacing the posterior vaginal fornix

1.14 Location and Attachments of the Pelvic Organs: Comparison of Transverse Sections in the Male and Female

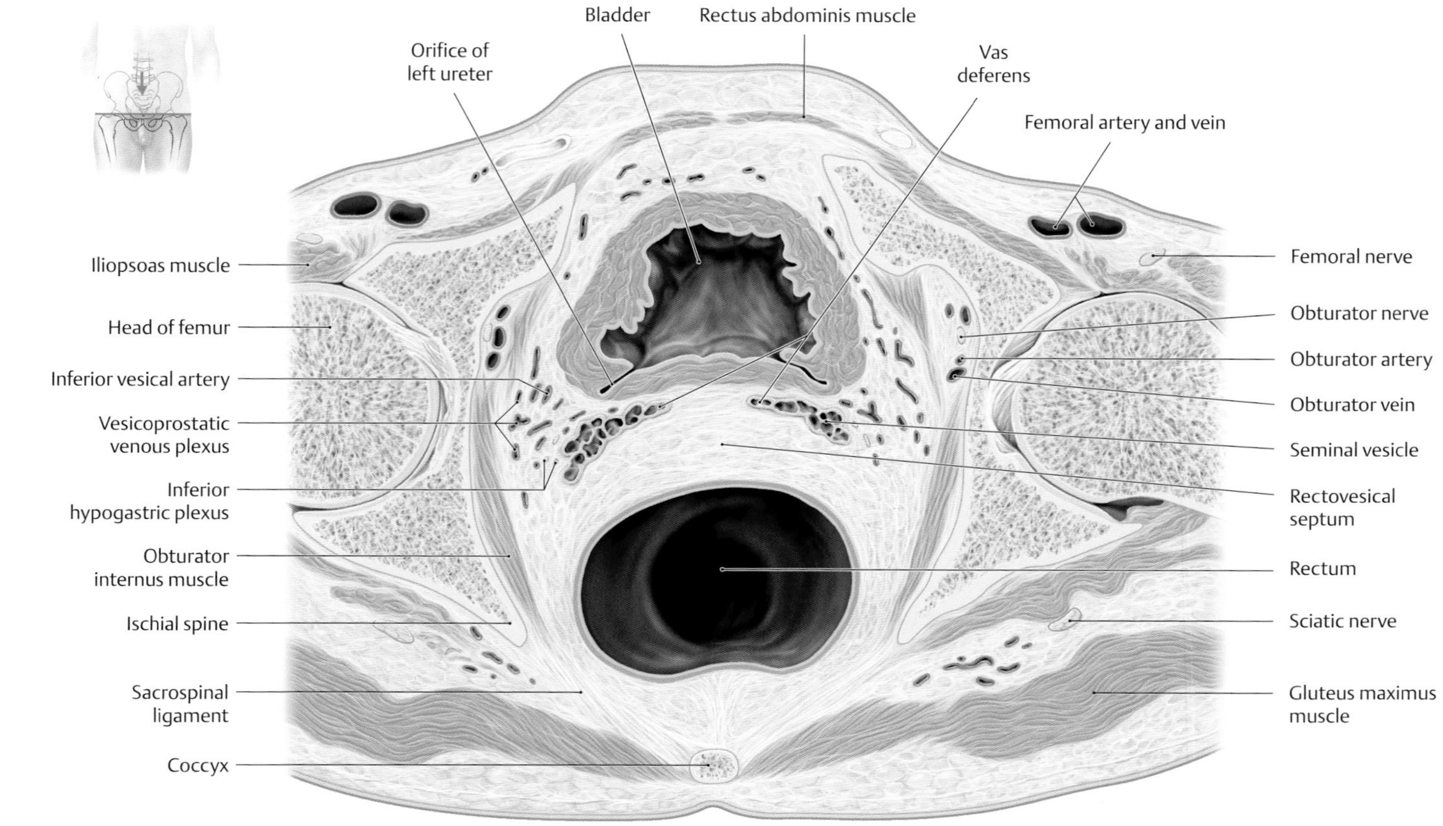

Bladder   Rectus abdominis muscle

Orifice of
left ureter

Vas
deferens

Femoral artery and vein

Iliopsoas muscle

Head of femur

Inferior vesical artery

Vesicoprostatic
venous plexus

Inferior
hypogastric plexus

Obturator
internus muscle

Ischial spine

Sacrospinal
ligament

Coccyx

Femoral nerve

Obturator nerve

Obturator artery

Obturator vein

Seminal vesicle

Rectovesical
septum

Rectum

Sciatic nerve

Gluteus maximus
muscle

A Location of the male pelvic organs in transverse section

Section through the male pelvis at the level of the hip joints, viewed from above. The bladder lies anteriorly and has been sectioned at the level of the ureteral orifices. Just behind the bladder are the sectioned seminal vesicles. The posterior orifice is the rectum, which is separated from the bladder by the connective tissue of the rectovesical septum. The connective tissue around the bladder and rectum allows them to change their shape and volume as they become distended. The connective tissue *lateral* to the bladder (the lateral vesicular ligament) contains multiple sections of an extensive venous network, the vesical venous plexus, which drains venous blood from the bladder and prostate (as the vesicoprostatic venous plexus) to the vesical veins (not visible here) and then to the internal iliac vein.

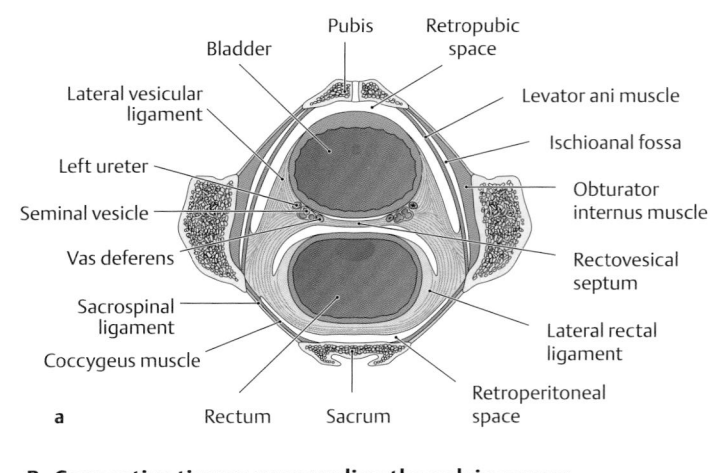

Pubis   Retropubic
space
Bladder

Lateral vesicular
ligament

Left ureter

Seminal vesicle

Vas deferens

Sacrospinal
ligament

Coccygeus muscle

Levator ani muscle

Ischioanal fossa

Obturator
internus muscle

Rectovesical
septum

Lateral rectal
ligament

Retroperitoneal
space

a   Rectum   Sacrum

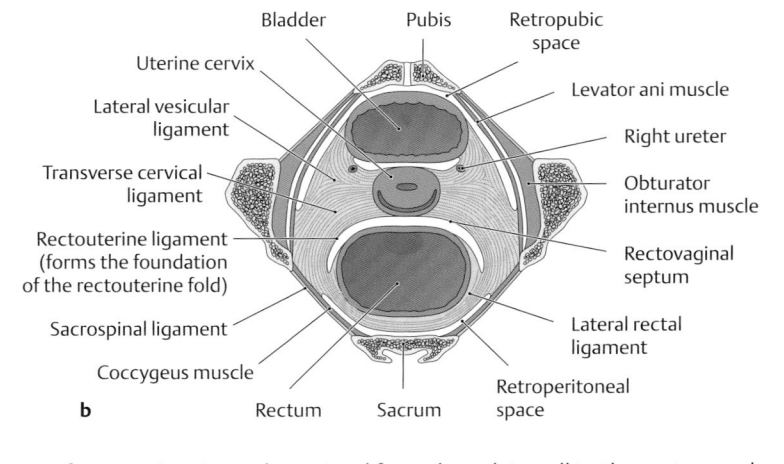

Bladder   Pubis   Retropubic
space

Uterine cervix

Lateral vesicular
ligament

Transverse cervical
ligament

Rectouterine ligament
(forms the foundation
of the rectouterine fold)

Sacrospinal ligament

Coccygeus muscle

Levator ani muscle

Right ureter

Obturator
internus muscle

Rectovaginal
septum

Lateral rectal
ligament

Retroperitoneal
space

b   Rectum   Sacrum

B Connective tissues surrounding the pelvic organs

Superior view. **a** Male pelvis, **b** female pelvis.

Most of the connective tissue in the extraperitoneal space of the male and female pelvis consists of loose connective tissue. Its function is to impart a certain mobility to the pelvic organs. Another function of this connective tissue, however, is to give attachment and stability to the pelvic organs. This purpose is served by two large supporting columns of connective tissue that extend from the pelvic wall to the rectum and to the bladder. These columns not only provide structural support but also transmit neurovascular bundles to the organs. The connective tissue is also condensed to form a coronally-oriented connective-tissue plate that is called the *rectovesical septum* in the male (see p. 170) and the *rectovaginal septum* in the female.

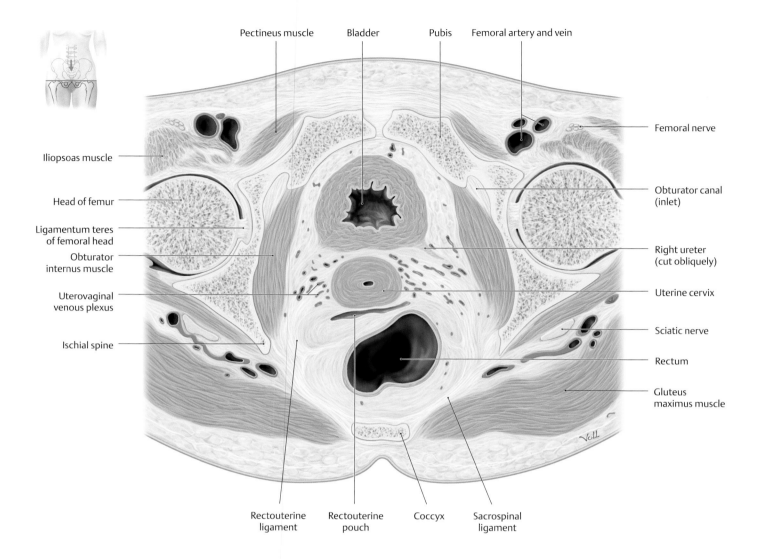

Pectineus muscle — Bladder — Pubis — Femoral artery and vein

Iliopsoas muscle

Head of femur

Ligamentum teres
of femoral head

Obturator
internus muscle

Uterovaginal
venous plexus

Ischial spine

Femoral nerve

Obturator canal
(inlet)

Right ureter
(cut obliquely)

Uterine cervix

Sciatic nerve

Rectum

Gluteus
maximus muscle

Rectouterine
ligament — Rectouterine
pouch — Coccyx — Sacrospinal
ligament

C Location of the female pelvic organs in transverse section
Section through the female pelvis at the superior border of the pubic symphysis. The section cuts the bladder just above the ureteral orifices. Posterior to the bladder is a section of the uterine cervix, and behind that is the rectum (separated from the cervix by the base of the rectouterine pouch). As in the male pelvis, connective tissue is distributed around the bladder and rectum. Additional connective tissue is found around the cervix, representing a downward prolongation of the transverse cervical ligament. A venous network, the uterovaginal venous plexus, is embedded in the connective tissue and is cut at numerous sites in the section above. This plexus provides venous drainage for the uterus and vagina.

Note: Peritoneal pouches exist in front of and behind the uterus: the vesicouterine pouch anteriorly and the rectouterine pouch posteriorly. The section shown here cuts the pelvis at the level of the rectouterine pouch (cul-de-sac). The vesicouterine pouch does not extend as inferiorly and terminates above the plane of section. As a result, the area between the cervix and bladder in this section is occupied by connective tissue (formerly called the "vesicovaginal septum").

2.1 Embryonic Development of the Gastrointestinal Tract: The Foregut

A Embryonic development of the gastrointestinal canal

The gastrointestinal canal and its associated organs (liver and pancreas) develop from the endoderm. The peritoneum develops from the mesoderm and covers the organs of the gastrointestinal tract. During the early phase of embryonic development (fifth week), the organs rotate and change their position while the visceral peritoneum fuses at selected sites to the parietal peritoneum. The following processes are important in understanding the topographical anatomy of the abdominal cavity:

- Rotation of the stomach and formation of the liver and pancreas (see **C**, **D**, and **E**)
- Development of the pancreas and its migration to the dorsal wall of the peritoneal cavity behind the peritoneum ("retroperitonealization," see **E** and **G**)
- Formation of the omental bursa (see **F**)
- Rotation of the intestinal loop and the disposition of the small and large intestine (see p. 180)
- Development of the cecum and vermiform appendix (see p. 180)
- Migration of the ascending and descending colon to the dorsal body wall and attachment of the mesocolon (retroperitonealization, see p. 181)
- Formation of the greater omentum (see p. 181).

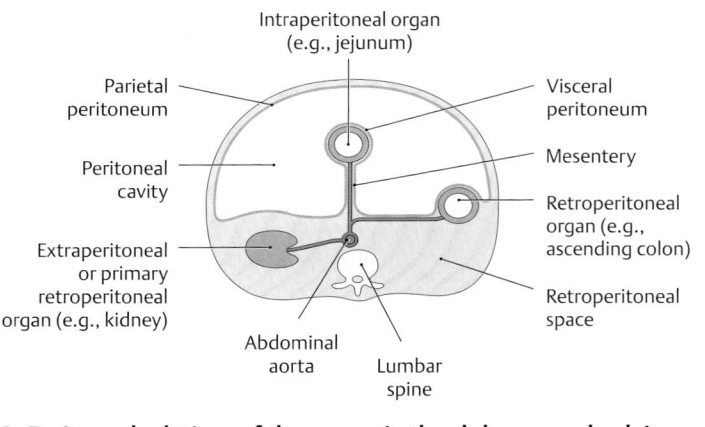

B Peritoneal relations of the organs in the abdomen and pelvis

Transverse section through the embryonic abdomen at the level of the lumbar spine, viewed from above. A knowledge of the embryonic development of the alimentary tract can yield important topographical and functional insights. All organs can be classified based on their relationship to the peritoneal cavity.

Intraperitoneal organs lie *within* the peritoneal cavity and are covered by *visceral* peritoneum. This allows them to glide relative to one another and relative to the wall of the peritoneal cavity. Neurovascular structures are distributed to these organs through a mesentery, which passes from the wall of the peritoneal cavity to the organ and is also covered by peritoneum on both sides (examples: jejunum and ileum).

Extraperitoneal organs are located in a connective-tissue space that is *behind* or *below* the peritoneal cavity (retro- or subperitoneal). Organs that are primarily extraperitoneal from the outset do not have a peritoneal covering. Organs that are secondarily extraperitoneal (become extraperitoneal during the course of embryonic development) are covered by peritoneum anteriorly, while their posterior surface is fused to the parietal peritoneum. The neurovascular structures that supply the extraperitoneal organs course within the (retroperitoneal) connective-tissue space and do not require a mesentery (example: the kidneys).

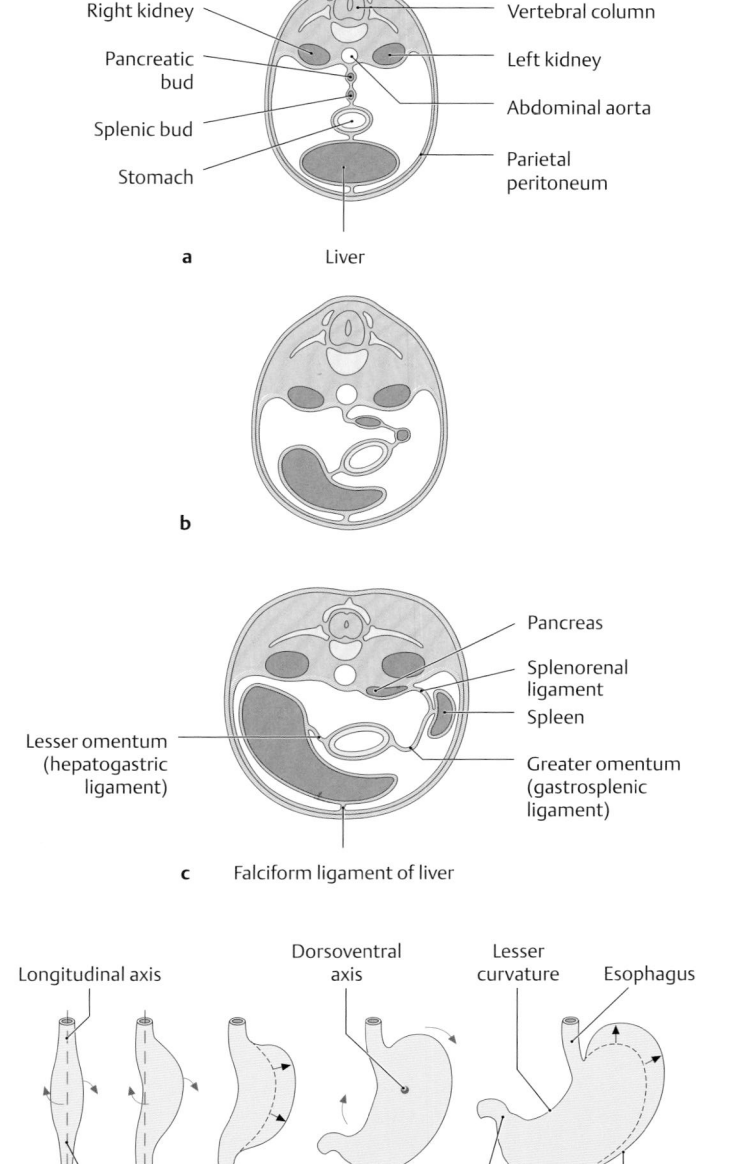

C Rotation of the stomach (after Sadler)
a–c Abdomen in transverse section, viewed from above.
a At the end of the 5th week of development, **c** in the 11th week of development (the pancreas is already retroperitoneal).

a Liver, stomach, spleen, and pancreas displayed on one axis.
b,c As the stomach rotates (details in **d**), the liver gradually moves to the right while the spleen and pancreas are carried to the left. The stomach, liver, and spleen remain intraperitoneal, while the pancreas becomes retroperitoneal.

d Stomach viewed from the anterior side.
The stomach rotates around its longitudinal axis (by approximately 90°) and also around a dorsoventral axis (see arrows). As a result, the ventral wall of the stomach moves to the right while the dorsal wall moves to the left. The dorsal wall grows faster than the ventral wall, forming the *greater curvature* on the left side of the stomach and the *lesser curvature* on the right side.

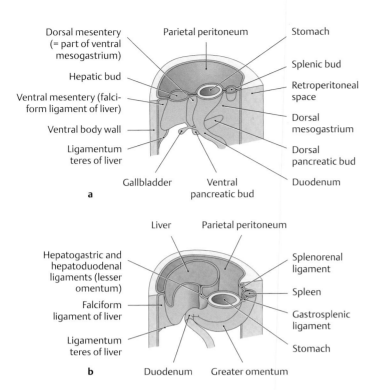

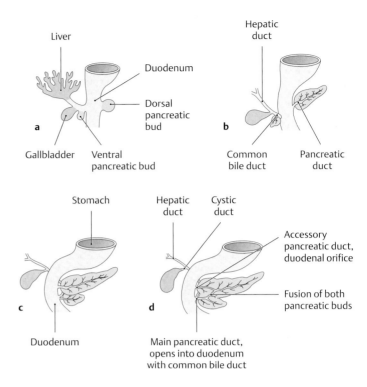

D Formation of the ventral and dorsal mesogastrium and migration of the organs in the upper abdomen
Transverse section of the abdomen, left superior view.

a Fifth week of development: By this stage the liver, gallbladder, and *ventral* pancreatic bud have developed in the *ventral* mesogastrium. The spleen and *dorsal* pancreatic bud have developed in the *dorsal* mesogastrium.

b Eleventh week of development: With the rotation of the stomach, the ventral mesogastrium becomes the *lesser omentum* while the dorsal mesogastrium becomes the *greater omentum*. The ventral mesentery develops into the *falciform ligament* with the *ligamentum teres* of the liver in the free margin. The mesenteric expansions ventral and dorsal to the spleen become the gastrosplenic and splenorenal ligaments.

E Dorsal and ventral pancreatic buds (after Sadler)
Embryonic gut viewed from the left side. The two pancreatic buds form as endodermal outgrowths from the duodenum in the ventral and dorsal mesentery. The ventral bud develops in close association with the common bile duct. It migrates around the duodenum and assumes a position slightly caudal to the dorsal bud (**c**). The two buds fuse, and a communication is established between their ducts (**d**). The duct of the ventral bud generally opens jointly with the common bile duct into the duodenum at the major duodenal papilla (of Vater), while the duct of the dorsal bud may open higher at the minor duodenal papilla (the papillae are inside the duodenum, hence they are not visible here).

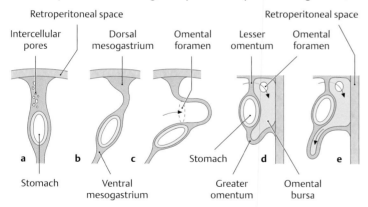

F Development of the omental bursa (after Sadler)
a–c Transverse sections through the abdomen, viewed from above.
d, e Sagittal sections, viewed from the left side.

Between the fourth and fifth weeks of embryonic development, isolated clefts or spaces develop in the dorsal mesogastrium at the same time the stomach is undergoing rotation. As the stomach rotates and displaces the dorsal mesogastrium, these clefts coalesce into a large open space behind the rotated stomach: the omental bursa. This bursa terminates blindly on its cranial, caudal, and left sides. A single physiological opening, the omental foramen, remains on the right side (see arrow in **d**; the lower arrow in **e** shows the deepening pouch formed by the greater omentum).

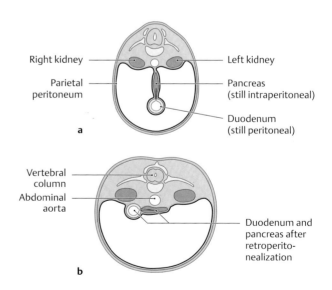

G Retroperitonealization of the pancreas and duodenum
(after Sadler)
Superior view, simplified schematic. The liver, stomach, and spleen in the dorsal mesogastrium are not shown. As a result of gastric rotation, the pancreas migrates dorsally while the duodenum swings dorsally toward the right side. Both organs fuse to the dorsal wall of the peritoneal cavity, becoming secondarily retroperitoneal.

179

2.2 Embryonic Development of the Gastrointestinal Tract: Rotation of the Primary Intestinal loop

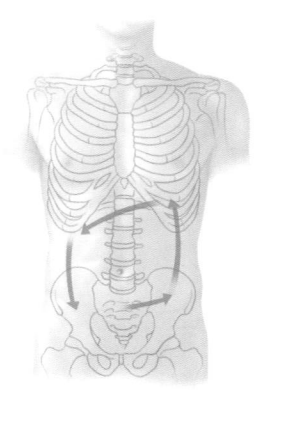

A Rotation of the primary intestinal loop
Projected onto the anterior trunk wall and skeleton.
Note: The primary intestinal loop rotates *counter*clockwise when viewed from the front, contrasting with the *clockwise* rotation of the stomach (see p. 178). This is important in understanding how the organs reach their final positions.
The frame-like shape of the colon and the location of the junction between the small intestine and cecum in the right lower abdomen (the ileocecal junction) result from the normal rotation of the intestinal loop. Incomplete rotation of the intestinal loop (less than 270°) or rotation in the *clockwise* direction results in an abnormal position of the colon segments. This condition may remain asymptomatic or may cause twisting and occlusion of intestinal segments.

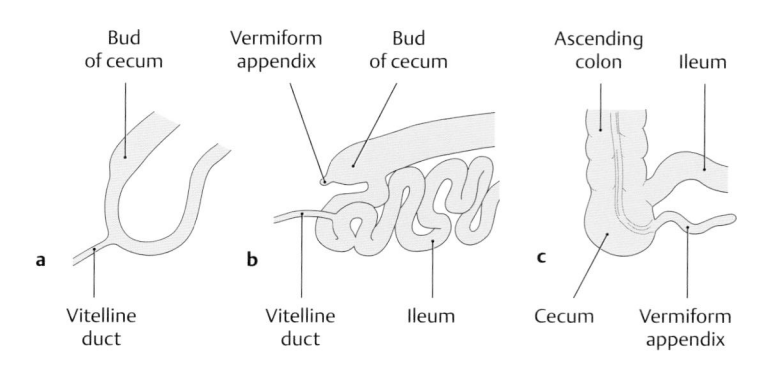

B Development of the cecum and vermiform appendix
(after Sadler)
Anterior view.

a In approximately the 6th week of development, the rudiment of the cecum appears at the junction of the small intestine and large intestine.
b In the 7 th to 8 th week, the rudiment of the vermiform appendix appears on the cecum.
c The ileum, cecum, and vermiform appendix shown in their normal relationship at the conclusion of embryonic development. The cecum at this stage forms a blind sac at the commencement of the large intestine. The ileum opens into the cecum from the left side. The vermiform appendix extends inferomedially from the cecum.

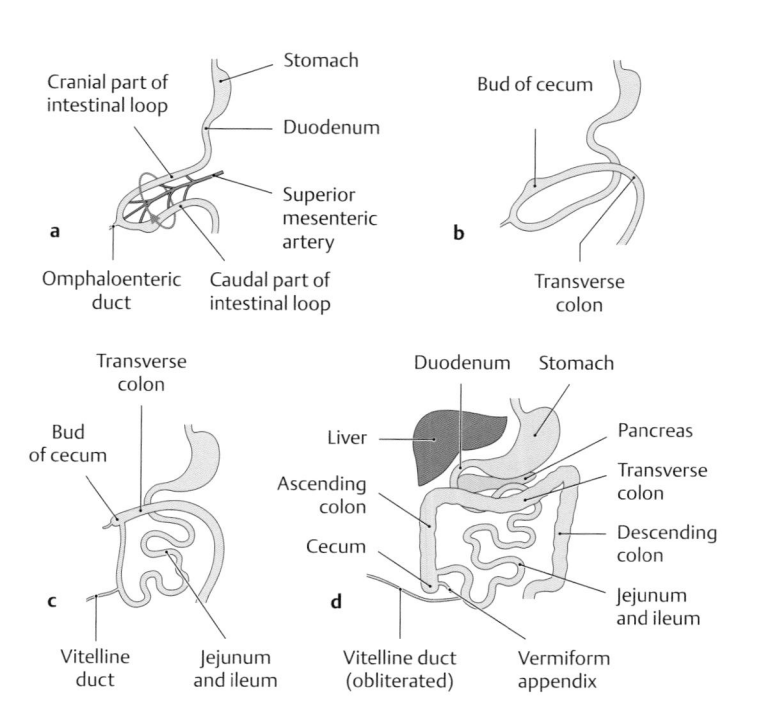
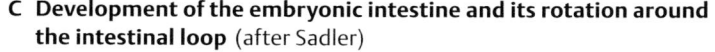

C Development of the embryonic intestine and its rotation around the intestinal loop (after Sadler)
Gastrointestinal canal viewed from the left side. The rotation of the primary intestinal (midgut) loop is an extremely complex process lasting approximately from the 5th to 11 th week of embryonic development.

a, b Viewed from the left, the intestinal loop goes through a total rotation of 270° in the counterclockwise direction (the axis of rotation is the superior mesenteric artery). After an initial rotation of 180°, the transverse colon lies in anterior to the duodenum.
c The cecum is located in the right upper quadrant. The small intestine already shows definite coiling, and the bowel loops have reached their final position.
d When the rotation of the stomach and intestinal loop is complete, the organs have assumed their typical adult positions:

- The liver is in the right epigastrium (attached to the duodenum and stomach by the lesser omentum).
- The lesser curvature of the stomach is directed upward to the right, the greater curvature downward to the left.
- The pancreas and most of the duodenum are retroperitoneal.
- The cecum, vermiform appendix, and ileocecal junction are in the right lower quadrant, and the vitelline duct is obliterated.
- The colon forms a frame around the jejunum and ileum, the transverse colon lying anterior to the duodenum.

At this stage the ascending and descending colon become secondarily retroperitoneal (see **D**).
Note: Due to space limitations, the rotation of the intestinal loop occurs partly *outside* the embryonic body cavity (extracorporeal). The rotated midgut then retracts back into the abdomen. Failure of this retraction may lead to an omphalocele, in which part of the small intestine protrudes through the abdominal wall at the umbilicus.

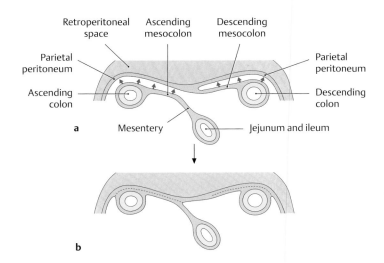

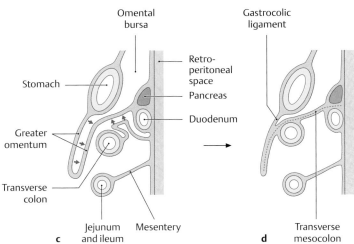

D Retroperitonealization of the ascending and descending colon and fusion of the greater omentum (after Moore and Persaud)
a, b Transverse sections, viewed from above. Following rotation of the intestinal loop, the colon segments have assumed their definitive positions with their mesenteries on the posterior wall of the peritoneal cavity. The ascending and descending mesocolon fuse completely to the parietal peritoneum, allowing the ascending and descending colon to become secondarily retroperitoneal.

c, d Sagittal sections, viewed from the left side. The greater omentum is draped over the transverse colon, which remains intraperitoneal. As the two layers of the greater omentum fuse together, the inferior recess of the omental bursa becomes smaller. When the greater omentum also fuses secondarily to the mesentery of the transverse colon, it assumes its final conformation and creates the definitive transverse mesocolon.

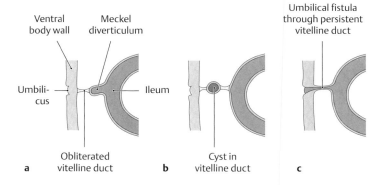

E Remnants of the vitelline duct (after Sadler)
Generally the vitelline duct, initially patent in the embryo, is completely obliterated and is lost as a connection between the ileum and trunk wall. Occasionally, however, the obliteration is incomplete or leaves an intact cord of connective tissue that tethers the ileum to the anterior trunk wall. This can have various manifestations:

a The wall of the ileum is outpouched at the fibrous cord, forming a **Meckel diverticulum** (usually located 40–60 cm cranial to the ileocecal valve). This protrusion is subject to inflammatory changes and often contains ectopic gastric or pancreatic tissue.
b A cyst remains within the fibrous cord. This **cyst** may cause complaints and requires differentiation from a tumor.
c The vitelline duct remains patent over its entire length, resulting in an **umbilical fistula**. In extreme cases, portions of the small intestine may herniate at the umbilicus and become inflamed. If a remnant of the vitelline duct persists as a fibrous cord between the ileum and umbilicus, mobile loops of small intestine may wrap around it and become strangulated (intestinal paralysis or "ileus," which often has a fatal outcome if untreated).

F Developmental anomalies of the gastrointestinal canal
The anomalies listed here, some quite rare except for Meckel diverticula, vary considerably in their pathological significance: A complete or near-complete occlusion in the gastrointestinal tract is usually fatal without treatment, whereas mild degrees of narrowing may remain asymptomatic. The twisting of bowel segments often causes strangulation and obstruction leading to a life-threatening condition.

Duodenal atresia	Solid duodenum without a lumen
Duodenal stenosis	Narrowing of the duodenal lumen (e.g., by an anular pancreas)
Biliary atresia	Congenital or acquired obstruction of some or all of the extrahepatic bile ducts
Anular pancreas	Duodenal stenosis (see above) caused by a ring of pancreatic tissue (see p. 214)
Omphalocele	Extracorporeal protrusion of small intestine at the umbilicus, caused by a failure of the rotated intestinal loop to retract (see **C**)
Malrotation	Abnormal or failed rotation of the intestinal loop (see **A** and **C**)
Volvulus	Twisting of small intestine on its mesentery, with risk of bowel obstruction or necrosis
Intestinal stenosis	Narrowing of the intestinal lumen
Intestinal atresia	Complete occlusion of the intestinal lumen, usually incompatible with life
Meckel diverticulum	Failure of regression of the vitelline duct with an associated ileal diverticulum (see **E**)

181

2.3 Stomach: Location, Peritoneal Relationships, and Relationship to Adjacent Organs

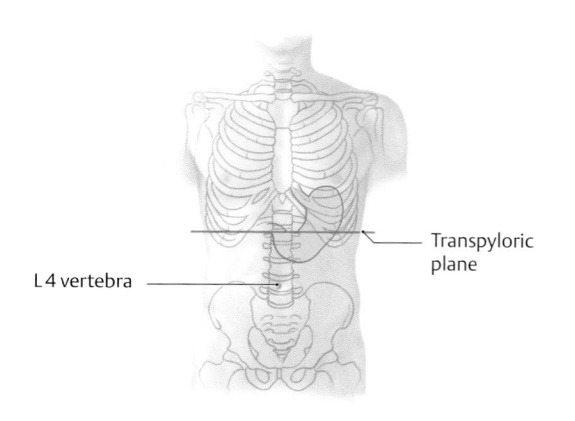

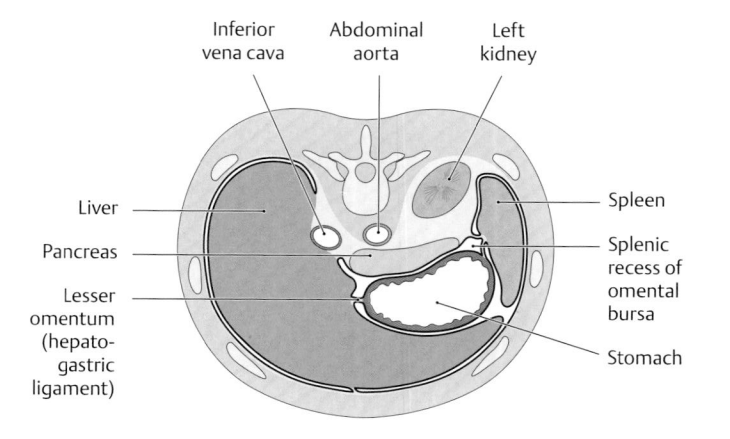

A Projection onto the trunk

Anterior view.

Note the position of the transpyloric plane (halfway between the superior border of the pubic symphysis and the superior border of the manubrium sterni, see p. 150). It provides an important landmark in physical examinations, for example, as the pylorus is located at or slightly below the transpyloric plane, hence its name. Unlike other parts of the stomach, the pylorus maintains a constant position because it is connected to the duodenum, which is retroperitoneal and therefore relatively immobile.

B Topographical relationships

Transverse section at approximately the T 12 / L 1 level, viewed from above.

Note the relationship of the stomach to the spleen, pancreas, liver, and omental bursa: The greater curvature of the stomach extends to the spleen. The left lobe of the liver extends in front of the stomach and into the left upper quadrant (LUQ). Thus when the abdomen is opened, very little of the stomach is visible, most of it is obscured by the mass of the liver. The omental bursa is a narrow peritoneal space located directly behind the stomach. The pancreas forms most of the posterior wall of the bursa. With its peritoneal covering, the stomach is very mobile relative to the surrounding organs, and this is an important factor in facilitating its intrinsic peristaltic movements. The stomach has direct peritoneal attachments to the spleen and liver owing to its embryonic placement in the dorsal and ventral mesogastrium (see p. 179).

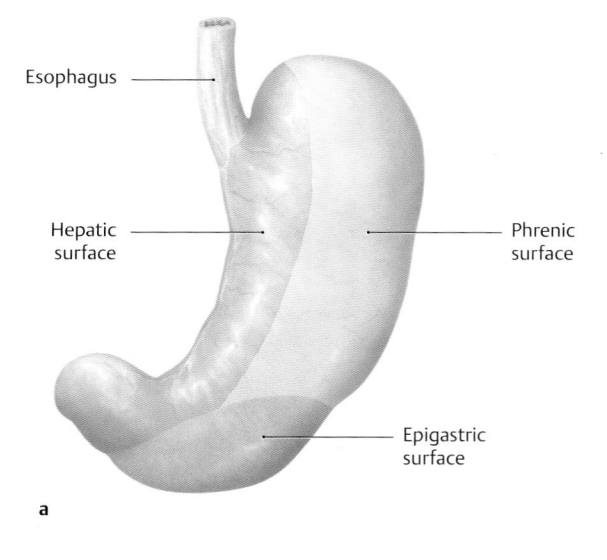

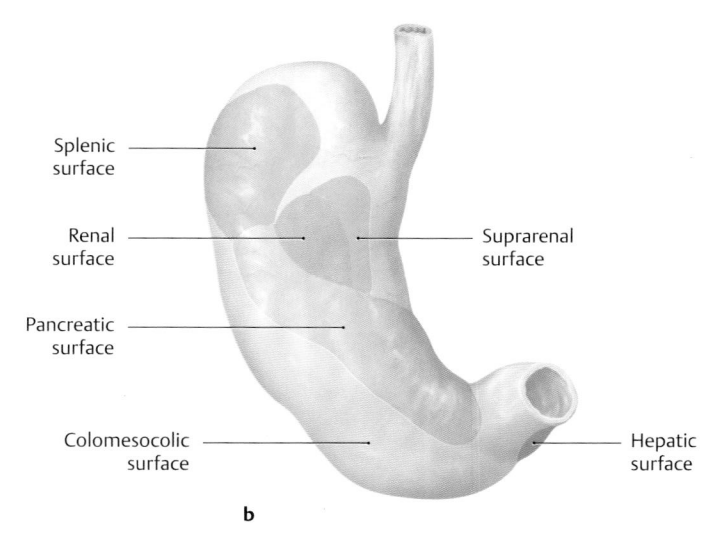

C Areas of contact with adjacent organs

a, b Anterior and posterior views of the stomach walls. Because the stomach is intraperitoneal, it is very mobile relative to adjacent organs. But since the stomach is in close contact with other organs, lesions that penetrate the stomach wall (ulcers, malignant tumors) may spread to nearby organs or may cause adhesions to develop between the stomach and adjacent organs.

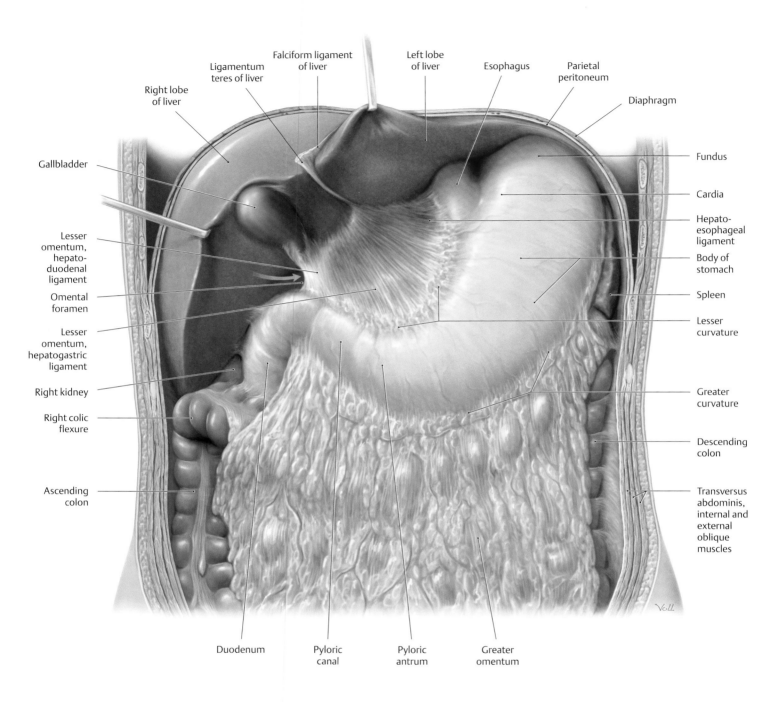

Right lobe of liver	Ligamentum teres of liver
Falciform ligament of liver	Left lobe of liver
Esophagus	Parietal peritoneum
Diaphragm	

Gallbladder

Lesser omentum, hepato-duodenal ligament

Omental foramen

Lesser omentum, hepatogastric ligament

Right kidney

Right colic flexure

Ascending colon

Fundus

Cardia

Hepato-esophageal ligament

Body of stomach

Spleen

Lesser curvature

Greater curvature

Descending colon

Transversus abdominis, internal and external oblique muscles

Duodenum   Pyloric canal   Pyloric antrum   Greater omentum

D The stomach in situ

Anterior view of the opened upper abdomen. The liver has been retracted superolaterally, and the esophagus has been pulled slightly downward for better exposure. The arrow points to the omental foramen, the opening in the omental bursa behind the lesser omentum. Peritoneal adhesions are visible between the liver and the descending part of the duodenum. The lesser omentum is visibly subdivided into a relatively thick hepatoduodenal ligament (transmitting neurovascular structures to the porta hepatis) and a thinner hepatogastric ligament, which is attached to the lesser curvature of the stomach. A hepato-esophageal ligament can also be identified. The greater curvature of the stomach is closely related to the spleen in the left upper quadrant (LUQ). The greater omentum is a duplication of peritoneum that covers the transverse colon and drapes over the loops of small intestine (not visible here).

2.4 Stomach: Shape and Interior

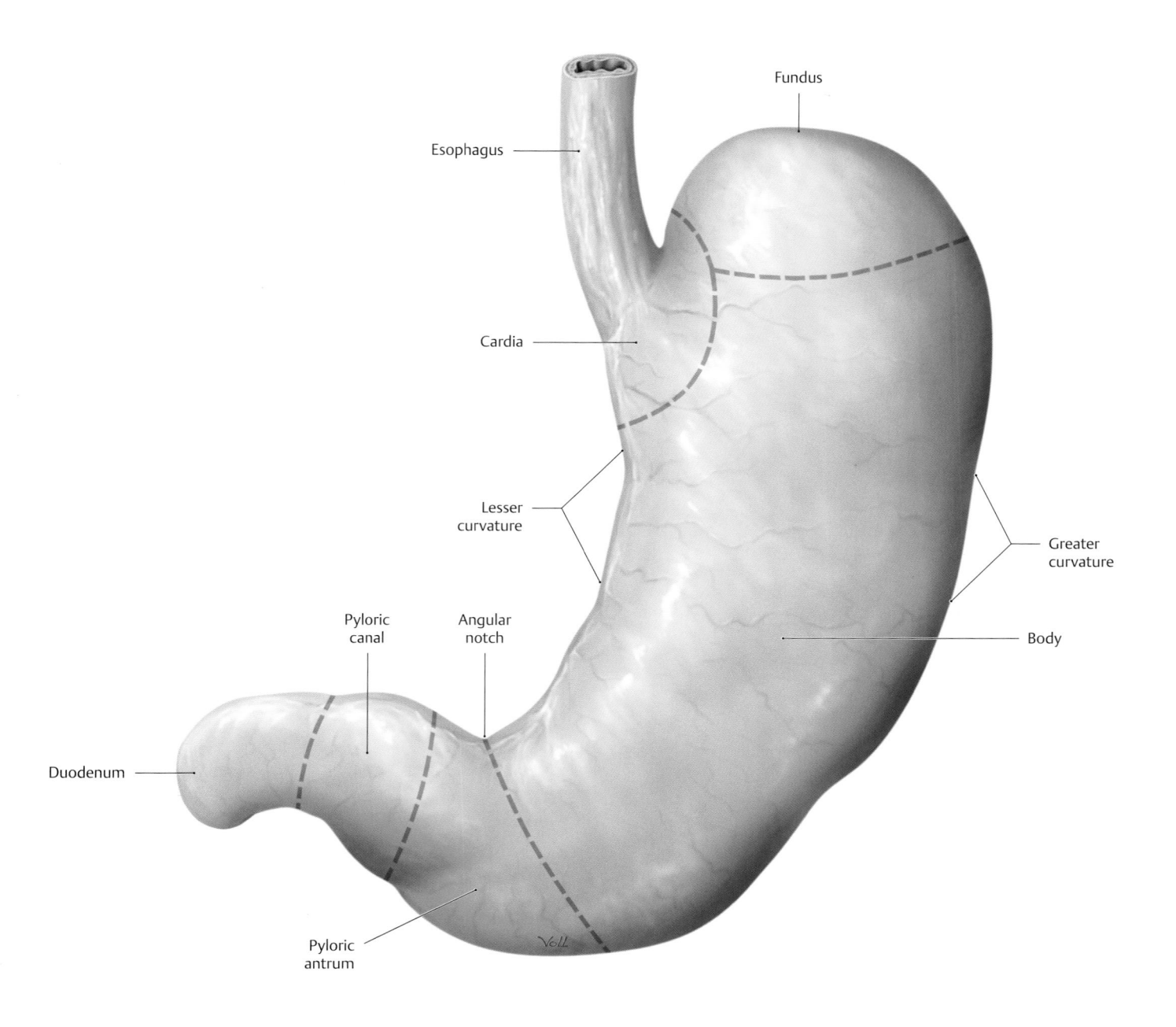

Fundus

Esophagus

Cardia

Lesser curvature

Greater curvature

Pyloric canal

Angular notch

Body

Duodenum

Pyloric antrum

A Shape and anatomical divisions

Anterior view of the anterior wall. The body (corpus) of the stomach is the largest part of the stomach. It terminates blindly at the gastric fundus, which in the standing patient is the highest part of the stomach and is usually filled with air (visible on radiographs as the "gastric bubble"). *Note:* The cardia is the area of the gastric inlet where the esophagus opens into the stomach (at the cardiac orifice). While the esophagus is invested by adventitial connective tissue, the stomach has a visceral peritoneal covering or serosa. The transition from adventitia to serosa is sharply defined, and occasionally the serosa continues a short distance onto the lower end of the esophagus.

The part of the stomach that opens into the duodenum, the pyloric part, consists of a broad pyloric antrum, a narrow pyloric canal, and the pylorus itself (pyloric orifice). The circular muscle layer of the stomach is markedly thickened at the end of the pyloric canal to form the pyloric sphincter (not visible here), which produces a visible external constriction of the pyloric canal.

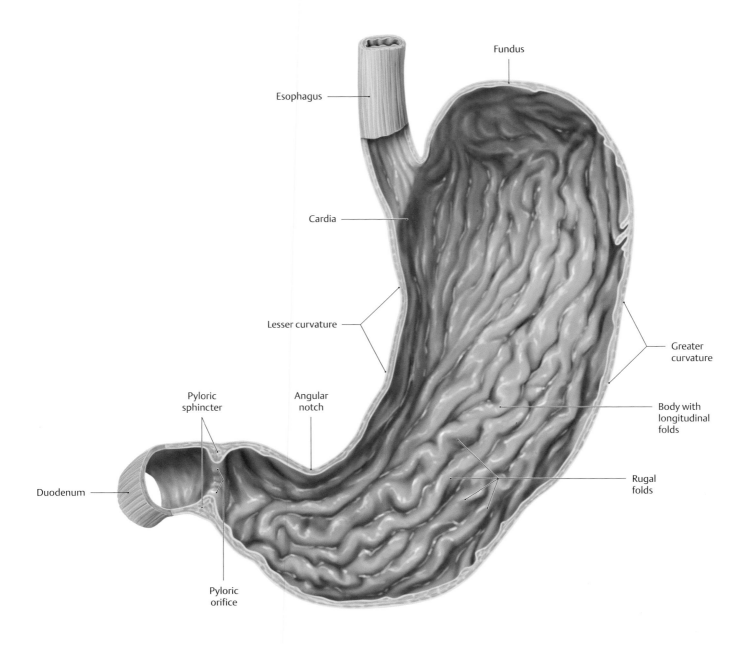

Esophagus

Fundus

Cardia

Lesser curvature

Greater curvature

Pyloric sphincter

Angular notch

Body with longitudinal folds

Duodenum

Rugal folds

Pyloric orifice

B Interior of the stomach

Anterior view of the stomach with the anterior wall removed. For clarity, small portions of the esophagus and duodenum are also shown. The gastric mucosa forms prominent folds (rugal folds) that serve to increase its surface area. These folds are directed longitudinally toward the pylorus, forming "gastric canals." The rugal folds are most promi-

nent in the body of the stomach and along the greater curvature and diminish in size toward the pyloric end. The mucosa imparts a glossy sheen to the stomach lining.

Note: The pyloric orifice is quite large in this dissection. Normally, the orifice usually opens to a luminal diameter of only 2–3 mm.

2.5 Stomach: Wall Structure and Histology

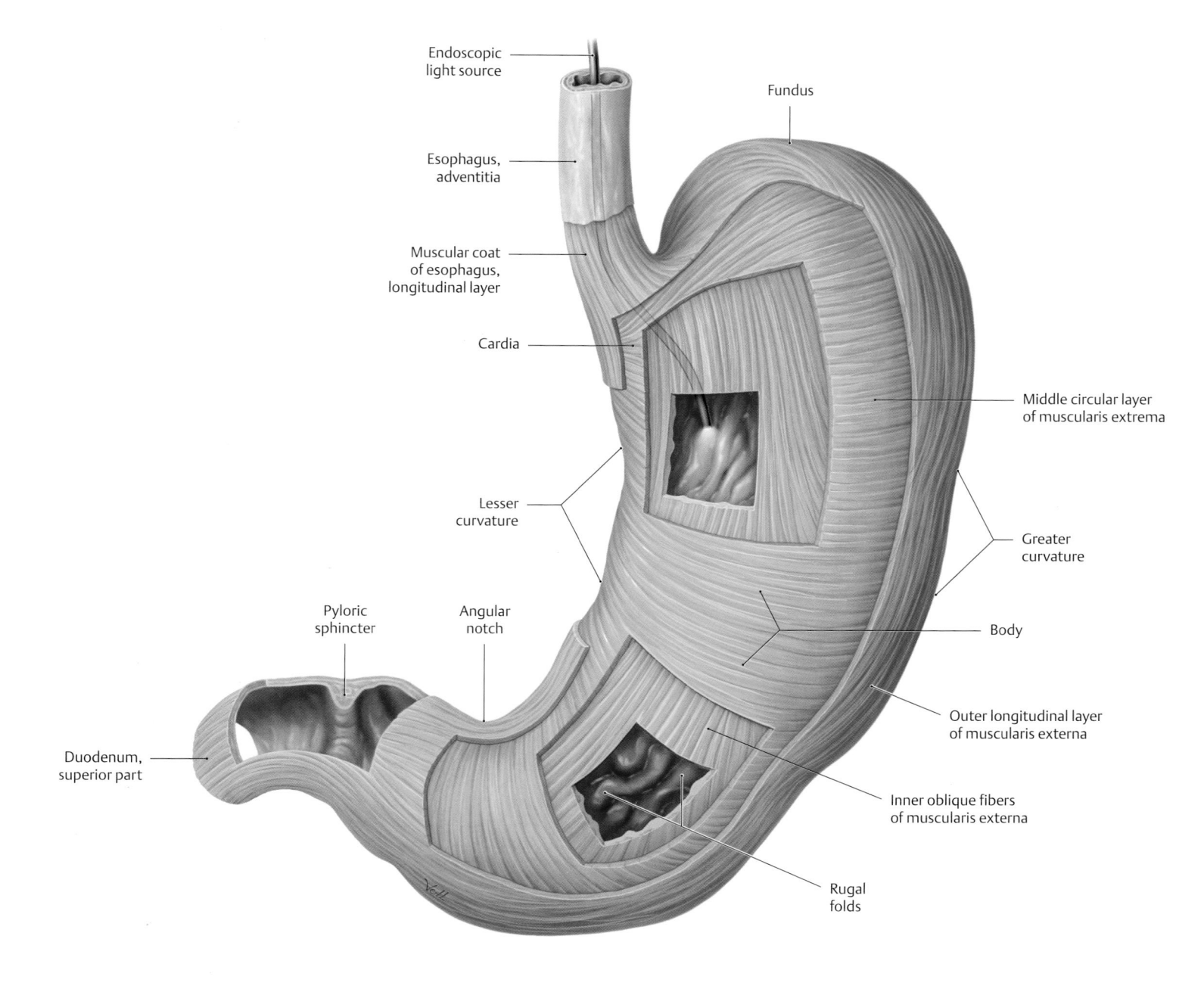

Endoscopic light source

Fundus

Esophagus, adventitia

Muscular coat of esophagus, longitudinal layer

Cardia

Middle circular layer of muscularis extrema

Lesser curvature

Greater curvature

Pyloric sphincter

Angular notch

Body

Duodenum, superior part

Outer longitudinal layer of muscularis externa

Inner oblique fibers of muscularis externa

Rugal folds

A Muscular layers

Anterior view of the anterior stomach wall with the serosa and subserosa removed. The muscular coat of the stomach has been windowed at several sites. The *entire stomach wall* ranges from 3 mm to approximately 10 mm in thickness (see **B** for individual layers). Most of its muscular coat consists not of two layers (as in other hollow organs of the gastrointestinal tract) but of *three* muscular layers:

- An outer longitudinal layer, which is most pronounced along the greater curvature (greatest longitudinal expansion)
- A middle circular layer, which is well developed in the body of the stomach and most strongly developed in the pyloric canal (anular sphincter, see p. 184)

- An innermost layer of oblique fibers, which is derived from the circular muscle layer and is clearly visible in the body of the stomach

The three-layered structure of its muscular wall enables the stomach to undergo powerful churning movements. The muscles can forcefully propel solid food components against the stomach wall in the acidic gastric juice, breaking the material up into particles approximately 1 mm in size that can pass easily through the pylorus. The longitudinally-oriented rugal folds (reserve folds that disappear when the stomach is distended) form channels, called gastric canals, that rapidly convey liquids from the gastric inlet to the pylorus.

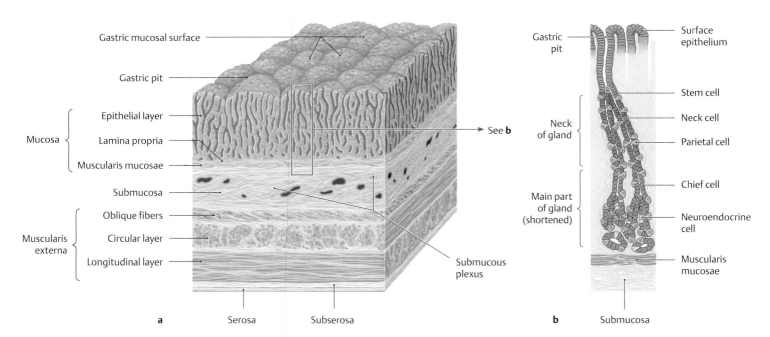

a Serosa   Subserosa   **b**   Submucosa

B Structure of the stomach wall and gastric glands

a The **structure of the stomach wall** illustrates the layered wall structure that is typical of the hollow organs throughout the gastrointestinal tract. The stomach is unique, however, in that its muscular coat consists of three rather than two layers (see **A**).

Note: The serosa (visceral layer of the peritoneum) and subserosa (connective-tissue layer giving attachment to the serosa and transmitting neurovascular structures for the muscular coat) are present only in areas where the organ in question is covered by visceral peritoneum. In wall areas that lack a peritoneal covering (e.g., large portions of the duodenum and colon), the serosa and subserosa are replaced by a fibrous adventitia, which connects the wall of the organ to the connective tissue of surrounding structures.

The *mucosa* contains specialized cells that are aggregated into *glands* (visible microscopically). The glandular *orifices* open at the base of the gastric pits (see **b**). In the body and pylorus of the stomach these glands extend down to the muscular layer of the mucosa, the muscularis mucosae (deeper glands = more cells = higher secretory output). The *submucosa* (layer of connective tissue transmitting neurovascular structures for the muscular coat) contains the *submucous*

plexus for visceromotor and viscerosensory control of the hollow organs in the gastrointestinal tract. This plexus, like the *myenteric plexus* (located in the muscular coat for visceromotor control of the visceral muscle, not shown here), is part of the *enteric* nervous system, which contains, in total, millions of scattered ganglion cells.

b **Structure of the gastric glands** (after Lüllmann-Rauch) (simplified schematic of a gland from the body of the stomach). Several types of cells are distinguished in the fundus and body of the stomach:
- Surface epithelial cells: cover the surface of the mucosa and secrete a mucous film
- Neck cells: produce mucin to strengthen the mucous film (make it more anionic)
- Parietal cells: produce HCl and intrinsic factor, which is necessary for vitamin B_{12} absorption in the ileum
- Chief cells: produce pepsinogen, which is converted to pepsin (for protein breakdown) in the stomach
- Neuroendocrine cells: different subtypes producing gastrin (G cells), somatostatin (D cells), or other factors controlling motility and secretion.
- Stem cells: reservoir for replenishing the surface epithelial cells and gland cells

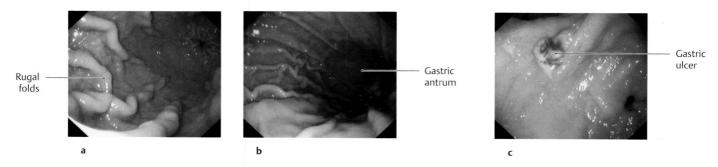

a   **b**   **c**

C Endoscopic appearance of the gastric mucosa

a, b Healthy gastric mucosa with a glistening surface **c** Gastric ulcer.

a View into the body of the stomach, which has been moderately distended by air insufflation. The mucosa is raised into prominent, tortuous rugal folds that form the gastric canals.

b Inspection of the pyloric antrum shows less prominent folds than in the body of the stomach.

c Fibrin-covered gastric ulcer with hematin spots. A gastric ulcer is defined as a tissue defect that extends at least into the muscularis mucosae, but many ulcers extend much deeper into the stomach wall. Most gastric ulcers are caused by infection with *Helicobacter pylori,* a bacterium that is resistant to stomach acid (from Block, Schachschal and Schmidt: *The Gastroscopy Trainer.* Stuttgart: Thieme, 2004).

2.6 Small Intestine: Duodenum

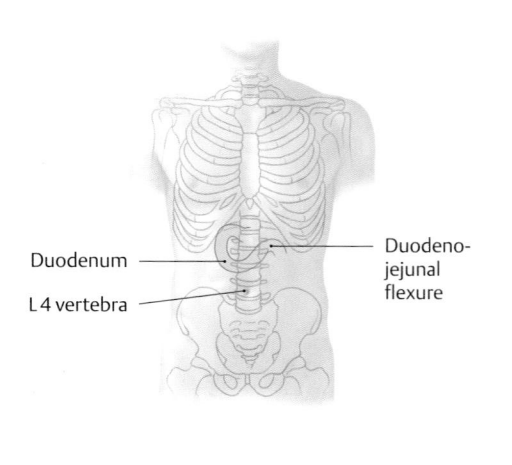

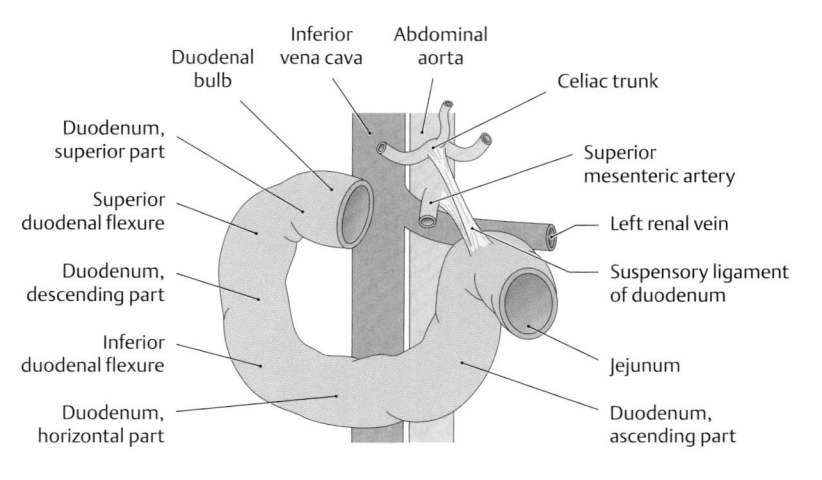

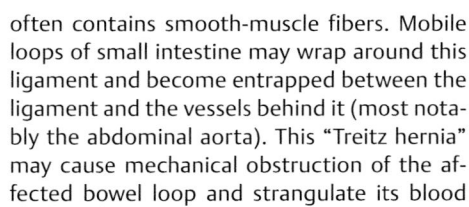

A Projected onto the vertebral column

The duodenum is a C-shaped loop of small intestine lying predominantly on the right side of the vertebral column in the right upper quadrant (RUQ) and encompassing the L 1 through L 3 vertebrae and occasionally extending to L 4. The concavity of the duodenum normally encloses the head of the pancreas at the L 2 level (see **D**).

B Parts of the duodenum

Anterior view. The anatomical parts of the duodenum (superior, descending, horizontal, and ascending parts with intervening flexures) have a total length of approximately 12 finger-widths (L. *duodeni* = "twelve at a time").
Note the suspensory ligament of the duodenum (called also the ligament of Treitz), which

often contains smooth-muscle fibers. Mobile loops of small intestine may wrap around this ligament and become entrapped between the ligament and the vessels behind it (most notably the abdominal aorta). This "Treitz hernia" may cause mechanical obstruction of the affected bowel loop and strangulate its blood supply.

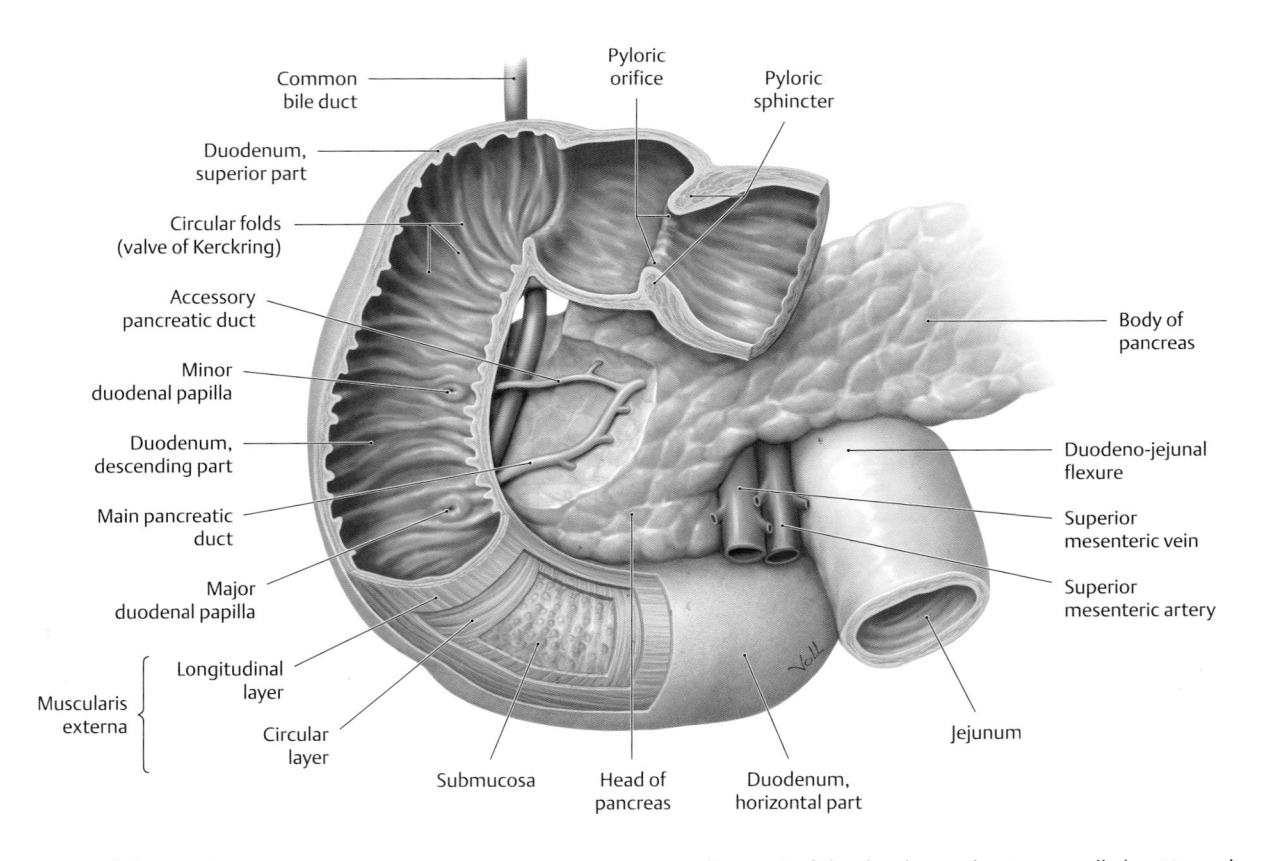

C Wall structure and duct orifices

Anterior view. Most of the duodenum has been opened. The pyloric orifice (here greatly dilated) opens to a luminal diameter of only about 2–3 mm for the passage of chyme. The duodenum has basically the same wall structure as the other hollow organs of the gastrointestinal tract (see **B**, p. 187). The structure of the mucosa is shown in **F**. The de-

scending part of the duodenum has two small elevations along its inner curve: the minor duodenal papilla, which bears the orifice of the accessory pancreatic duct, and the major duodenal papilla (called also the papilla of Vater), which has a common orifice for the pancreatic duct and common bile duct. Thus, the release of bile and pancreatic juice to aid digestion takes place in the upper part of the duodenum.

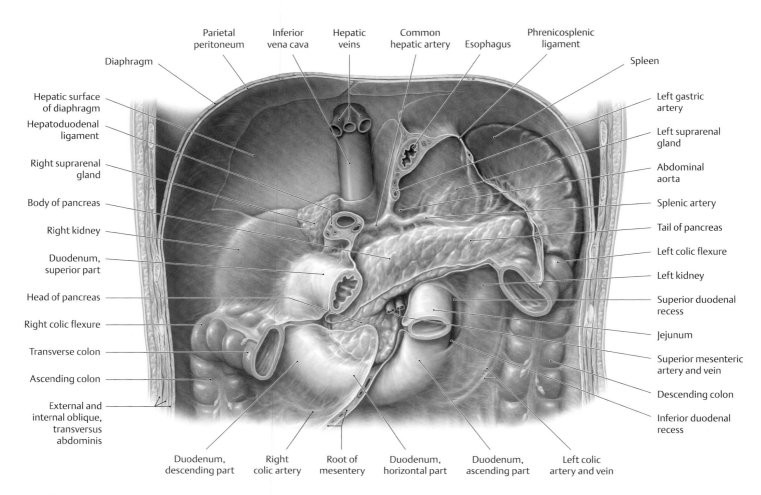

Parietal peritoneum — Inferior vena cava — Hepatic veins — Common hepatic artery — Esophagus — Phrenicosplenic ligament — Spleen

Diaphragm

Hepatic surface of diaphragm — Left gastric artery

Hepatoduodenal ligament — Left suprarenal gland

Right suprarenal gland — Abdominal aorta

Body of pancreas — Splenic artery

Right kidney — Tail of pancreas

Duodenum, superior part — Left colic flexure

Head of pancreas — Left kidney

Right colic flexure — Superior duodenal recess

Transverse colon — Jejunum

Ascending colon — Superior mesenteric artery and vein

External and internal oblique, transversus abdominis — Descending colon

Inferior duodenal recess

Duodenum, descending part — Right colic artery — Root of mesentery — Duodenum, horizontal part — Duodenum, ascending part — Left colic artery and vein

D The duodenum in situ

Anterior view. The stomach, liver, small intestine, and large portions of the transverse colon have been removed. The retroperitoneal fat and connective tissue, including the perirenal fat capsule, have been substantially thinned. The head of the pancreas lies in the concavity of the C-shaped loop of the duodenum. The first 2 cm of the superior part of the duodenum is still intraperitoneal (attached to the liver by the hepatoduodenal ligament), but most of the duodenum is retroperito-neal. Owing largely to the proximity of the duodenum and the head of the pancreas, lesions of the pancreas (tumors) or malformations (anular pancreas, see p. 214) may cause duodenal obstruction. The peritoneum at the duodeno-jejunal junction forms the superior and inferior duodenal recesses. Mobile loops of small intestine may enter these peritoneal recesses and become entrapped there (*internal hernia*), causing a potentially life-threatening bowel obstruction.

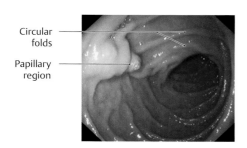

Circular folds

Papillary region

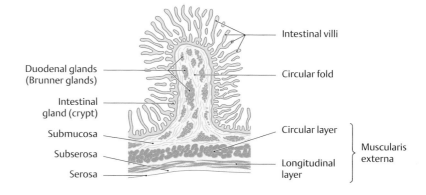

Intestinal villi

Duodenal glands (Brunner glands) — Circular fold

Intestinal gland (crypt)

Submucosa — Circular layer

Subserosa — Muscularis externa

Serosa — Longitudinal layer

E Endoscopic view

The endoscope is pointing down into the descending part of the duodenum. The papillary region where the bile duct and pancreatic duct open into the duodenum is visible on the left side of the image at approximately the 10 o'clock position. The circular folds (valves of Kerckring) are typical of those found in the small intestine, diminishing in size in the proximal to distal direction (from Block, Schachschal and Schmidt: *Endoscopy of the Upper GI Tract.* Stuttgart: Thieme, 2004).

F Histological structure

Longitudinal section through the duodenal wall. The duodenum has basically the same histological structure as the other hollow organs of the gastrointestinal tract (see **B**, p. 187), with some notable differences such as the presence of duodenal (Brunner) glands (secrete mucins and bicarbonate to neutralize the acidic gastric juice) and valves of Kerckring (specialized circular folds). Other features that distinguish the duodenum from the jeju-num and ileum are its more prominent mucosal folds, which diminish in size toward the end of the small intestine.

Note: The muscularis externa of *all* portions of the intestine, unlike that of the stomach, consists of only two layers: an inner layer of circular muscle fibers and an outer layer of longitudinal muscle fibers.

2.7 Small Intestine: Jejunum and Ileum

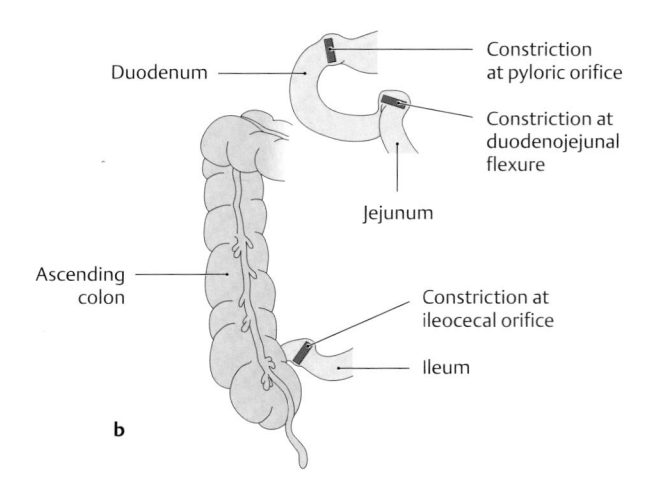

a

Duodenum
Right colic flexure
Jejunum
Ascending colon
Cecum
Vermiform appendix
Ileum
Left colic flexure
Transverse colon
Descending colon
Sigmoid colon
Rectum

Duodenum
Constriction at pyloric orifice
Constriction at duodenojejunal flexure
Jejunum
Ascending colon
Constriction at ileocecal orifice
Ileum

b

A Parts of the small intestine: overview (a) and anatomical constrictions (b)
Anterior view. The large intestine surrounds the loops of small intestine like a frame. Because the small bowel loops are intraperitoneal and therefore very mobile, it is not possible to define their location by reference to skeletal landmarks . If the intestinal loop rotates normally during embryonic development (see p. 180), the duodenum lies *behind* the transverse colon. If the intestinal loop rotates in the wrong direction, the duodenum will come to lie *in front of* the transverse colon.
Note the following normal anatomical constrictions:

- Junction of the pylorus and duodenum (luminal diameter of the pyloric orifice is only about 2–3 mm)
- Duodenojejunal flexure
- Ileocecal orifice

Swallowed foreign bodies may become lodged at these sites, obstructing intestinal transit and causing mechanical intestinal paralysis (*mechanical ileus*, a life-threatening condition that is an absolute indication for surgical treatment).

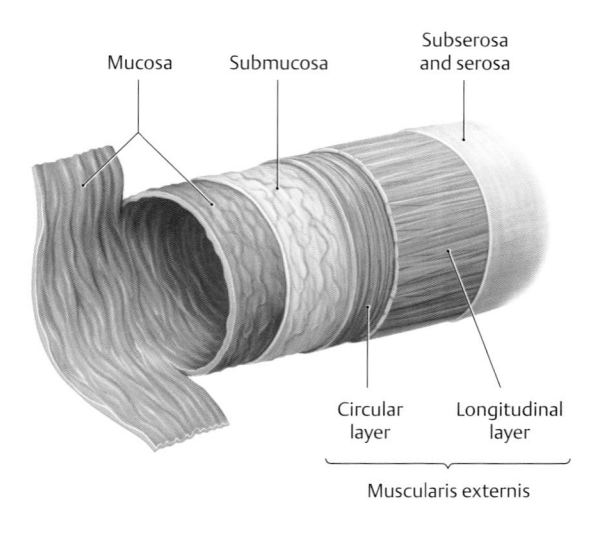

Mucosa Submucosa Subserosa and serosa
Circular layer Longitudinal layer
Muscularis externis

B Wall structure of the jejunum and ileum
The wall layers of the small intestine are displayed in a "telescoped" cross-section. The mucosal layer has been incised longitudinally and opened. The jejunum and ileum have basically the same wall structure as the other hollow organs of the gastrointestinal tract (see **B**, p. 187), but local differences are observed in the circular folds (see **C**) and vascular supply (see p. 268).

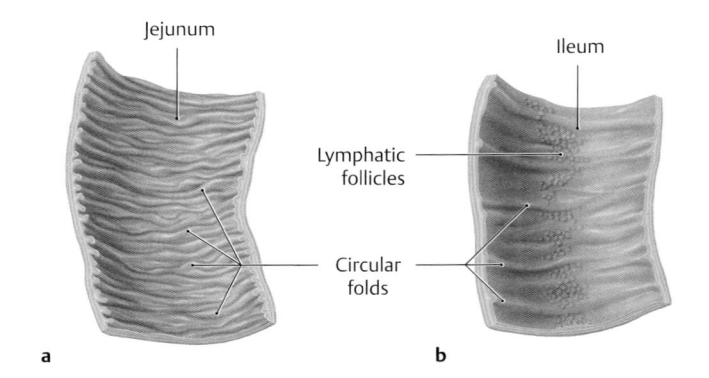

Jejunum Ileum
Lymphatic follicles
Circular folds

a **b**

C Differences in the wall structure of the jejunum and ileum
Macroscopic views of the jejunum (**a**) and ileum (**b**), which have been opened longitudinally to display their mucosal surface anatomy.
Note: The transversely oriented circular folds in the jejunum (see **D**) are spaced much closer together than in the ileum. Lymphatic follicles are particularly abundant in the wall of the ileum (from the lamina propria to the submucosa) for mounting an immune response to antigens in the intestinal contents ("aggregated lymph nodules," Peyer's patches).

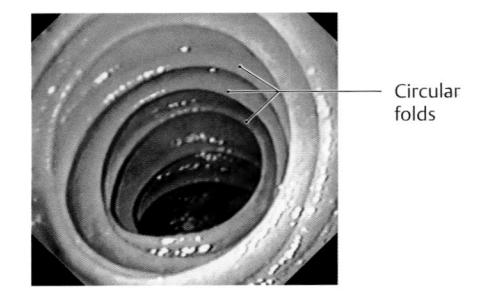

Circular folds

D Endoscopic view of the jejunum
View in the distal direction reveals the numerous circular folds along the jejunum (from Block, Meier and Manns: *Lehratlas der Gastroskopie*. Thieme, 1997).

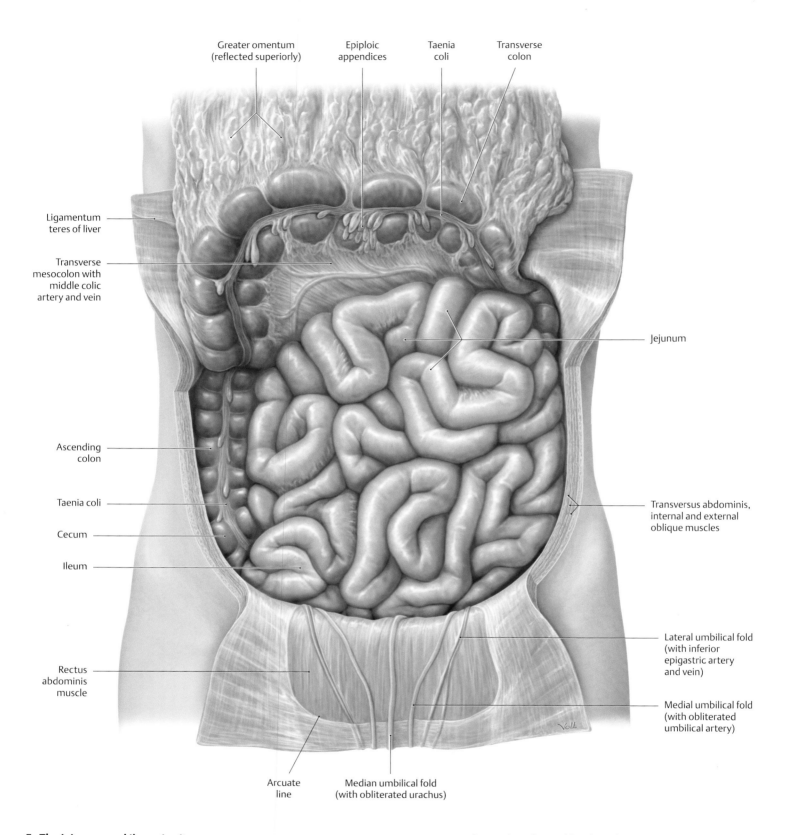

Greater omentum (reflected superiorly)

Epiploic appendices

Taenia coli

Transverse colon

Ligamentum teres of liver

Transverse mesocolon with middle colic artery and vein

Jejunum

Ascending colon

Transversus abdominis, internal and external oblique muscles

Taenia coli

Cecum

Ileum

Lateral umbilical fold (with inferior epigastric artery and vein)

Rectus abdominis muscle

Medial umbilical fold (with obliterated umbilical artery)

Arcuate line

Median umbilical fold (with obliterated urachus)

E The jejunum and ileum in situ
Anterior view. The abdominal wall has been opened and the transverse colon has been reflected upward. Coils of jejunum and ileum completely fill the four quadrants of the peritoneal cavity below the transverse mesocolon and are framed by the colon segments. In this dissection the loops of small intestine have been displaced slightly to the left in front of the descending colon, hiding it from view. The ascending colon and cecum are visible along the right flank of the abdomen.

2.8 Large Intestine: Colon Segments

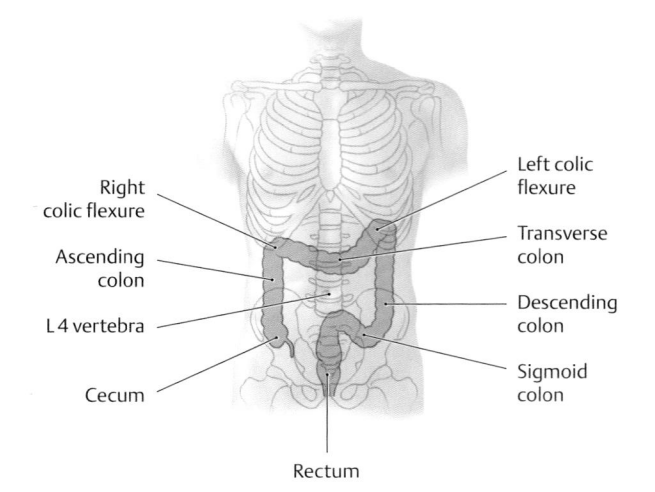

A Projection of the large intestine onto the skeleton

Because of the embryonic rotation of the primary intestinal (midgut) loop, the large intestine typically forms a frame encompassing the small intestine. The position and length of the colon segments may vary, however, depending on the course of intestinal rotation. For example, when the intestinal loop rotates normally, the ascending colon acquires a "normal" length (as shown here). If intestinal rotation is incomplete, the ascending colon is shortened. The transverse colon is particularly mobile owing to its mesocolon, while the ascending and descending colon are less mobile because they are fixed to the posterior wall of the peritoneal cavity. The left colic flexure usually occupies a somewhat higher level than the right colic flexure due to the space occupied by the large right lobe of the liver. Also, the descending colon is usually more posterior than the ascending colon.

B Distinctive morphological features of the large intestine

There are four morphological features — three visible externally and one internally — that distinguish the large intestine from the small intestine. It should be noted that these features do not occur equally in all parts of the large intestine and are absent in the cecum, vermiform appendix, and rectum.

Taeniae coli	In most portions of the large intestine, the longitudinal muscle fibers do not form a continuous layer around the intestinal wall but are concentrated to form three longitudinal bands, the taeniae (see **C**). Taeniae are not present in the rectum or vermiform appendix. The three taenia converge to form the muscularis externa of the appendix.
Epiploic appendices	Fat-filled protrusions of the serosa, scattered over the surface of the large intestine except on the cecum (absent or sparse) and rectum (absent).
Haustra (haustrations)	Saccular wall protrusions between the transverse folds of the large intestine (see p. 195), absent in the rectum
Semilunar folds	Visible only *internally*, in contrast to the external features above. They are functional features caused by contraction of the muscular coat. The internal folds correspond to external constrictions that separate the haustra.

D Anatomical divisions of the large intestine

The large intestine consists of the following divisions in the proximal-to-distal direction:

- Cecum with the vermiform appendix
- Colon, consisting of four parts:
  - Ascending colon
  - Transverse colon
  - Descending colon
  - Sigmoid colon
- Rectum

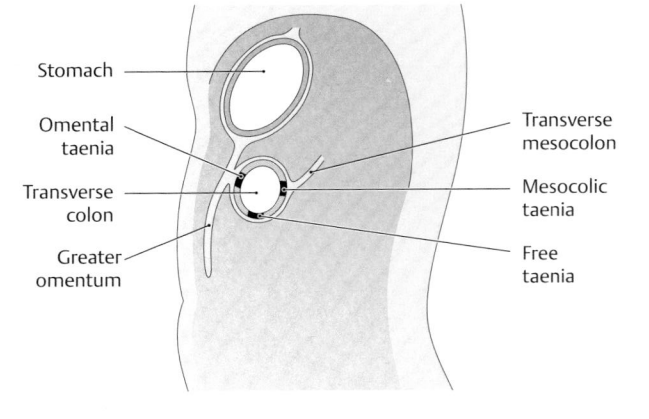

C The three taeniae of the colon

Sagittal section, viewed from the left side. The three taeniae are named for their position on the colon:

- Free taenia (Taenia libera)
- Omental taenia (the taenia at the attachment of the greater omentum)
- Mesocolic taenia (the taenia at the attachment of the mesocolon)

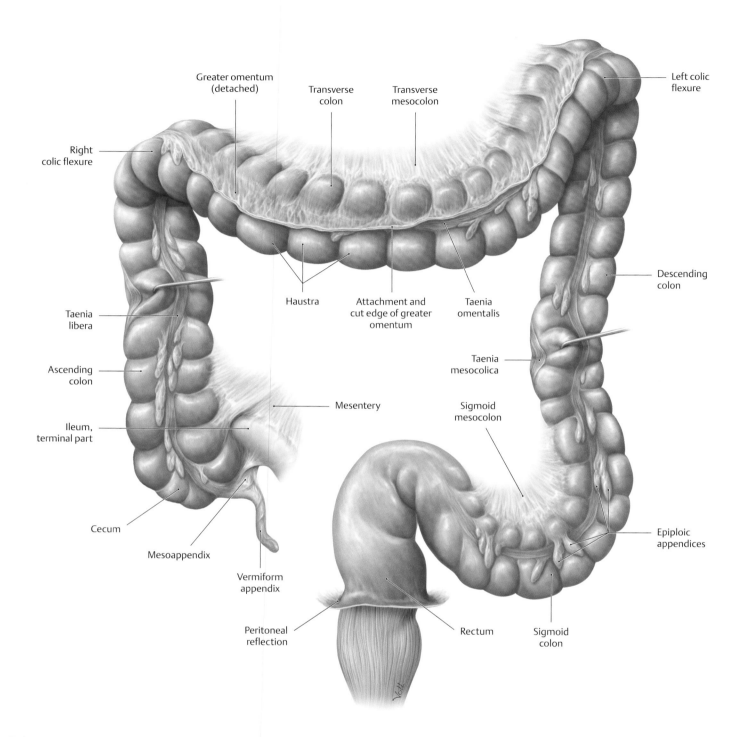

Greater omentum (detached)

Transverse colon

Transverse mesocolon

Left colic flexure

Right colic flexure

Haustra

Attachment and cut edge of greater omentum

Taenia omentalis

Descending colon

Taenia libera

Taenia mesocolica

Ascending colon

Mesentery

Sigmoid mesocolon

Ileum, terminal part

Cecum

Mesoappendix

Sigmoid colon

Epiploic appendices

Vermiform appendix

Peritoneal reflection

Rectum

Sigmoid colon

E Large intestine: segments, shape, and distinctive features

Anterior view, large intestine. The terminal part of the ileum and portions of the transverse and sigmoid mesocolon are shown. The ascending and descending colon have been rotated to display their taeniae.

Note: Colorectal cancer, which has become one of the most common cancers in industrialized countries, has a special predilection for the rectosigmoid junction and the rectum itself (i.e., sites on the anal side of the left colic flexure).

The various colon segments possess all the morphological characteristics of the large intestine (haustra, taeniae, epiploic appendices, see **B**). Typically these features disappear past the junction of the sigmoid colon and rectum. As the taeniae disappear, they are replaced on the rectum by a continuous layer of longitudinal muscle fibers. Instead of haustra, the rectum has three permanent constrictions that are produced by internal transverse folds (see p. 198). The peritoneal reflection on the anterior rectal wall represents the site where the peritoneum is reflected onto the posterior wall of the uterus (in the female) or onto the upper surface of the bladder (in the male).

Note: The ascending and descending colon are (secondarily) retroperitoneal and therefore, unlike the sigmoid and transverse colon, they do *not* have a mesocolon and are covered only anteriorly by peritoneum. The rectum is extraperitoneal in the lesser pelvis, lacks a "suspensory ligament," and bears other unique features (see p. 196).

2.9 Large Intestine: Wall Structure, Cecum, and Vermiform Appendix

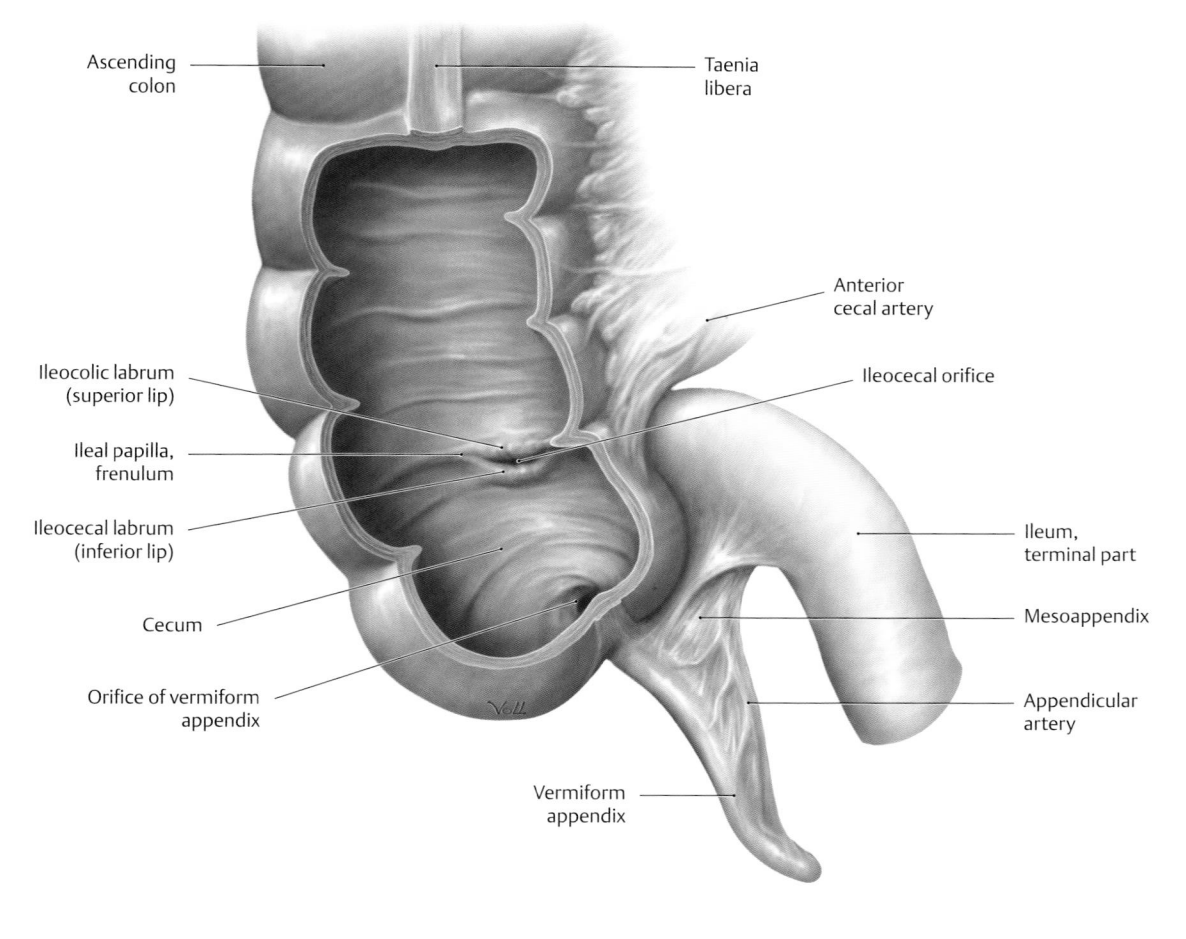

Labels: Ascending colon · Taenia libera · Anterior cecal artery · Ileocolic labrum (superior lip) · Ileocecal orifice · Ileal papilla, frenulum · Ileocecal labrum (inferior lip) · Ileum, terminal part · Cecum · Mesoappendix · Orifice of vermiform appendix · Appendicular artery · Vermiform appendix

A Cecum and terminal ileum

Anterior view. The cecum is unique owing to its end-to-side connection with the terminal part of the small intestine (ileum) and the presence of the vermiform appendix. As a result, there are two openings in the wall of the cecum: the *ileocecal orifice* on a small papilla (ileal papilla) and, below that, the *orifice of the vermiform appendix*. The ileocecal orifice is approximately round in the living individual but is often slit-like in the postmortem condition. It is bounded by superior and inferior flaps or "lips," the ileocolic labrum (= superior lip) and the ileocecal labrum (= inferior

lip). Both are continued as a narrow ridge of mucosa, the frenulum of the ileocecal orifice.

Note: Inflammation of the vermiform appendix (appendicitis) is one of the most common surgically treated diseases of the gastrointestinal tract. If acute appendicitis goes untreated, the inflammation may perforate into the free peritoneal cavity (a "ruptured appendix" in popular jargon). This creates a route by which bacteria in the bowel lumen can enter the peritoneal cavity and gain access to the large peritoneal surface, quickly inciting a life-threatening inflammation of the peritoneum (peritonitis).

B Ileocecal orifice

Anterior view of a longitudinal coronal section of the cecum and ileum. The ileocecal orifice hermetically seals the terminal ileum from the cecum and prevents the reflux of material from the large intestine into the ileum (structural constriction, see **A**, p. 190). The end of the ileum evaginates the circular muscle layer of the large intestine into the cecal lumen. All layers of the ileal wall except the longitudinal muscle and peritoneum contribute to the structure of the ileocecal orifice. The combined circular muscle layers of the ileum and cecum function as a sphincter which periodically opens the orifice, allowing the contents of the small intestine to enter the large Intestine while effectively preventing reflux. The function of this sphincter is similar to that of the pylorus.

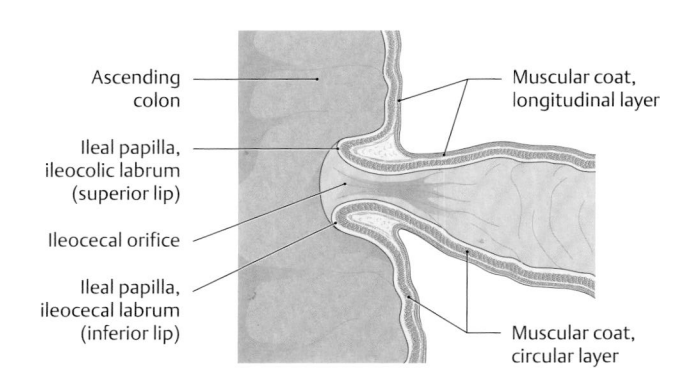

Labels: Ascending colon · Muscular coat, longitudinal layer · Ileal papilla, ileocolic labrum (superior lip) · Ileocecal orifice · Ileal papilla, ileocecal labrum (inferior lip) · Muscular coat, circular layer

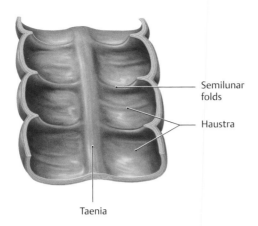

Semilunar folds

Haustra

Taenia

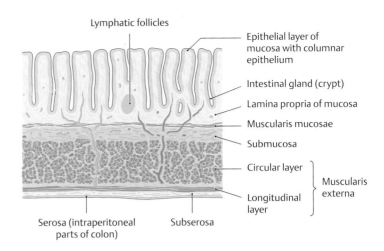

Lymphatic follicles

Epithelial layer of mucosa with columnar epithelium

Intestinal gland (crypt)

Lamina propria of mucosa

Muscularis mucosae

Submucosa

Circular layer

Longitudinal layer

Muscularis externa

Serosa (intraperitoneal parts of colon)   Subserosa

C Interior of the colon

The interior of the colon is marked by transversely oriented folds called semilunar folds. They are formed by the shortness of the muscular taenia of the colon wall and are visible externally as anular constrictions. The sacculations between the folds are the colonic haustra. The semilunar folds are inconstant features that depend on the muscular tension in the taenia. The folds and haustra move slowly down the colon with waves of peristaltic activity.

D Wall structure of the colon and cecum

Longitudinal section through the bowel wall. All the typical wall layers of the gastrointestinal canal are present: the mucosa, submucosa, muscularis externa, and serosa (or adventitia in the retroperitoneal parts of the colon, see **B**, p. 187, and **D**, p. 153). There are several features, however, that distinguish the wall structure of the colon and cecum from that of the stomach and small intestine:

- The mucosa is *devoid* of villi (i.e., the total surface area is not enlarged as much as in the small intestine). Instead of villi, there are large numbers of deep *crypts* (Lieberkühn crypts), more numerous than in the small intestine.
- The epithelial layer of the mucosa contains large numbers of goblet cells (for clarity, not shown here).
- The colonic mucosal surface undulates in large-scale, crescent-shaped, semilunar folds (see **C**).
- The muscularis externa consists of an inner circular layer and an outer longitudinal layer, which is concentrated in three longitudinal bands, the taeniae (see p. 192).

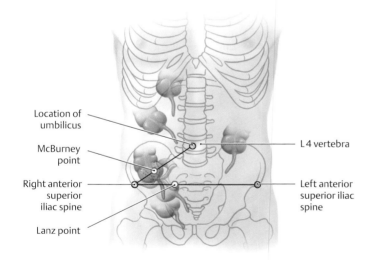

Location of umbilicus

McBurney point

Right anterior superior iliac spine

Lanz point

L 4 vertebra

Left anterior superior iliac spine

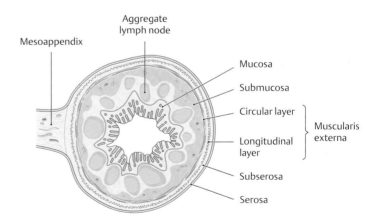

Mesoappendix

Aggregate lymph node

Mucosa

Submucosa

Circular layer

Longitudinal layer

Muscularis externa

Subserosa

Serosa

E Variants in the position of the vermiform appendix

Disturbances in the rotation of the embryonic gut can result in numerous positional variants of the cecum and vermiform appendix. The appendix may even come to lie in the left side of the abdomen. The inflammation of an appendix in the *typical position* is characterized by tenderness at two points:

- McBurney point: Position on a line connecting the umbilicus and the right anterior superior iliac spine. The McBurney point is one-third of the distance along this line from the iliac spine.
- Lanz point: Position on a line connecting the the anterior superior iliac spines. The Lanz point is one third of the distance along this line from the right spine.

Although very useful, these are not definitive clinical signs. Tenderness may be felt at other abdominal sites, especially if the appendix is in an atypical position.

F Wall structure of the vermiform appendix

The vermiform appendix has the typical wall structure of an intraperitoneal intestinal tube. One striking feature is the abundance of lymphatic follicles in the submucosa (also present in the colon and cecum, but in much smaller numbers). With its high degree of immunological activity, the appendix has been characterized as the "intestinal tonsil." The mucosa has numerous deep crypts that are in intimate contact with the lymphatic follicles in the lamina propria and the submucosa (crypts and lymphatic follicles are not visible here). Since the vermiform appendix is intraperitoneal, it possesses a small mesentery, the mesoappendix, which transmits neurovascular structures.

2.10 Large Intestine: Location and Shape of the Rectum

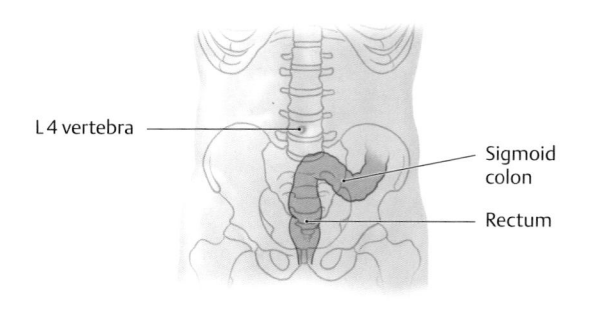

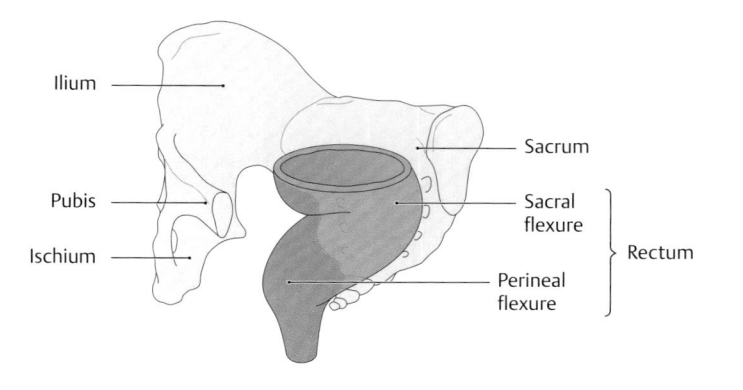

A Projection of the rectum onto the bony pelvis
Anterior view. The rectum extends approximately from the superior border of the third sacral vertebra to the perineum and is 15–16 cm long. It is "straight" only in the frontal projection (as shown here); it presents two flexures in the sagittal projection (see **B**).

B Curves of the rectum
Left anterior view. Two curves can be identified: the sacral flexure (retroperitoneal) and the perineal flexure (extraperitoneal), which represents the start of the anal canal. The *sacral flexure* is anteriorly concave, following the curvature of the sacrum. The more distal *perineal flexure* is anteriorly convex. It is an important functional component of rectal continence (see pp. 199–201). The rectum shown in the diaphragm is largely empty. The rectum is still more or less straight in a small child. In the adult, it straightens only when the rectal ampulla is grossly distended with feces.

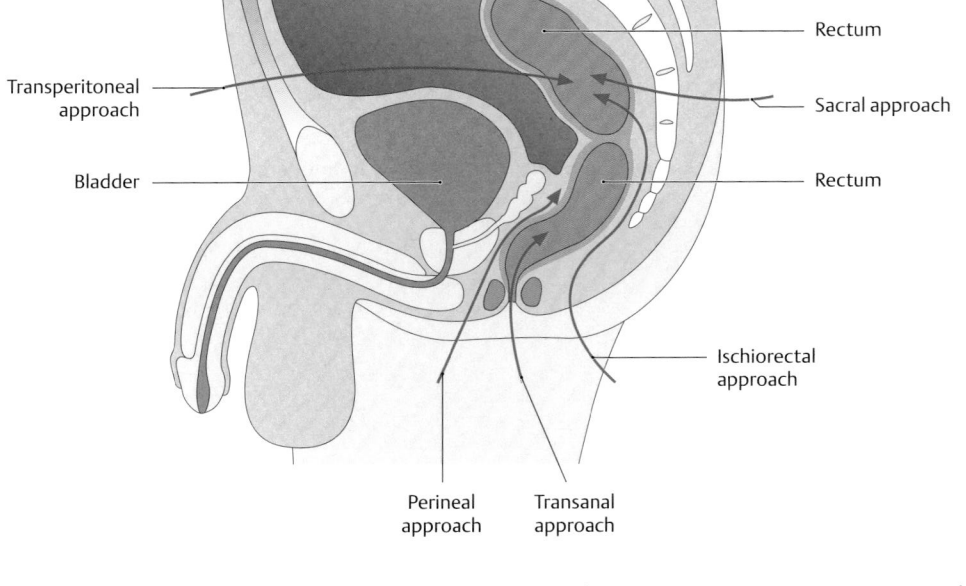

C Surgical approaches to the rectum
Sagittal section through a male pelvis, left lateral view.
Note: With a posterior or caudal approach, it is unnecessary to open the peritoneal cavity because the rectum is retro- or extraperitoneal. The major advantage of these approaches is that they do not risk spreading microorganisms from the rectum into the peritoneal cavity.

D Distinctive morphological features of the rectum

Although the rectum is considered part of the colon, it differs from the large intestine by the *absence* of several colonic characteristics:

- Longitudinal muscle bands (taeniae). The rectum has a continuous longitudinal muscle layer.
- Fatty epiploic appendages
- Haustra
- Semilunar mucosal folds. The rectum has deep, large transverse folds (see p. 198).

In addition, the rectum has a compound embryonic origin. Above the anorectal line, it is derived, like the colon, from embryonic endoderm. The anal canal, however, develops from ectoderm.

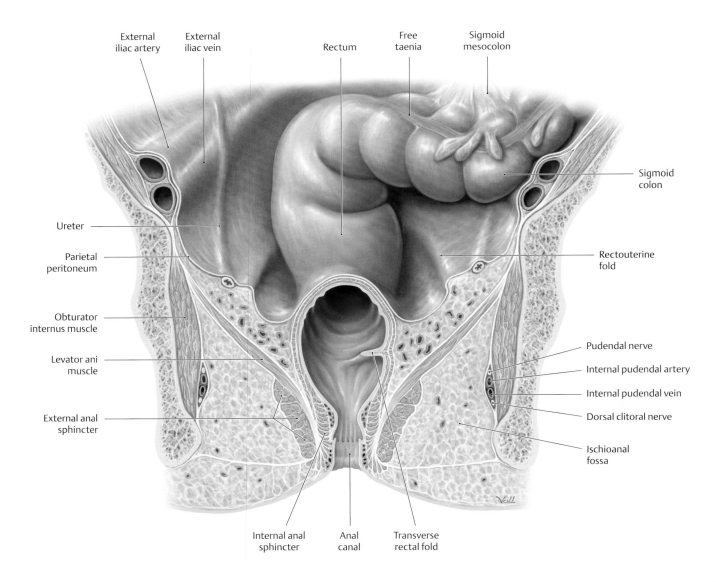

External iliac artery

External iliac vein

Rectum

Free taenia

Sigmoid mesocolon

Sigmoid colon

Ureter

Parietal peritoneum

Rectouterine fold

Obturator internus muscle

Levator ani muscle

Pudendal nerve

Internal pudendal artery

Internal pudendal vein

External anal sphincter

Dorsal clitoral nerve

Ischioanal fossa

Internal anal sphincter

Anal canal

Transverse rectal fold

E The rectum in situ

Coronal section of the female pelvis, anterior view, with the rectum opened from about the level of the middle transverse rectal fold. The taeniae of the sigmoid colon are not continued onto the rectum. The constrictions in the outer wall of the rectum correspond to the transverse folds on the inner wall. The rectum (which would appear in this form only if the ampulla were full) is shown in a slightly raised position. Below the levator ani muscle is the powerful external anal sphincter, the muscular component of the rectal continence organ. The pararectal connective tissue below the peritoneal cavity contains numerous vessels that supply the rectum.

This drawing was made from the dissection of a female cadaver. Thus, the peritoneum would be reflected from the anterior wall of the rectum onto the posterior wall of the uterus. Although both the anterior rectal wall and uterus are not visible here (anterior to this plane of section), parts of the rectouterine folds are still visible.

197

2.11 Large Intestine: Wall Structure of the Rectum and Mechanism of Defecation

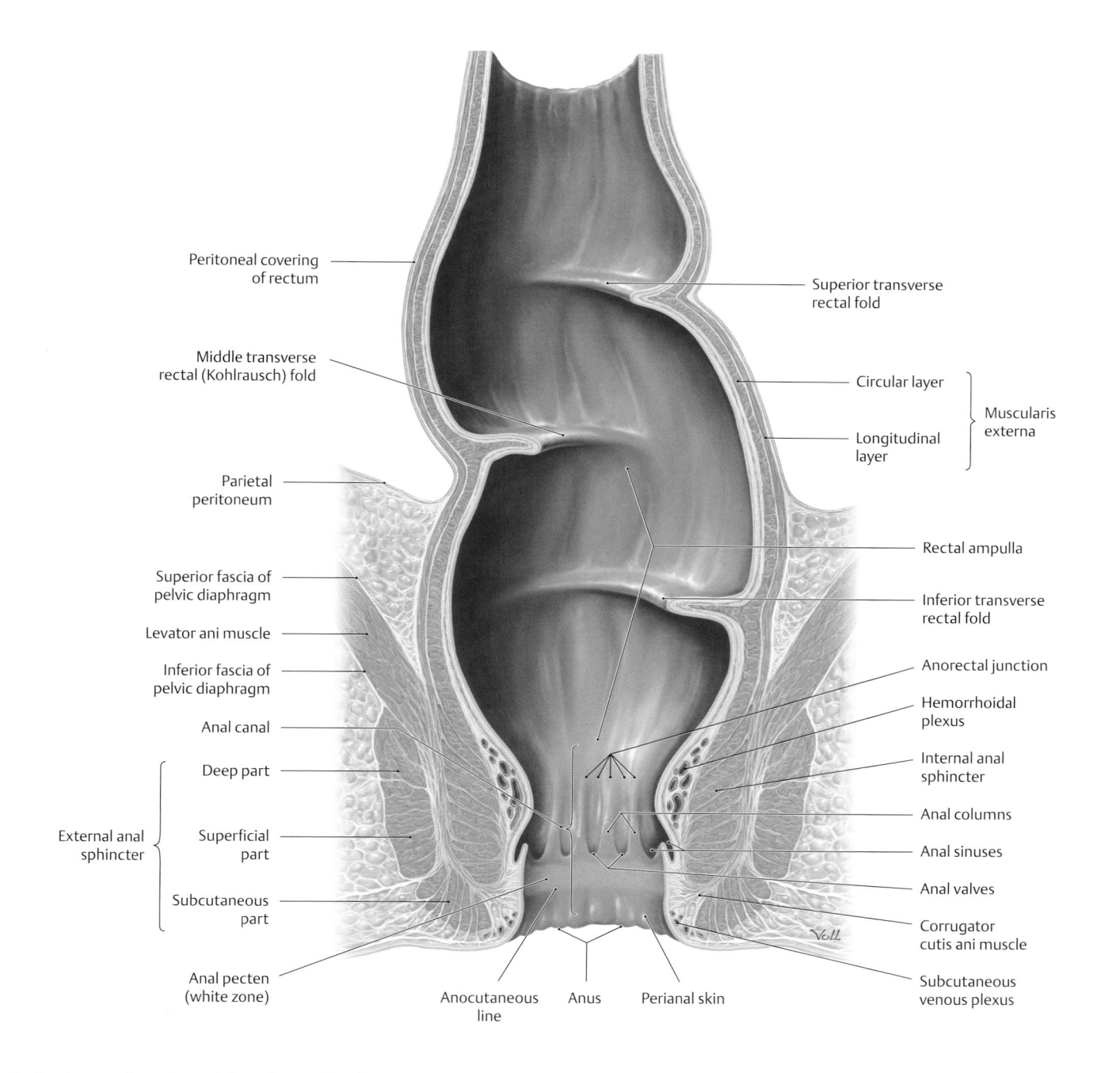

Peritoneal covering of rectum

Middle transverse rectal (Kohlrausch) fold

Parietal peritoneum

Superior fascia of pelvic diaphragm

Levator ani muscle

Inferior fascia of pelvic diaphragm

Anal canal

External anal sphincter
- Deep part
- Superficial part
- Subcutaneous part

Anal pecten (white zone)

Anocutaneous line

Anus

Perianal skin

Superior transverse rectal fold

Circular layer

Longitudinal layer

Muscularis externa

Rectal ampulla

Inferior transverse rectal fold

Anorectal junction

Hemorrhoidal plexus

Internal anal sphincter

Anal columns

Anal sinuses

Anal valves

Corrugator cutis ani muscle

Subcutaneous venous plexus

A Rectum and anal canal: interior and wall structure

Anterior view of the rectum in coronal section with the anterior wall removed. Instead of semilunar folds, the rectum contains three permanent transverse folds. The terminal part of the gastrointestinal tract is divided into two segments based on its mucosal surface anatomy (anorectal line)*:

- Rectal ampulla: the lowest portion of the rectum between the middle transverse rectal fold *(Kohlrausch fold)* and the anorectal junction. The ampulla is the most distensible part of the rectum. The middle transverse fold, which projects into the rectum from its right posterior wall, is approximately 6–7 cm from the anus and can just be reached with the palpating finger. Rectal tumors located below the Kohlrausch fold may therefore be palpable.

- Anal canal: developmentally, a pelvic floor derivative located below the anorectal junction and terminating at the anus. The anal canal is surrounded by the internal and external anal sphincters and the levator ani muscle. The hemorrhoidal plexus is a network of cavernous tissue with an arterial blood supply. The muscles and hemorrhoidal plexus combine with other structures to form the continence organ (see **C**), which provides for fecal continence and flatus control. The peritoneum covers the rectum laterally and anteriorly to approximately the level of the middle transverse rectal fold.

* The anal canal may be considered the lowest segment of the rectum based on functional clinical considerations as well as functional anatomical criteria (neurovascular supply, lymphatic drainage). In this interpretation the anorectal junction separates two rectal segments: the (upper) rectal ampulla and the (lower) anal canal.

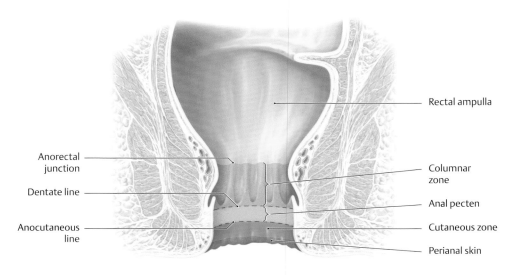

	Rectal ampulla
Anorectal junction	
Dentate line	Columnar zone
	Anal pecten
Anocutaneous line	Cutaneous zone
	Perianal skin

Region	Boundary	Epithelium
Rectum		Colon-type epithelium with crypts and goblet cells
	Anorectal junction (formerly: anorectal line)	
Anal canal with three levels		
• Columnar zone		Stratified, nonkeratinized squamous epithelium
	Dentate line	
• Anal pecten		Stratified, nonkeratinized squamous epithelium
	Anocutaneous line	
• Cutaneous zone		Stratified, keratinized squamous epithelium with sebaceous glands
Perianal skin (pigmented)		Stratified, keratinized squamous epithelium with sebaceous glands, hairs, and sweat glands

B Epithelial regions of the anal canal
(after Lüllmann-Rauch)

The anal canal is the terminal part of the alimentary canal. It can be divided into three levels based on the characteristics of its epithelium. These levels reflect a transition from the rectal epithelium above the anal canal to the external perineal skin below the anal canal. The three levels of the anal canal are separated by two indistinct lines that mark the epithelial junctions.

Note: The anal pecten has a whitish appearance ("white zone") because the mucosa at that level is intimately attached to the internal anal sphincter by connective tissue. The pecten is endowed with numerous stretch and pain receptors (reflex zone for continence and defecation). Just above the dentate line, anal glands (*proctodeal glands*, not present in all individuals) open into the anal canal, especially posteriorly. They may become infected, and the pus collection (abscess) may break through to the outer skin of the anus, forming an *anal fistula*. These lesions often require surgical treatment.

C Structure of the continence organ and mechanism of defecation

The continence organ provides for gas-tight closure of the rectum and consists of the distensible hollow organ, vascular and muscular (see pp. 200, 201) continence mechanisms, and their neural control. These angiomuscular continence mechanisms are integrated into a structurally narrow segment that results from the tightness and angulation (perineal flexure) of the anal canal:

- Distensible hollow organ:
  - Rectum with its stretch receptors, most numerous in the rectal ampulla (viscerosensory innervation)
  - Anus with distensible skin in the anal canal (somatosensory innervation)
- Muscular continence:
  - Internal anal sphincter (visceromotor innervation)
  - External anal sphincter (somatomotor innervation)
  - Levator ani complex, especially the puborectalis muscle (somatomotor innervation)
- Vascular continence:
  - Hemorrhoidal plexus (permanently distended cavernous tissue that subsides only during defecation)
- Neural control:
  - Visceral and somatic nervous system (mainly from S2 – S4) with the pelvic splanchnic nerves, pudendal nerve, and rectal plexus

The hollow organ, continence mechanisms, and neural control (see p. 201) interact as follows during defecation:

→ Filling of the rectal ampulla
→ Stimulation of local stretch receptors in the ampullary wall
→ Urge to defecate
→ Contraction of the rectal longitudinal muscle, shortening the rectum
→ Relaxation of the anal sphincters (increases blood drainage from the hemorrhoidal plexus, which detumesces) and the puborectalis muscle
→ Widening of the anal canal plus straightening of the rectum

Defecation is also assisted by straining, which raises the intra-abdominal pressure. The control center for defecation lies in the S2 – S4 segments of the sacral spinal cord. After early childhood (when hygienic habits are acquired), defecation and fecal incontinence are also subject to voluntary central nervous control.

2.12 Large Intestine:
Innervation of the Rectum and Continence Mechanisms

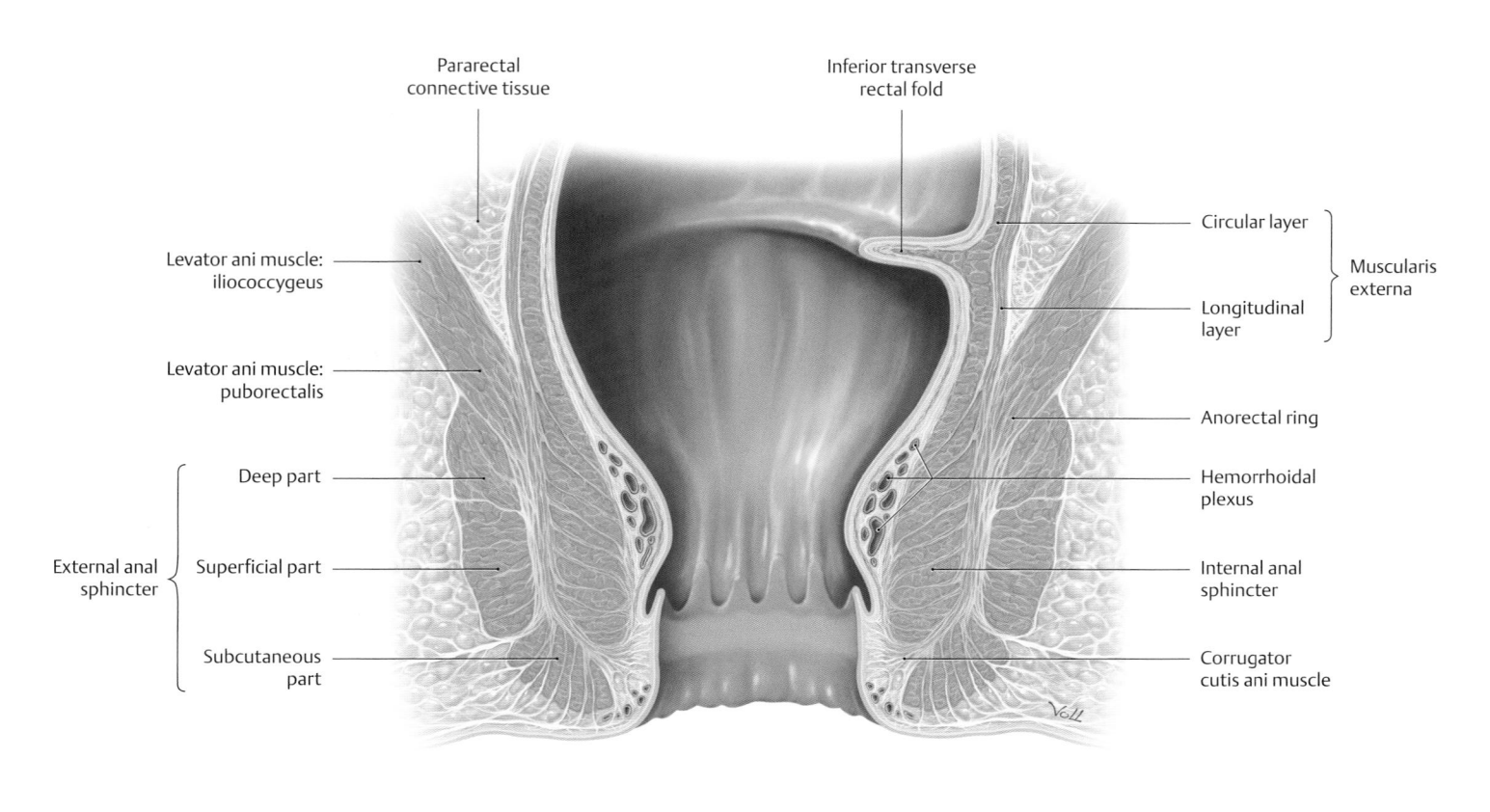

A Continence organ: structure of the muscular continence mechanism

Anterior view of the rectum in coronal section with the anterior wall removed. The continence organ consists of four functional components:

- A structurally narrow segment (chiefly the internal anal sphincter)
- The "anorectal angle" created by the puborectalis muscle (= component of the levator ani muscle, see **B**)
- The constricting function of the external anal sphincter

- The expansive and constricting properties of the hemorrhoidal plexus (located beneath the mucosa in the rectal wall, see **D**)

Note: Fibers from the internal anal sphincter pass through the external anal sphincter and blend with the subcutaneous tissue of the perianal skin; thus, a visceral smooth muscle projects into the subcutaneous connective tissue. This expansion of the internal sphincter, whose tonus tightens and wrinkles the skin around the anus, bears the specific name of "corrugator cutis ani" muscle.

B Continence organ: closure by the puborectalis muscle

The puborectalis muscle is a component of the levator ani complex. It arises from the posterior surface of the pubic bone and loops around the rectum to form an anteriorly open sling. By drawing the rectum anterosuperiorly, it increases the angle of the rectal "kink" (part of the perineal flexure) above the anal canal and helps to prevent fecal expulsion.

Note: The puborectalis is the most important muscle for maintaining fecal continence; injury to that muscle (e.g., during an operation) results in more severe incontinence than injury to both of the sphincter muscles.

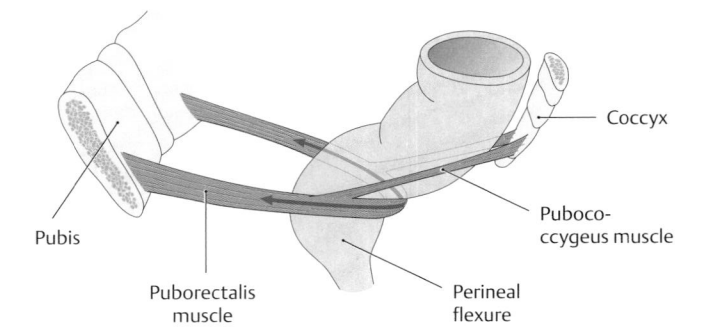

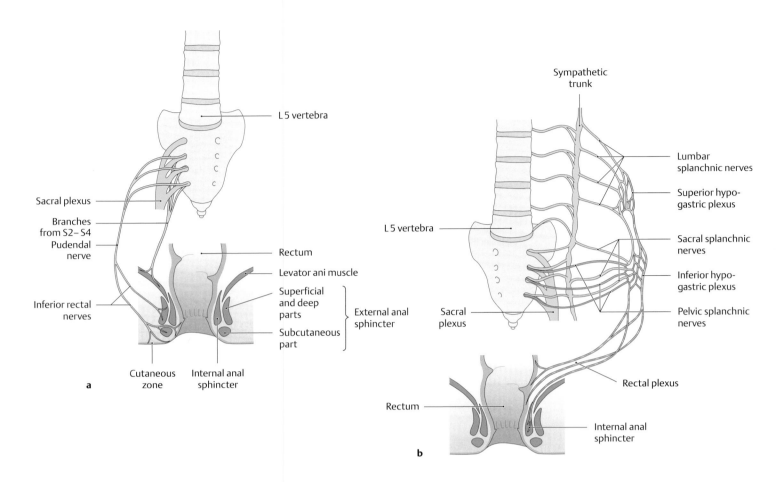

a

- L 5 vertebra
- Sacral plexus
- Branches from S2– S4
- Pudendal nerve
- Inferior rectal nerves
- Rectum
- Levator ani muscle
- Superficial and deep parts
- Subcutaneous part
- External anal sphincter
- Cutaneous zone
- Internal anal sphincter

b

- Sympathetic trunk
- Lumbar splanchnic nerves
- Superior hypogastric plexus
- L 5 vertebra
- Sacral splanchnic nerves
- Inferior hypogastric plexus
- Sacral plexus
- Pelvic splanchnic nerves
- Rectal plexus
- Rectum
- Internal anal sphincter

C Innervation of the continence organ (after Stelzner)
a Somatomotor and somatosensory innervation, **b** visceromotor and viscerosensory innervation.

- Somatomotor: pudendal nerve for the external anal sphincter, levator nerves for the levator ani muscle (especially the puborectalis). They provide active, partially voluntary innervation of the external anal sphincter and levator ani.
- Somatosensory: inferior rectal nerves for the anus and perianal skin. Arising from the pudendal nerve, they transmit touch and especially pain sensation. The skin of the anus is extremely sensitive to pain. Even small tears in the anal skin, which often show inflammatory changes, tend to be extremely painful.

- Visceromotor: pelvic splanchnic nerves (S2 – S4) for the internal anal sphincter. The resting tone of the internal sphincter helps to maintain closure of the anal canal and inhibits venous drainage from the hemorrhoidal plexus; the cavernous body remains distended, contributing to fecal continence and flatus control. Topographically, the pelvic splanchnic nerves are closely related to the rectal plexuses.
- Viscerosensory: pelvic splanchnic nerves (S2 – S4) supply the wall of the rectum, particularly the stretch receptors in the rectal ampulla. Stretching of the ampulla by the fecal column triggers a subjective awareness of the need to defecate.

D Continence organ: arterial supply to the vascular continence mechanism (hemorrhoidal plexus)
External and caudal view of the perineum (supine patient in the lithotomy position). The hemorrhoidal plexus is a permanently distended cavernous body at the anorectal junction. It is supplied by the superior rectal artery, and sustained contraction of the muscular sphincter apparatus in a continent individual inhibits venous drainage from the hemorrhoidal plexus, which remains full and ensures gas-tight closure of the rectum. The hemorrhoidal plexus is supplied by arterial branches at the 3, 7 and 11 o'clock positions (noteworthy for ligation of the superior rectal artery). When the sphincter apparatus relaxes during defecation, it removes tension from the hemorrhoidal plexus and allows blood to drain from the cavernous tissue.
Note: The condition known colloqially as *hemorrhoids* results from abnormal, excessive dilation and consequent abrasion of the hemorrhoidal plexus.

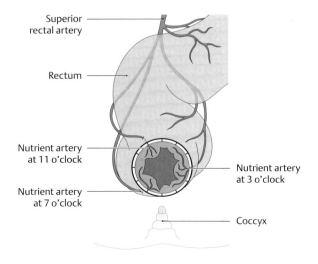

- Superior rectal artery
- Rectum
- Nutrient artery at 11 o'clock
- Nutrient artery at 7 o'clock
- Nutrient artery at 3 o'clock
- Coccyx

2.13 Radiography of the Small and Large Intestine

Circular folds   Jejunum

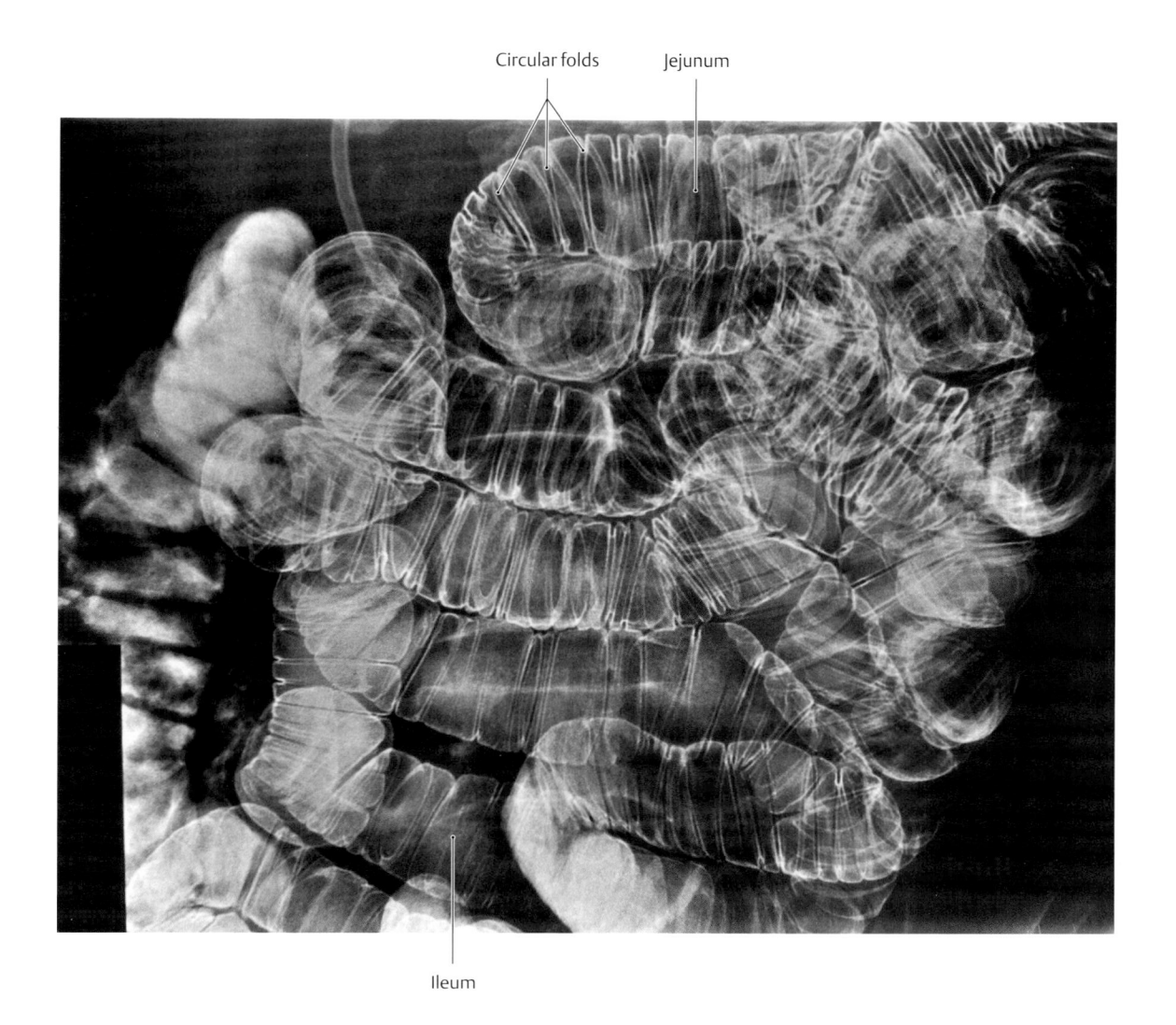

Ileum

A Double-contrast radiograph of the small intestine
Double-contrast radiograph of the small intestine in the anteroposterior projection (x-ray source in front of the patient, film-screen combination behind the patient). Anterior view. In a double-contrast study, air is instilled into the bowel through a tube and a radiopaque liquid con- trast medium is administered to provide an exceptionally high-contrast image. This technique guarantees high morphological resolution and is sensitive in detecting mucosal changes. The image above illustrates a normal double-contrast study. The transversely oriented circular folds of the small intestine are defined with great clarity.

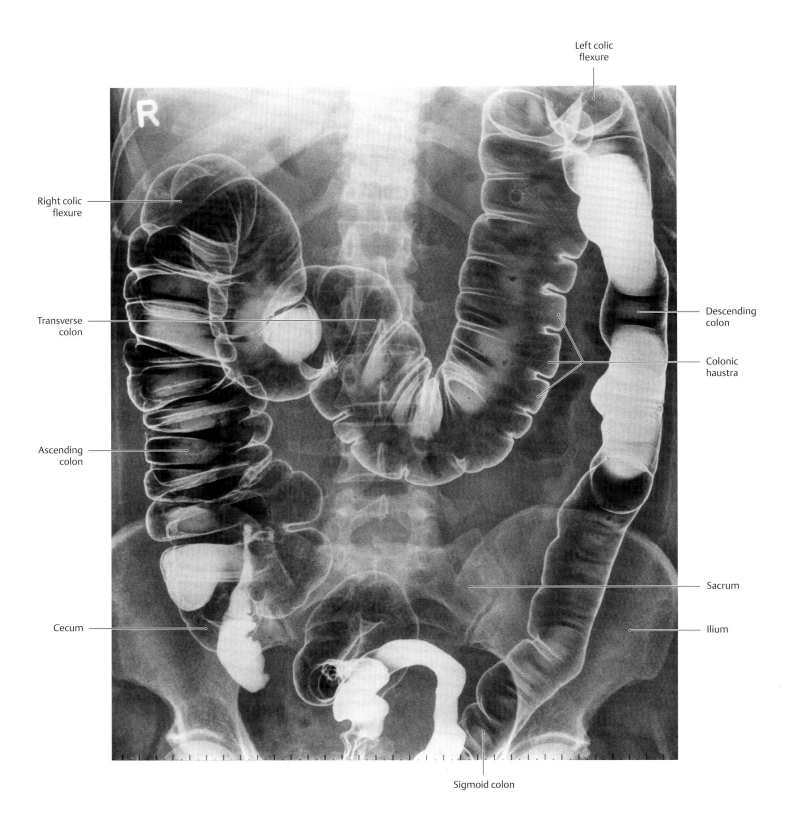

Left colic flexure

Right colic flexure

Transverse colon

Ascending colon

Cecum

Descending colon

Colonic haustra

Sacrum

Ilium

Sigmoid colon

B Double-contrast radiograph of the large intestine
Double-contrast radiograph of a normal large intestine in the antero-posterior projection, anterior view. The film clearly demonstrates the different parts of the large intestine and their haustra. The radiopaque contrast medium is not evenly distributed, and opaque areas of variable size indicate sites where the contrast medium has pooled.

Note the variability in the shape and position of the colon segments compared with the diagrams in **A**, p. 192, and in **E**, p. 193. The image above shows considerable sagging of the transverse colon in the standing patient, but this finding is well within the normal range of variation. Because the transverse colon is intraperitoneal, it has a mesentery (transverse mesocolon) that gives it considerable mobility.

2.14 Liver: Position and Relationship to Adjacent Organs

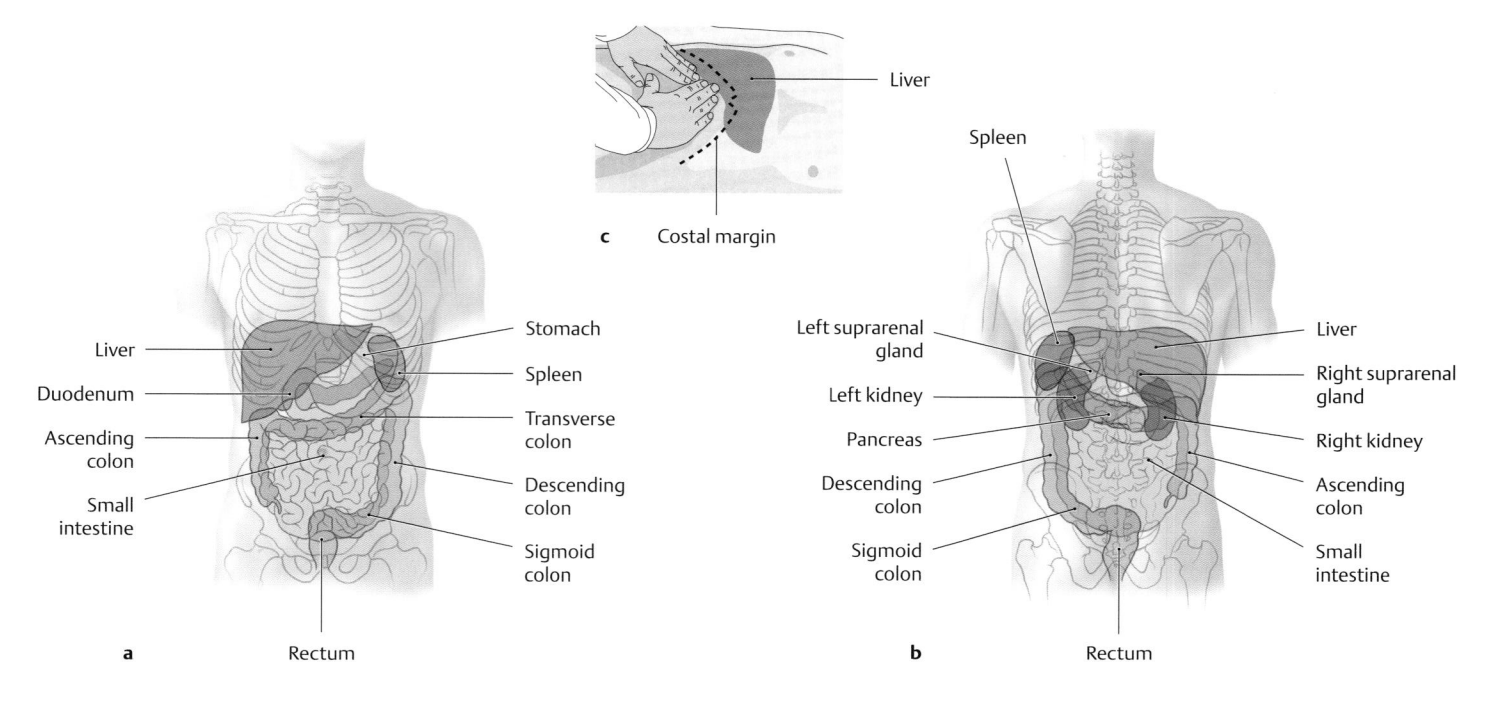

c   Costal margin

Liver
Stomach
Duodenum
Spleen
Ascending colon
Transverse colon
Small intestine
Descending colon
Sigmoid colon

a   Rectum

Spleen
Left suprarenal gland
Liver
Left kidney
Right suprarenal gland
Pancreas
Right kidney
Descending colon
Ascending colon
Sigmoid colon
Small intestine

b   Rectum

A   Projection of the liver onto the trunk and adjacent organs; palpation of the liver

a Anterior view, **b** posterior view, **c** palpation of the liver.

The liver is situated mainly in the right upper quadrant but extends across the epigastrium into the left upper quadrant, lying anterior to the stomach. The right lobe of the liver is closely related to the right kidney and right colic flexure. Owing to the dome of the hemidiaphragm, the pleural cavity overlaps the anterior and posterior surfaces of the liver. Because the liver is attached to the inferior surface of the diaphragm,

its position is significantly affected by respiratory excursions. It also depends on posture and age: The liver descends in the standing position, and it is also affected by the gradual settling of organs that occurs with aging. The liver is palpated (**c**) most easily by having the patient lie supine with the abdominal wall relaxed (legs drawn up) and exhale fully (the liver rises with the diaphragm), followed by a full inhalation. This causes the liver to fall, and its sharp inferior border (see **D**) can be palpated at the margin of the ribs. If the liver is abnormally enlarged (hepatomegaly), it may occasionally extend to the pelvic brim.

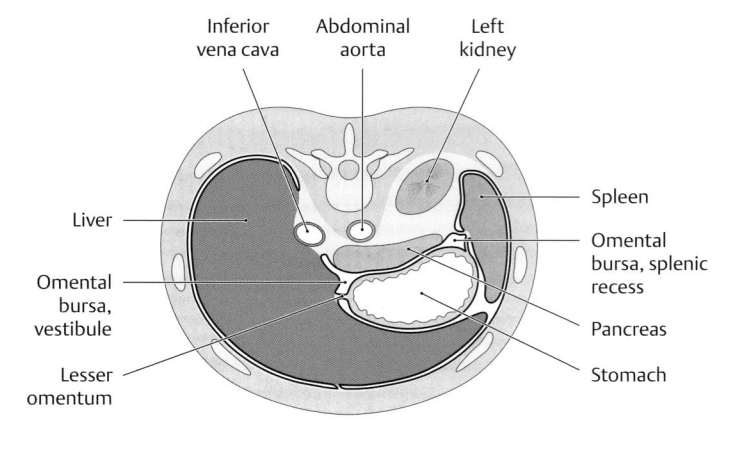

Inferior vena cava
Abdominal aorta
Left kidney
Liver
Spleen
Omental bursa, splenic recess
Omental bursa, vestibule
Pancreas
Lesser omentum
Stomach

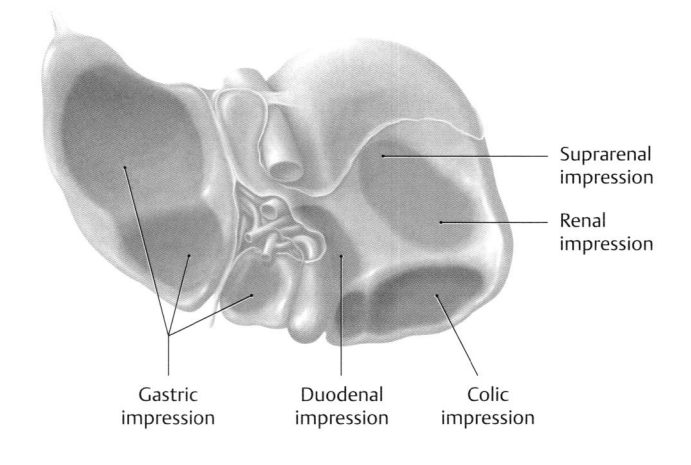

Suprarenal impression
Renal impression
Gastric impression
Duodenal impression
Colic impression

B   Position of the liver

Transverse section through the abdomen at approximately the T12/L1 level, viewed from above. The liver is intraperitoneal except for the "bare area," which is not visible here. The left lobe of the liver extends into the LUQ, where it is anterior to the stomach. The peritoneal fold between the liver and the lesser curvature of the stomach (lesser omentum) can be seen. Portions of the liver form the right boundary of the omental bursa.

C   Areas of contact with other organs

View of the visceral surface of the liver.

Note: Impressions from organs that are in direct contact with the liver are visible only on a liver that has been hardened in place by a chemical preservative ("fixation"). An unfixed liver from a cadaver that has not been chemically preserved is so soft that generally it will not show organ impressions. Diseases of the liver may easily spread to other organs, and vice versa, at areas of contact with adjacent organs (extensive owing to the size and topography of the liver).

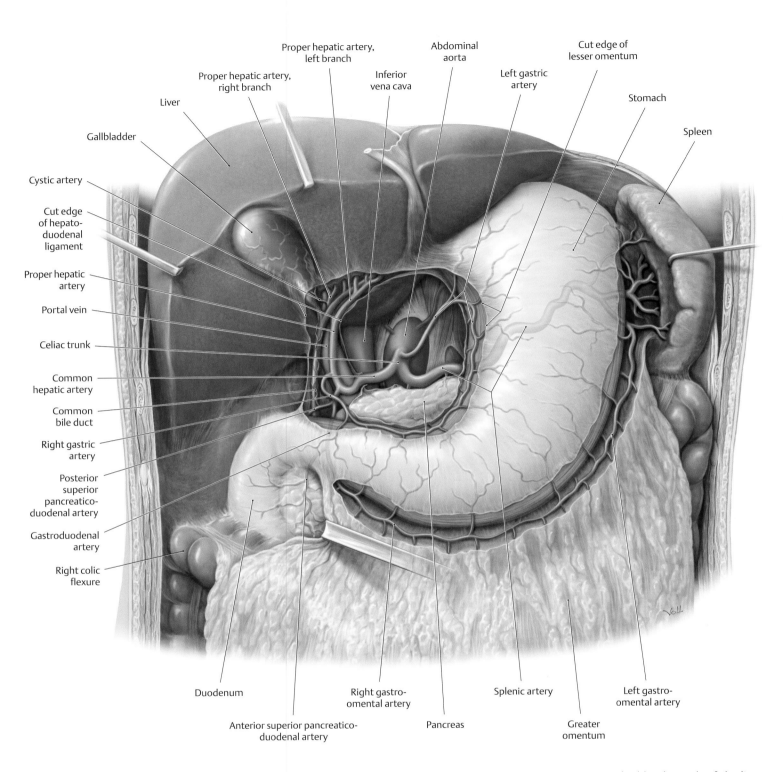

Proper hepatic artery, left branch

Abdominal aorta

Cut edge of lesser omentum

Proper hepatic artery, right branch

Inferior vena cava

Left gastric artery

Stomach

Liver

Spleen

Gallbladder

Cystic artery

Cut edge of hepato-duodenal ligament

Proper hepatic artery

Portal vein

Celiac trunk

Common hepatic artery

Common bile duct

Right gastric artery

Posterior superior pancreatico-duodenal artery

Gastroduodenal artery

Right colic flexure

Duodenum

Anterior superior pancreatico-duodenal artery

Right gastro-omental artery

Pancreas

Splenic artery

Greater omentum

Left gastro-omental artery

D The liver in situ

Anterior view of the opened upper abdomen. Retractors have been placed on the liver and spleen to improve the exposure. The lesser omentum has been opened, allowing a direct view into the omental bursa. A small section of pleural cavity can be seen immediately to the right and slightly above the right lobe of the liver (see p. 207). The anterior border of the liver, which points downward in situ, has a sharp edge that is clearly palpable when the liver is enlarged. The inferior surface of the liver bears a fossa for the gallbladder (see p. 210), whose fundus is directed anteriorly toward the abdominal wall and extends slightly past the inferior hepatic border. The right portion of the lesser omentum,

the hepatoduodenal ligament, transmits the blood vessels of the liver (proper hepatic artery and portal vein) and the common bile duct. The contour of the right kidney can be seen on the inferior surface of the right lobe of the liver.

Note: The opening of the hepatic veins into the inferior vena cava is located just below the diaphragm (see pp. 276, 277), just a few centimeters from the right atrium of the heart. Thus, in cases where the right side of the heart has lost pumping power (right-sided heart failure), blood may engorge the liver, causing palpable hepatic enlargement. When palpating the liver, the examiner should take into account the variable position of the organ (see **Ac**).

2.15 Liver: Peritoneal Relationships and Shape

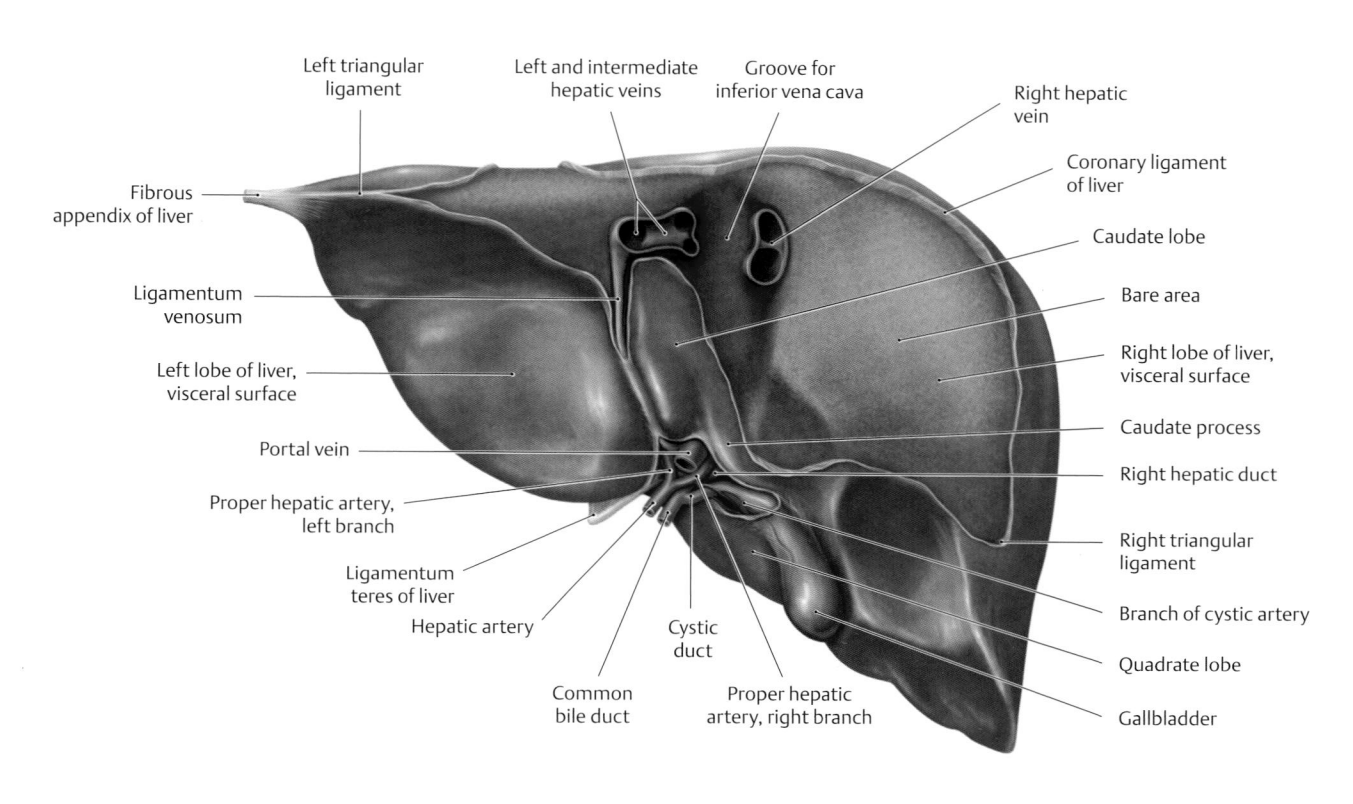

Left triangular ligament

Left and intermediate hepatic veins

Groove for inferior vena cava

Right hepatic vein

Coronary ligament of liver

Fibrous appendix of liver

Ligamentum venosum

Caudate lobe

Bare area

Left lobe of liver, visceral surface

Right lobe of liver, visceral surface

Caudate process

Portal vein

Right hepatic duct

Proper hepatic artery, left branch

Right triangular ligament

Ligamentum teres of liver

Branch of cystic artery

Hepatic artery

Cystic duct

Quadrate lobe

Common bile duct

Proper hepatic artery, right branch

Gallbladder

A Peritoneal covering of the liver

Posterior view of the upper part of the diaphragmatic surface of the liver. The liver is surrounded by a fibrous capsule with extensions that pass into the liver and transmit neurovascular structures. Most of the *surface* of the liver is covered by glistening visceral peritoneum, which is external to the fibrous capsule. Only the bare area, which is highly variable in extent, *lacks a peritoneal covering*; it has a rough appearance because the fibrous capsule forms its surface. The hepatic veins (usually three in number) leave the liver in the bare area, and thus *outside* the peritoneal covering. This is different from all other intraperitoneal organs, which have mesenteric structures for transmitting their veins and arteries. In the case of the liver, only the *afferent* artery, *afferent* portal vein, and common bile duct course in the hepatoduodenal ligament (see **Cb**), while the efferent veins do not. At sites where the visceral peritoneum is reflected into the parietal peritoneum on the inferior surface of the diaphragm, the delicate peritoneal epithelium is often backed by connective tissue to form a ligamentous band (coronary ligament, see **Ca**). This connective tissue is drawn out into a tapered band at the extremity of the left lobe (the fibrous appendix of the liver).

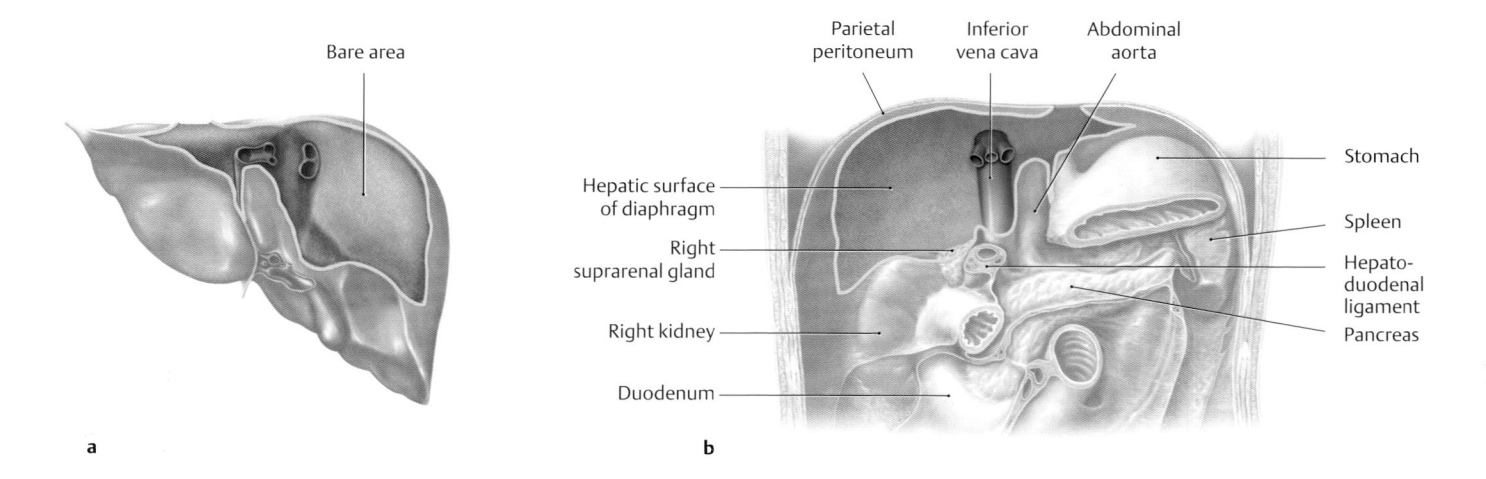

Bare area

Parietal peritoneum

Inferior vena cava

Abdominal aorta

Stomach

Hepatic surface of diaphragm

Spleen

Right suprarenal gland

Hepato-duodenal ligament

Right kidney

Pancreas

Duodenum

a

b

B Bare area of the liver and the hepatic surface of the diaphragm

Posterior view of the diaphragmatic surface of the liver (**a**) and the inferior surface of the diaphragm (**b**). The lines of peritoneal reflection on the liver and diaphragm demonstrate the mirror-image correspondence of the bare area with the hepatic surface of the diaphragm. The bare area is firmly attached to the inferior surface of the diaphragm by peritoneal reflection (coronary ligaments), rendering the liver immobile despite its intraperitoneal location.

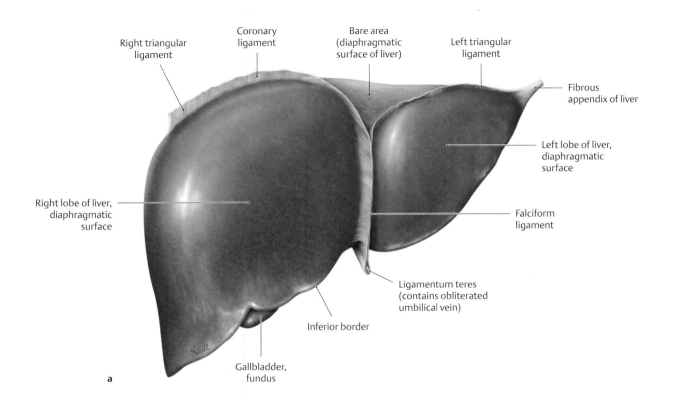

Right triangular ligament

Coronary ligament

Bare area (diaphragmatic surface of liver)

Left triangular ligament

Fibrous appendix of liver

Right lobe of liver, diaphragmatic surface

Left lobe of liver, diaphragmatic surface

Falciform ligament

Ligamentum teres (contains obliterated umbilical vein)

Inferior border

Gallbladder, fundus

a

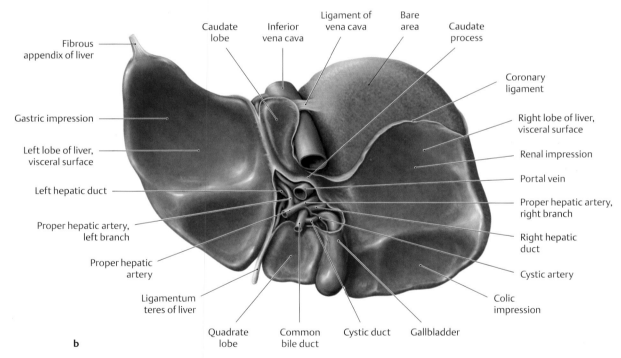

Fibrous appendix of liver

Caudate lobe

Inferior vena cava

Ligament of vena cava

Bare area

Caudate process

Coronary ligament

Gastric impression

Right lobe of liver, visceral surface

Left lobe of liver, visceral surface

Renal impression

Left hepatic duct

Portal vein

Proper hepatic artery, left branch

Proper hepatic artery, right branch

Proper hepatic artery

Right hepatic duct

Ligamentum teres of liver

Cystic artery

Colic impression

Quadrate lobe

Common bile duct

Cystic duct

Gallbladder

b

C Liver: diaphragmatic and visceral surfaces

a Anterior view of the diaphragmatic surface. Two lobes are visible in this view: the larger right lobe and the smaller left lobe. Between the two lobes is the falciform ligament of the liver, a "ventral mesentery" that extends to the anterior abdominal wall.

b Inferior view of the visceral surface. Two more of the four hepatic lobes are visible in this view: the caudate lobe and quadrate lobe. The visceral surface also contains the porta hepatis where neurovascular structures enter and leave the liver (common hepatic duct, proper hepatic artery, portal vein). Topographically, the hepatoduodenal ligament is a component of the lesser omentum. The extent of the hepatoduodenal ligament can be appreciated by noting the cut edge of visceral peritoneum surrounding the portal triad. Along with the hepatogastric ligament, it creates a "dorsal mesentery" for the liver. The numerous impressions from adjacent organs are seen this plainly only in a liver that has been chemically preserved. The gallbladder is closely applied to the visceral surface of the liver. Its fundus extends slightly past the inferior hepatic border, and its neck is directed toward the porta hepatis, where it comes into contact with the extrahepatic bile ducts.

207

2.16 Liver: Segmentation and Histology

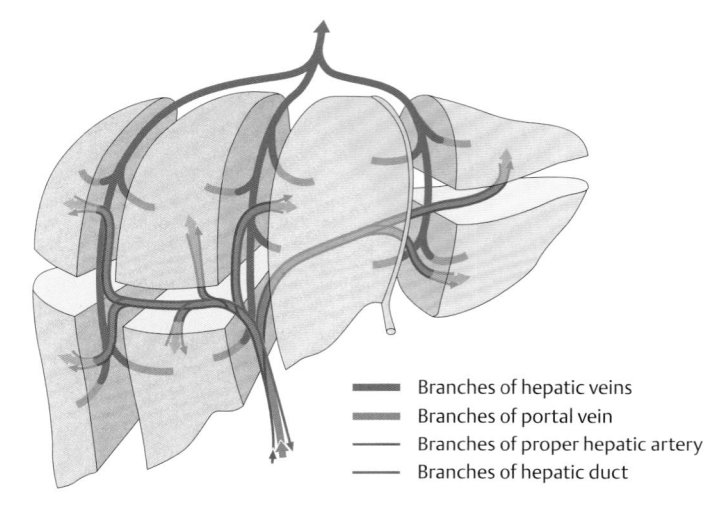

— Branches of hepatic veins
▬ Branches of portal vein
— Branches of proper hepatic artery
— Branches of hepatic duct

A Segmentation of the liver

Anterior view. The proper hepatic artery, portal vein, and common hepatic duct enter / exit the liver at the porta hepatis as the "portal triad." The central branch first divides into two larger branches, functionally subdividing the liver into left parts (yellow) and right parts (purple). The boundary between the left and right parts of the liver is an imaginary line that roughly connects the gallbladder bed to the inferior vena cava (caval-gallbladder line, see **Cb**). Thus it is not identical to the externally visible boundary formed by the falciform ligament (see p. 207). The portal triad continue to ramify within the liver, forming a total of eight segments that are more or less functionally independent of one another. This allows the surgeon to resect one or more hepatic segments without damaging the liver as a whole. Additionally, the remaining hepatic segments have a high regenerative potential. In the diagram above, the liver has been "exploded" at its virtual segmental boundaries to demonstrate the position and shape of its segments (numerical designations are shown in **B** and **C**).

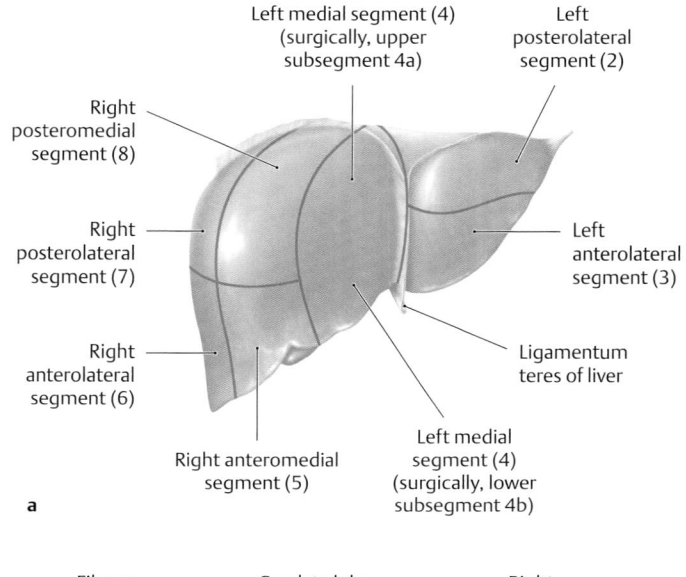

Left medial segment (4) (surgically, upper subsegment 4a)
Left posterolateral segment (2)
Right posteromedial segment (8)
Right posterolateral segment (7)
Left anterolateral segment (3)
Right anterolateral segment (6)
Ligamentum teres of liver
Right anteromedial segment (5)
Left medial segment (4) (surgically, lower subsegment 4b)

a

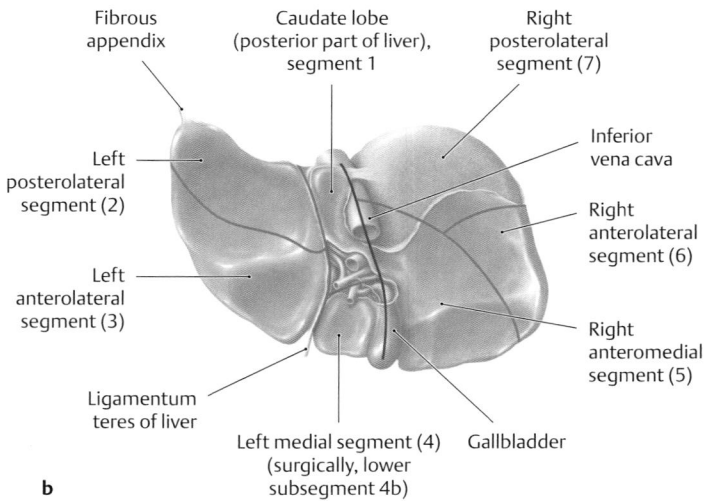

Fibrous appendix
Caudate lobe (posterior part of liver), segment 1
Right posterolateral segment (7)
Left posterolateral segment (2)
Inferior vena cava
Right anterolateral segment (6)
Left anterolateral segment (3)
Right anteromedial segment (5)
Ligamentum teres of liver
Left medial segment (4) (surgically, lower subsegment 4b)
Gallbladder

b

B Hepatic segments grouped by parts and divisions

Left part of the liver	• Posterior part, caudate lobe	• Segment 1
	• Left lateral division	• Left posterolateral segment (= segment 2) • Left anterolateral segment (= segment 3)
	• Left medial division	• Left medial segment (= segment 4), subdivided into subsegment 4a (above) and 4b (below)
Right part of the liver	• Right medial division	• Right anteromedial segment (= segment 5) • Right posteromedial segment (= segment 8)
	• Right lateral division	• Right anterolateral segment (= segment 6) • Right posterolateral segment (= segment 7)

C Projection of segmental boundaries onto the surface of the liver

Views of the diaphragmatic surface (**a**) and visceral surface of the liver (**b**).* The segments defined by the divisions of the portal vascular triad (see **A**) are projected onto the surface of the liver with their virtual boundaries. In this way the pattern of hepatic segmentation, which is based on vascular distribution, can be directly compared with the traditional division of the liver into four lobes based on external morphological criteria. For surgical purposes, it is useful to group the segments by parts and divisions (see **B**) because the portion of the liver selected for surgical resection may encompass not just one segment but two neighboring segments or the entire right or left part of the liver. Surgeons can positively identify the hepatic segments by ligating the feeding vessels until the segment or segments become discolored due to loss of blood supply.

* Blue line in **b**: caval-gallbladder line

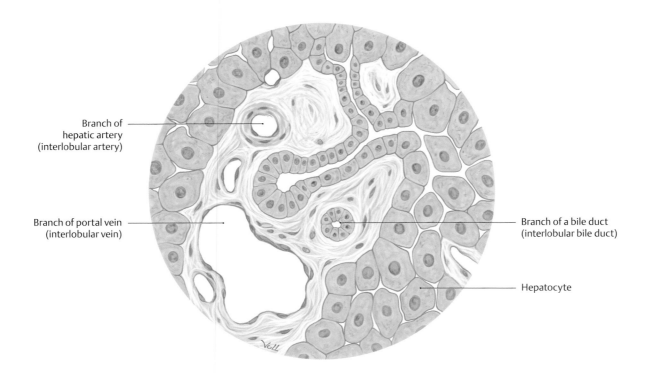

D Histological appearance of a portal area
Hematoxylin and eosin stain, magnification approximately 540 x. The portal triad of the liver, while grossly visible at the porta hepatis, ramifies into a network of microscopic branches embedded in connective tissue: the portal area. The portal triad at this level consists of the hepatic artery, which becomes the interlobular artery (situated between several lobules), the portal vein, which becomes the interlobular vein, and the common hepatic duct, which becomes the interlobular bile duct. These structures are easily distinguished from one another by differences in their calibers, wall thickness, and wall structure:

- Interlobular artery: thick wall, squamous endothelium, small lumen
- Interlobular vein: thin wall, squamous epithelium, large lumen
- Interlobular bile duct: cuboidal epithelium and very small lumen

Cirrhosis of the liver is characterized by a proliferation of connective tissue in the liver that is most conspicuous in the portal area and about the central veins. Necrotic hepatocytes are permanently replaced by scar tissue. The sinuses — the capillary bed of the liver — are obliterated in the scarred areas, progressively diminishing the blood flow through the liver. The afferent blood vessels are still carrying the same amount of blood to the liver, however. This causes obstruction of portal venous flow and an abnormal pressure increase (portal hypertension). In many cases the blood is returned to the right heart by an alternate route (portosystemic collaterals, see p. 293).

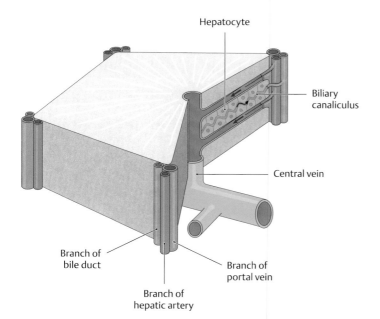

E Structure of a central venous lobule (hepatic lobule)
This is a *three-dimensional structural model* of a hepatic lobule based on studies of numerous histological sections (see **D**). It shows that each polyhedral hepatic lobule is composed of hepatocytes that are arrayed around a central vein (hence the term "central venous lobule"). Ultimately the central veins return their blood to the hepatic veins. The portal area (see **D**) in this model is located *between* adjacent lobules at the points where the lobules interconnect (hence the term "interlobular" for the artery, vein and bile duct).
While the interlobular artery and vein convey their blood into sinusoids that have a stable wall (see **D**), the biliary canaliculi that transfer bile to the interlobular bile duct do not have their own walls. They also course between the hepatocytes, but on the opposite side from the sinusoids. If biliary stasis develops between adjacent hepatocytes (e.g., due to hepatitis), the hepatocytes may separate and lose their intercellular contacts. Abnormally large interspaces may form, allowing the bile to escape from the biliary canaliculi and seep to the opposite side of the cells, where it can enter the sinusoids and bloodstream, causing a yellowish discoloration of the skin and mucous membranes (jaundice).

2.17 Gallbladder and Bile Ducts: Location and Relationship to Adjacent Organs

A Projection of the extrahepatic bile ducts onto the skeleton

Viewed from the front, the gallbladder is projected at a point where the mid-clavicular line intersects the inferior border of the ninth rib. The orifice of the common bile duct (which generally opens jointly with the pancreatic duct on the major duodenal papilla) lies approximately at the level of the L2 vertebral body. The gallbladder emerges beneath the right costal arch at approximately the L1/L2 level. In certain diseases (e.g., cholecystitis), tenderness to pressure may be noted at this location.

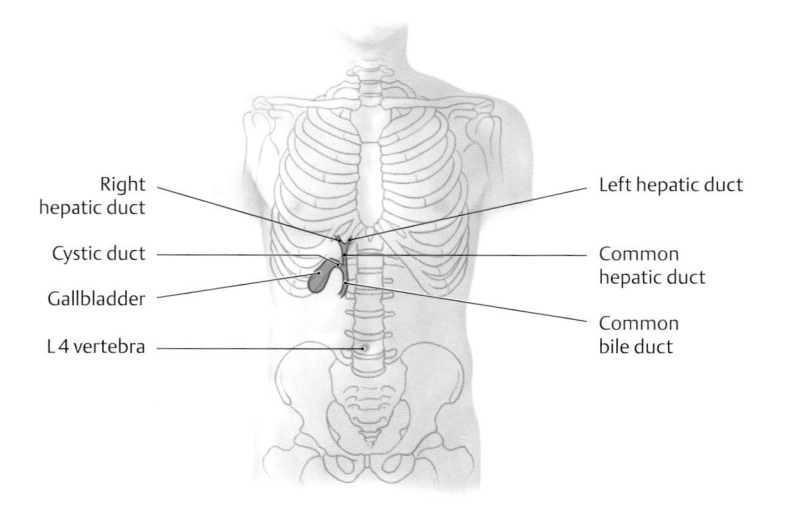

Right hepatic duct
Cystic duct
Gallbladder
L4 vertebra
Left hepatic duct
Common hepatic duct
Common bile duct

B Projection of the intra- and extrahepatic bile ducts onto the surface of the liver

Anterior view. Bile flows through the biliary canaliculi (microscopic) into the small interlobular bile ducts in the portal area (see p. 209). These ducts coalesce to form increasingly larger units that drain a hepatic segment. The bile from all the segments ultimately drains into two large collecting vessels, the left and right hepatic ducts, which receive the small left and right ducts of the caudate lobe, respectively, while still inside the liver. The right and left hepatic ducts unite to form the common hepatic duct. Almost immediately the excretory duct of the gallbladder, the cystic duct, enters the side of the common hepatic duct, which then becomes the common bile duct.

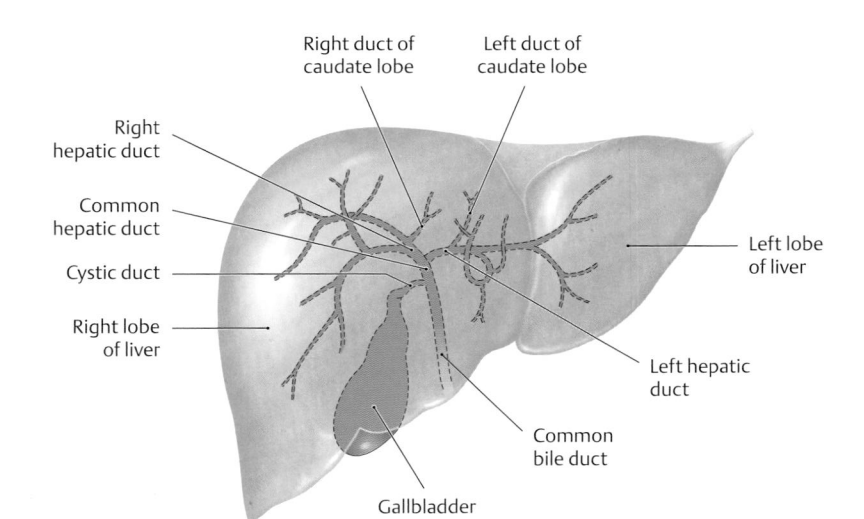

Right duct of caudate lobe
Left duct of caudate lobe
Right hepatic duct
Common hepatic duct
Cystic duct
Right lobe of liver
Left lobe of liver
Left hepatic duct
Common bile duct
Gallbladder

C Position of the gallbladder at the porta hepatis

Inferior view with the common bile duct divided. The peritoneal covering of the liver is reflected onto the gallbladder, which therefore is intraperitoneal.

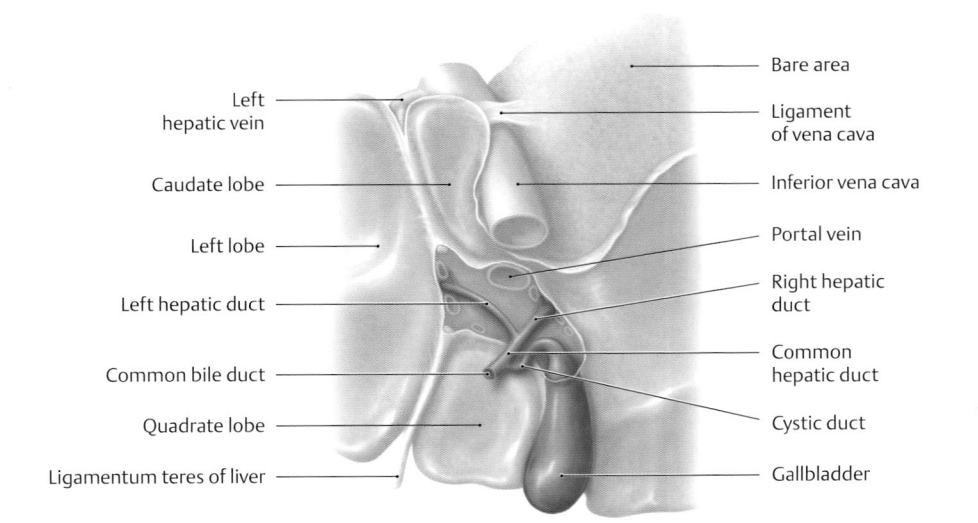

Left hepatic vein
Caudate lobe
Left lobe
Left hepatic duct
Common bile duct
Quadrate lobe
Ligamentum teres of liver
Bare area
Ligament of vena cava
Inferior vena cava
Portal vein
Right hepatic duct
Common hepatic duct
Cystic duct
Gallbladder

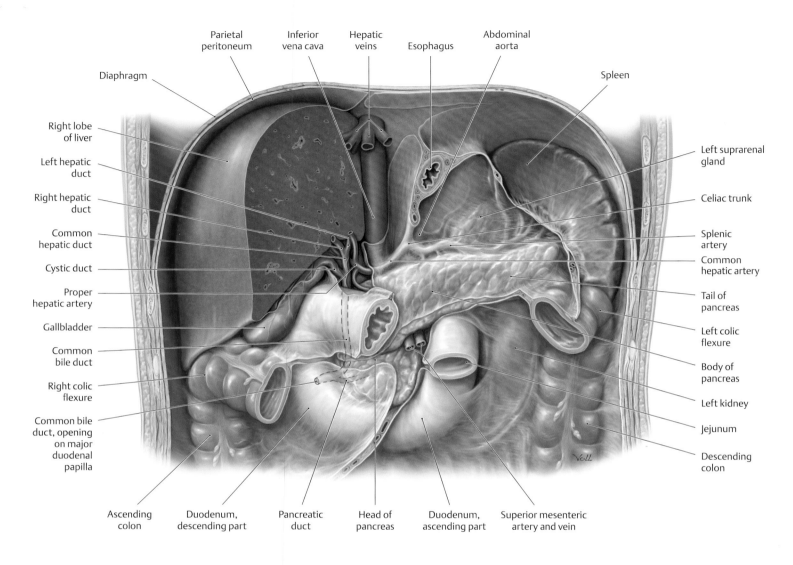

D Relationship of the biliary tract to adjacent organs

Anterior view of the opened abdomen. The stomach, small intestine, transverse colon, and large portions of the liver have been removed, and the peritoneum has been divided in the area of the hepatoduodenal ligament. The gallbladder is partially contained in a fossa on the visceral surface of the liver. The common bile duct passes behind the duodenum toward the head of the pancreas. After passing through the head of the pancreas, the bile duct frequently unites with the pancreatic duct, as shown here. Both ducts then open together at the major duodenal papilla in the descending part of the duodenum (see p. 188).

2.18 Gallbladder and Extrahepatic Bile Ducts: Structure and Sphincter System

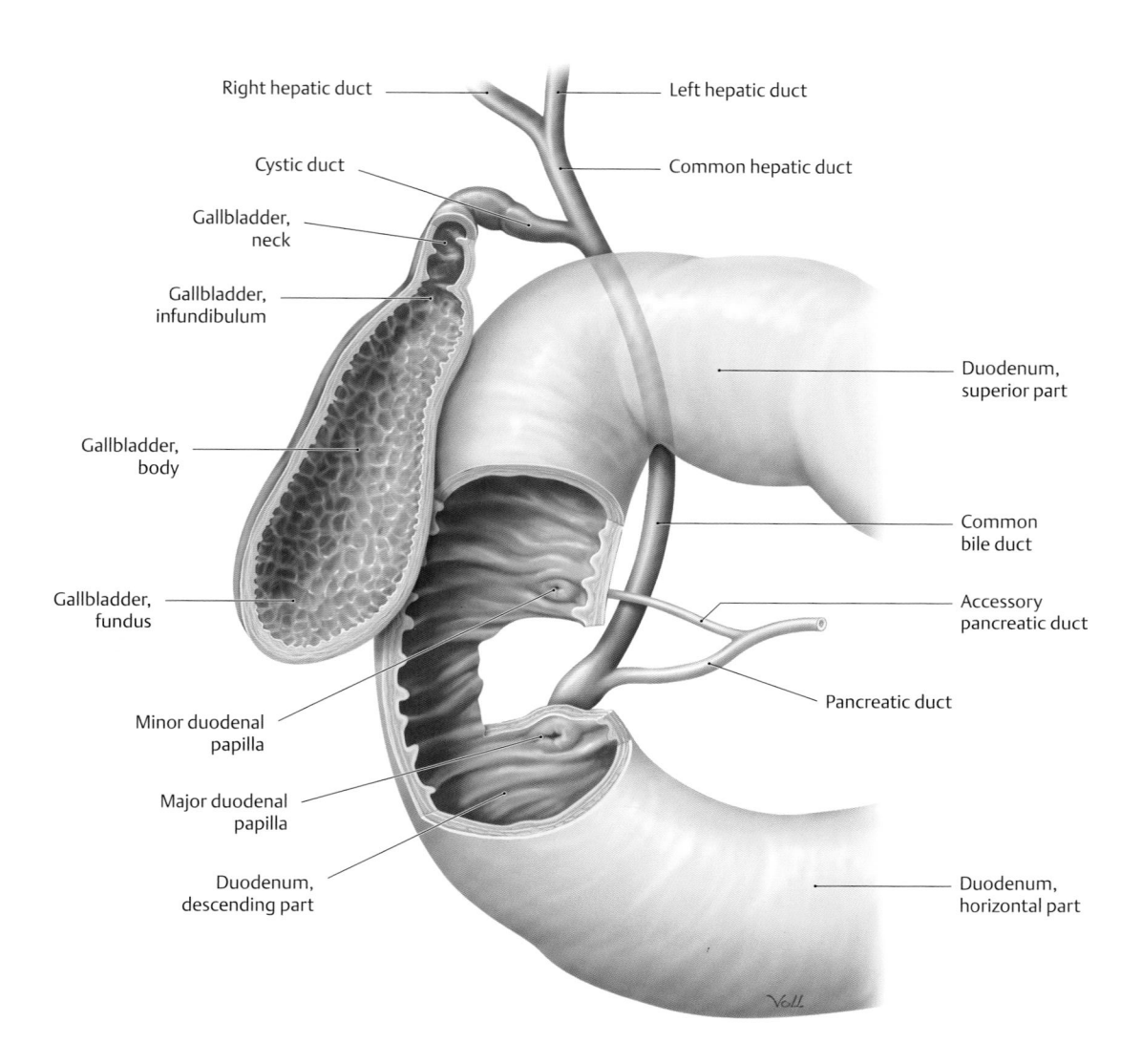

Right hepatic duct

Left hepatic duct

Cystic duct

Common hepatic duct

Gallbladder, neck

Gallbladder, infundibulum

Duodenum, superior part

Gallbladder, body

Common bile duct

Gallbladder, fundus

Accessory pancreatic duct

Minor duodenal papilla

Pancreatic duct

Major duodenal papilla

Duodenum, descending part

Duodenum, horizontal part

A Divisions of the extrahepatic bile ducts

Anterior view. The gallbladder has been opened, and the duodenum has been opened and windowed. The web-like pattern of folds in the gallbladder mucosa is plainly seen. The mucosa between the folds may be deepened to form crypts that can trap bacteria (with risk of cholecystitis). The largest part of the gallbladder is the *body*, which is joined to the neck by the funnel-shaped infundibulum. The neck leads to the cystic duct, which opens end-to-side into the common hepatic duct, formed by the union of the *right* and *left hepatic ducts*. The large duct formed by the union of the cystic duct and common hepatic duct is called the *common bile duct*. This duct often receives the pancreatic duct, both of which then discharge their secretions into the duodenum at the major duodenal papilla (of Vater). A short distance superior to the major papilla is the minor duodenal papilla, whose associated duct (accessory pancreatic duct) crosses in front of the common bile duct. The diagram illustrates a normal pattern of development in which the common hepatic and pancreatic ducts unite to form an ampulla (variants are shown in **C**).

Note: The combined termination of the common bile duct and pancreatic duct has two important implications: A tumor in the head of the pancreas may obstruct the common bile duct (causing biliary reflux into the liver with jaundice), and a gallstone that has migrated from the gallbladder into the common bile duct may obstruct the terminal part of the pancreatic duct. The obstruction of pancreatic secretions may incite a life-threatening pancreatitis.

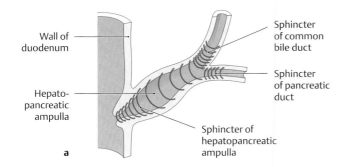

Wall of duodenum

Sphincter of common bile duct

Sphincter of pancreatic duct

Hepato-pancreatic ampulla

Sphincter of hepatopancreatic ampulla

a

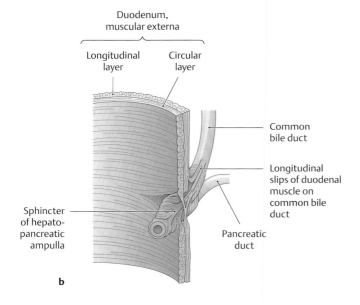

Duodenum, muscular externa

Longitudinal layer

Circular layer

Common bile duct

Longitudinal slips of duodenal muscle on common bile duct

Sphincter of hepato-pancreatic ampulla

Pancreatic duct

b

B Function and structure of the biliary sphincter system

a Sphincters of the common bile duct and pancreatic duct. Each duct has its own sphincter system. Typically both of the ducts unite to form a large ampulla, the hepatopancreatic ampulla, which also has its own sphincter. The sphincter mechanism is supported by adjacent venous pads (not shown here) in the walls of the ducts.

b Integration of the sphincter system in the duodenal wall. The muscles of both ducts blend with the sphincter muscle of the hepatopancreatic ampulla, which passes through the duodenal wall.

Note: The ampullary sphincter system works independently of the circular muscle layer of the duodenal wall, allowing the sphincters to function even during fasting when the duodenum is relaxed. In this state the ductal sphincters are contracted and bile is stored. When food is ingested, the sphincter system opens and allows bile to flow into the duodenum. The sphincter system forms a normal anatomical constriction where a gallstone may become lodged, obstructing the outflow of bile and pancreatic juice (pancreatitis, see **A**). The function of the sphincters, the discharge of bile by the gallbladder, and the production of bile by the liver are controlled partially by the autonomic nervous system (especially the parasympathetic system) and partially by gastrointestinal hormones (e.g., cholecystokinin and secretin).

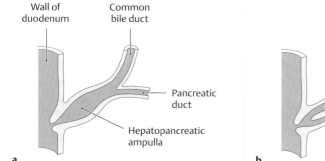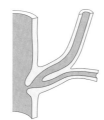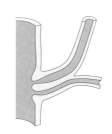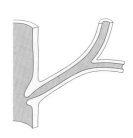

Wall of duodenum

Common bile duct

Pancreatic duct

Hepatopancreatic ampulla

a   b   c   d

C Extrahepatic bile ducts: typical anatomy and variants
Variants in the termination of the common bile duct and pancreatic duct.

a Typical anatomy: Both ducts open at the major duodenal papilla by way of a common ampulla (the most common form).

b–d Variants:
b Varying degrees of septation of the common ampulla.
c Complete septation of the ampulla, with a separate opening for each duct.
d The ducts unite without forming a true ampulla.

2.19 Pancreas: Location and Relationship to Adjacent Organs

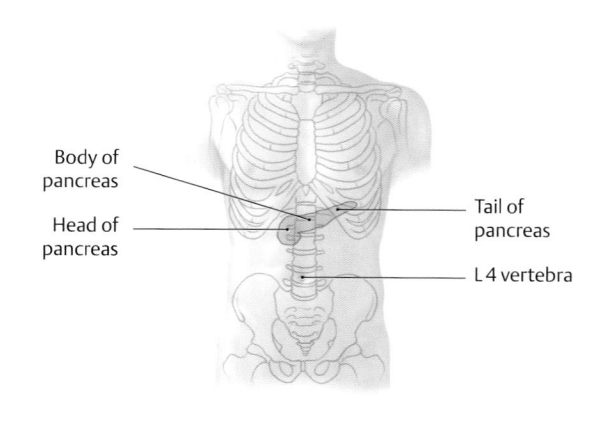

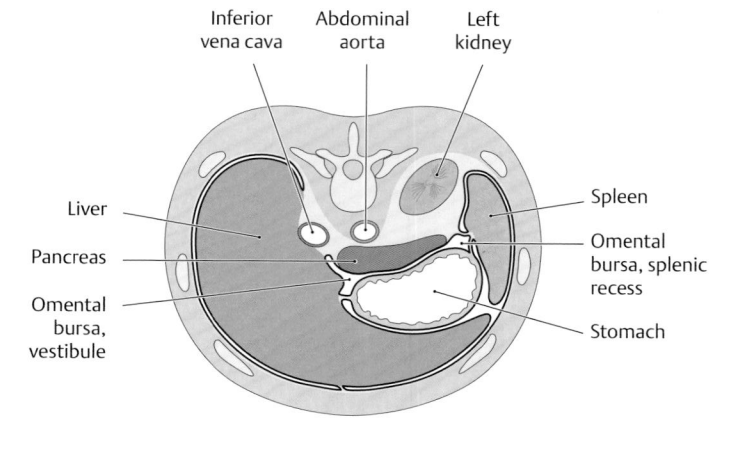

A Projection of the pancreas onto the vertebral column
The pancreas is an elongated organ that is oriented transversely in the right and left upper quadrants, lying mainly in the epigastric region. The body of the pancreas crosses the midline at the L1/L2 level. The head of the pancreas is directed to the right and extends to the L2/L3 level. The tail of the pancreas may closely approach the spleen in the LUQ. The pain associated with diseases of the pancreas is often a "girdling pain" that encircles the upper abdomen and even the lower thorax (see p. 310).

B Location of the pancreas
Transverse section through the abdomen at approximately the T12/L1 level, viewed from above. The pancreas is a secondarily retroperitoneal organ located on the posterior wall of the omental bursa. It extends almost to the spleen on the left side.
Note: The pancreas appears shortened at this level because its head is below the plane of section.

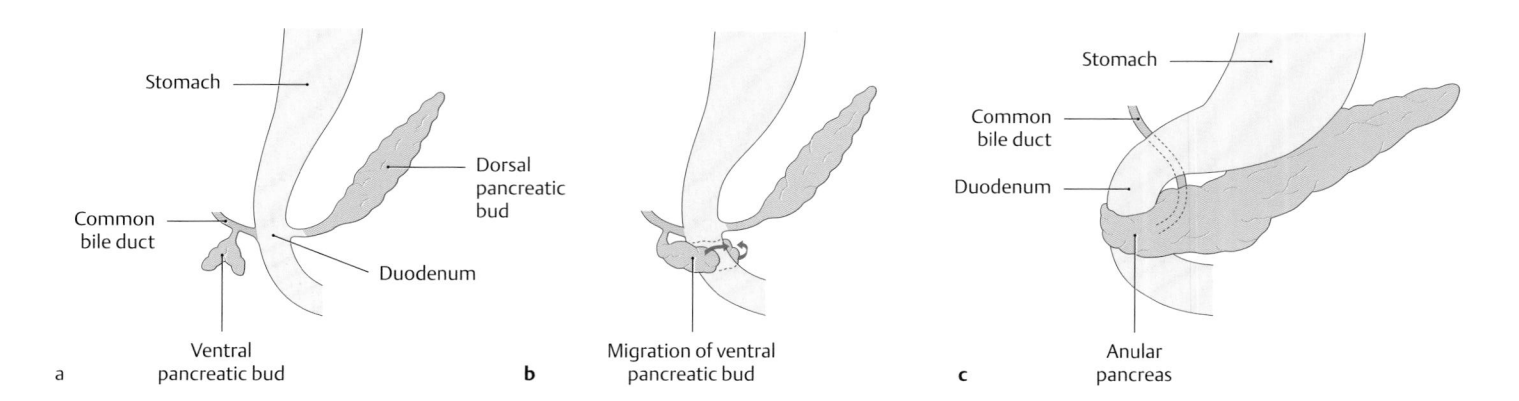

C Anomalous development of the pancreas (anular pancreas)
Embryologically, the pancreas develops from a dorsal and ventral bud that grow into the dorsal and ventral mesoduodenum. The ventral pancreatic bud consists of a left and right part. Normally only the *right* part of the ventral bud migrates back around the duodenum to the future convex right side of that organ, coming to lie *behind* the duodenum when its development is completed (see p. 179). The future com-mon bile duct migrates in the same direction, also coming to lie behind the duodenum. The *left* part of the ventral bud generally regresses at an early stage. But if it persists, both the anterior and posterior sides of the duodenum will be encircled by a ring of pancreatic tissue: an *anular pancreas*. This rare anomaly may cause obstruction of the duodenum (duodenal stenosis) immediately after birth, but it can also be asymptomatic.

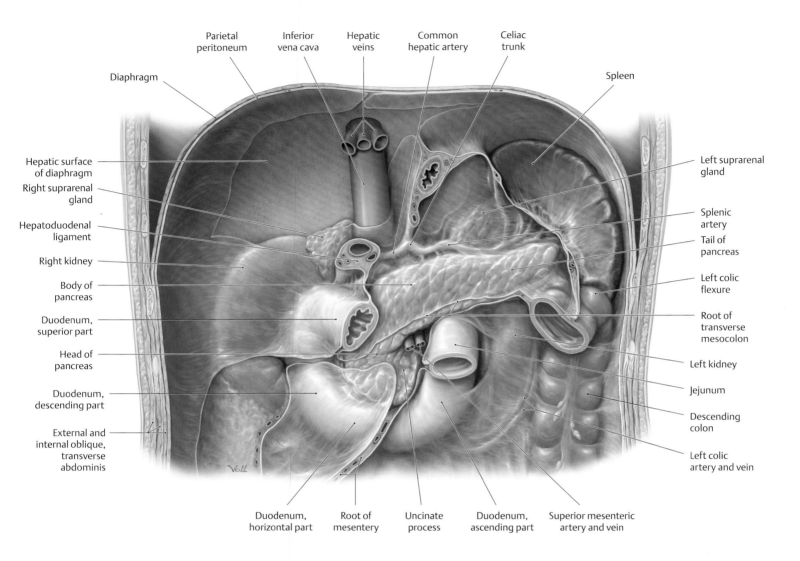

Parietal peritoneum — Inferior vena cava — Hepatic veins — Common hepatic artery — Celiac trunk — Spleen

Diaphragm

Hepatic surface of diaphragm

Right suprarenal gland

Hepatoduodenal ligament

Right kidney

Body of pancreas

Duodenum, superior part

Head of pancreas

Duodenum, descending part

External and internal oblique, transverse abdominis

Left suprarenal gland

Splenic artery

Tail of pancreas

Left colic flexure

Root of transverse mesocolon

Left kidney

Jejunum

Descending colon

Left colic artery and vein

Duodenum, horizontal part — Root of mesentery — Uncinate process — Duodenum, ascending part — Superior mesenteric artery and vein

D The pancreas in situ

Anterior view. The liver, stomach, small intestine, and large intestine have been removed proximal to the left colic flexure. The retroperitoneal fat and connective tissue and the perirenal fat capsule have been greatly thinned to better demonstrate the structures in the retroperitoneum. Surgical access to the pancreas is difficult due to overlying organs and the proximity of large vessels. The head of the pancreas is enclosed within the C-shaped loop of the duodenum. The line of attachment of the transverse mesocolon runs along the anterior surface of the pancreas. Malignant tumors of the pancreas may spread to nearby blood vessels (most notably the superior mesenteric artery and vein) and may surround and constrict them, reducing blood flow to dependent organs. Similarly, inflammations and tumors of the head of the pancreas may constrict the common bile duct, leading to obstructive jaundice.

2.20 Pancreas: Ductal Anatomy and Histology

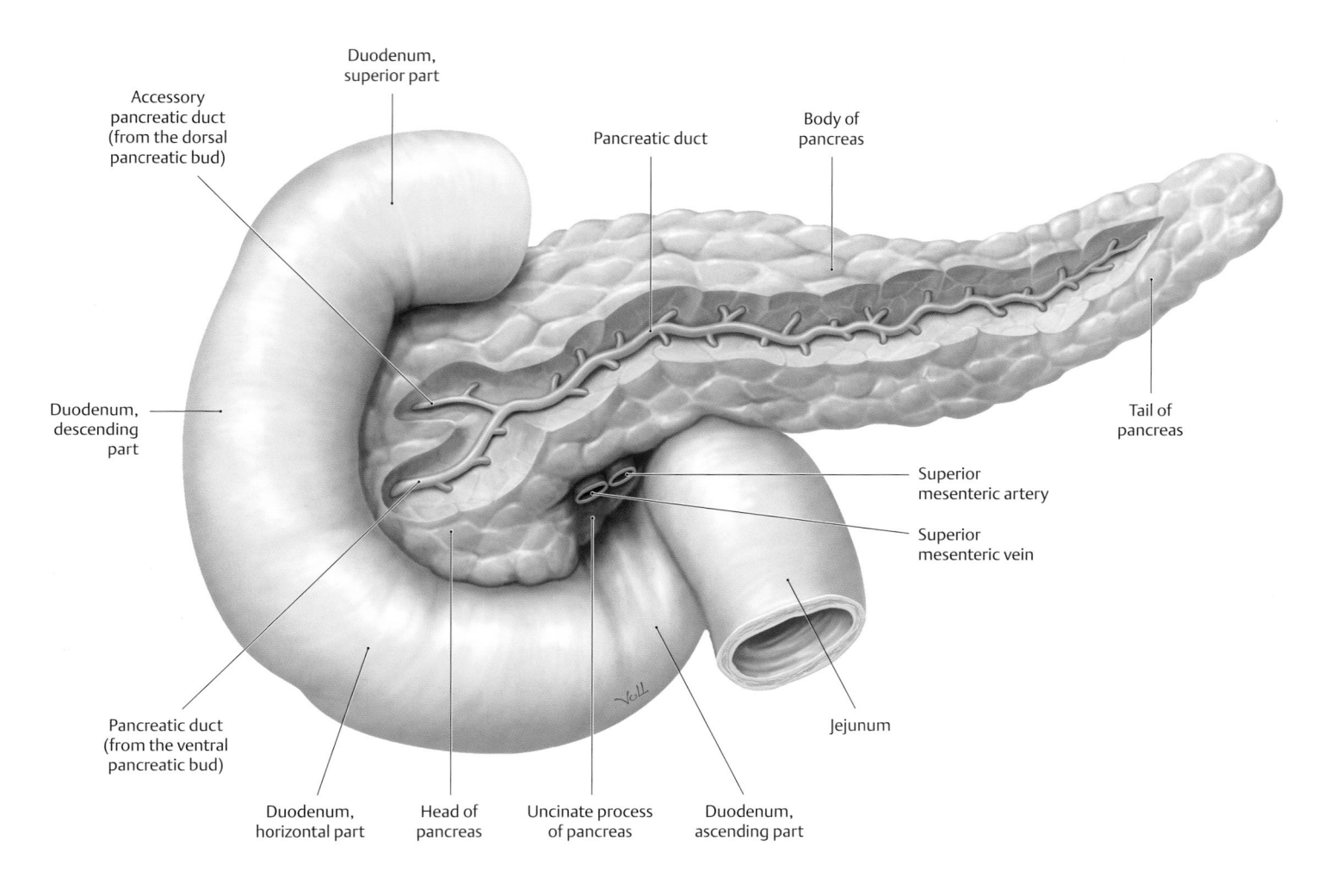

Accessory
pancreatic duct
(from the dorsal
pancreatic bud)

Duodenum,
superior part

Pancreatic duct

Body of
pancreas

Duodenum,
descending
part

Tail of
pancreas

Superior
mesenteric artery

Superior
mesenteric vein

Pancreatic duct
(from the ventral
pancreatic bud)

Jejunum

Duodenum,
horizontal part

Head of
pancreas

Uncinate process
of pancreas

Duodenum,
ascending part

A Location and course of the pancreatic duct

Anterior view. The anterior side of the pancreas has been partially dissected. This drawing illustrates the most common form: The ducts from the former ventral and dorsal pancreatic buds have united to form a common duct. The main pancreatic duct is formed from the distal portion of the dorsal pancreatic duct. The proximal portion of the main duct is derived from the ventral pancreatic duct. The main pancreatic duct opens into the descending part of the duodenum (usually sharing an orifice with the common bile duct) on the *major* duodenal papilla (see p. 188). The remaining small segment of the former dorsal pancre-

atic duct, now called the *accessory pancreatic duct*, is found only in the head of the pancreas and opens into the duodenum on its own papilla, the *minor* duodenal papilla, which is slightly cranial to the major papilla (see p. 188). Several variants of ductal anatomy may be encountered:

- Both ducts remain separate and open on two separate papillae.
- Both ducts are united, forming a single duct that opens on only one papilla.
- In both cases (though rarely), the common bile duct may open into the duodenum by a separate orifice.

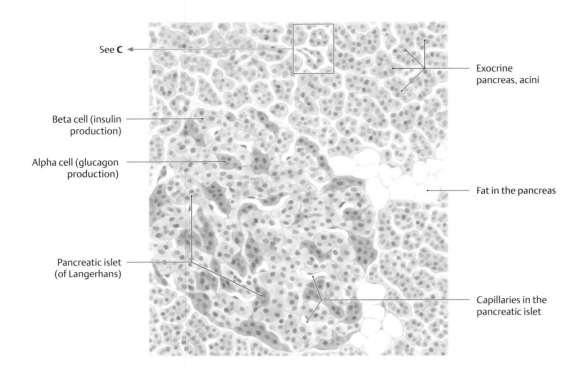

See **C**	Exocrine pancreas, acini
Beta cell (insulin production)	
Alpha cell (glucagon production)	Fat in the pancreas
Pancreatic islet (of Langerhans)	Capillaries in the pancreatic islet

B Histological structure of the pancreas

Histologically, the pancreas consists of two functionally distinct types of glandular tissue:

- The **exocrine pancreas** (98 % of the organ mass, light pink in the upper part of the figure) consists of myriad berry-shaped glands (*acini*, see **C**), which secrete an enzyme-rich fluid through the pancreatic duct into the duodenum. Produced at a rate of approximately 2 liters / day, this fluid contains enzymes that assist numerous digestive processes in the bowel. Insufficiency of the exocrine pancreas leads to impaired digestive function.
- The **endocrine pancreas** (2 % of the organ mass) consists of the pancreatic islets (of Langerhans) — approximately 1 million clusters of endocrine cells scattered throughout the exocrine pancreatic tissue.

Specialized staining methods (as depicted here) can be used to distinguish two types of islet cells—the much more numerous beta (B) cells, which produce insulin, and a minority population of cells somewhat more concentrated on the islet periphery, alpha (A) cells, which produce glucagon. Other islet cell types, distinguishable only by immunohistochemical methods, include delta (D) cells, which produce somatostatin, and others that make pancreatic polypeptide or additional neuroendocrine factors. Pancreatic islets are well-vascularized, providing direct, efficient release of these substances into the bloodstream. Glucagon mobilizes hepatic stores of glycogen and raises blood glucose levels; insulin promotes glucose utilization and lowers blood glucose levels. Destruction of pancreatic B cells is the hallmark of (type I) diabetes mellitus.

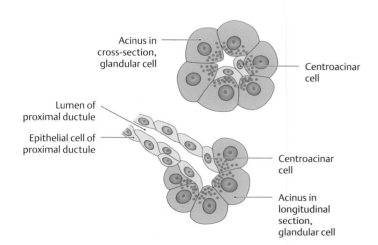

Acinus in cross-section, glandular cell	Centroacinar cell
Lumen of proximal ductule	
Epithelial cell of proximal ductule	Centroacinar cell
	Acinus in longitudinal section, glandular cell

C Histological structure of the pancreas: the acinus

These drawings represent higher-magnification views of an acinus from the exocrine pancreas shown in cross-section and in longitudinal section (detail from **B**). The acinar cells, which produce the enzyme-rich secretion (numerous proteins), stain intensely with conventional techniques, causing them to appear dark in the histological section.

Note: It is characteristic of the pancreas that the proximal ductule — the initial part of the system that transports secretions — is invaginated into the center of the acinus. The ductule cells stain less intensely than the acinar cells. Because of this, the cells that lie morphologically at the center of the acinus, and are conspicuous in histological sections as the relatively light-staining *centroacinar cells*. The pancreas is the only exocrine gland that contains centroacinar cells.

2.21 Spleen

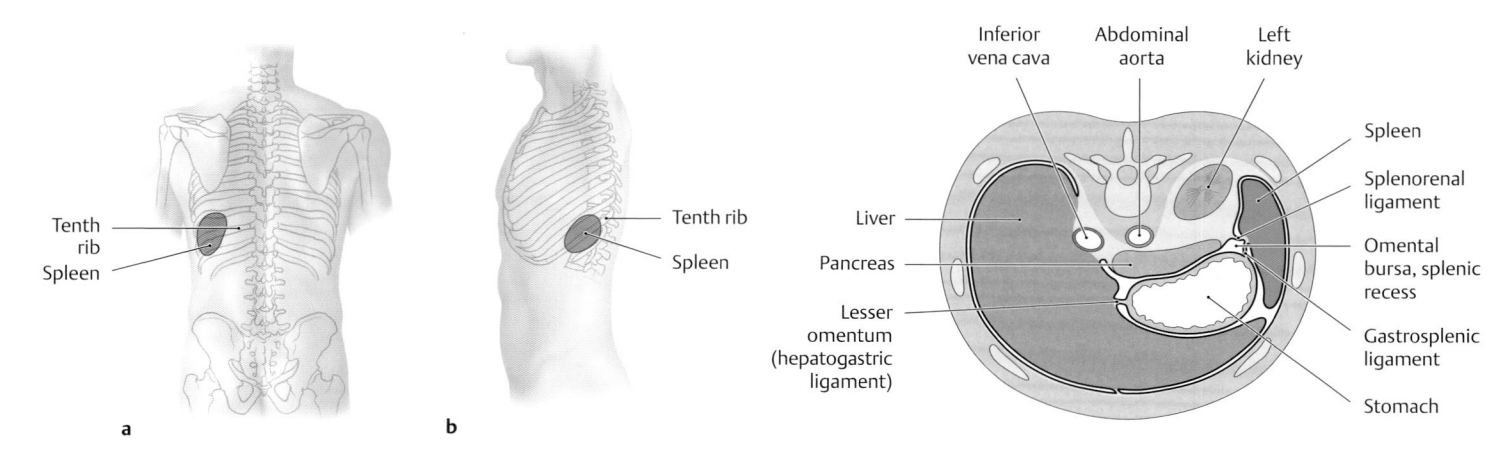

A Projection of the spleen onto the skeleton

Posterior view (**a**) and left lateral view (**b**). The spleen is located in the left upper quadrant. Its position varies considerably with respiration because it lies just below the diaphragm and is directly affected by its movements, even though (unlike the liver) it is not attached to the diaphragm. At functional residual capacity (the resting position between inspiration and expiration), the hilum of the spleen crosses the tenth rib on the left side. Generally a healthy, unenlarged spleen is not palpable on physical examination.

B Location of the spleen

Transverse section through the abdomen, viewed from above. This section demonstrates the relationship of the spleen to neighboring organs. The intraperitoneal spleen lies in its own compartment and is attached by folds of peritoneum to the posterior trunk wall (splenorenal ligament) and to the stomach (gastrosplenic ligament). A recess of the omental bursa (splenic recess) extends to the spleen.

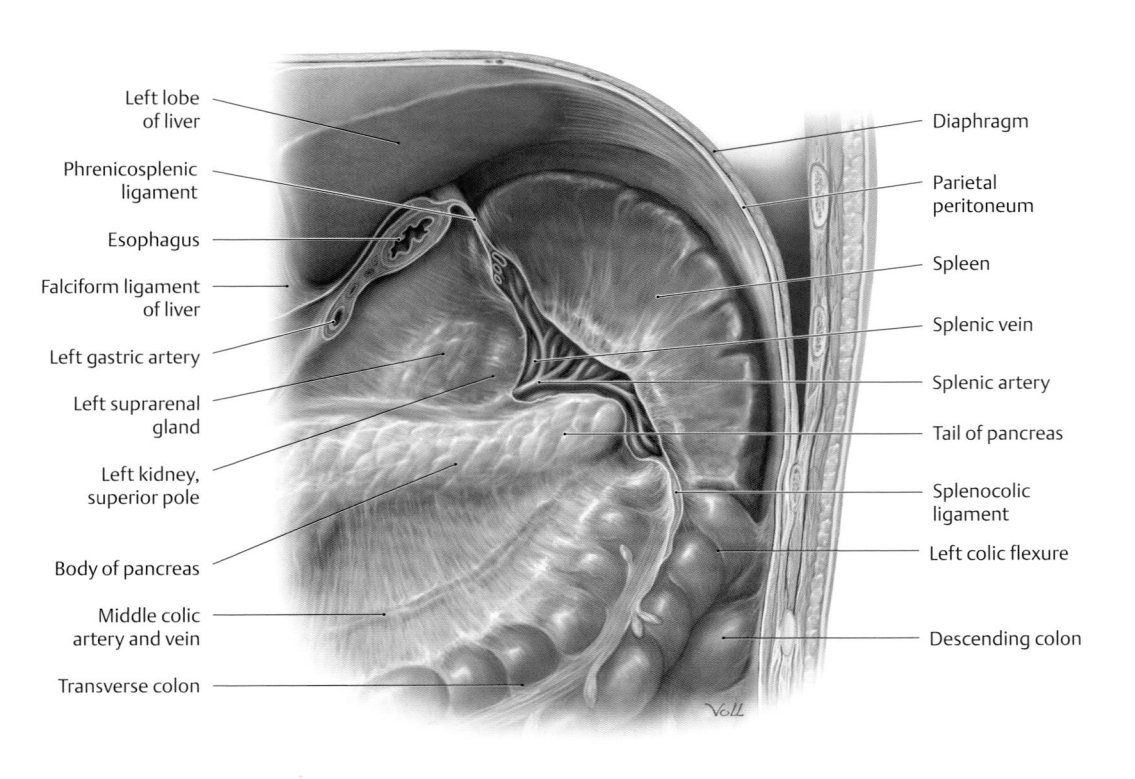

C The spleen in situ: peritoneal relationships

Anterior view into the LUQ with the stomach removed. When the spleen is abnormally enlarged, it may press heavily upon the stomach and colon, causing pain. The drawing illustrates the close proximity of the spleen to the tail of the pancreas and left colic flexure, which is also called the splenic flexure.

Note the peritoneal attachment between the spleen and transverse colon (splenocolic ligament, part of the greater omentum). Embryologi-cally, the greater omentum is a dorsal mesentery in which the spleen develops. During rotation of the stomach in the embryo, the spleen moves from its original position posterior to the gut into the LUQ. A "side stitch" (piercing sensation felt below the rib cage during exercise) is believed to be caused by stretching of the peritoneal covering and splenocolic ligament due to swelling of the spleen during physical exercise.

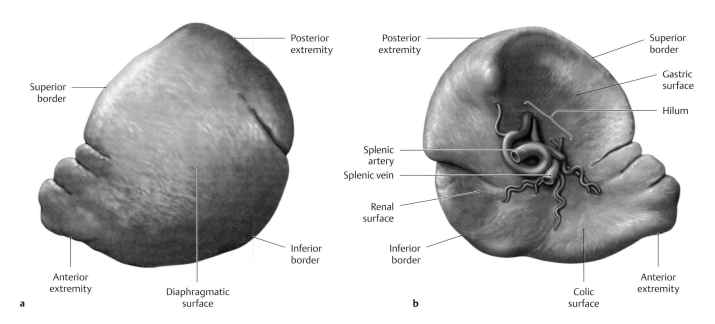

Superior border

Posterior extremity

Posterior extremity

Superior border

Gastric surface

Hilum

Splenic artery

Splenic vein

Renal surface

Inferior border

Inferior border

Anterior extremity

Diaphragmatic surface

a

Colic surface

Anterior extremity

b

D Spleen: shape and surface anatomy

Views of the costal surface (**a**) and visceral surface (**b**) of the organ. The spleen is highly variable in its conformation in different people, but because this very soft organ is covered by a firm fibrous capsule, it maintains a relatively constant external shape ("coffee bean"). Since it is very difficult to suture the soft splenic tissue, it is not uncommon to treat splenic injuries by splenectomy, which eliminates a potential source of severe intraperitoneal bleeding. The blood vessels that enter and leave the organ at the splenic hilum are usually tortuous and form multiple coils.

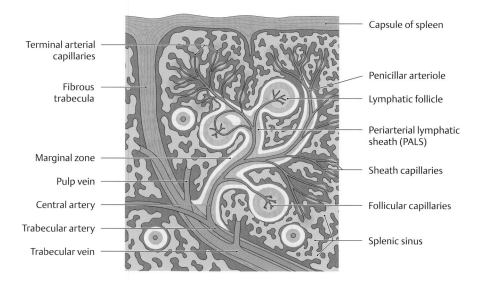

Terminal arterial capillaries

Fibrous trabecula

Marginal zone

Pulp vein

Central artery

Trabecular artery

Trabecular vein

Capsule of spleen

Penicillar arteriole

Lymphatic follicle

Periarterial lymphatic sheath (PALS)

Sheath capillaries

Follicular capillaries

Splenic sinus

E Structure of the spleen

The spleen is the single largest lymphoid organ and the only lymphatic organ that is incorporated directly into the bloodstream (to screen out abnormal cells, see below). Strands of connective tissue called trabeculae extend from the firm fibrous capsule toward the hilum of the spleen, subdividing the splenic tissue into small chambers. The branches of the fibrous trabeculae and the vessels they transmit (*trabecular arteries and veins*) determine the architecture of the spleen. Between the fibrous trabeculae is a meshwork of fine reticular connective tissue, the splenic pulp. On entering the pulp, the blood vessels become known as the *pulp arteries* and *pulp veins*. The terminal arterial branches have the appearance of the mycelia of bread mold (*penicillium*), and are thus named "penicillar" arterioles. Two types of splenic pulp are distinguished: red pulp and white pulp.

• The *red pulp* consists of cavities (splenic sinuses) that are engorged with blood in the living organism (aggregation of large masses of red blood cells), accounting for its red color and its name (in the section shown here, the pulp is devoid of blood and is colorless). The function of the red pulp is to screen out aging and defective erythrocytes from the bloodstream. The numerous sinuses within the reticular meshwork give the spleen its soft, spongy consistency.

• The *white pulp* consists of splenic nodules (malpighian bodies) — variable-sized aggregations of lymphocytes (periarterial lymphatic sheaths, lymphatic follicles) that consist of clones of beta cells that are proliferatory in response to antigens.

The lymphatic aggregations of the white pulp ensheath the pulp arteries in varying degrees to ensure close contact between the blood and lymphocytes. The pulp arteries ramify extensively before delivering their blood to the sinuses of the red pulp. From there the blood is conveyed by pulp veins to the trabecular veins, which in turn empty into the splenic vein.

2.22 Suprarenal Glands

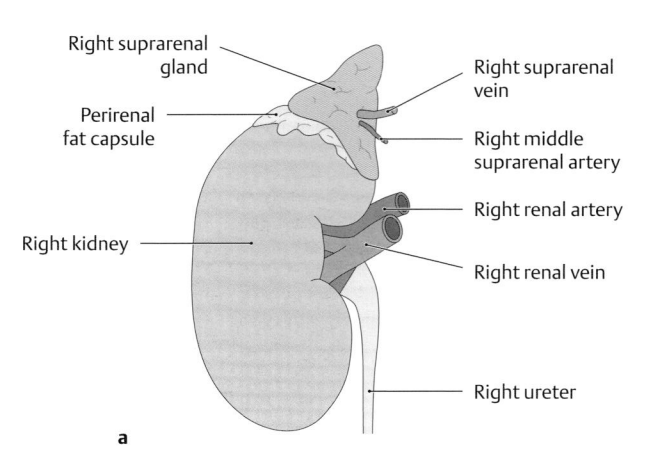

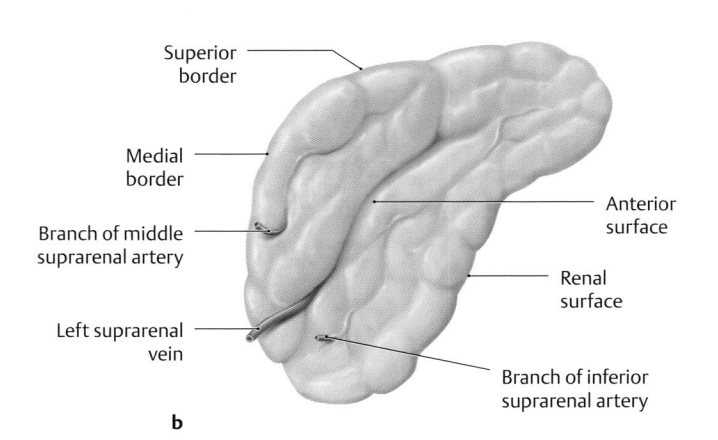

a

b

A Location and shape
a Location of the suprarenal gland on the right kidney. **b** Isolated left suprarenal gland, anterior view.
The renal surface of each suprarenal gland lies upon the superior pole of the associated kidney. A thin layer of fat separates the suprarenal gland from the *renal* fibrous capsule (making it easy to dissect the gland from

the kidney). The *perirenal* fat capsule, however, encompasses both the kidney and the suprarenal gland.
Note: The entire suprarenal gland cannot be seen while in situ, and its true size is not appreciated until it has been detached from the kidney. Portions descend on the posterior surface of the kidney and are not visible in situ.

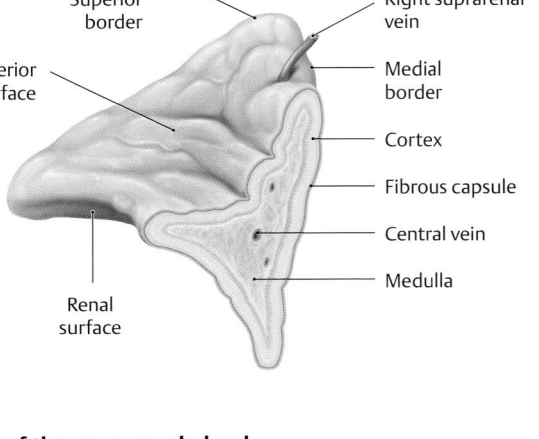

a

B Structure of the suprarenal gland
a Right suprarenal gland, cut open. **b** Histological section from a suprarenal gland.
The suprarenal gland consists of an outer cortex and an inner medulla (see **a**). The **cortex** is covered by a thin fibrous capsule and consists of three morphologically distinct zones (see **b**) in which adrenocortical hormones are produced and secreted into the bloodstream. These zones are, from outside to inside:

- Zona glomerulosa: mainly secretes mineralocorticoids (aldosterone)
- Zona fasciculata: mainly secretes glucocorticoids (hydrocortisone)
- Zona reticularis: sex hormones (estrogens and androgens)

Note: Loss or deficiency of both suprarenal cortices leads to Addison disease, while hyperfunction of the suprarenal cortex (or adrenocortical tumors) leads to Cushing syndrome.
The **suprarenal medulla** is essentially a completely different endocrine gland, of different origin, that happens to be anatomically (but also functionally) associated with the suprarenal cortex. The cortex is derived embryonically from mesoderm lining the posterior abdominal wall. The suprarenal medulla is, by contrast, a neural crest derivative, and thus has an ectodermal origin. The catecholamines epinephrine

and norepinephrine are produced in the suprarenal medulla and are released into the bloodstream. From a (neuro)functional standpoint, the suprarenal medulla is less a gland than a *sympathetic ganglion*: presynaptic sympathetic neurons pass from the greater and lesser splanchnic nerves into the suprarenal medulla. Because the suprarenal glands are endocrine glands and sympathetic ganglia in one, they can secrete both epinephrine and glucocorticoids (cortisone) in response to stress.

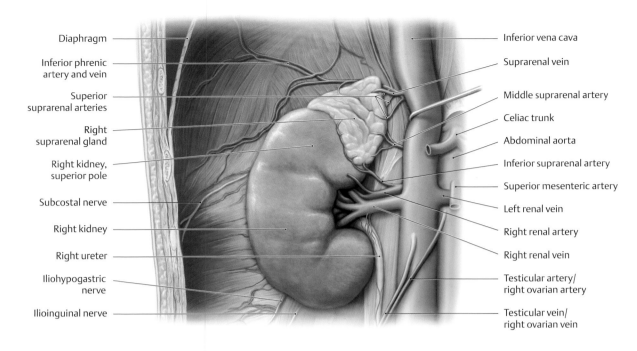

Diaphragm
Inferior phrenic artery and vein
Superior suprarenal arteries
Right suprarenal gland
Right kidney, superior pole
Subcostal nerve
Right kidney
Right ureter
Iliohypogastric nerve
Ilioinguinal nerve

Inferior vena cava
Suprarenal vein
Middle suprarenal artery
Celiac trunk
Abdominal aorta
Inferior suprarenal artery
Superior mesenteric artery
Left renal vein
Right renal artery
Right renal vein
Testicular artery/ right ovarian artery
Testicular vein/ right ovarian vein

a

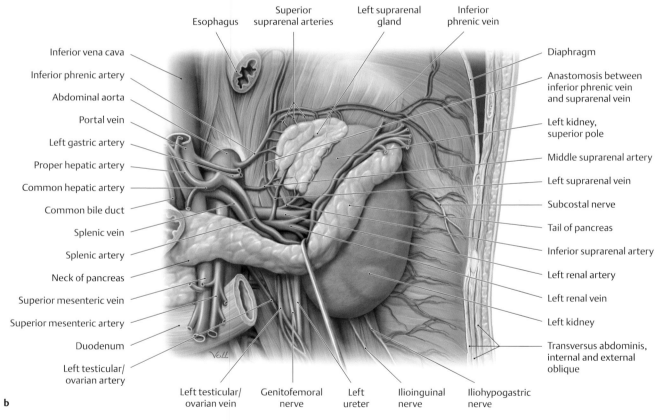

Esophagus
Superior suprarenal arteries
Left suprarenal gland
Inferior phrenic vein

Inferior vena cava
Inferior phrenic artery
Abdominal aorta
Portal vein
Left gastric artery
Proper hepatic artery
Common hepatic artery
Common bile duct
Splenic vein
Splenic artery
Neck of pancreas
Superior mesenteric vein
Superior mesenteric artery
Duodenum
Left testicular/ ovarian artery

Diaphragm
Anastomosis between inferior phrenic vein and suprarenal vein
Left kidney, superior pole
Middle suprarenal artery
Left suprarenal vein
Subcostal nerve
Tail of pancreas
Inferior suprarenal artery
Left renal artery
Left renal vein
Left kidney
Transversus abdominis, internal and external oblique

Left testicular/ ovarian vein
Genitofemoral nerve
Left ureter
Ilioinguinal nerve
Iliohypogastric nerve

b

C Right and left suprarenal glands in situ

Anterior view of the right (**a**) and left (**b**) kidney and suprarenal gland with the perirenal fat capsule removed. To demonstrate the vessels behind the suprarenal gland, the vena cava has been retracted medially in **a** and the pancreas has been retracted inferiorly in **b**. The principal differences between the two suprarenal glands are as follows:

- The right suprarenal gland is often somewhat smaller than the left suprarenal gland, which frequently extends inferiorly to the renal hilum.
- The right suprarenal gland is pyramid-shaped while the large left suprarenal gland is more oblong.

- The right suprarenal gland is normally in contact with the inferior vena cava (retracted medially here), but the left suprarenal gland is *not* in contact with the abdominal aorta.
- The right suprarenal vein usually opens *directly* into the inferior vena cava, unlike the left suprarenal vein, which opens into the left renal vein.

Note: The suprarenal glands are richly vascularized because, as endocrine organs, they release their hormones directly into the bloodstream.

221

2.23 Overview of the Urinary Organs

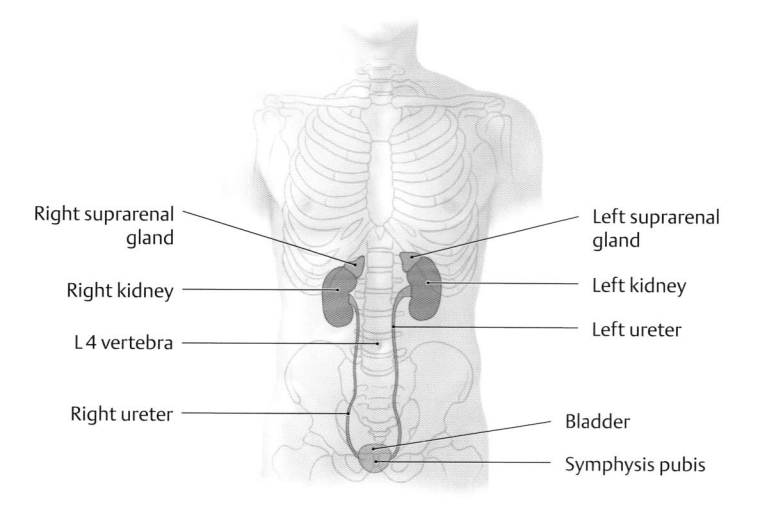

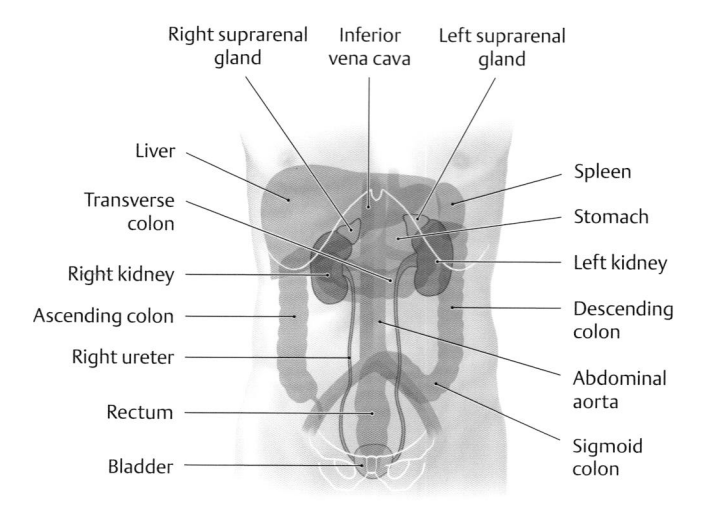

A Projection of the kidneys and other urinary organs onto the skeleton

Anterior view. The suprarenal glands are also shown to aid orientation. The kidneys are located next to the vertebral column and are high enough that they overlap the eleventh and twelfth ribs. The renal hilum is situated at the L 1/L 2 level. Usually the right kidney is somewhat lower than the left kidney due to the space occupied by the liver (see p. 204). The bladder is shown fully distended in the diagram. When empty, it is considerably smaller and is hidden behind the symphysis pubis. The ureters descend in the retroperitoneum and open into the bladder from the posterior side.

B Projection of the urinary organs onto the organs of the abdomen and pelvis

Anterior view. Owing to its large size, the liver displaces the right kidney slightly inferiorly. The bladder is shown in a fully distended state. It is anterior to the rectum in the male and anterior to the uterus (not shown here) in the female. Because of this relationship, marked distention of the rectal ampulla or enlargement of the uterus due to pregnancy exerts greater pressure on the bladder, creating an urge to urinate even when the bladder is not full. Urinary incontinence may develop due to pathological processes of longer duration, such as muscular tumors of the uterus (fibroids), or due to weakening of the bladder closure mechanism as a result of previous vaginal deliveries (descent of the muscular pelvic floor).

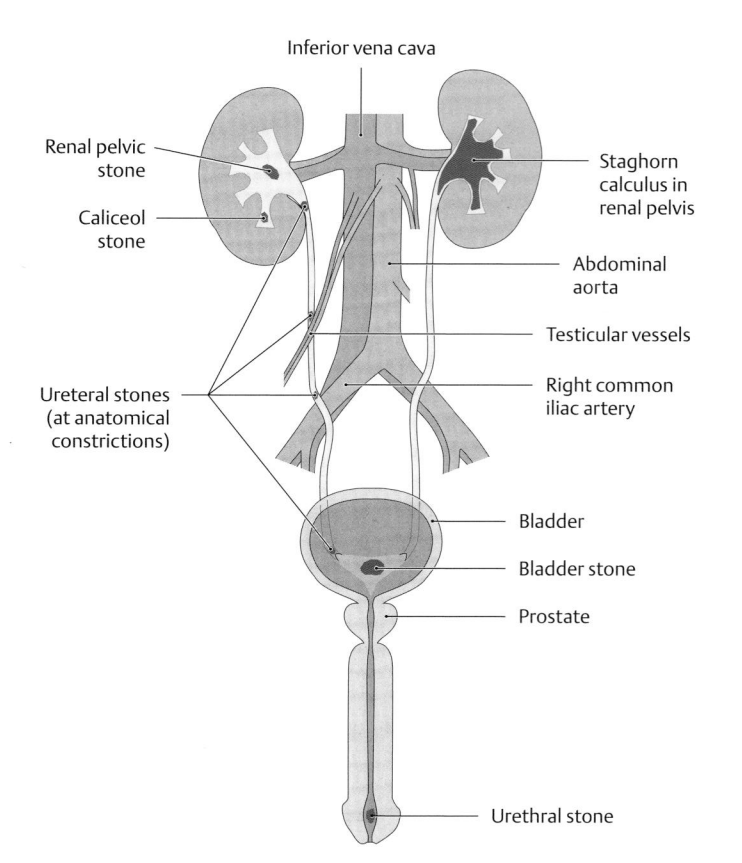

C Common sites of occurrence of urinary stones

When the solubility limit of certain compounds in the urine (e.g., uric acid) is exceeded, the compounds do not remain in solution but are precipitated to form crystallization nuclei. These calculi ("stones") may develop anywhere in the upper urinary tract and may migrate to various sites in any of the urinary organs (renal and renal pelvic stones, ureteral stones, bladder stones, urethral stones). Larger stones are particularly apt to become lodged in the ureter, often stimulating powerful waves of muscular contractions to expel the stone and causing excruciating pain (renal colic, ureteral colic).

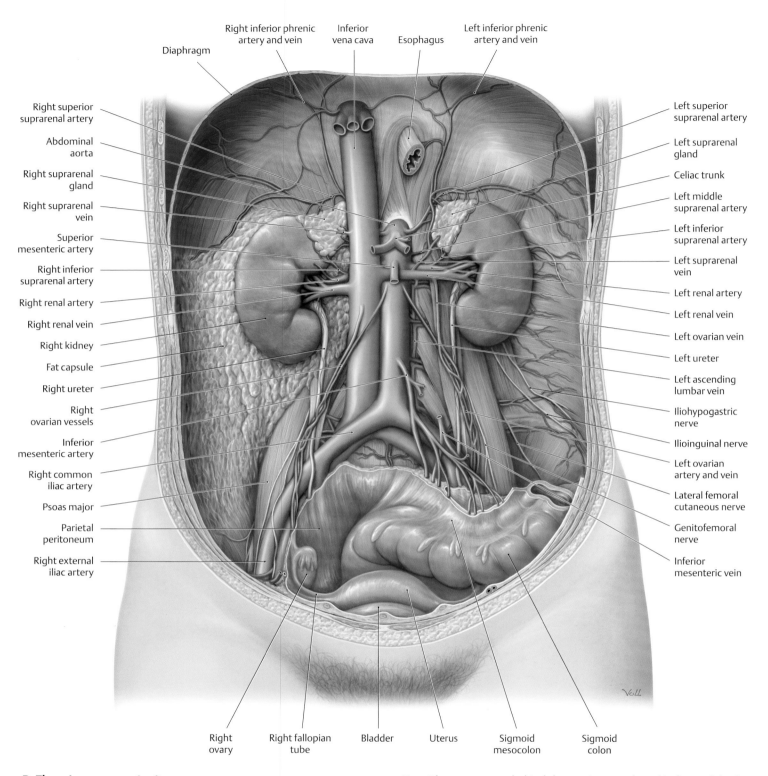

Right inferior phrenic
artery and vein

Inferior
vena cava

Esophagus

Left inferior phrenic
artery and vein

Diaphragm

Right superior
suprarenal artery

Abdominal
aorta

Right suprarenal
gland

Right suprarenal
vein

Superior
mesenteric artery

Right inferior
suprarenal artery

Right renal artery

Right renal vein

Right kidney

Fat capsule

Right ureter

Right
ovarian vessels

Inferior
mesenteric artery

Right common
iliac artery

Psoas major

Parietal
peritoneum

Right external
iliac artery

Left superior
suprarenal artery

Left suprarenal
gland

Celiac trunk

Left middle
suprarenal artery

Left inferior
suprarenal artery

Left suprarenal
vein

Left renal artery

Left renal vein

Left ovarian vein

Left ureter

Left ascending
lumbar vein

Iliohypogastric
nerve

Ilioinguinal nerve

Left ovarian
artery and vein

Lateral femoral
cutaneous nerve

Genitofemoral
nerve

Inferior
mesenteric vein

Right
ovary

Right fallopian
tube

Bladder

Uterus

Sigmoid
mesocolon

Sigmoid
colon

D The urinary organs in situ

Anterior view of an opened female abdomen. The spleen and gastrointestinal organs have been removed to the sigmoid colon, and the
esophagus has been pulled slightly inferiorly. The fat capsule remains
partially intact on the right side, removed on the left side. The kidneys
and suprarenal glands are incorporated into the retroperitoneum by
the structural fat of this capsule. The moderately distended bladder is
just visible above the symphysis pubis in front of the uterus. The parietal peritoneum has been removed to provide a clear view into the
retroperitoneum.

Note: The ureters pass behind the ovarian vessels and in front of the iliac
vessels as they descend in the retroperitoneum. These sites represent
clinically important constrictions of the ureter where a stone from the
renal pelvis may become lodged (see **C**).

In most cases the kidneys are not oriented parallel to the coronal plane.
The renal hilum, where the blood vessels and ureter enter and leave the
kidneys, is directed anteromedially (see **B**, p. 224, and **B**, p. 226). Also,
the renal superior poles are closer together than the inferior poles, so
that the kidneys appear slightly "tilted" toward the midline. Thus the
renal hilum also points slightly downward.

2.24 Kidneys: Topographical Anatomy

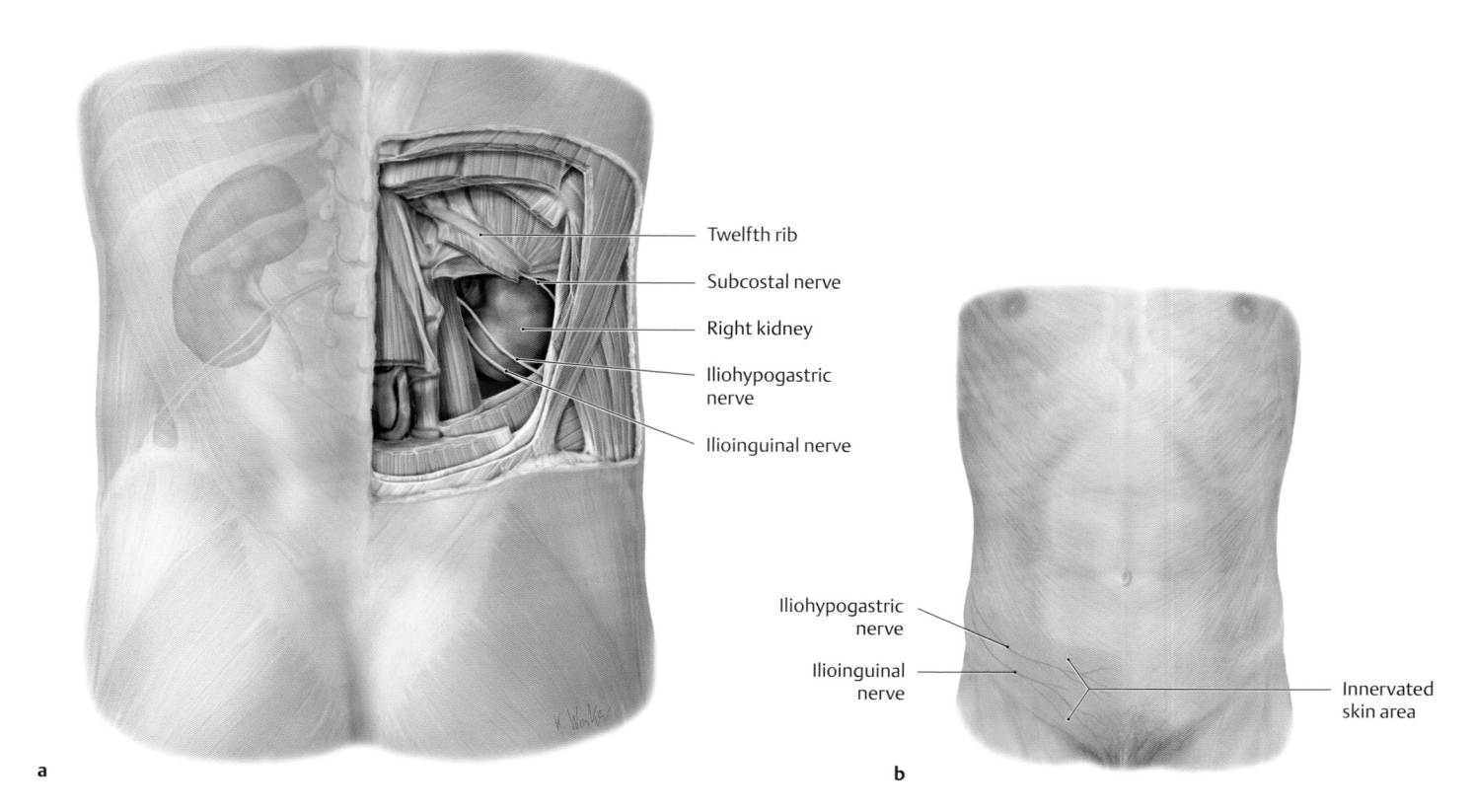

Twelfth rib

Subcostal nerve

Right kidney

Iliohypogastric nerve

Ilioinguinal nerve

Iliohypogastric nerve

Ilioinguinal nerve

Innervated skin area

a

b

A Proximity of the kidneys to the iliohypogastric and ilioinguinal nerves

a When all layers of the trunk wall have been divided and the fat capsule removed (see p. 223), it can be seen how close the kidneys are to the iliohypogastric and ilioinguinal nerves (branches of the lumbar plexus from T 12 and especially L 1). These nerves supply motor inner-

vation to the muscles of the trunk wall and sensory innervation to skin areas on the lateral and anterior abdominal wall. Thus, when an abnormally enlarged kidney exerts pressure on the iliohypogastric and ilioinguinal nerves, pain may be referred to the skin area shown in **b**. The subcostal nerve (also from T 12) usually lies far enough from the kidneys that it is not compressed by renal enlargement.

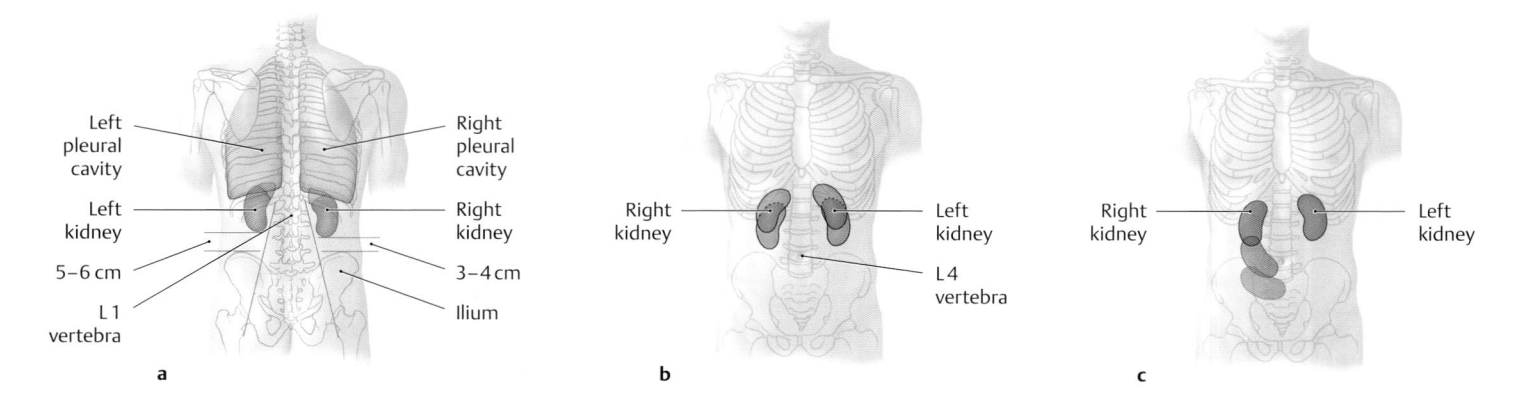

Left pleural cavity

Right pleural cavity

Left kidney

Right kidney

5–6 cm

3–4 cm

L 1 vertebra

Ilium

Right kidney

Left kidney

L 4 vertebra

Right kidney

Left kidney

a

b

c

B Location of the kidneys, normal vs. pathological mobility

a **Posterior view.** The pleural cavities overlap the kidneys posteriorly owing to the convexity of the diaphragm.

Note that the right kidney is lower than the left kidney and is closer to the palpable iliac crest (see **C**, p. 150).

b, c **Anterior view.** The kidneys are located in the retroperitoneum just below the diaphragm. Hence they move passively with the diaphragm during respiratory excursions, moving inferiorly and slightly laterally during inspiration because of their oblique position (their inferior poles point away from the spine, see oblique red lines in **a**). These

passive movements may cause respiration-dependent pain in patients with renal disease. A *pathological* increase in renal mobility ("floating kidney," see **c**) results from atrophy of the fat capsule that normally surrounds the kidneys and keeps them in a stable position. A wasting illness (e.g., metastatic tumors of varying origin) may cause such severe fatty atrophy that the kidneys descend to a lower level in the abdomen. As they are still tethered by the ureter and vascular stalk, this descent may kink the renal vessels or ureter and interfere with renal blood flow or urinary outflow.

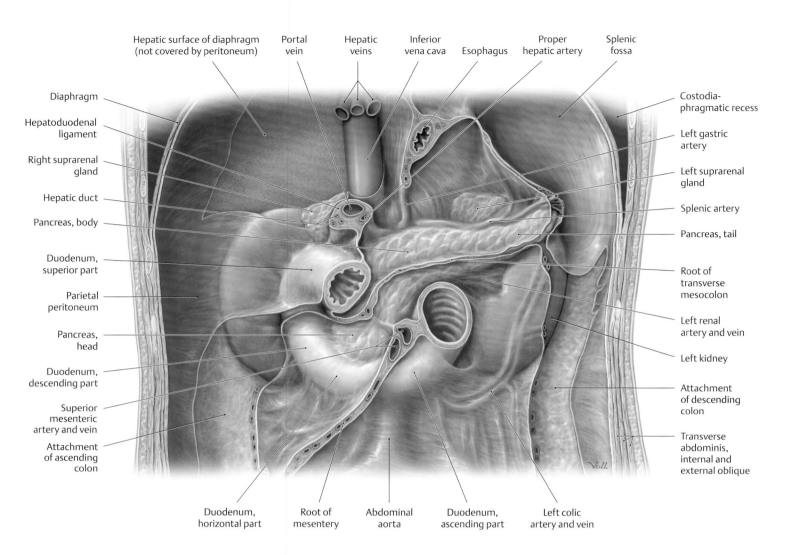

Hepatic surface of diaphragm (not covered by peritoneum)

Portal vein

Hepatic veins

Inferior vena cava

Esophagus

Proper hepatic artery

Splenic fossa

Diaphragm

Hepatoduodenal ligament

Right suprarenal gland

Hepatic duct

Pancreas, body

Duodenum, superior part

Parietal peritoneum

Pancreas, head

Duodenum, descending part

Superior mesenteric artery and vein

Attachment of ascending colon

Costodia-phragmatic recess

Left gastric artery

Left suprarenal gland

Splenic artery

Pancreas, tail

Root of transverse mesocolon

Left renal artery and vein

Left kidney

Attachment of descending colon

Transverse abdominis, internal and external oblique

Duodenum, horizontal part

Root of mesentery

Abdominal aorta

Duodenum, ascending part

Left colic artery and vein

C Topographical relations of the kidneys in the retroperitoneum
Anterior view. All of the intraperitoneal organs and secondarily retroperitoneal portions of the colon (ascending and descending colon) have been removed, leaving the duodenum and pancreas in place. Most of the fat capsule anterior to the kidneys has also been removed. Both kidneys are overlapped by the attachments of the ascending and descend-

ing colon on the posterior wall of the peritoneal cavity and by the root of the transverse mesocolon. Because the pancreas, parts of the duodenum, and the left and right colic flexures are *secondarily* retroperitoneal, they are in close proximity to the *primarily* retroperitoneal kidneys but are still separated from them by the fat and connective tissue of the fat capsule (see **D**).

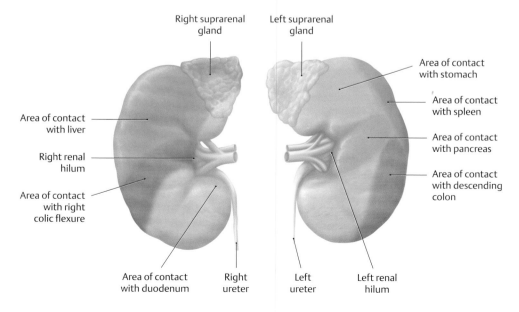

Right suprarenal gland

Left suprarenal gland

Area of contact with stomach

Area of contact with spleen

Area of contact with pancreas

Area of contact with descending colon

Area of contact with liver

Right renal hilum

Area of contact with right colic flexure

Area of contact with duodenum

Right ureter

Left ureter

Left renal hilum

D Areas of renal contact with abdominal and pelvic organs
Anterior view. The suprarenal glands (also shown for clarity) are very close to the kidneys but do not touch them, being separated from the renal surface by the perirenal fat capsule. The *anterior surfaces* of the kidneys are related to numerous abdominal organs. The *retroperitoneal* organs are separated from the kidneys (also retroperitoneal) by the fasciae of the renal bed. The kidneys are additionally separated from the *intraperitoneal* organs by the peritoneum (see p. 226). As a result, surrounding organs do not form impressions on the kidneys, which are relatively firm and stable in their dimensions, and the areas of renal contact with other organs are important in terms of topographical anatomy but have little clinical importance.

2.25 Kidneys: Fasciae and Capsules; Shape and Structure

A Position of the kidneys in the renal bed

Right renal bed. **a** Sagittal section at approximately the level of the renal hilum, viewed from the right side. **b** Transverse section through the abdomen at approximately the L1/L2 level, viewed from above.

The renal bed is located on each side of the spine in the retroperitoneum. It contains the kidneys, which are invested by a thin **organ capsule** (renal fibrous capsule), and the suprarenal glands, which are surrounded by the **perirenal fat capsule** that also encloses the kidneys. The fat capsule is thicker posteriorly than anteriorly.

Note: Swelling of the kidney (usually due to inflammation) may cause severe pain due to stretching of the fibrous capsule.

The fat capsule is surrounded by the **renal fascia**, which separates it from its surroundings by two layers:

- The anterior layer behind the parietal peritoneum (to which it is fused at some sites)
- The posterior layer, which is partially attached to the transversalis fascia and muscular fasciae on the posterior trunk wall

The renal fascia, and thus the renal bed, is open inferiorly and medially to allow passage of the ureter and renal vessels. It is closed laterally and superiorly by fusion of the fascial layers. Because of this arrangement, inflammatory processes that are adjacent to the kidney but within the renal fascia tend to spread to the contralateral side or inferiorly and may spread into the pelvis.

Note: The entire renal bed moves downward during inspiratory depression of the diaphragm, *indirectly* causing the kidney and suprarenal gland to move as well. This differs from the liver, which is attached to the diaphragm (bare area) and is *directly* moved by diaphragm excursions.

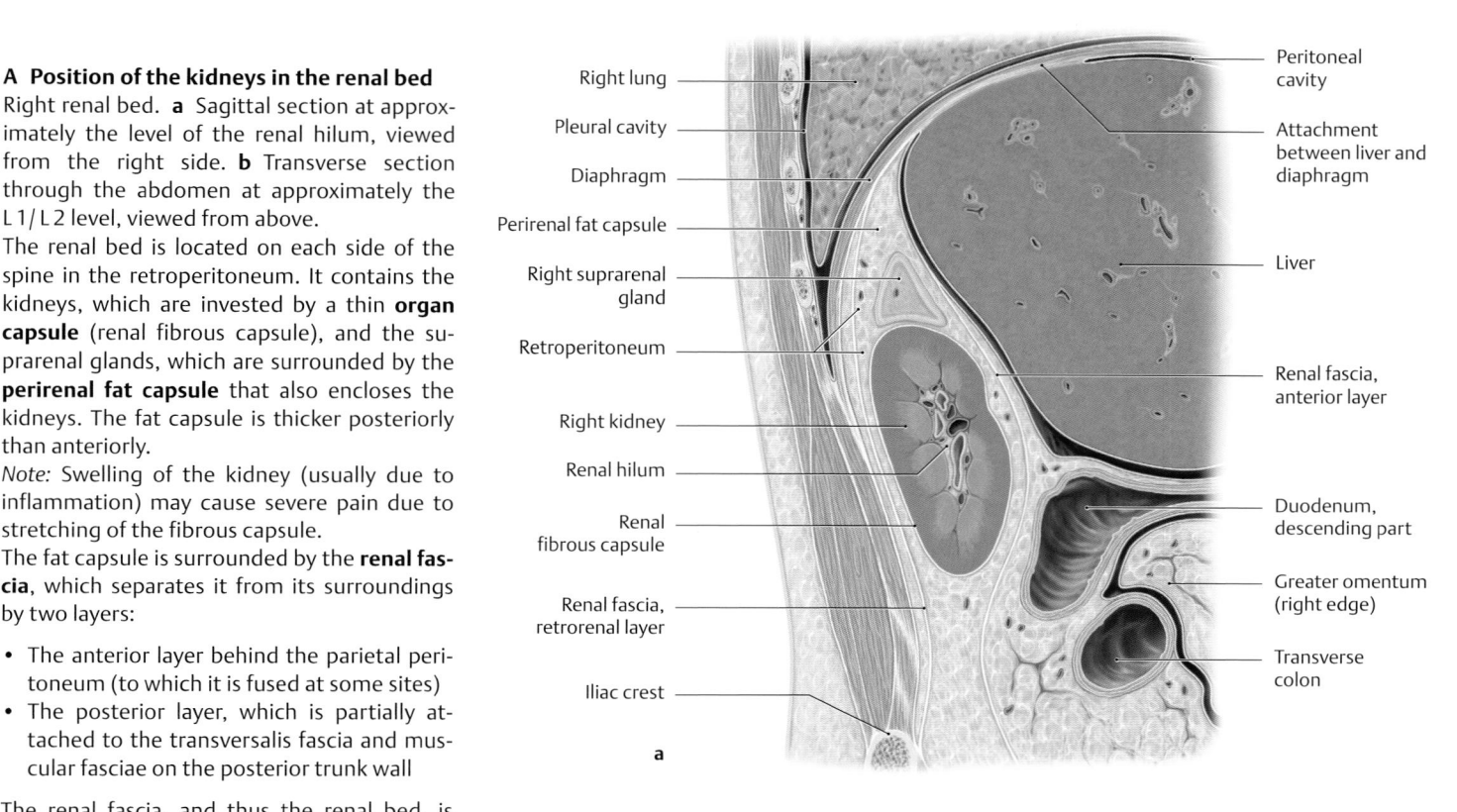

Right lung — Pleural cavity — Diaphragm — Perirenal fat capsule — Right suprarenal gland — Retroperitoneum — Right kidney — Renal hilum — Renal fibrous capsule — Renal fascia, retrorenal layer — Iliac crest

Peritoneal cavity — Attachment between liver and diaphragm — Liver — Renal fascia, anterior layer — Duodenum, descending part — Greater omentum (right edge) — Transverse colon

a

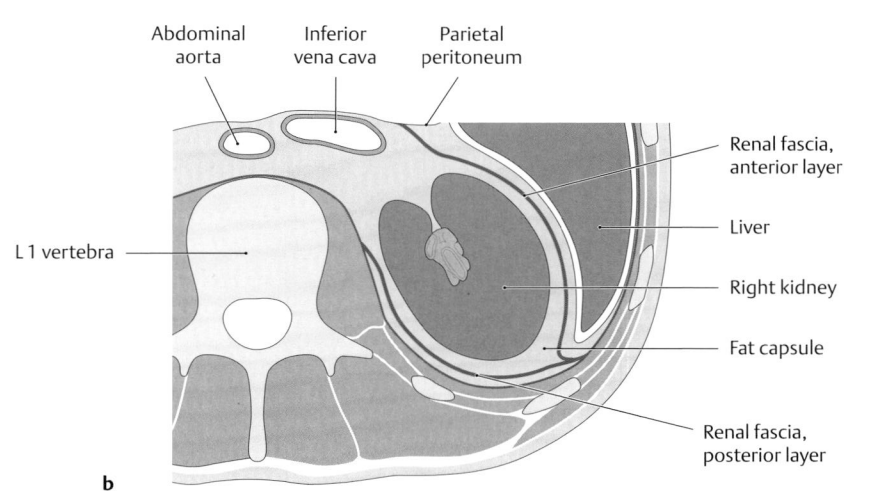

Abdominal aorta — Inferior vena cava — Parietal peritoneum

L1 vertebra

Renal fascia, anterior layer — Liver — Right kidney — Fat capsule — Renal fascia, posterior layer

b

B Renal bed: fasciae and capsules of the kidneys

Renal fibrous capsule	Thin, firm connective-tissue capsule that closely invests each kidney
Perirenal fat capsule	Mass of fat that surrounds the kidneys and suprarenal glands *and* completely occupies the renal bed; it is thickest lateral and posterior to the kidneys
Renal fascia	Connective-tissue fascial sac that encloses the perirenal fat, portions of the abdominal aorta and inferior vena cava close to the kidney (see **Ab**), and the proximal ureter; subdivided into a thin anterior layer and a thick posterior layer (see **Aa**)

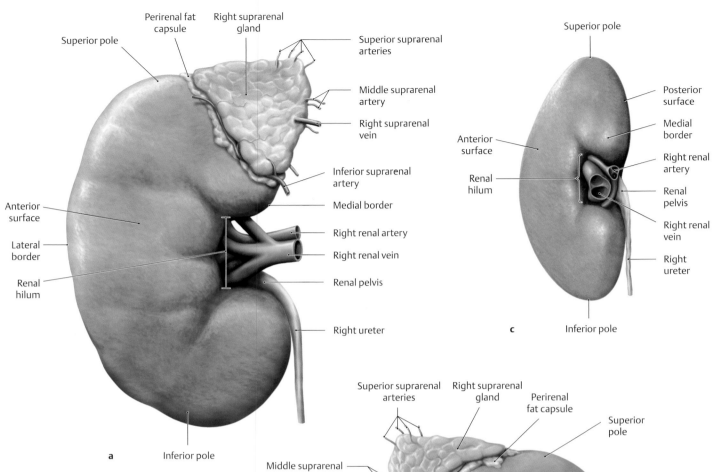

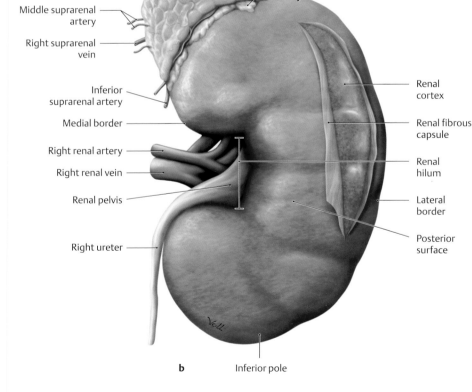

C Structure and shape of the kidney

Anterior view (**a**), posterior view (**b**), and medial view (**c**) of the right kidney. The suprarenal gland is left intact in **a** and **b**, and the ureter has been cut at the level of the inferior renal pole. The fibrous capsule that directly invests the kidney is intact in **a** and **c** and has been partially opened in **b** to display the underlying renal parenchyma. The renal sinus (the deep space into which the hilum opens) generally contains a certain amount of structural fat, and so the vascular structures and renal pelvis are not exposed to view intraoperatively as they are in these drawings. The normal kidney measures an average of 12 x 6 x 3 cm (L x W x T) and weighs 150–180 g. It has:

- two poles (superior and inferior),
- two surfaces (anterior and posterior), and
- two borders (lateral and medial).

The medial border bears the renal hilum, where vascular structures and the ureter enter and leave the kidney. The shallow surface grooves result from the embryonic lobulation of the kidney. The hilar structures are usually arranged as follows from anterior to posterior (as shown in **c**): right renal vein, right renal artery, and right ureter.

Note: The renal artery is usually posterior to the renal vein because the right renal artery passes to the right kidney *behind* the inferior vena cava (where the renal veins terminate), while the left renal vein passes to the left kidney *in front of* the abdominal aorta (which gives origin to the renal arteries). The left renal artery may also loop around the left renal vein from above to occupy an anterior position. The ureter leaves the renal pelvis (see p. 230) below the vessels and is usually somewhat posterior in relation to the blood vessels.

2.26 Kidneys: Architecture and Microstructure

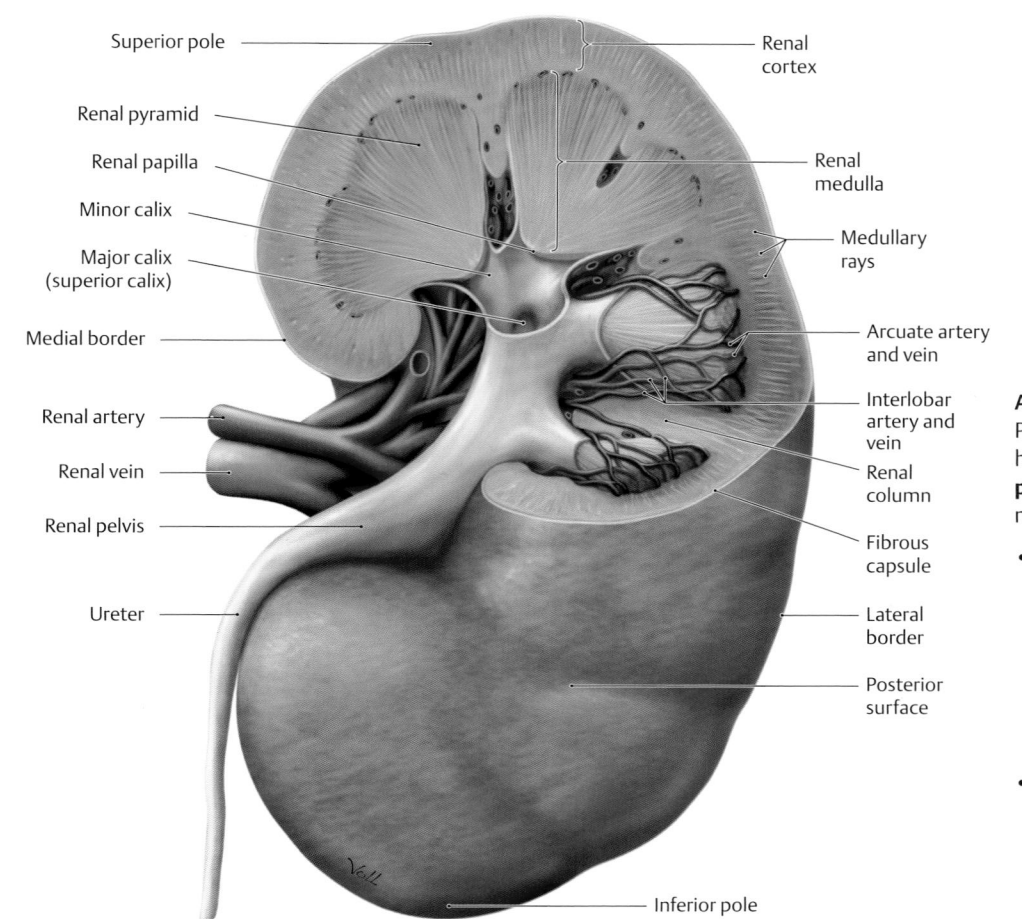

Superior pole

Renal pyramid

Renal papilla

Minor calix

Major calix (superior calix)

Medial border

Renal artery

Renal vein

Renal pelvis

Ureter

Renal cortex

Renal medulla

Medullary rays

Arcuate artery and vein

Interlobar artery and vein

Renal column

Fibrous capsule

Lateral border

Posterior surface

Inferior pole

A Macroscopic structure of the kidney

Posterior view of a right kidney with the upper half of the kidney partially removed. The **renal parenchyma** consists of an outer cortex and inner medulla:

- The *renal cortex* is a relatively thin layer that lies beneath the fibrous capsule and forms columns (renal columns) that extend between the pyramids of the medulla. The cortex and columns contain approximately 2.4 million renal corpuscles (which contain the glomeruli, see **B**) as well as the proximal and distal renal tubules (see **C**).
- The *renal medulla* consists of approximately 10–12 renal pyramids. The bases of the pyramids are directed toward the cortex and capsule, while their apices converge toward the renal pelvis. The medulla mainly contains the ascending and descending limbs of the renal tubules.

The **renal pelvis** is described on p. 230.

Distal tubule, straight portion

Macula densa

Afferent glomerular arteriole

Juxtaglomerular cells (modified smooth-muscle cells in afferent arteriole)

Vascular pole of glomerulus

Capillary loops with podocytes (visceral layer of Bowman's capsule)

Urinary pole of glomerulus

Efferent glomerular arteriole

Extraglomerular mesangial cells

Glomerular capsule (parietal layer of Bowman's capsule)

Urinary space

Initial part of proximal convoluted tubule

a

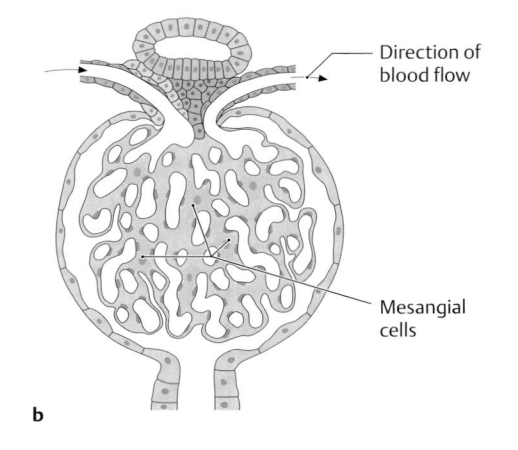

Direction of blood flow

Mesangial cells

b

B Renal corpuscle

a With the capsule opened, **b** in section.

The renal corpuscle is the interface between the blood vessels and the excretory portion of the urinary tract (see **C**). It consists of a central convoluted vascular loop, the glomerulus, and a bulbous envelope lined by squamous epithelial cells, the *glomerular capsule* (Bowman's capsule). Blood enters the *glomerulus* at the vascular pole of the renal corpuscle by flowing through the *afferent* glomerular arteriole, and it leaves the

glomerulus through the *efferent* glomerular arteriole. The primary urine is formed within the renal corpuscle and drains through a tubular system at the urinary pole of the glomerulus. The initial portion of this tubular system that is connected to the glomerular capsule is the proximal convoluted tubule (see **C**).

Note: Specialized cells at the vascular pole of the renal corpuscle regulate the blood pressure that is necessary for ultrafiltration.

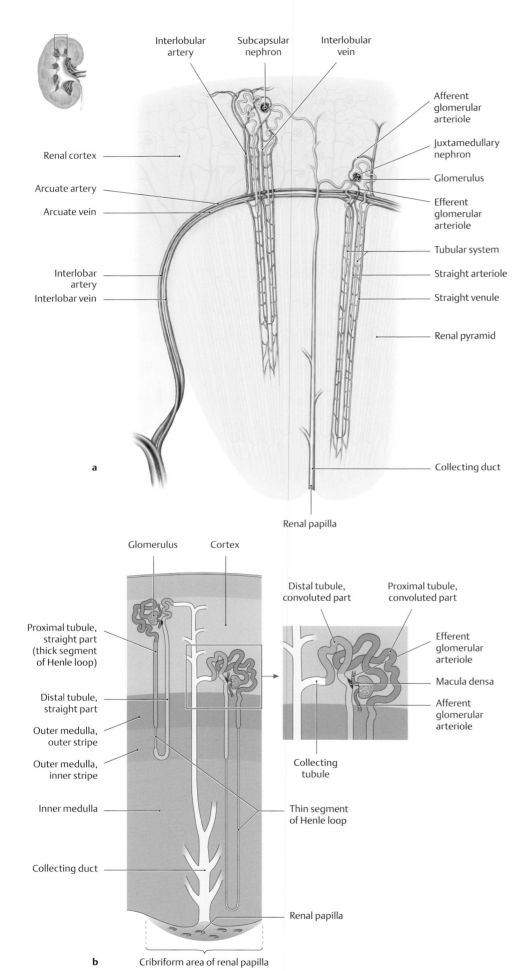

Interlobular artery

Subcapsular nephron

Interlobular vein

Renal cortex

Arcuate artery

Arcuate vein

Interlobar artery

Interlobar vein

a

Afferent glomerular arteriole

Juxtamedullary nephron

Glomerulus

Efferent glomerular arteriole

Tubular system

Straight arteriole

Straight venule

Renal pyramid

Collecting duct

Renal papilla

Glomerulus   Cortex

Proximal tubule, straight part (thick segment of Henle loop)

Distal tubule, straight part

Outer medulla, outer stripe

Outer medulla, inner stripe

Inner medulla

Collecting duct

b   Cribriform area of renal papilla

Distal tubule, convoluted part

Proximal tubule, convoluted part

Efferent glomerular arteriole

Macula densa

Afferent glomerular arteriole

Collecting tubule

Thin segment of Henle loop

Renal papilla

C Architecture of the renal vessels and intrarenal collecting system

a Renal vessels: Sectional view of a medullary pyramid with adjacent cortical areas. The intrarenal vascular and collecting systems are closely interrelated spatially and functionally. An ultrafiltrate from the blood (primary urine) drains into a microscopically small system of renal tubules. *Blood flow to the kidney* (**a**) is supplied by interlobar arteries that pass along the sides of the medullary pyramids from the renal hilum. Each interlobar artery supplies two adjacent medullary pyramids and the associated cortical zones (these branches are not shown). At the base of the pyramid, the interlobar artery gives rise to the arcuate artery, from which the interlobular arteries are distributed into the cortex as far as the fibrous renal capsule. The *afferent* glomerular arterioles that arise from an interlobular artery each supply one glomerulus. The *efferent* glomerular arterioles that emerge from the glomerulus are still carrying blood at a high oxygen tension; they supply the renal cortex or medulla.

b Intrarenal collecting system: The smallest functional unit of the kidney is the nephron, which consists of the renal corpuscle (see **B**), renal tubules, and collecting ducts. There are approximately one to two million nephrons in each kidney. They process approximately 1700 liters of blood daily, which is filtered by the countercurrent mechanism to form approximately 170 liters of *primary urine*. This primary filtrate enters the tubular system at the urinary pole of the renal corpuscle and reaches the renal papilla as the *final urine*, which drains into the calyceal system (approximately 1.7 liters / day). The *tubular system* consists of the proximal and distal tubules (each with a convoluted and straight portion) and an intermediate tubule (with descending and ascending limbs). The intermediate tubule and the adjacent straight portions of the proximal and distal tubules comprise the *loop of Henle*. While passing through the tubular system, substances contained in the filtrate (mainly water) are reabsorbed while other substances (e.g., ions) are secreted into the filtrate. This process yields the final urine, which passes through a collecting tubule into a collecting duct and drains through the renal papilla into the *caliceal system*. It is conveyed from the calices and renal pelvis to the ureter by peristalsis.

2.27 Kidneys: Renal Pelvis and Urinary Transport

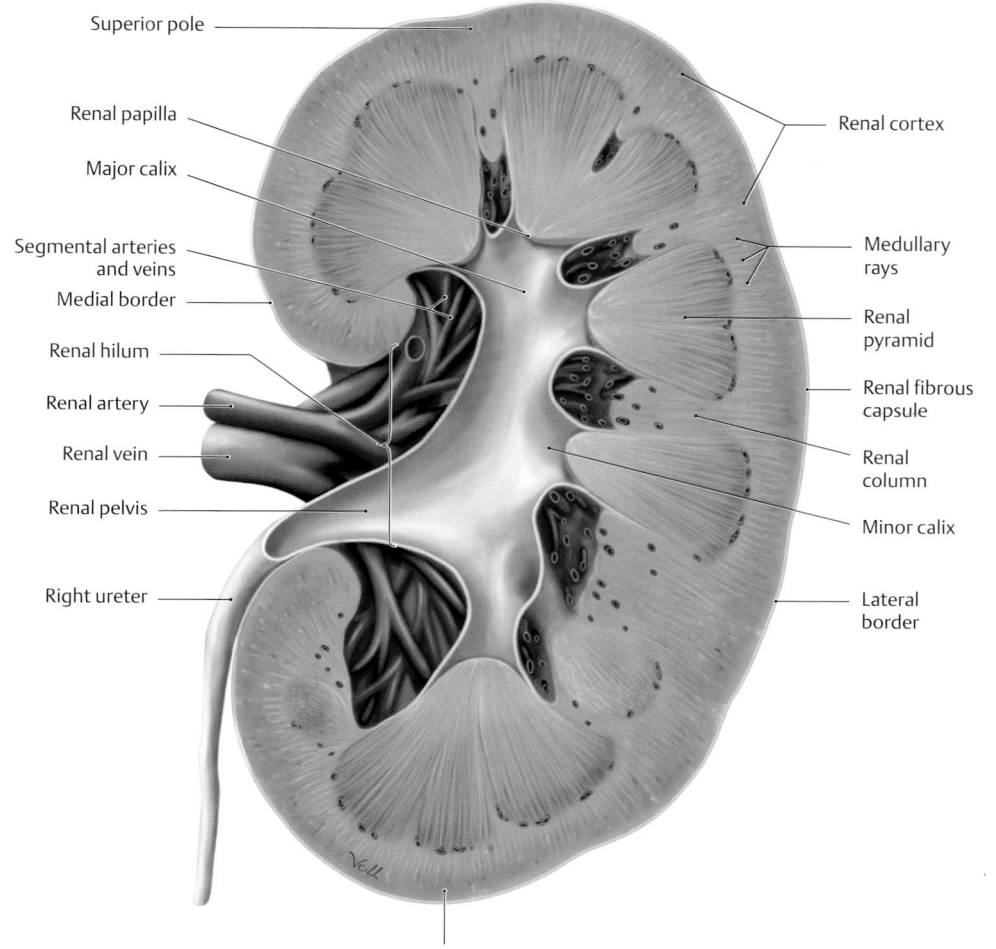

Superior pole

Renal papilla

Major calix

Segmental arteries and veins

Medial border

Renal hilum

Renal artery

Renal vein

Renal pelvis

Right ureter

Renal cortex

Medullary rays

Renal pyramid

Renal fibrous capsule

Renal column

Minor calix

Lateral border

Inferior pole

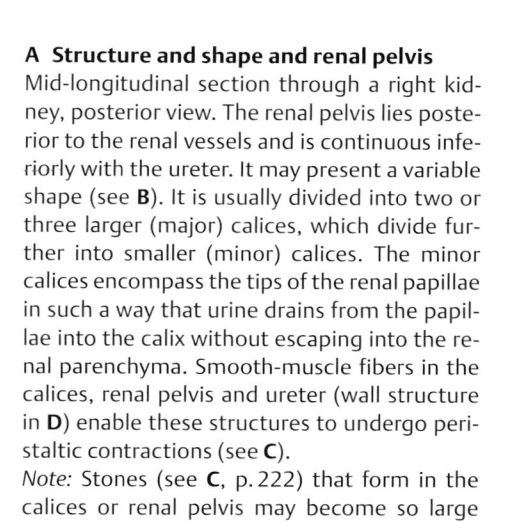

A Structure and shape and renal pelvis

Mid-longitudinal section through a right kidney, posterior view. The renal pelvis lies posterior to the renal vessels and is continuous inferiorly with the ureter. It may present a variable shape (see **B**). It is usually divided into two or three larger (major) calices, which divide further into smaller (minor) calices. The minor calices encompass the tips of the renal papillae in such a way that urine drains from the papillae into the calix without escaping into the renal parenchyma. Smooth-muscle fibers in the calices, renal pelvis and ureter (wall structure in **D**) enable these structures to undergo peristaltic contractions (see **C**).

Note: Stones (see **C**, p. 222) that form in the calices or renal pelvis may become so large that they fill the cavity lumen and assume its shape (caliceal stone, staghorn calculus).

B Variations in the shape of the renal pelvis

Anterior view of the left renal pelvis. The renal pelvis and ureter develop from an outgrowth of the mesonephric duct. This "ureteral bud" grows superiorly from the pelvis toward the embryonic renal bud and unites with it. The calices subsequently form by branching from the renal pelvis. This branching occurs in various patterns with approximately equal frequency, and mixed forms are also seen:

- Linear pattern (**a**)
- Dendritic (ramified) pattern (**b**)
- Ampullary pattern (**c**)

Minor calix

Major calix

Renal pelvis

Ureter

a

Minor calix

Major calix

Renal pelvis

Ureter

b

Minor calix

Renal pelvis

Ureter

c

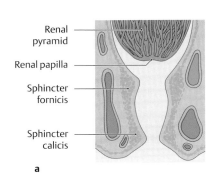

Renal
pyramid

Renal papilla

Sphincter
fornicis

Sphincter
calicis

a

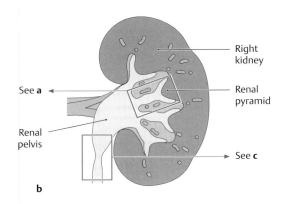

Right
kidney

See **a**

Renal
pyramid

Renal
pelvis

See **c**

b

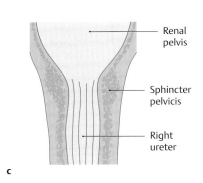

Renal
pelvis

Sphincter
pelvicis

Right
ureter

c

C Closure mechanisms of the renal calices and renal pelvis; urinary transport
(after Rauber and Kopsch)

Schematic representation of a kidney (**b**) with magnified sections of a calix (**a**) and renal pelvis (**c**) and a dynamic functional diagram of the calix and pelvis during urinary transport (**d**). Urine is transported by an active mechanism. The smooth musculature of the sphincter fornicis and calicis (**a**) and the sphincter pelvicis (**c**) (the functional sphincter system) enables the wall of the renal calices and pelvis to contract in segments. These contractions are continuous with the peristaltic waves of the ureter, with the result that the urinary tract is never patent over its entire length but is patent in some portions and closed in others (**d**). This

maintains a distal flow of urine from the tip of the renal papilla into the calix, through the renal pelvis, into the ureter, and on toward the bladder while preventing the reflux of urine into the kidneys.

Note: If this active transport process is impaired (e.g., by renal stones or drugs that inhibit the ureteral muscles), urine may reflux into the kidney and incite an inflammatory process in the renal pelvis. The papillae, calices and pelvis are often affected jointly by disease (e.g., inflammation) because of their close proximity to one another. One of the most common diseases is suppurative bacterial pyelonephritis (*pyelo-*, referring to the [renal] pelvis, from Gr. *pyelos*—trough, tub, or vat).

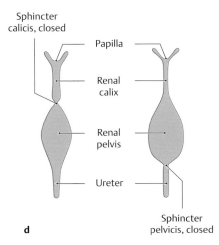

Sphincter
calicis, closed

Papilla

Renal
calix

Renal
pelvis

Ureter

Sphincter
pelvicis, closed

d

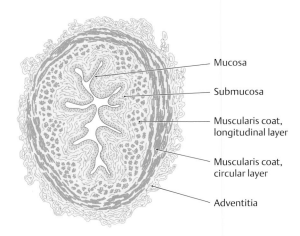

Mucosa

Submucosa

Muscularis coat,
longitudinal layer

Muscularis coat,
circular layer

Adventitia

D Wall structure of the ureter

Transverse section through a ureter. A characteristic feature is the stellate lumen that appears in cross-section due to the longitudinal mucosal folds. As in the urethra and bladder, the ureteral mucosa consists of a transitional epithelium of varying height (see p. 237). The smooth muscle consists basically of a longitudinal and a circular layer. It is powerfully developed and shows a functionally spiral architecture (see **E**). When a renal stone enters the ureter, the smooth muscle in the uterine wall undergoes powerful contractions in an effort to expel the stone, causing very severe pain (renal or ureteral colic). The colic may be relieved by drugs that suppress the activity of the parasympathetic nervous system, though this will also inhibit normal urinary transport to the bladder. The renal pelvis is structurally analogous to the ureter, including the stellate shape of its lumen.

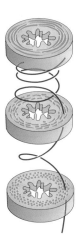

E Arrangement of the ureteral musculature (after Graumann, von Keyserlingk, and Sasse)

Schematic cross-sections at various levels of the ureter. The longitudinal and circular muscle layers of the ureter wall have a slightly oblique arrangement, forming a kind of spiral that propels urine toward the bladder by peristaltic contractions. Although the ureters are richly innervated (see pp. 316–317), the peristaltic contractions are instigated by spontaneously depolarizing smooth-muscle cells in the walls of the renal pelvis. Peristaltic waves of contraction (with a speed of 2–3 cm / s) are propagated through direct electrical connections (gap junctions) between adjacent smooth-muscle cells. Autonomic motor innervation and local sensory reflexes serve to modulate this intrinsic activity. This mechanism may thus have some superficial similarities to the system that controls heartbeat.

231

2.28 Ureters and Bladder in the Male: Topographical Anatomy

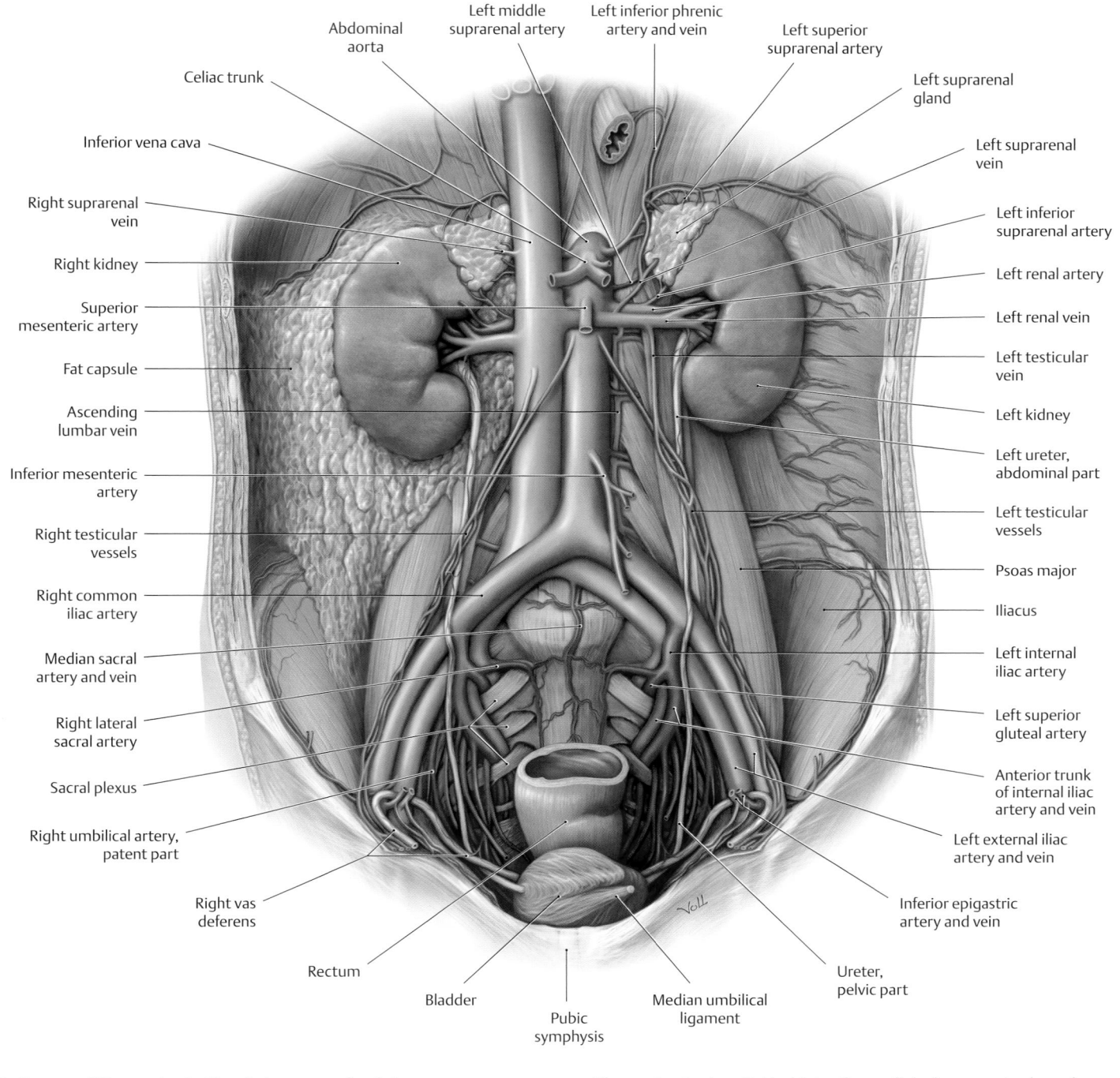

Left middle suprarenal artery

Abdominal aorta

Left inferior phrenic artery and vein

Left superior suprarenal artery

Celiac trunk

Left suprarenal gland

Inferior vena cava

Left suprarenal vein

Right suprarenal vein

Left inferior suprarenal artery

Right kidney

Left renal artery

Superior mesenteric artery

Left renal vein

Fat capsule

Left testicular vein

Ascending lumbar vein

Left kidney

Inferior mesenteric artery

Left ureter, abdominal part

Right testicular vessels

Left testicular vessels

Right common iliac artery

Psoas major

Median sacral artery and vein

Iliacus

Right lateral sacral artery

Left internal iliac artery

Sacral plexus

Left superior gluteal artery

Right umbilical artery, patent part

Anterior trunk of internal iliac artery and vein

Right vas deferens

Left external iliac artery and vein

Rectum

Inferior epigastric artery and vein

Bladder

Ureter, pelvic part

Pubic symphysis

Median umbilical ligament

A Course of the ureter in the abdomen and pelvis
Anterior view, male abdomen. All organs have been removed except the urinary organs, suprarenal glands, and a rectal stump. The esophagus has been pulled slightly downward, and the fat capsule of the right kidney has been partially preserved. A prolongation of the renal pelvis, the ureter passes inferiorly and slightly anterior in the retroperitoneum for a length of approximately 26–29 cm. It opens into the posterior aspect of the bladder. *Anatomically*, the ureter consists of three parts:

- Abdominal part (from the renal pelvis to the linea terminalis of the bony pelvis)
- Pelvic part (from the linea terminalis to the bladder wall)
- Intramural part (passes through the bladder wall)

The ureter is also divided into three *clinical* segments, based more on the presence of a free segment and two organ-bound segments than on the anatomical boundary between the abdominal and pelvic parts:

- Renal segment (connected to the kidney)
- Lumbar segment (between the kidney and bladder)
- Vesical segment (in the bladder wall, corresponds anatomically to the intramural part)

The most common *congenital anomalies* of the ureter are duplication anomalies and clefts. They may allow urine to back up to the kidney (e.g., a cleft may allow reflux due to deficient vesicoureteral closure), producing an infection that ascends from the bladder to the renal pelvis (bacterial pyelonephritis).

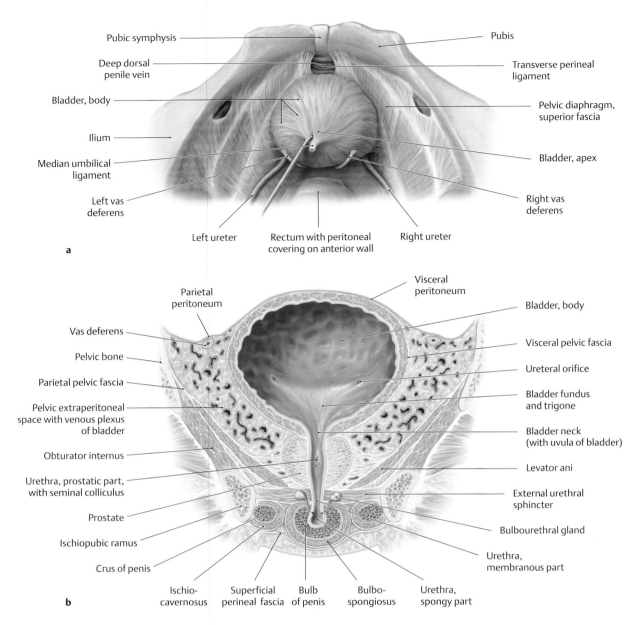

Pubic symphysis

Deep dorsal
penile vein

Bladder, body

Ilium

Median umbilical
ligament

Left vas
deferens

Left ureter

Rectum with peritoneal
covering on anterior wall

Right ureter

Pubis

Transverse perineal
ligament

Pelvic diaphragm,
superior fascia

Bladder, apex

Right vas
deferens

a

Parietal
peritoneum

Visceral
peritoneum

Vas deferens

Pelvic bone

Parietal pelvic fascia

Pelvic extraperitoneal
space with venous plexus
of bladder

Obturator internus

Urethra, prostatic part,
with seminal colliculus

Prostate

Ischiopubic ramus

Crus of penis

Ischio-
cavernosus

Superficial
perineal fascia

Bulb
of penis

Bulbo-
spongiosus

Urethra,
spongy part

Bladder, body

Visceral pelvic fascia

Ureteral orifice

Bladder fundus
and trigone

Bladder neck
(with uvula of bladder)

Levator ani

External urethral
sphincter

Bulbourethral gland

Urethra,
membranous part

b

B Location of the bladder in the pelvis and on the pelvic floor

a Superior view with the bladder pulled slightly posteriorly and the urogenital peritoneum removed. When the bladder is distended (as shown here), it has an almost spherical shape. It is located in the lesser pelvis on the muscular sheet of the pelvic diaphragm, lying principally upon the levator ani and its fascia (superior fascia of the pelvic diaphragm). This area of contact is smaller in the male than in the female (see p. 235) because the lesser pelvis also contains the prostate.

b Anterior view of a coronal section angled slightly posteriorly with the bladder and urethra opened. The portions of the bladder not covered by peritoneum are integrated into the pelvis by a connective-

tissue space, which has a well-developed venous plexus. This plexus and the mobile visceral peritoneum allow for considerable changes in bladder size. The urethra, whose initial portion is surrounded by connective tissue like the bladder itself, pierces the external urethral spincter, which forms the external urethral sphincter. In the male, the initial part of the urethra is also surrounded by the prostate, which lies upon the levator ani of the pelvic diaphragm.

C Anatomical constrictions of the ureter

There are three normal *anatomical constrictions* where a stone from the renal pelvis is apt to become lodged:

- Origin of the ureter from the renal pelvis (ureteropelvic junction)
- Site where the ureter crosses over the external or common iliac vessels
- Passage of the ureter through the bladder wall (uretovesicular junction)

Occasionally a *fourth constriction* can be identified where the testicular or ovarian artery and vein pass in front of the ureter.

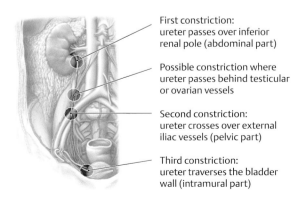

First constriction:
ureter passes over inferior
renal pole (abdominal part)

Possible constriction where
ureter passes behind testicular
or ovarian vessels

Second constriction:
ureter crosses over external
iliac vessels (pelvic part)

Third constriction:
ureter traverses the bladder
wall (intramural part)

2.29 Ureters and Bladder in the Female: Topographical Anatomy

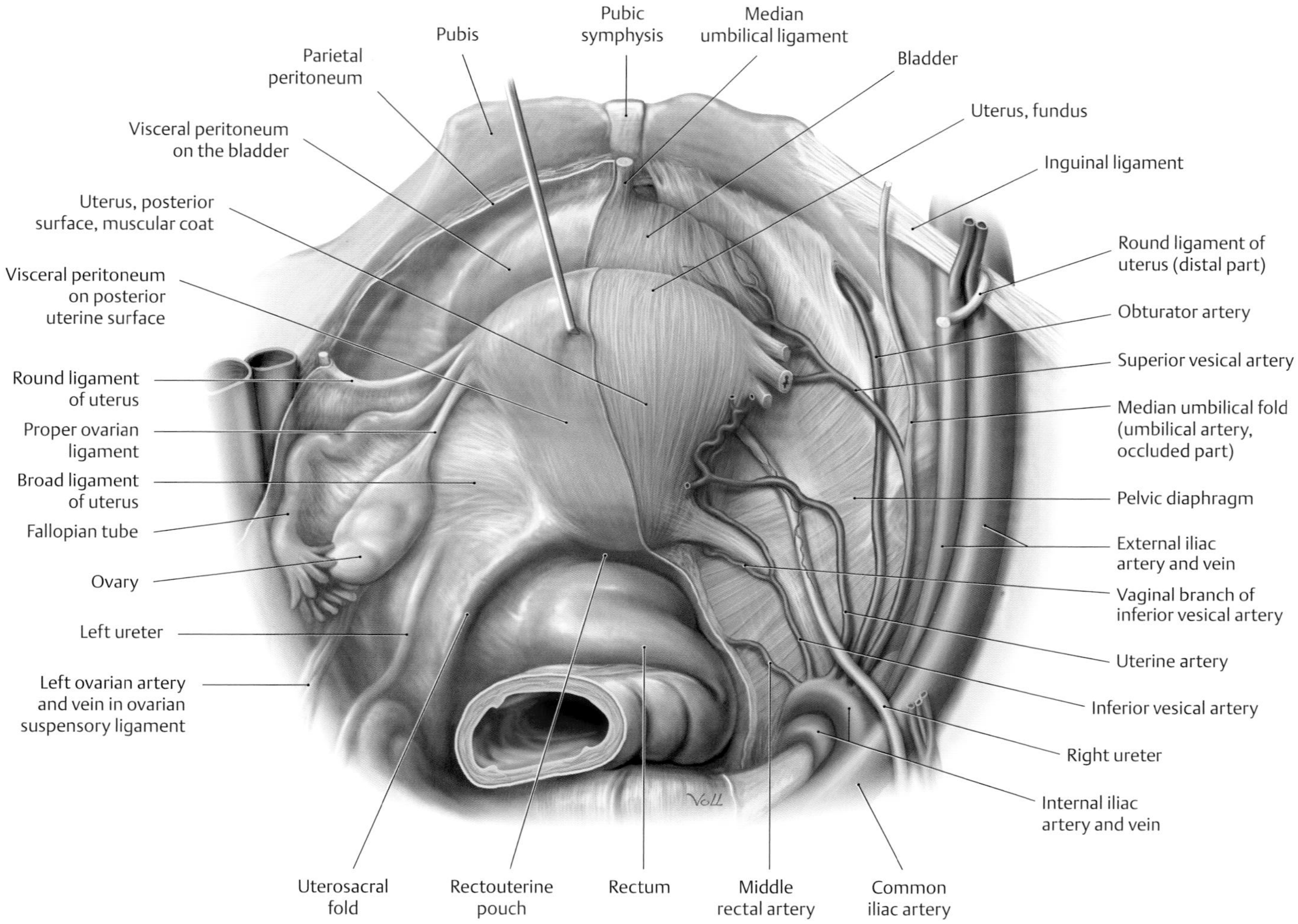

Pubis

Pubic symphysis

Median umbilical ligament

Bladder

Parietal peritoneum

Visceral peritoneum on the bladder

Uterus, fundus

Uterus, posterior surface, muscular coat

Inguinal ligament

Visceral peritoneum on posterior uterine surface

Round ligament of uterus (distal part)

Obturator artery

Round ligament of uterus

Superior vesical artery

Proper ovarian ligament

Median umbilical fold (umbilical artery, occluded part)

Broad ligament of uterus

Pelvic diaphragm

Fallopian tube

External iliac artery and vein

Ovary

Vaginal branch of inferior vesical artery

Left ureter

Uterine artery

Left ovarian artery and vein in ovarian suspensory ligament

Inferior vesical artery

Right ureter

Internal iliac artery and vein

Uterosacral fold

Rectouterine pouch

Rectum

Middle rectal artery

Common iliac artery

A Course of the ureter in the female pelvis
Superior view. Most of the peritoneum has been removed on the right side, and the large intestine has been removed down to a rectal stump. *Note:* The ureter takes the following course in the female abdomen and pelvis:

- Passes behind the ovarian vessels.
- Crosses in front of the iliac vessels (usually the external iliac vessels on the right side, also the common iliac vessels on the left side).
- Passes inferior to the uterine artery (see p. 291).

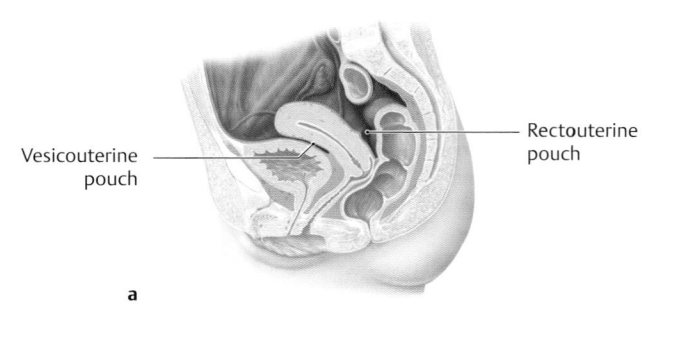

Vesicouterine pouch

Rectouterine pouch

a

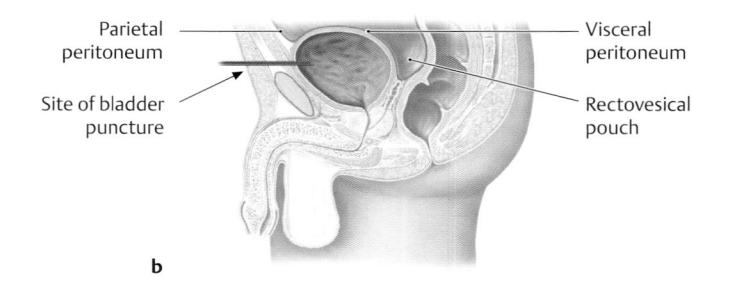

Parietal peritoneum

Visceral peritoneum

Site of bladder puncture

Rectovesical pouch

b

B Location and peritoneal covering of the female (a) and male (b) bladder
Midsagittal section, viewed from the left side. The bladder is shown slightly distended, raising the uterus to a slightly higher position. The peritoneum extends from the posterior surface of the anterior abdominal wall to the superior surface of the bladder and is reflected onto the organ posterior to the bladder, forming a peritoneal pouch. In the female, it forms the vesicouterine pouch; in the male, it forms the recto-

vesical pouch. Most of the bladder is loosely embedded in pelvic connective tissue.
Note: A well-distended bladder pushes the visceral peritoneum superiorly, creating an area that is devoid of peritoneum anterior to the bladder. This provides an access route for percutaneous puncture of the distended bladder above the symphysis without having to enter the peritoneal cavity with the needle.

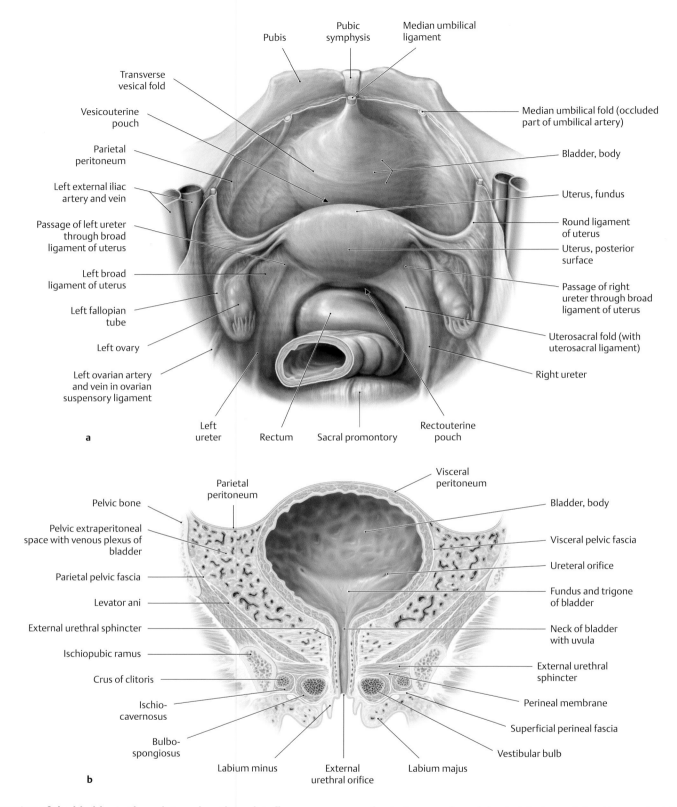

a

Pubis

Pubic symphysis

Median umbilical ligament

Transverse vesical fold

Vesicouterine pouch

Parietal peritoneum

Left external iliac artery and vein

Passage of left ureter through broad ligament of uterus

Left broad ligament of uterus

Left fallopian tube

Left ovary

Left ovarian artery and vein in ovarian suspensory ligament

Left ureter

Rectum

Sacral promontory

Median umbilical fold (occluded part of umbilical artery)

Bladder, body

Uterus, fundus

Round ligament of uterus

Uterus, posterior surface

Passage of right ureter through broad ligament of uterus

Uterosacral fold (with uterosacral ligament)

Right ureter

Rectouterine pouch

b

Parietal peritoneum

Pelvic bone

Pelvic extraperitoneal space with venous plexus of bladder

Parietal pelvic fascia

Levator ani

External urethral sphincter

Ischiopubic ramus

Crus of clitoris

Ischio-cavernosus

Bulbo-spongiosus

Labium minus

External urethral orifice

Labium majus

Visceral peritoneum

Bladder, body

Visceral pelvic fascia

Ureteral orifice

Fundus and trigone of bladder

Neck of bladder with uvula

External urethral sphincter

Perineal membrane

Superficial perineal fascia

Vestibular bulb

C Location of the bladder in the pelvis and on the pelvic floor

a Superior view. The uterus is shown upright for clarity. Most of the large intestine has been removed, leaving the urogenital peritoneum intact. The transverse vesical fold, a peritoneal fold on the surface of the bladder, is effaced when the bladder is full (as shown here). In the female, the bladder lies inferior to the uterus and elevates it when distended. When the structures of the pelvic floor (levator ani and its

fasciae) are weakened due to injuries sustained in a vaginal delivery, for example, they may allow the bladder to descend, resulting in incontinence.

b Coronal section tilted slightly posteriorly, anterior view. The bladder and urethra have been opened. The attachments of the bladder to the connective tissue and muscular structures of the pelvic floor are described on p. 168

2.30 Bladder and Urethra: Wall Structure and Function

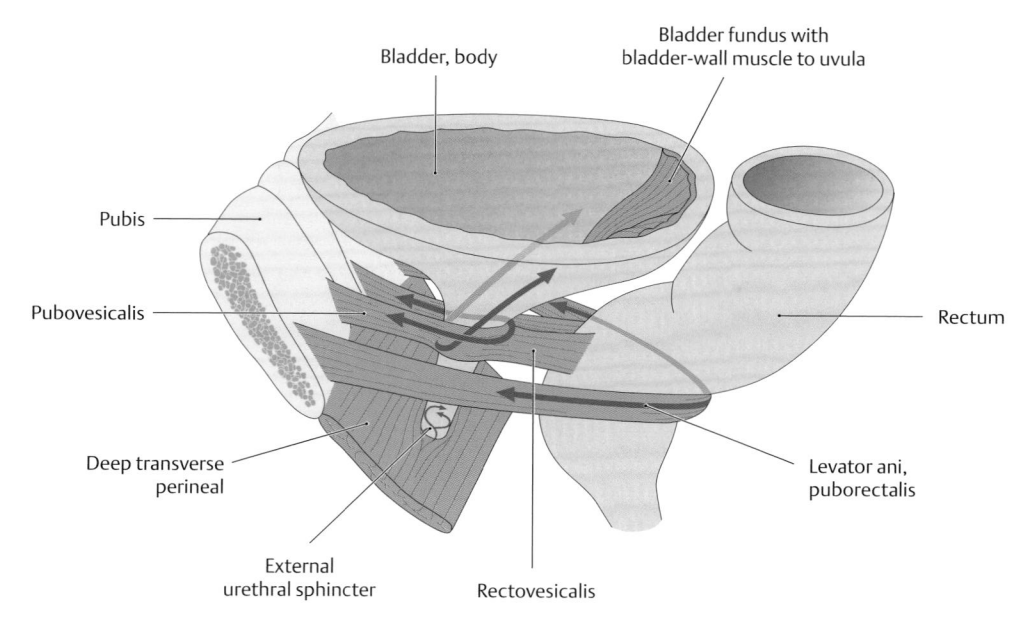

Bladder, body

Bladder fundus with bladder-wall muscle to uvula

Pubis

Pubovesicalis

Rectum

Deep transverse perineal

Levator ani, puborectalis

External urethral sphincter

Rectovesicalis

A Muscular mechanisms for opening and closing the bladder: micturition and continence

The muscular apparatus of the bladder and urethra performs three functions:

- Empties the bladder completely during micturition
- Protects the ureteral orifices from reflux
- Maintains urinary continence with a full bladder.

Involuntary (autonomic) and voluntary (somatic, by the pudendal nerve) muscle control interact as follows in opening and closing the bladder:

- **Involuntary mechanism for opening the bladder (controlling micturition).** The sequence of events is as follows: The sacral micturition center is activated by a center in the brainstem (pontine micturition center) → The detrusor vesicae muscle contracts, raising the pressure within the bladder → The bladder trigone is raised, and a groove forms at the bladder outlet → The uvula of the bladder retracts from the internal urethral orifice, and the ureteral orifice narrows (to prevent reflux) → The pubovesicalis and rectovesicalis smooth muscles contract, dilating the urethra (fibers to the anterior and posterior urethral walls), and blood drains from the venous plexus beneath the uvular mucosa → The sphincters relax → Voiding occurs.

- **Muscular mechanisms for closing the bladder (maintaining continence):**
  - Involuntary closure mechanism: Loops of muscle fibers in the bladder wall encircle the urethral orifice. They are supported by the looped fibers of the pubovesicalis.
  - Voluntary closure mechanism: Descending fibers from the pelvic floor muscle (deep transverse perineal) encircle the urethra (external urethral sphincter). With a structural weakness of the pelvic floor, which may develop after multiple vaginal deliveries, this closure mechanism may fail. When combined with descent of the pelvic floor and bladder, this failure may lead to urinary incontinence.

The maximum bladder capacity is approximately 700 mL in the female and 500 mL in the male (it may exceed 4000 mL in patients with abnormal urinary retention). Urgency may be felt, however, when the bladder contains as little as 150–200 mL of urine, and even smaller volumes may cause urgency during pregnancy due to pressure from the gravid uterus. A normal bladder contains no residual urine after voiding.

B Attachments of the bladder

Most of the bladder is loosely attached to the connective tissue of the pelvis via the visceral pelvic fascia. Only its superior surface is covered by visceral peritoneum. The "lateral vesicular ligament" refers to the connective tissue located mainly around the bladder (see **A**, p. 168). The ligaments listed here are basically condensations of connective tissue that surround the entire bladder. Individual strands of connective tissue may contain smooth muscle.

Anterior ligaments		
Pubovesical ligament		
Puboprostatic ligaments	Posterior surface of symphysis → bladder, prostate	
Posterior ligaments		
Rectovesical ligaments		
Rectoprostatic ligaments	Rectum → bladder, prostate	
Cranial ligament	Median umbilical fold with urachus	

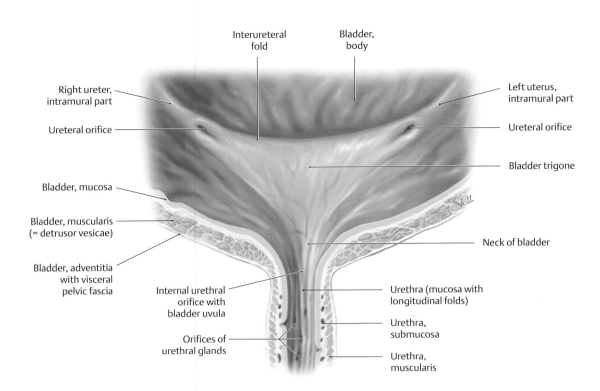

C Wall structure and interior of the bladder and urethra

Anterior view. Controlled by autonomic innervation, the smooth muscle of the bladder wall consists mainly of the three layers of the detrusor vesicae: the inner longitudinal layer and the outer circular and longitudinal layers (the individual layers are not shown here). The outermost layer sends longitudinal slips posteriorly to the vesicoprostaticus or vesicovaginalis and anteriorly to the pubovesicalis (see **A**). The detrusor vesicae consists of one layer in the bladder trigone, its elliptical slips forming a functional smooth-muscle sphincter that surrounds the internal urethral orifice (the "internal urethral sphincter," see **A**; more pronounced in the male). Fibers of deep transverse perineal profundus (see **A**) form a loop of striated muscle (with voluntary, somatic innervation) that encircles the external urethral orifice: the external urethral sphincter.

Note the slit-like ureteral orifice and the oblique transit of the ureter through the bladder wall. This obliquity creates a normal constriction in the intramural part of the ureter (see p. 233). The oblique course, the ureteral muscle, and the bladder-wall muscle provide for functional closure of the ureteral orifice and guard against reflux.

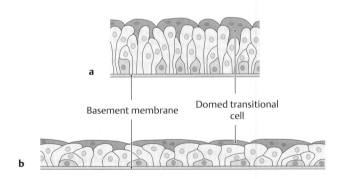

D Epithelium of the bladder mucosa

a Bladder empty: tall epithelium. **b** Bladder full: flattened epithelium. Like almost all portions of the urinary tract (except the distal urethra), the bladder is lined by transitional epithelium whose height and stratification depend on the degree of distention of the urinary tract segment. The transitional epithelium basically consists of multiple cell layers. The conspicuous cells in the surface layer are called "transitional cells" because they change shape.

Note: The total thickness of the bladder wall (muscle plus mucosa) ranges from 2 to 5 mm in the full bladder and from 8 to 15 mm in the empty bladder.

E Innervation of the bladder

Autonomic innervation (visceromotor and viscerosensory)	
Parasympathetic nervous system	Pelvic splanchnic nerves (S2–S4) via the inferior pelvic plexus
Sympathetic nervous system	Lumbar splanchnic nerves via the inferior mesenteric ganglion and inferior hypogastric plexus, and sacral splanchnic nerves

Autonomic innervation includes the motor innervation of the bladder smooth muscle for controlling continence and micturition (both systems) and the perception of visceral pain due to excessive distention (chiefly the parasympathetic system).

Somatic innervation
Pudendal nerve (S2–S4)

This consists mainly of innervation to the voluntary external urethral sphincter but also includes the sensory innervation to portions of the urethra.

2.31 Urethra: Location and Structure

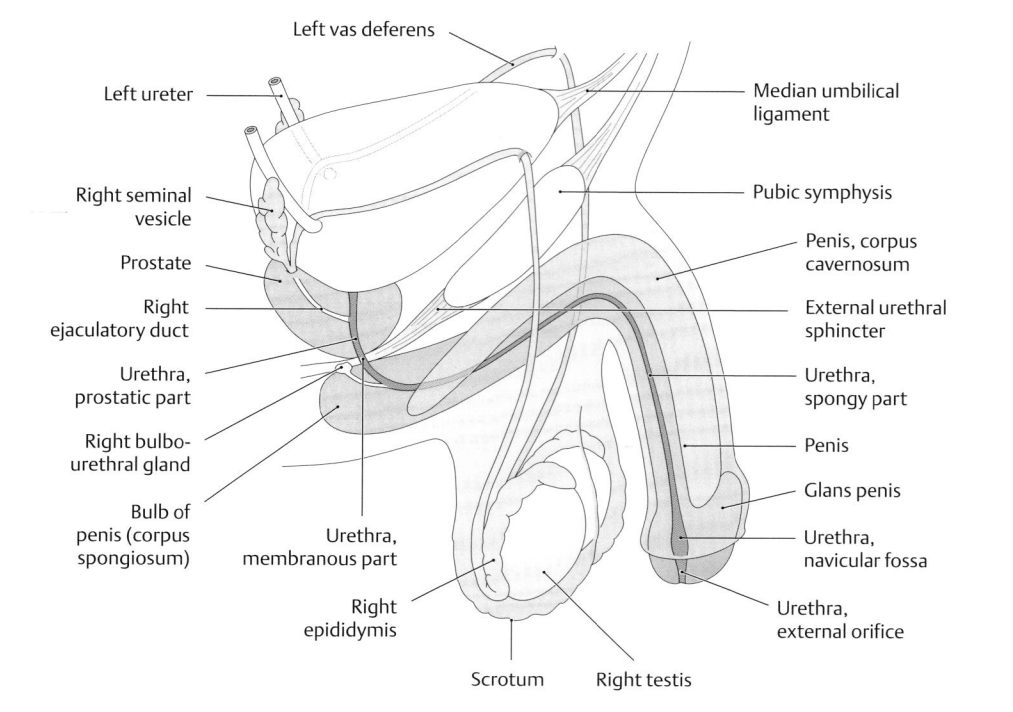

Wall segments	Constrictions and expansions
Internal urethral orifice	
Intramural part	First constriction: internal urethral sphincter
Prostatic part	First expansion
Membranous part	Second constriction: external urethral sphincter
Spongy part	Second expansion: ampulla Third expansion: navicular fossa
External urethral orifice	Third constriction

A Parts of the male urethra

Male urogenital system in the pelvis, viewed from the right side. Unlike the female urethra, the male urethra functions as a common urinary *and* genital passage. It has an average length of 20 cm and consists of four parts with three constrictions and three expansions (see **B**). The intramural part of the urethra in the bladder wall is not shown here. While the female urethra is essentially straight (see **E**), the male urethra presents two curves: an *infrapubic curve* and a *prepubic curve*. These curves are important in transurethral bladder catheterization (see **F**).

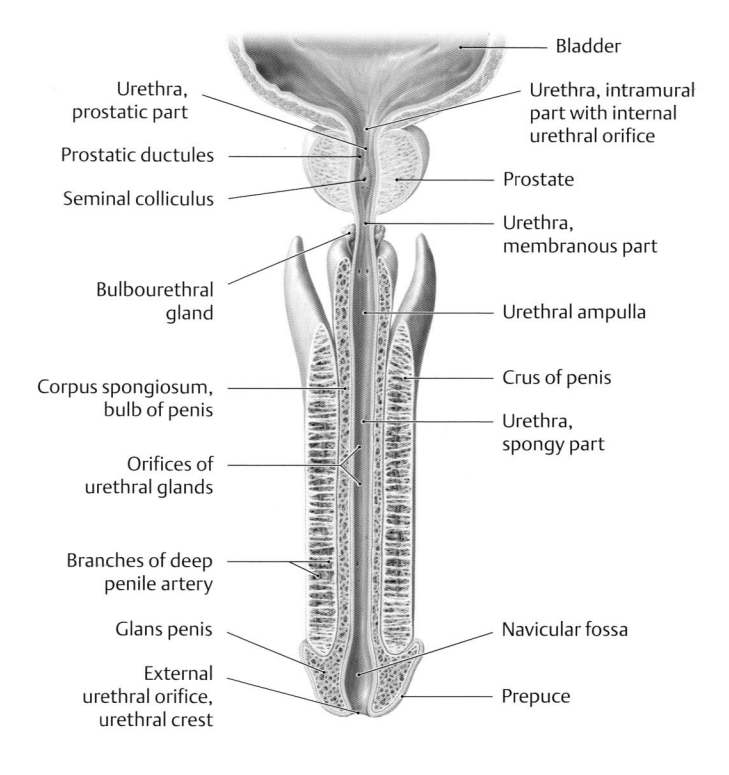

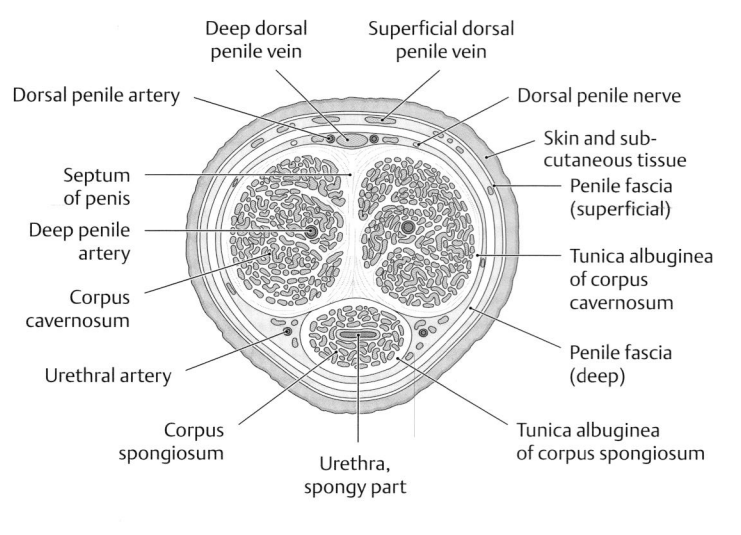

C Location of the male urethra in the penis

Transverse section through the penile shaft. The spongy part of the urethra is contained in the corpus spongiosum of the penis. The corpus spongiosum does not become completely hard even at maximum erection, ensuring that the urethra remains patent during ejaculation. The urethral lumen often presents a flattened rather than circular shape in cross-section, with the upper and lower walls touching.

D Male urethra in longitudinal section

The whole length of the urethra has been cut open and displayed without curves, and all of the pelvic floor muscles have been removed. The four parts of the male urethra can be identified. The male urethra extends distally in the corpus spongiosum to its external orifice on the glans penis. The *prostatic part* of the urethra may be greatly narrowed in patients with benign prostatic enlargement (*prostatic hyperplasia*). This condition is often marked by incomplete voiding and the dribbling of urine after micturition. The residual urine left in the bladder may incite an (often bacterial in nature) inflammation of the bladder (cystitis).

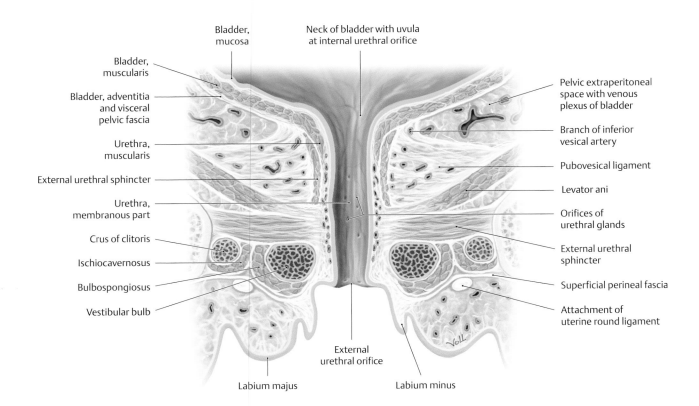

Bladder, mucosa

Bladder, muscularis

Bladder, adventitia and visceral pelvic fascia

Urethra, muscularis

External urethral sphincter

Urethra, membranous part

Crus of clitoris

Ischiocavernosus

Bulbospongiosus

Vestibular bulb

Neck of bladder with uvula at internal urethral orifice

Pelvic extraperitoneal space with venous plexus of bladder

Branch of inferior vesical artery

Pubovesical ligament

Levator ani

Orifices of urethral glands

External urethral sphincter

Superficial perineal fascia

Attachment of uterine round ligament

External urethral orifice

Labium majus

Labium minus

E Female urethra in longitudinal section

Coronal section tilted slightly posterior, anterior view. Unlike the male urethra, the female urethra is straight and only about 3–5 cm long.

Thus it is much easier to catheterize than in the male. At the same time, the short length of the female urethra inereases susceptibility to urinary tract infections.

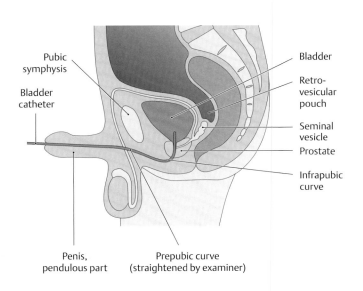

Pubic symphysis

Bladder catheter

Penis, pendulous part

Prepubic curve (straightened by examiner)

Bladder

Retro-vesicular pouch

Seminal vesicle

Prostate

Infrapubic curve

F Transurethral bladder catheterization in the male

The two curves of the male urethra (infrapubic and prepubic) and its three constrictions may pose an obstacle to transurethral catheterization. The prepubic curve can be straightened out somewhat by straightening the penile shaft.

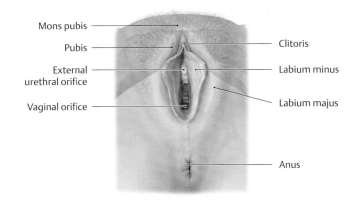

Mons pubis

Pubis

External urethral orifice

Vaginal orifice

Clitoris

Labium minus

Labium majus

Anus

G External orifice of the female urethra

Viewed from below. The pubic bone (pubis) is shown in shadow to aid orientation. The external urethral orifice is located between the labia minora, anterior to the vagina. Despite its proximity to the female external genitalia, the female urethra functions exclusively as a urinary passage. The close topographical relationship of the urethra and external genitalia is important during embryonic development, however: both the urethra and the vagina initially have a common opening at the urogenital sinus and become separated only after further development. Failure of this separation results in an abnormal fistulous connection between the vagina and urethra, a *urethrovaginal fistula*. Even with normal embryonic development, the proximity of the urethra (which is physiologically germ-free) to the vagina (which is not a sterile zone) predisposes to bacterial inflammation of the urethra (*urethritis*). Given the short length of the female urethra, the infection can easily ascend to the bladder (*cystitis*).

2.32 Overview of the Genital Tract

Classification of the genital organs

The genital organs of the male and female can be classified in various ways:

- Topographically (**A**) as:
  - internal genital organs (internal genitalia) or
  - external genital organs (external genitalia)
- Functionally (**B, C**) as:
  - organs for germ-cell and hormone production (gonads) or
  - organs of transport, incubation and copulation, plus accessory sex glands
- Ontogenically (see pp. 242, 243) as:
  - the undifferentiated gonad primordium (develops into the gonads)
  - two undifferentiated duct systems (develop into the male and female transport organs, the female uterus, a portion of the female copulatory organ, and one of the accessory sex glands in the male)
  - the urogenital sinus and its derivatives (giving rise to the external genitalia of both sexes, the accessory sex glands, and portions of the copulatory organs)

A Male and female internal and external genitalia *

	Male	Female
Internal genitalia	Testis Epididymis Vas deferens Prostate Seminal vesicle Bulbourethral gland	Ovary Uterus Fallopian tube Vagina (upper portion)
External genitalia	Penis and urethra Scrotum and coverings of the testis	Vagina (vestibule only) Labia majora and minora Mons pubis Greater and lesser vestibular glands Clitoris

* The *female* external genitalia (pudend) are known clinically as the *vulva*.

B Functions of the male genital organs

Organ	Function
Testis	Germ-cell production Hormone production
Epididymis	Reservoir for sperm (sperm maturation)
Vas deferens	Transport organ for sperm
Urethra	Transport organ for sperm and urinary organ
Accessory sex glands (prostate, seminal vesicles, and bulbourethral glands)	Production of secretions (semen)
Penis	Copulatory and urinary organ

C Functions of the female genital organs

Organ	Function
Ovary	Germ-cell production Hormone production
Fallopian tube	Site of conception and transport organ for zygote
Uterus	Organ of incubation and parturition
Vagina	Organ of copulation and parturition
Labia majora and minora	Copulatory organ
Greater and lesser vestibular glands	Production of secretions

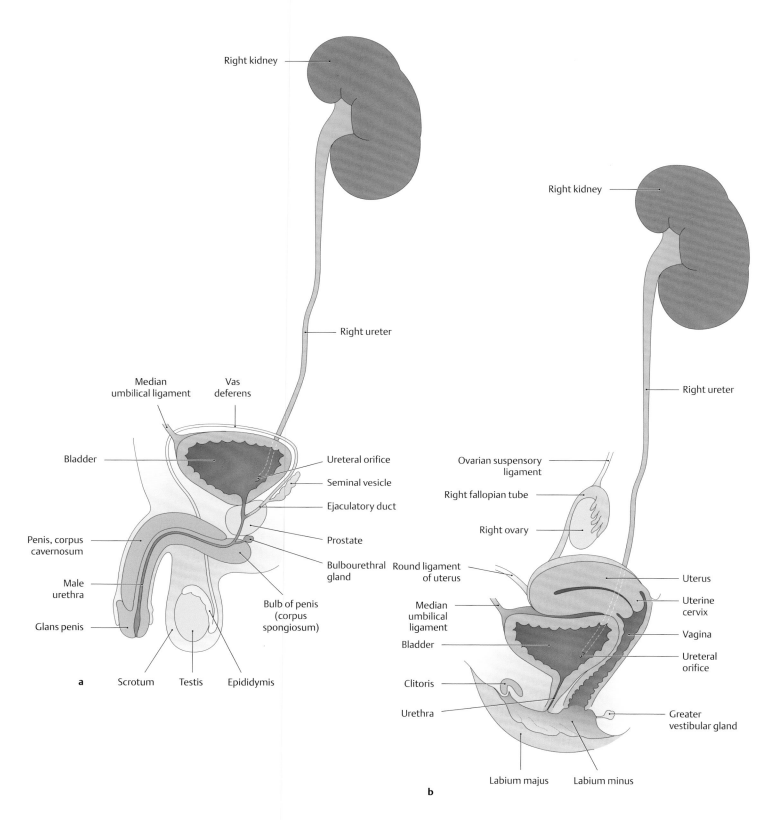

D Overview of the urogenital system
Schematic representation of the urogenital apparatus in the male and female, viewed from the left side. Unpaired pelvic organs and the external genitalia are shown in midsagittal section.

a In the **male**, the urinary and genital organs are closely interrelated functionally and topographically. The urethra passes through the prostate, which is derived embryologically from the urethral epithelium. All of the accessory sex glands (prostate, seminal vesicles, and bulbourethral glands) ultimately discharge their secretions into the urethra

b In the **female**, the urinary and genital tracts are *functionally* separate from each other. *Topographically*, however, the anterior wall of the uterus is closely related to the urinary bladder. In the external genital region as well, the urethra is embedded in the anterior wall of the vagina.

For these reasons, the collective term *urogenital system* is generally used.

2.33 Embryology of the Genital Organs

A Development of embryonic rudiments in the male and female
Although the gonad primordium (future ovary or testis) is genetically determined, it is "colonized" only secondarily by primordial germ cells. Once this has taken place, the primordial gonad begins its sex-specific hormone production, laying the foundation for further development.

The *ureteral bud* develops from the perivesical portions of the mesonephric ducts in both sexes, doing so independently of sex and hormones. Embryonic remnants of the duct systems are often still present in the mature male and female. They have no functional importance, but in rare cases they may lead to disease (e.g., cysts or malignant tumors).

Rudiment	Definitive structure in the male	Definitive structure in the female	Nonfunctioning remnants in the male	Nonfunctioning remnants in the female
Undifferentiated gonad with • cortex • medulla	Testis with • Seminiferous tubules • Rete testis	Ovary with • follicle • ovarian stroma		
Mesonephric ductule	Efferent ductules of testis		Paradidymis	Epo- and paroophoron
Mesonephric (wolffian) duct	• Epididymal duct • Vas deferens • Ejaculatory duct • Seminal vesicle • *Ureter* • *Renal pelvis and calices, collecting ducts*	• *Ureter* • *Renal pelvis and calices, collecting ducts*	Appendix of epididymis	Vesicular appendix, Gartner duct
Paramesonephric (müllerian) duct		• Fallopian tube • Uterus • Superior portion of vagina	Appendix of testis	Morgagni hydatids
Urogenital sinus	• Prostate • Bulbourethral gland • *Bladder* • *Male urethra*	• Inferior portion of vagina • Greater and lesser vestibular glands • *Bladder* • *Female urethra*	Prostatic utricle	
Phallus (genital tubercle)	Corpus cavernosum of penis	Clitoris, glans of clitoris		
Genital folds	• Glans of penis	• Labia minora • Vestibular bulb	Penile raphe	
Labioscrotal swellings	Scrotum	Labia majora		
Gubernaculum		• Proper ovarian ligament • Round ligament of uterus	Gubernaculum of testis	
Genital tubercle (of Müller)			Seminal colliculus	Hymen

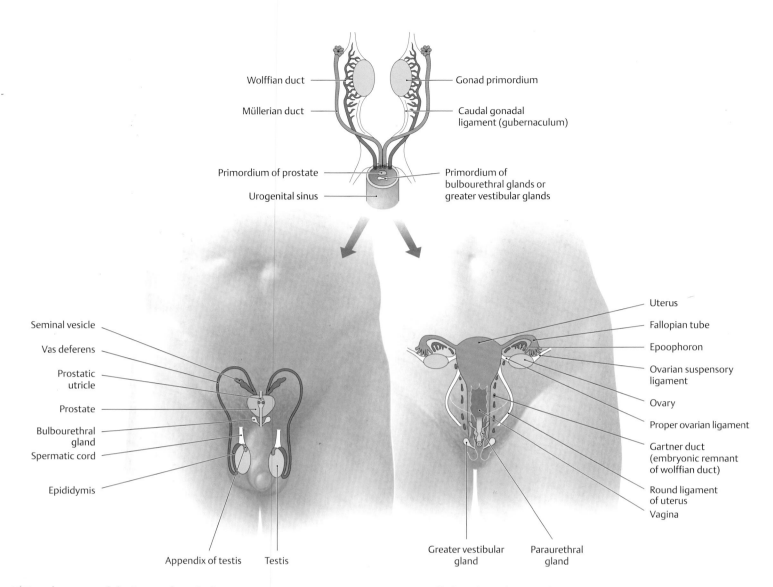

Wolffian duct

Müllerian duct

Primordium of prostate

Urogenital sinus

Gonad primordium

Caudal gonadal ligament (gubernaculum)

Primordium of bulbourethral glands or greater vestibular glands

Seminal vesicle

Vas deferens

Prostatic utricle

Prostate

Bulbourethral gland

Spermatic cord

Epididymis

Appendix of testis   Testis

Uterus

Fallopian tube

Epoophoron

Ovarian suspensory ligament

Ovary

Proper ovarian ligament

Gartner duct (embryonic remnant of wolffian duct)

Round ligament of uterus

Vagina

Greater vestibular gland   Paraurethral gland

B Development of the internal genitalia
Genetically male embryo with testicular primordium: Under the influence of testosterone produced in the testis, the *wolffian ducts* develop into the vas deferens and epididymis. The müllerian ducts regress in response to anti-müllerian hormone, which is also produced in the testis.

Genetically female embryo with ovarian primordium: Under the influence of ovarian hormones, the *müllerian ducts* develop into the fallopian tubes (uterine tubes) and also fuse to form the uterus and part of the vagina. The wolffian ducts, which can develop only in response to testosterone, regress almost completely.

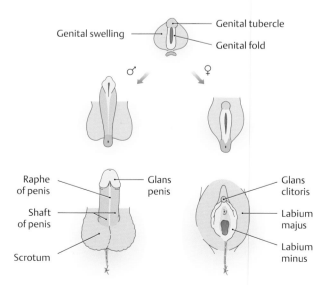

Genital swelling

Genital tubercle

Genital fold

♂   ♀

Raphe of penis

Shaft of penis

Scrotum

Glans penis

Glans clitoris

Labium majus

Labium minus

C Development of the external genitalia
The external genital organs and accessory sex glands in both sexes develop from the urogenital sinus, which gives rise to the urethra and urinary bladder. As a result, developmental abnormalities in this region often lead to anomalies involving the urinary tract *and* genital tract such as fistulae (abnormal connecting ducts) between the vagina and urethra.

Note: In the male, the terminal portion of the urinary tract functions as a urinary *and* genital passageway. In the female, the urinary and genital organs are functionally separate and therefore the female urethra functions exclusively as a urinary passage. In both sexes, however, the urinary and genital organs are so closely related topographically that they are often referred to collectively as the urogenital organs.

2.34 Female Internal Genitalia: Overview

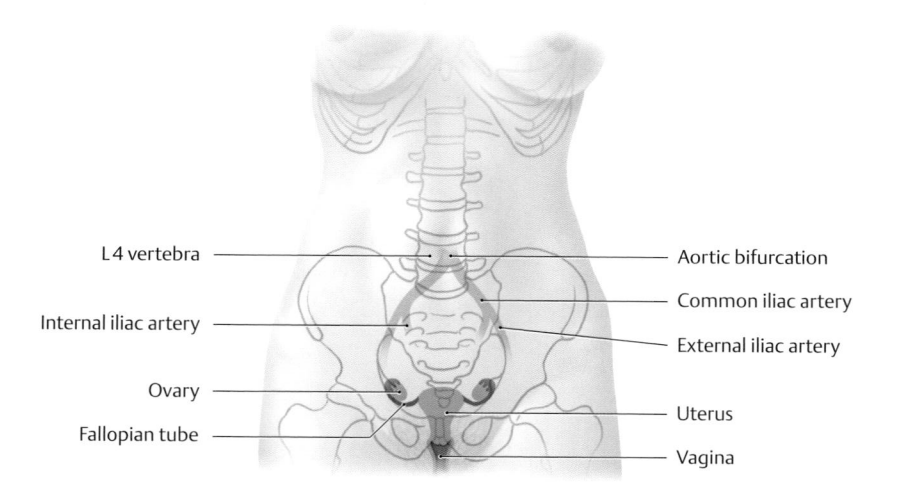

A Projection of the female internal genitalia onto the pelvis

Anterior view. The bifurcation of the abdominal aorta into the common iliac arteries is also shown to aid orientation. The uterus, like the vagina, is located in the pelvic midline while the ovaries are superior, lateral, and posterior to the uterus in the RLQ and LLQ. Each ovary occupies a fossa located just inferior to the division of the common iliac artery. The fallopian tubes do not pass to the ovaries by the shortest route but circle around them from the lateral side, because both of the müllerian ducts (which develop into the fallopian tubes) run lateral to the gonadal ridge in which the ovaries develop.

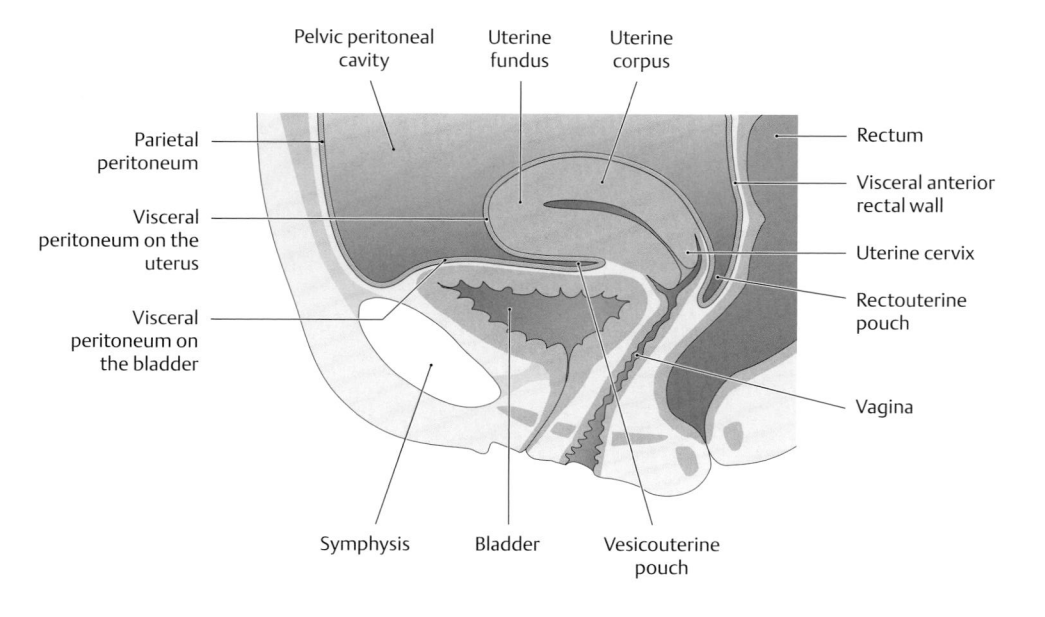

B Uterus and vagina: relationship to the pelvic organs

Midsagittal section through a female pelvis, viewed from the left side. The peritoneum has been outlined in color. The uterus directly overlies the bladder (see also p. 169), and the rectum is posterior to the uterus. The fundus and corpus (body) of the uterus are covered by visceral peritoneum, which is reflected onto the bladder and rectum to form the vesicouterine pouch and rectouterine pouch. The peritoneum extends farther down the posterior wall of the uterus than its anterior wall, with the result that the *posterior* part of the uterine cervix and upper vagina is covered by peritoneum while the anterior part is not. The vagina is surrounded on all sides by pelvic connective tissue. This tissue is thickened anteriorly and posteriorly to form the vesicovaginal and rectovaginal septa.

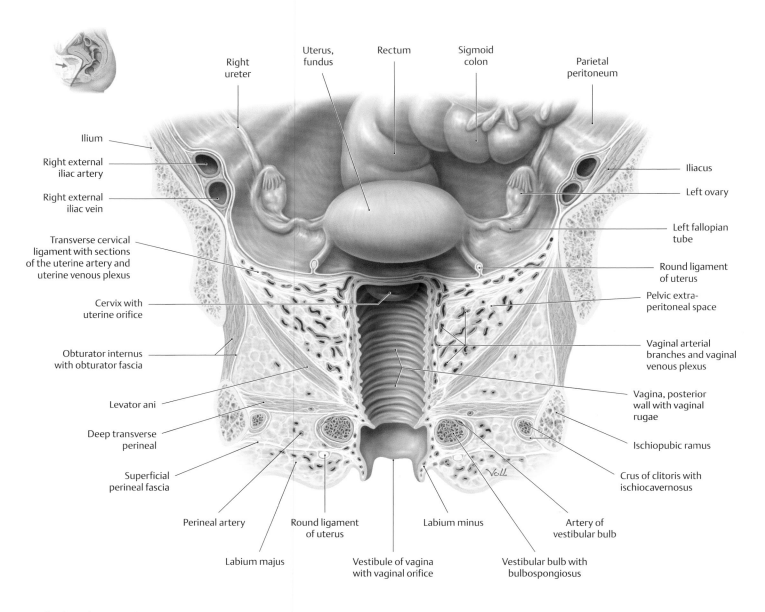

Right ureter

Uterus, fundus

Rectum

Sigmoid colon

Parietal peritoneum

Ilium

Right external iliac artery

Right external iliac vein

Iliacus

Left ovary

Left fallopian tube

Transverse cervical ligament with sections of the uterine artery and uterine venous plexus

Round ligament of uterus

Pelvic extra-peritoneal space

Cervix with uterine orifice

Vaginal arterial branches and vaginal venous plexus

Obturator internus with obturator fascia

Vagina, posterior wall with vaginal rugae

Levator ani

Ischiopubic ramus

Deep transverse perineal

Superficial perineal fascia

Crus of clitoris with ischiocavernosus

Perineal artery

Round ligament of uterus

Labium minus

Artery of vestibular bulb

Labium majus

Vestibule of vagina with vaginal orifice

Vestibular bulb with bulbospongiosus

C The female genital organs in situ

Slightly angled coronal section, anterior view. The bladder, which lies anterior to the vagina and inferior to the uterine fundus (see **B**), is not shown. This illustration represents a compilation of multiple sections to provide a single integrated view. The uterine fundus, which is directed anteriorly owing to its anteverted and anteflexed position (see p. 251), projects out of the deeper plane of section toward the observer. Around the vagina is a connective-tissue space containing an elaborate venous plexus. This loose connective tissue allows for considerable expansion of the vagina during childbirth. The sections of arterial vessels are arterial branches to the vagina as well as sections of the inferior vesical arteries.

2.35 Female Internal Genitalia: Topographical Anatomy and Peritoneal Relationships; Shape and Structure

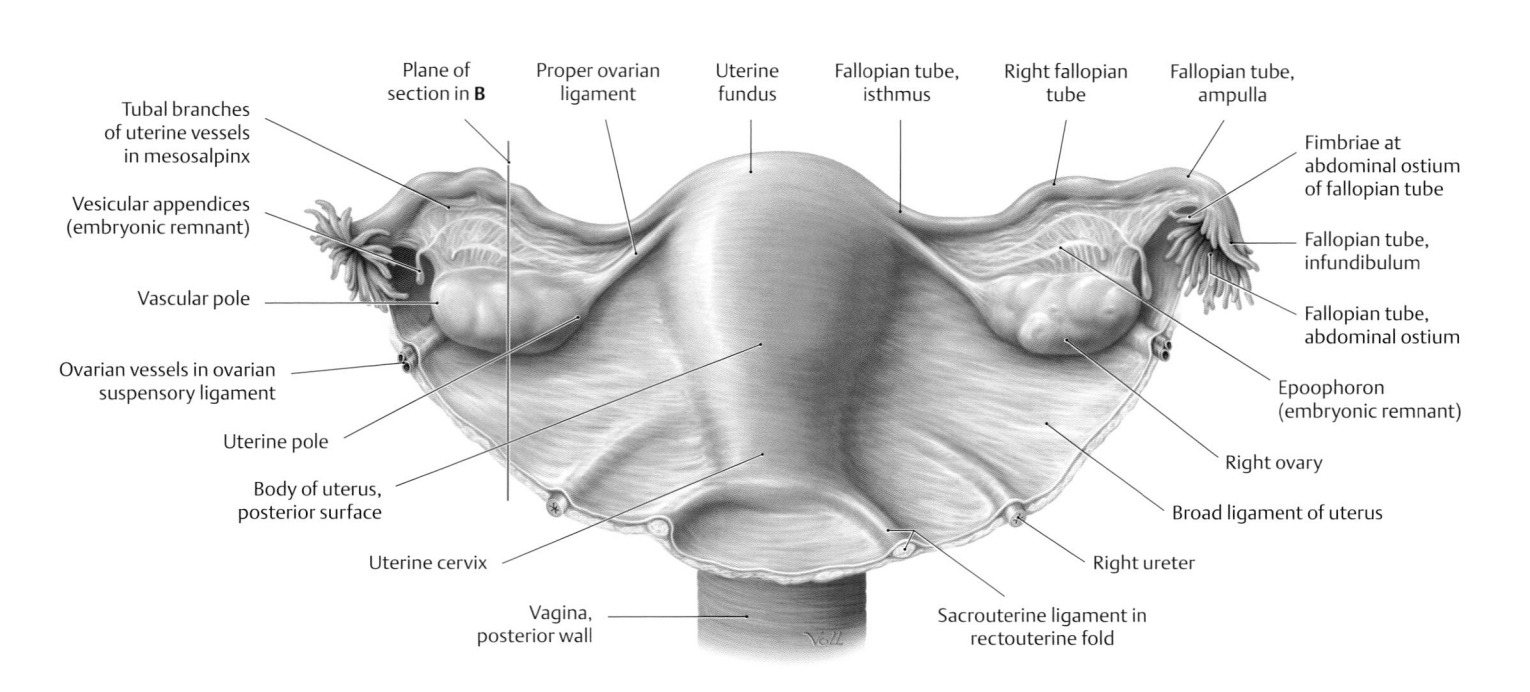

A Uterus and adnexa: topography and peritoneal relationships

Posterosuperior view of the uterus, adnexa, and the posterior surface of the uterine broad ligament. The uterine adnexa (ovary and fallopian tube) are attached to the superior border and posterior surface of the broad ligament by folds of peritoneum (mesovarium and mesosalpinx, see **B**). The mesometrium, which follows the anteflexed position of the uterus, attaches the uterus to the pelvic sidewall and transmits the *uterine* vascular structures. The *ovary* receives its vascular supply through the ovarian suspensory ligament (these and other ligaments are reviewed in **C**).

Note: The ureters descend in the retroperitoneum to the base of the broad ligament and run forward between its layers to the bladder, passing inferior to the uterine artery (not visible here, see p. 175). This relationship must be duly noted in operations on the uterus and broad ligament (risk of ureteral injury).

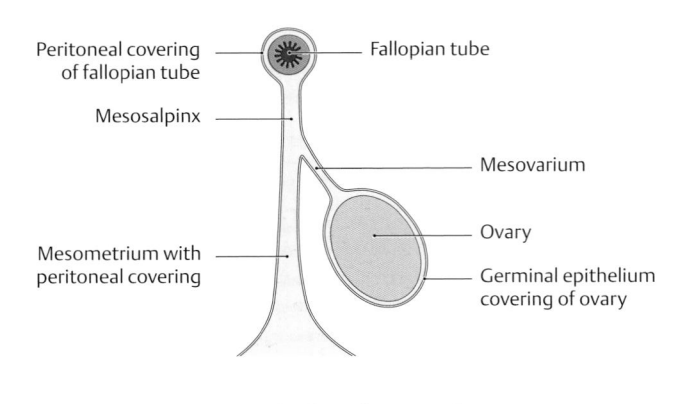

B Folds of peritoneum on the female genital organs

(after Graumann, von Keyserlinkg, and Sasse)

Sagittal section through the broad ligament of the uterus. The ovary, fallopian tube, and much of the uterus (see **A**) are covered by peritoneum. The fallopian tube is attached to the superior margin of the broad ligament by the mesosalpinx. The ovary is attached to the posterosuperior surface of the broad ligament by its own peritoneal structure, the mesovarium. These peritoneum-covered bands of connective tissue perform the same functions for the genital organs as the mesenteries do for the bowel and are named accordingly (see **C**): the mesovarium for the ovary, the mesosalpinx for the fallopian tube (salpinx), and the mesometrium for the uterus. Collectively they form the broad ligament.

C Ligaments and peritoneal structures of the female genital organs

Broad ligament of uterus	Broad fold of peritoneum extending from the lateral pelvic wall to the uterus (transmits vascular structures to the internal genital organs). The ligament has three main parts that extend to specific organs: • Mesometrium = to the uterus • Mesosalpinx = to the fallopian tube • Mesovarium = to the ovary The connective-tissue space between the two peritoneal layers of the broad ligament is known clinically as the parametrium
Transverse cervical ligament (cardinal ligament)	Transverse bands of connective tissue between the uterine cervix and pelvic wall (paracervix)
Round ligament of uterus	Distal remnant of the gubernaculum (= embryonic cord in both sexes, guides the descent of the testis or ovary). Extends from the lateral angle of the uterus through the inguinal canal into the subcutaneous connective tissue of the labium majus
Rectouterine fold	Peritoneum-covered fold of connective tissue between the uterus and rectum; often contains smooth muscle (rectouterine muscle)
Proper ovarian ligament	Proximal remnant of gubernaculum passing from the uterine pole of the ovary to the angle of the uterus with the fallopian tube
Ovarian suspensory ligament	Fold of peritoneum stretching from the pelvic wall to the ovary; transmits the ovarian vessels

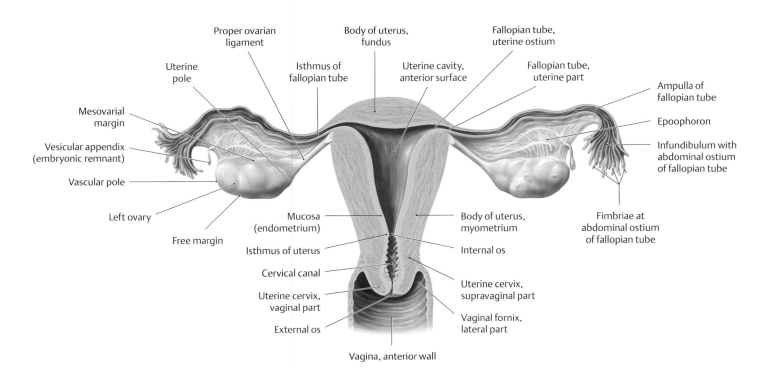

D Uterus and fallopian tubes: shape and structure
Posterior view of a coronal section with the uterus straightened and the mesometrium removed. The uterus consists basically of the corpus (with the fundus) and cervix, the corpus being joined to the cervix by a narrow isthmus approximately 1 cm long. Macroscopically, the uterine isthmus is classified as part of the cervix but histologically it is lined by endometrium. The junction of the body of the uterus and cervix is located at the *internal os* of the uterus. The lumen of the uterus, called the uterine cavity, communicates with the vaginal lumen through the isthmus and cervical canal. It has a total length ("probe length") of 7–8 cm. The *uterine cavity* presents a triangular shape in coronal section. The

uterine cervix is subdivided into a supravaginal part and vaginal part. The *external os* of the uterus is the opening in the vaginal part of the cervix that is directed toward the vagina. The vaginal part of the cervix projects into the vagina, forming recesses called the vaginal fornices.
The *fallopian tube* (uterine tube, total length approximately 10–18 cm) is subdivided from lateral to medial into the infundibulum, ampulla, isthmus, and uterine part. The abdominal ostium of the tube at the infundibulum is surrounded by fimbriae (the "fimbriated end") and opens into the peritoneal cavity. The ostium at the uterine end of the tube opens into the uterine cavity.

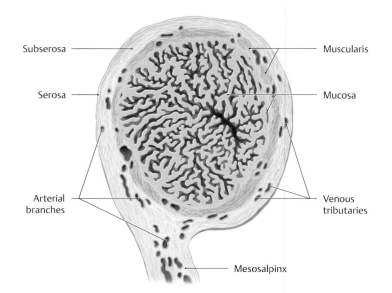

E Fallopian tube in cross-section: wall structure
Cross-sectional view of the ampullary portion of a right fallopian tube. The mesosalpinx extends inferiorly. The three wall layers are clearly distinguishable (wall thickness = 0.4–1.5 cm):

- The **mucosa** is raised into a great many folds that occupy most of the tubal lumen. These folds are of key importance in transporting the zygote to the uterus. Postinflammatory adhesions between the mucosal folds may hamper or even prevent transport of the fertilized ovum (see p. 254).
- The **muscularis** consists of several thin layers of smooth muscle that provide the fallopian tube with its motility (see **B**, p. 252) and propel the zygote toward the uterus by a ciliated epithelium.
- The **serosa** (peritoneal covering) of the fallopian tube is continuous with the mesosalpinx.

247

2.36 Female Internal Genitalia: Wall Structure and Function

Myometrium, supravascular layer

Myometrium, vascular layer

Myometrium, subvascular layer

Uterine cervix

a

Fallopian tube, mostly circular muscle fibers

Uterine fundus, mostly longitudinal muscle fibers

Body of uterus, longitudinal and oblique fibers

Uterine cervix, circular muscle fibers

b

A Layers (a) and functional principle (b) of the myometrium
(after Rauber and Kopsch)

The myometrium (muscular coat) of the uterus consists of three layers from outside to inside:

- **Supravascular layer:** thin outermost layer with criss-crossing lamellae; stabilizes the uterine wall
- **Vascular layer:** thick intermediate layer with a reticular pattern of muscle fibers; very vascular; the principal source for uterine contractions during labor
- **Subvascular layer:** thin innermost layer just below the endometrium; provides for functional closure of the uterine ostium of the fallopian tube. Its contraction promotes separation of the uterine mucosa (shedding of the functional layer) during menses and separation of the placenta after childbirth.

The myometrium performs two seemingly contradictory functions: It must keep the uterus *closed* during pregnancy, but it must *open* the cervix during childbirth. To fulfill these functions, the individual muscle layers (see above) are equipped with longitudinal, oblique, and transverse or circular fibers. The circular muscle fibers are most abundant in the cervical region and serve to maintain closure of the cervix during pregnancy. The longitudinal and oblique muscle fibers are most abundant in the uterine body and fundus; they shorten the uterus and lower the fundus during childbirth. The myometrium blends with the circular fibers of the fallopian tube muscles at the uterine fundus near the tubal ostium. Myometrial contractions are stimulated most effectively by the pituitary hormone oxytocin. These contractions occur not only during labor and delivery but also during menstruation, when they aid in expulsion of the uterine mucosa. Benign tumors of the myometrium (fibroids, myomas) may cause abnormalities of menstrual bleeding.

B Wall structure of the uterus

The uterine wall also consists of three layers from inside to outside:

- **Mucosa** or **endometrium** (see **C**):
  Single layer of columnar epithelium (epithelial layer) on a connective-tissue base (lamina propria)
- **Muscular coat** or **myometrium** (see **A**):
  Several smooth-muscle layers with a total thickness of approximately 1.5 cm
- **Serous coat** or **perimetrium:**
  Serosa covering the anterior and posterior sides of the uterine corpus and the posterior wall of the uterine cervix. The subserosa adjacent to the myometrium becomes adventitia in areas where the uterus lacks a peritoneal covering (e.g., at the attachment of the uterine broad ligament).

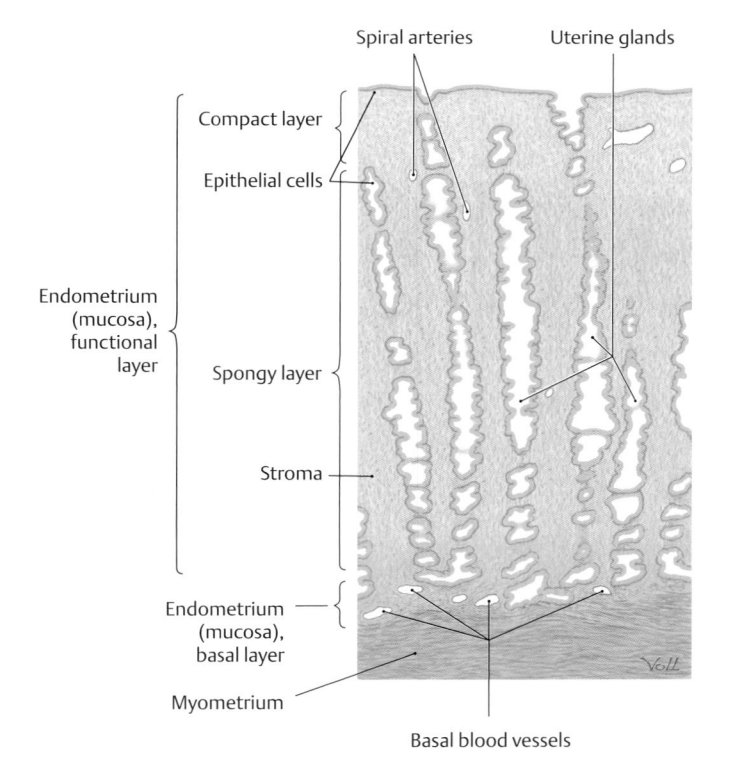

Spiral arteries — Uterine glands

Compact layer

Epithelial cells

Endometrium (mucosa), functional layer

Spongy layer

Stroma

Endometrium (mucosa), basal layer

Myometrium

Basal blood vessels

C Structure of the uterine mucosa (endometrium)

Structurally, the endometrium consists of a simple columnar epithelial cell layer and a lamina propria. The epithelial layer lines the uterine surface and encloses the tubular, coiled endometrial uterine glands. The lamina propria, which surrounds and supports the *uterine glands*, is made up of connective tissue (stroma) and the vessels embedded in it. The endometrium is *functionally* subdivided into a basal layer (stratum basale) and a functional layer (stratum functionale). The *basal layer* is approximately 1 mm thick, is largely exempt from the cyclical changes in the endometrium, and is not shed during menstruation. The *functional layer* varies in thickness at different phases of the ovarian cycle in women of reproductive age. It is shed at intervals of approximately 28 days during menstruation. It is thickest during the secretory phase of the ovarian cycle, at which time it consists of a superficial compact layer and a deeper spongy layer. It receives its blood supply from tortuous vessels called spiral arteries. While in this secretory state, the endometrium is most receptive to the implantation of a zygote. The mucosa of the uterine cervix does not participate in these cyclical changes.

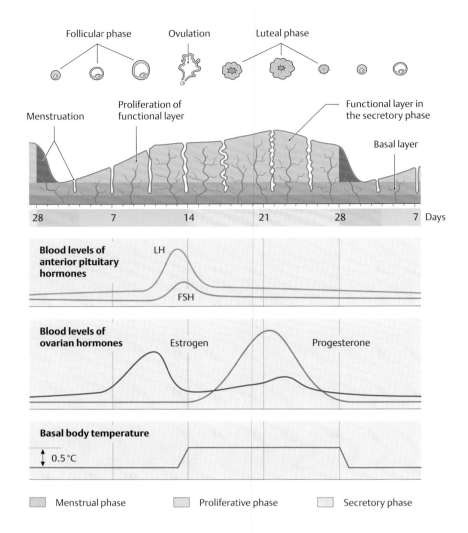

Follicular phase   Ovulation   Luteal phase

Menstruation   Proliferation of functional layer   Functional layer in the secretory phase   Basal layer

28   7   14   21   28   7 Days

Blood levels of anterior pituitary hormones
LH
FSH

Blood levels of ovarian hormones
Estrogen   Progesterone

Basal body temperature
0.5 °C

Menstrual phase   Proliferative phase   Secretory phase

D Cyclical changes in the endometrium

The ovary secretes estrogens (e.g., estradiol) and progestins (e.g., progesterone) on a cyclical basis. Estrogens stimulate proliferation of the endometrium, while progestins induce its secretory transformation. The release of both hormones is controlled chiefly by the hormones FSH (= follicle stimulating hormone) and LH (= luteinizing hormone), which are secreted cyclically by the pituitary gland. While estrogens are produced by the ovarian follicle, progestins are produced in significant amounts only by the corpus luteum. If conception does not take place, the corpus luteum regresses and stops producing hormones. As a result of this, the functional layer of the endometrium breaks down and is expelled during menstruation. Estrogen production by a new, pituitary-stimulated ovarian follicle initiates a new cycle, which lasts an average of 28 days (= 1 lunar month). Ovulation usually occurs on day 14 of the cycle. *Note:* For practical reasons, the first day of the menstrual period (which lasts about 4 days) is considered day 1 of the cycle, despite the fact that the cycle ends with menstruation. This is because the sudden onset of menstrual bleeding is easier to detect than its more gradual cessation. From the standpoint of the endometrium, however, the last day of the menstrual period (difficult to detect) marks the end of the cycle.

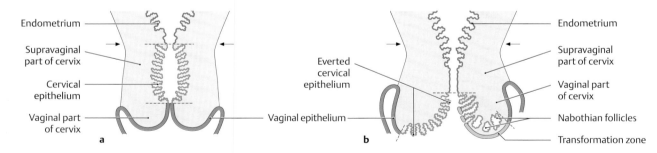

Endometrium
Supravaginal part of cervix
Cervical epithelium
Vaginal part of cervix
a
Vaginal epithelium

Everted cervical epithelium
Endometrium
Supravaginal part of cervix
Vaginal part of cervix
Nabothian follicles
Transformation zone
b

E Cervical epithelium and its changes
(after Lüllmann-Rauch)

Simplified schematic representation of the cervix and vagina in coronal section, anterior view. The arrows indicate the location of internal os, and the dashed lines mark the boundaries of the cervical epithelium. The cervical canal bears a single layer of columnar epithelium (cervical epithelium), while the vagina is lined by stratified, nonkeratinized squamous epithelium (vaginal epithelium). The boundary between the two epithelia varies in location according to the woman's hormonal status.

Before puberty (a): The vaginal part of the cervix is covered by vaginal epithelium, and the boundary with the cervical epithelium is not visible from the vagina (endocervical above the external os).

Reproductive age (b): In response to hormonal stimuli, the cervical epithelium is everted out of the cervical canal (ectropion), and so its boundary with the vaginal epithelium is visible from the vagina.

After menopause (epithelial relations same as before puberty, see **a**): The cervical epithelium has retracted, and its boundary with the vaginal epithelium is again endocervical.

Metaplastic transformation: In women of reproductive age, the single layer of everted cervical epithelium may undergo a transformation (metaplasia) to stratified, nonkeratinized squamous epithelium. If this squamous epithelium overgrows the orifices of the mucus-producing cervical glands, it may occlude them and incite the formation of mucus retention cysts (nabothian follicles).

Note: The squamous epithelium may also undergo malignant transformation, forming precancerous lesions that progress to cervical carcinoma. The precancerous changes can be detected early by a test in which smears of epithelial cells are taken from the vaginal part of the cervix and examined microscopically to assess their degree of differentiation (Papanicolaou or "Pap" smear). An iodine test can also be used to detect areas of greater or lesser differentiation on the vaginal part of the cervix: Normally differentiated surface epithelium is stained by the iodine solution owing to its glycogen content, whereas less differentiated (glycogen-deficient) epithelium remains unstained.

2.37 Female Internal Genitalia: Vagina, Uterine Positions

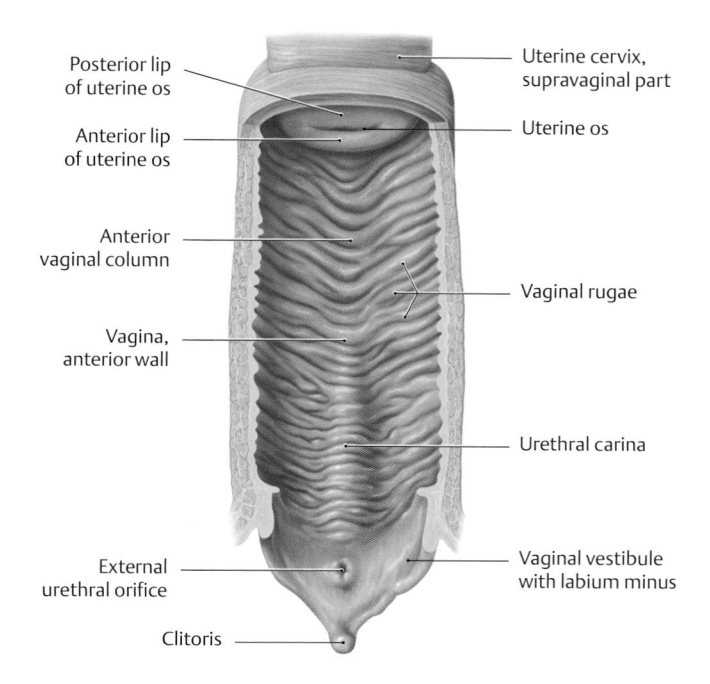

Posterior lip of uterine os

Anterior lip of uterine os

Anterior vaginal column

Vagina, anterior wall

External urethral orifice

Clitoris

Uterine cervix, supravaginal part

Uterine os

Vaginal rugae

Urethral carina

Vaginal vestibule with labium minus

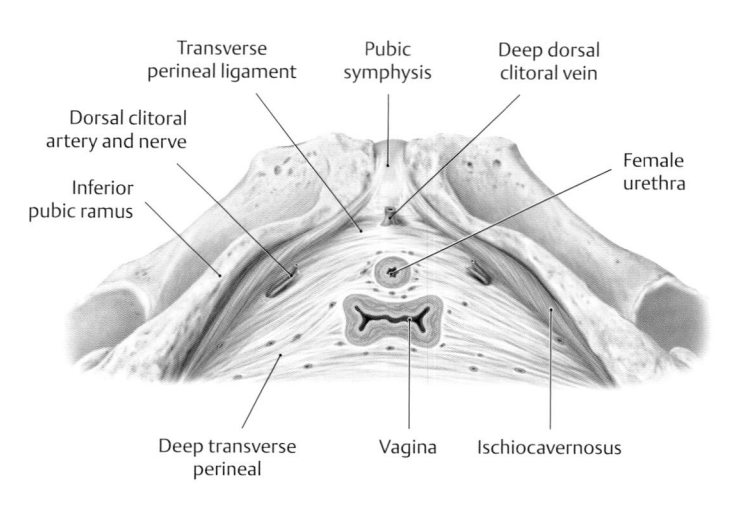

Transverse perineal ligament

Pubic symphysis

Deep dorsal clitoral vein

Dorsal clitoral artery and nerve

Inferior pubic ramus

Female urethra

Deep transverse perineal

Vagina

Ischiocavernosus

A Vagina

Posterior view. The vagina has been cut open along a coronal plane angled slightly posteriorly to display its anterior wall. The vaginal lumen presents an H-shaped cross section (see **B**), but the lumen in this dissection has been stretched open to a more circular shape (in situ the posterior and anterior walls are closely apposed). The vaginal mucosa has numerous transverse folds (rugae) as well as anterior and posterior ridges (vaginal columns) formed by the extensive venous plexus in the vaginal wall. The closely adjacent urethra raises the lower anterior wall of the vagina into a prominent longitudinal ridge (urethral carina).

B Location of the vagina in the pelvic floor

This drawing illustrates the close proximity of the vagina and urethra. Muscular fibers from the deep transverse perineal profundus encircle the vagina (see **G**, p. 239).

C Location of the vagina in the pelvis

Midsagittal section through a female pelvis, viewed from the left side. The longitudinal axis of the vagina is directed posterosuperiorly. The vagina is attached to the pelvic connective tissue anteriorly (vesicovaginal septum), posteriorly (rectovaginal septum), and laterally (not shown here). The vaginal fornix surrounds the vaginal part of the cervix, which itself is directed superiorly and anteriorly. As a result, the anterior fornix is considerably lower than the posterior fornix. The visceral peritoneum extends far down the posterior uterine wall, bringing the posterior part of the vaginal fornix into close proximity to the rectouterine pouch (cul-de-sac, the lowest part of the female peritoneal cavity).

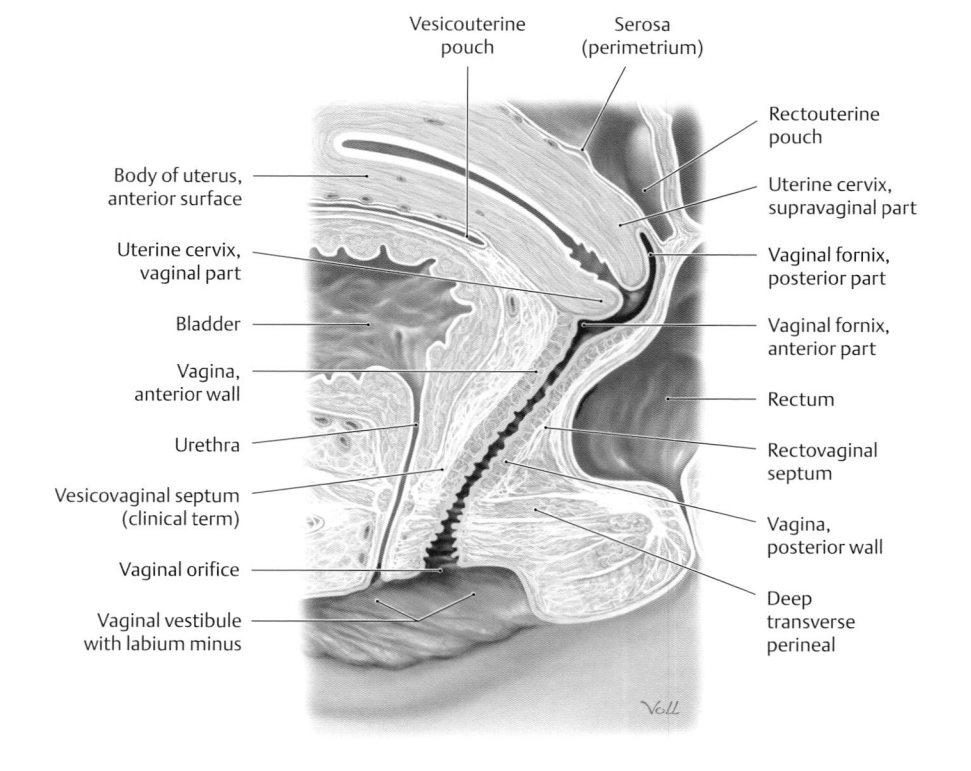

Vesicouterine pouch

Serosa (perimetrium)

Body of uterus, anterior surface

Uterine cervix, vaginal part

Bladder

Vagina, anterior wall

Urethra

Vesicovaginal septum (clinical term)

Vaginal orifice

Vaginal vestibule with labium minus

Rectouterine pouch

Uterine cervix, supravaginal part

Vaginal fornix, posterior part

Vaginal fornix, anterior part

Rectum

Rectovaginal septum

Vagina, posterior wall

Deep transverse perineal

D Curvature and position of the uterus

Midsagittal section of the uterus and upper vagina, viewed from the left side.

Note the two angles that determine the normal anteversion and anteflexion of the uterus (see **G**). Posterior angulation and curvature of the uterus (retroflexion, retroversion) are considered abnormal. A retroverted uterus is more susceptible to descent because it is more closely aligned with the longitudinal axis of the vagina. Moreover, a retroverted uterus that enlarges during pregnancy may become immobile below the sacral promontory (L 5 / S1 junction) and jeopardize the further course of the pregnancy by constraining uterine expansion.

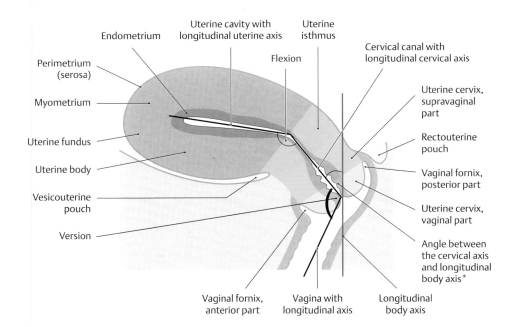

E Position and level of the uterus in the pelvis

Coronal section of the pelvis, anterior view. The uterus has been slightly straightened for clarity. Normally the uterus is located approximately in the median plane (**a**) with its vaginal part level with a line connecting the two ischial spines. The uterus may be displaced from this position to the left or right (sinistroposition or dextroposition, **b** and **c**) or may lie above or below the plane of the ischial spines (elevation or descent, see **d** and **e**). Anterior and posterior displacement (anteposition, retroposition) may also occur but are not illustrated here. Descent of the uterus usually results from a structural weakness of the pelvic floor (chiefly the levator ani, often after numerous vaginal deliveries). Displacement of the uterus may cause complaints and functional disturbances due to pressure on adjacent organs (bladder, rectum). Descent of the uterus may even cause the vaginal part of the uterus to protrude from the vagina (cervical prolapse).

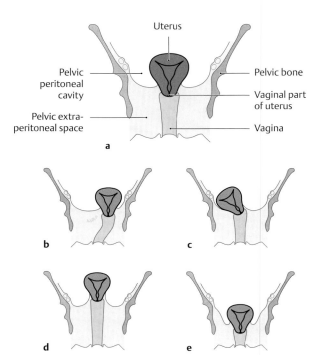
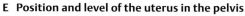

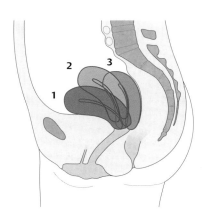

F Physiological changes in uterine position

Midsagittal section of the pelvis, viewed from the left side. Uterine position is directly affected by the varying degrees of bladder and rectal distention. **1** Bladder and rectum empty; **2** bladder and rectum full; **3** bladder full, rectum empty.

G Describing the position of the uterus in the pelvis

The position of the uterus in the pelvis can be described in terms of version, flexion, and position (angles are described in **D**).

Version	Inclination of the cervix in the pelvic cavity; defined by the angle between the cervical axis and the vagina; the normal condition is *anteversion*
Flexion	Inclination of the uterine corpus relative to the cervix; defined by the angle between the longitudinal axes of the cervix and uterine body; the normal condition is *anteflexion*
Position	Position of the vaginal part of the uterus in the pelvic cavity; physiologically, the vaginal part of the uterus is at the level of the interspinous line at the center of the pelvis

* The angle between the cervical axis and the longitudinal body axis is clinically relevant by certain conventions (see **D**).

2.38 Female Internal Genitalia: Ovary and Follicular Maturation

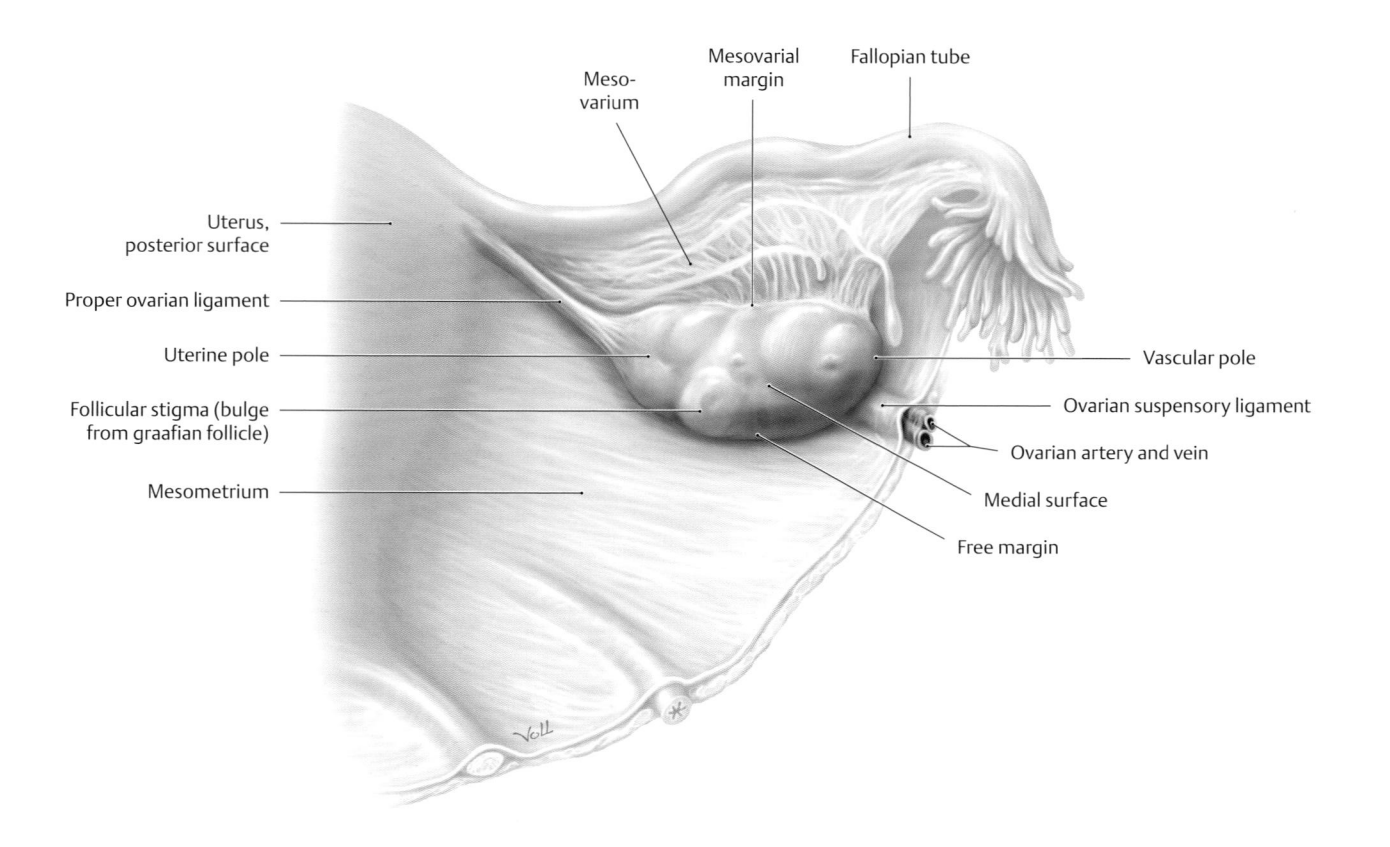

Mesovarium

Mesovarial margin

Fallopian tube

Uterus, posterior surface

Proper ovarian ligament

Uterine pole

Follicular stigma (bulge from graafian follicle)

Mesometrium

Vascular pole

Ovarian suspensory ligament

Ovarian artery and vein

Medial surface

Free margin

A Ovary
Posterior view of a right ovary, showing the peritoneal ligaments that transmit vessels to the ovary (ovarian suspensory ligament with the ovarian artery and vein, proper ovarian ligament with the ovarian branch of the uterine artery, and portions of the uterine venous plexus) along with part of the uterus, fallopian tube, and broad ligament. The ovary is positioned such that it lies in the iliac fossa of the lesser pelvis.
Note: Given the dual vascular supply to the ovary from the upper abdomen (the vessels accompany the ovary during its developmental descent) and the blood supply to the uterus (close to the ovary), both vascular systems should be ligated during a hysterectomy.
In a woman of reproductive age, the ovary is 3–5 cm long and has the size and shape of a plum. It consists of a cortical and medullary zone (see

C) and is surrounded by a tough collagenous capsule (tunica albuginea). The cortical zone contains follicles at varying stages of development. The follicles contain an oocyte surrounded by follicular epithelium and a connective-tissue mantle. Female hormones are not produced by the oocyte itself but by the cells that surround it. Although an intraperitoneal organ, the ovary is covered externally by germinal epithelium (on its tunica albuginea) and has a shiny surface.
Note: The visceral peritoneal covering of the ovary, a single-layered cuboidal epithelium that surrounds the tunica albuginea, has been referred to traditionally as "germinal epithelium," but it does not participate at all in the principal, reproductive function of the ovary—egg production—nor is it involved in replenishment of cells in the ovary itself. However, it is "germinal" in another, unfortunate way—90 % of all malignant ovarian tumors are thought to originate in this cell layer.

B Ovum collection mechanism
Posterior view of a right ovary and fallopian tube. Both the fallopian tube and the ovary are motile. The tube derives its motility from its muscular wall. Rotational and longitudinal movements of the tube make it easier for the fimbriated end of the tube to contact the entire ovary. The movements stop when the abdominal orifice of the tube has cupped the mound formed by a graafian follicle.

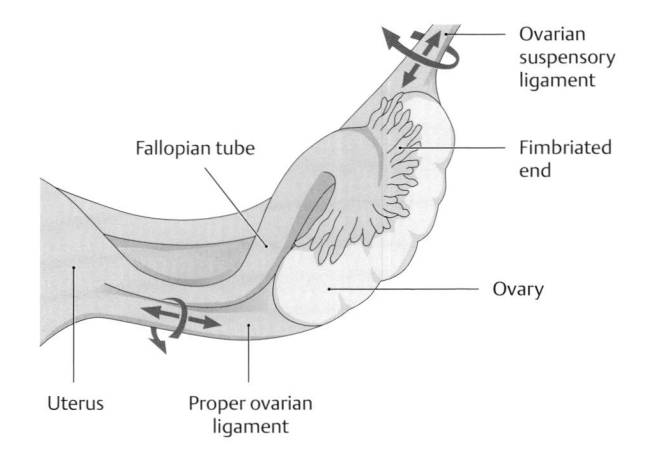

Ovarian suspensory ligament

Fallopian tube

Fimbriated end

Ovary

Uterus

Proper ovarian ligament

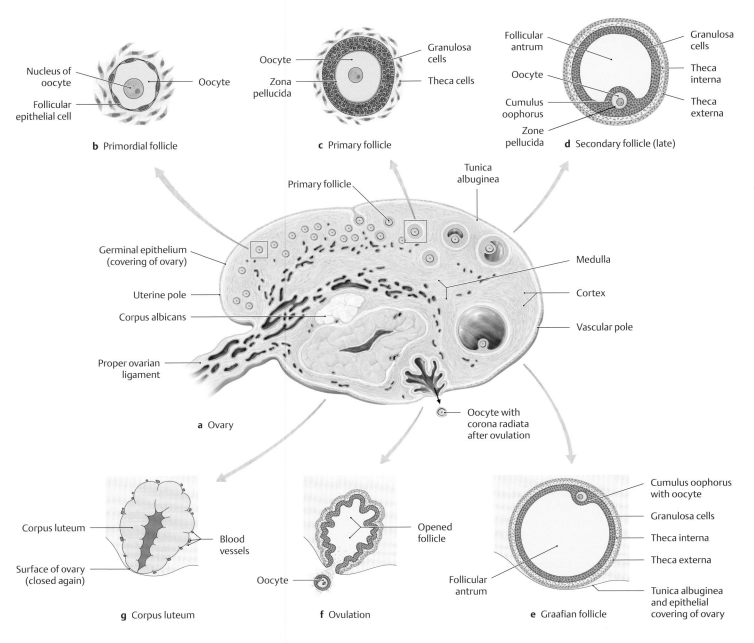

b Primordial follicle

Nucleus of oocyte
Oocyte
Follicular epithelial cell

c Primary follicle

Oocyte
Zona pellucida
Granulosa cells
Theca cells

d Secondary follicle (late)

Follicular antrum
Oocyte
Cumulus oophorus
Zone pellucida
Granulosa cells
Theca interna
Theca externa

a Ovary

Primary follicle
Tunica albuginea
Germinal epithelium (covering of ovary)
Uterine pole
Corpus albicans
Proper ovarian ligament
Medulla
Cortex
Vascular pole
Oocyte with corona radiata after ovulation

g Corpus luteum

Corpus luteum
Surface of ovary (closed again)
Blood vessels

f Ovulation

Opened follicle
Oocyte

e Graafian follicle

Cumulus oophorus with oocyte
Granulosa cells
Theca interna
Theca externa
Tunica albuginea and epithelial covering of ovary
Follicular antrum

C Follicular maturation in the ovary

The sequence of follicular maturation is illustrated in a clockwise direction around the ovary. The follicular stages are not drawn to scale.

- **Ovary:** Section through the ovary of an adult woman, demonstrating its structure and follicular stages. The central medulla is surrounded by a cortical region containing follicles at various stages of development. At the lower edge of the ovary, an oocyte is being released from a ruptured follicle (ovulation). After ovulation has taken place, the graafian follicle initially develops into a hormonally active corpus luteum and later regresses to form a white fibrous scar (corpus albicans) (see **a**).
- **Primordial follicle:** Oocyte surrounded by a single layer of flat epithelial cells (see **b**).
- **Primary follicle:** When the single layer of epithelium around the oocyte becomes multilaminar but without an atrium, the follicle is called a primary follicle (see **c**).
- **Secondary follicle:** The epithelium (composed of granulosa cells) becomes stratified with an antrum present, and the epithelium and oocyte are separated from each other by a conspicuous zona pellucida. The fluid-filled spaces between the epithelial cells coalesce to form a single cavity (follicular cavity or antrum) containing follicular

fluid. The connective tissue surrounding the follicular epithelium is organized into a theca externa and theca interna (hormone production), which are separated from the epithelium by a basement membrane.
- **Graafian follicle:** Preovulatory follicle with a large follicular cavity. The oocyte is located on an eccentric hillock, the cumulus oophorus, together with a large aggregation of epithelial cells, the corona radiata (see **e**).
  Note: The graafian follicle is approximately 2 cm in diameter — large enough to create a distinct bulge on the ovarian surface.
- **Ovulation:** The follicle ruptures, and the oocyte is expelled with the cumulus oophorus cells into the peritoneal cavity. Generally the oocyte is caught by the fimbriated end of the fallopian tube. Some spontaneous bleeding occurs into the follicular cavity (see **f**).
- **Corpus luteum:** This is a yellowish structure of very high hormonal activity formed by transformation of the graafian follicle. If the ovum is not fertilized, the corpus luteum involutes and degenerates during the menstrual cycle (becoming the corpus luteum of menstruation). If fertilization takes place, the corpus luteum persists (as the corpus luteum of pregnancy) during the first trimester in response to hormonal stimulation from the zygote, lasting until its hormonal function has been replaced by the placenta (see **g**).

2.39 Pregnancy and Childbirth

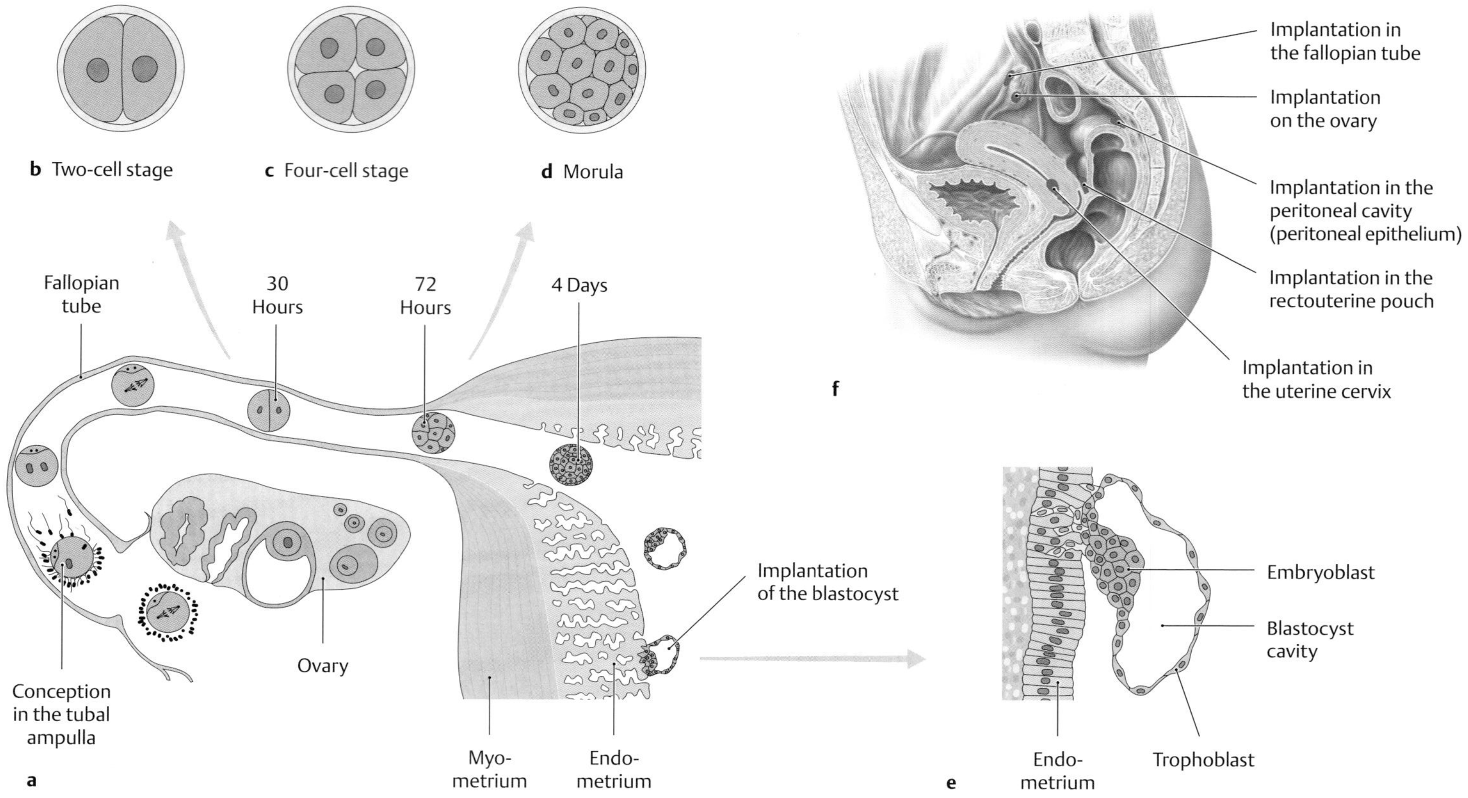

b Two-cell stage   **c** Four-cell stage   **d** Morula

Fallopian tube

30 Hours   72 Hours   4 Days

Conception in the tubal ampulla

Ovary

Myo-metrium   Endo-metrium

Implantation of the blastocyst

Endo-metrium   Trophoblast

Embryoblast

Blastocyst cavity

Implantation in the fallopian tube

Implantation on the ovary

Implantation in the peritoneal cavity (peritoneal epithelium)

Implantation in the rectouterine pouch

Implantation in the uterine cervix

a   **e**   **f**

A Phases in the migration of the fertilized ovum and sites of ectopic pregnancy

a Phases in the migration of the fertilized ovum: Normally the zygote migrates to the uterus. The ovum is fertilized in the fallopian tube, usually in its ampullary portion. Spermatozoa reach that site by a fla-gellating tail action that enables them to swim "upstream" against the flow of the ciliated epithelium (positive rheotaxis)—the same cur-rent that propels the zygote toward the uterine cavity. As it migrates through the fallopian tube, the zygote undergoes various stages of development. On approximately the sixth day after ovulation, the blastocyst implants in the endometrium, which has been prepared by secretory transformation (see close-up in **e**).

b–e show the two- and four-cell stages of development (30 hours), a morula with 16 cells (3 days), and the zygote after implantation (**e**).

f Sites of ectopic pregnancy. Under abnormal conditions, a fertilized ovum may become implanted at various sites outside the uterine cavity:

• at sites close to the uterus (tubal pregnancy) or
• within the peritoneal cavity (abdominal pregnancy).

In a tubal pregnancy (e.g., caused by postinflammatory adhesions of the tubal mucosa that hamper zygote migration), there is a risk of tubal wall rupture due to the close confines of the tubal lumen, possi-bly causing a life-threatening hemorrhage into the peritoneal cavity.

B Levels of the uterus during pregnancy

a Anterior view, **b** left lateral view.

The uterine fundus is palpable at different levels during the various lunar months of pregnancy (lunar month = a 28-day period).

Note: At the start of the 10th lunar month, the uterine fundus turns anteriorly and drops to a level that is slightly lower than in the 9th lunar month.

As term approaches, the greatly enlarged uterus presses against almost all the organs in the abdomen and pelvis. In the supine position the uterus may even compress the inferior vena cava, compromising ve-nous return to the heart. In emergency situations, therefore, a pregnant patient should always be placed in the *left lateral decubitus* position to avoid vascular compression.

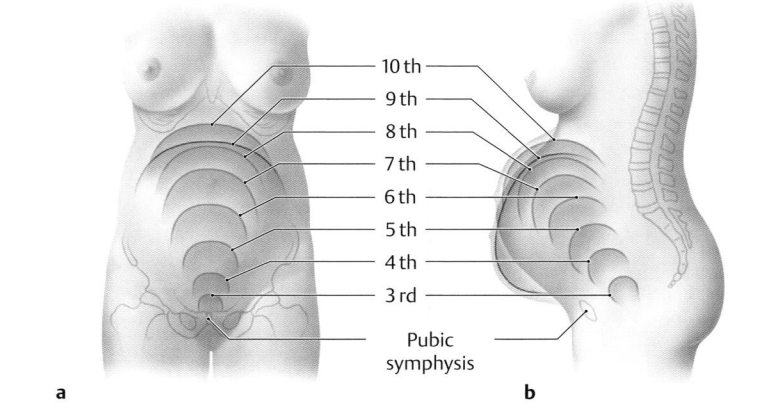

10th
9th
8th
7th
6th
5th
4th
3rd
Pubic symphysis

a   **b**

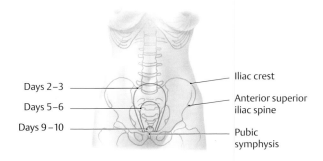

Days 2–3
Days 5–6
Days 9–10

Iliac crest
Anterior superior iliac spine
Pubic symphysis

C Postpartum involution of the uterus

Anterior view. With normal postpartum involution of the uterus, the uterine fundus can be palpated and physically examined at various levels. Three palpable bony landmarks (the iliac crest, anterior superior iliac spine, and pubic symphysis) can be helpful in evaluating the level of the uterine fundus.

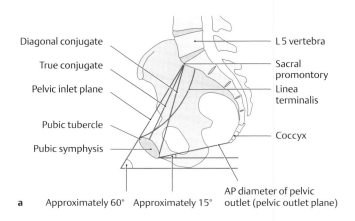

Diagonal conjugate
True conjugate
Pelvic inlet plane
Pubic tubercle
Pubic symphysis

L 5 vertebra
Sacral promontory
Linea terminalis
Coccyx

a Approximately 60° Approximately 15° AP diameter of pelvic outlet (pelvic outlet plane)

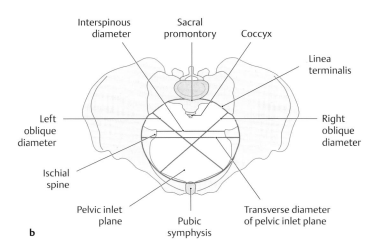

Interspinous diameter
Sacral promontory
Coccyx
Linea terminalis
Left oblique diameter
Right oblique diameter
Ischial spine
Pelvic inlet plane
Pubic symphysis
Transverse diameter of pelvic inlet plane

b

D Important obstetric pelvic dimensions: pelvic planes

a Midsagittal section of the female pelvis, viewed from the left side
b Superior view of a female pelvis.

During parturition, the fetus passes through various planes of the maternal pelvis. The pelvic dimensions of greatest clinical importance are sagittal (smallest anteroposterior diameter). The pelvis has its smallest

sagittal diameter at the "true conjugate," which is the shortest distance from the posterior surface of the pubic symphysis to the sacral promontory. That distance should be at least 11 cm; if not, a normal vaginal delivery may be difficult or impossible. The most important fetal dimensions are cranial, particularly the greatest sagittal head diameter. The principal pelvic dimensions are reviewed in **E**.

E Internal dimensions of the female pelvis

Designation	Definition	Length
Conjugate diameter (true conjugate)	Distance between the sacral promontory and the posterior border of the pubic symphysis	11 cm
Diagonal conjugate	Distance between the sacral promontory and the inferior border of the pubic symphysis	12.5–13 cm
AP diameter of pelvic outlet plane	Distance between the inferior border of the pubic symphysis and the tip of the coccyx	9 (+2) cm
Transverse diameter of pelvic inlet plane	Longest distance between the lineae terminales	13 cm
Interspinous diameter	Distance between the ischial spines	11 cm
Right (I) and left (II) oblique diameter	Distance between the sacroiliac joint at the level of the linea terminalis and the iliopectineal eminence on the opposite side	12 cm

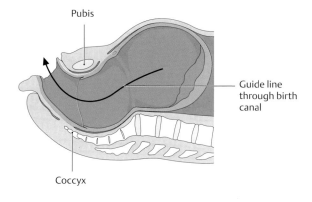

Pubis
Guide line through birth canal
Coccyx

F Birth canal in the expulsion phase of labor

(after Rauber and Kopsch)

The uterine cervix, vagina, and pelvic floor have been stretched open to form a "soft-tissue tube." The fetal head, which always rotates its greatest (sagittal) diameter to match the greatest diameter of the current pelvic plane, follows the line indicated. Most babies are delivered in the "occiput anterior" position, with the occiput pointing toward the pubic symphysis.

2.40 Male Genitalia: Accessory Sex Glands

A Accessory sex glands (prostate, seminal vesicles, and bulbo-urethral glands)

Posterior view of the bladder, prostate, seminal vesicles, and bulbourethral glands. The peritoneum and visceral pelvic fascia have been completely removed; stumps of both ureters and vasa deferentia have been left in place to aid orientation. Each of the **seminal vesicles** consists of a tube approximately 15 cm long that is coiled upon itself to a length of about 5 cm. The secretion from the seminal vesicles makes up approximately 70% of the volume of the ejaculate, is slightly alkaline (pH 7.4), and is very high in fructose (energy source for the spermatozoa). The term "seminal vesicle" is misleading in that the gland does not contain spermatocytes. The excretory duct of the seminal vesicle unites with the vas deferens to form the ejaculatory duct, which passes through the prostate. The seminal vesicles develop from the epithelium of the wolffian duct and are situated lateral to the vas deferens, which also develops from the wolffian duct. The **bulbourethral glands** are embedded in the deep transverse perineal, and their approximately 2- to 4-cm-long ducts open into the posterior aspect of the urethra. The secrete a clear, watery fluid that prepares the urethra for the passage of the sperm. The prostate is described in **B**.

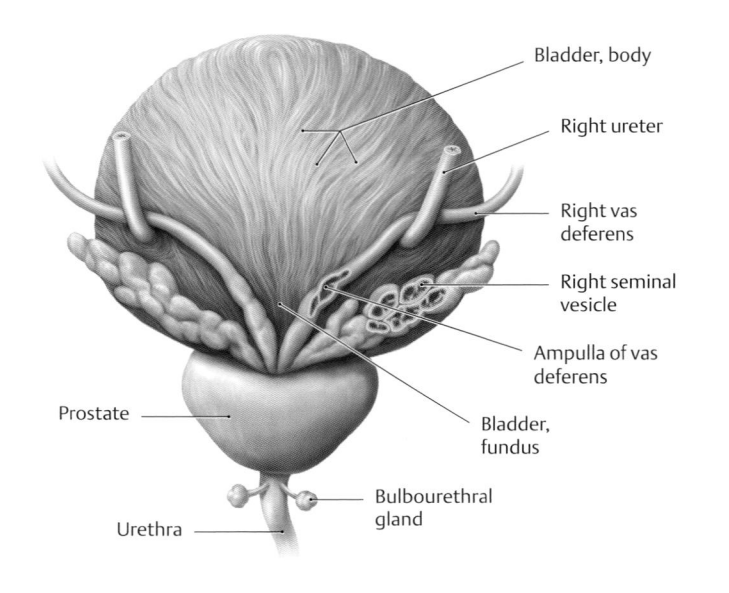

Bladder, body
Right ureter
Right vas deferens
Right seminal vesicle
Ampulla of vas deferens
Bladder, fundus
Bulbourethral gland
Prostate
Urethra

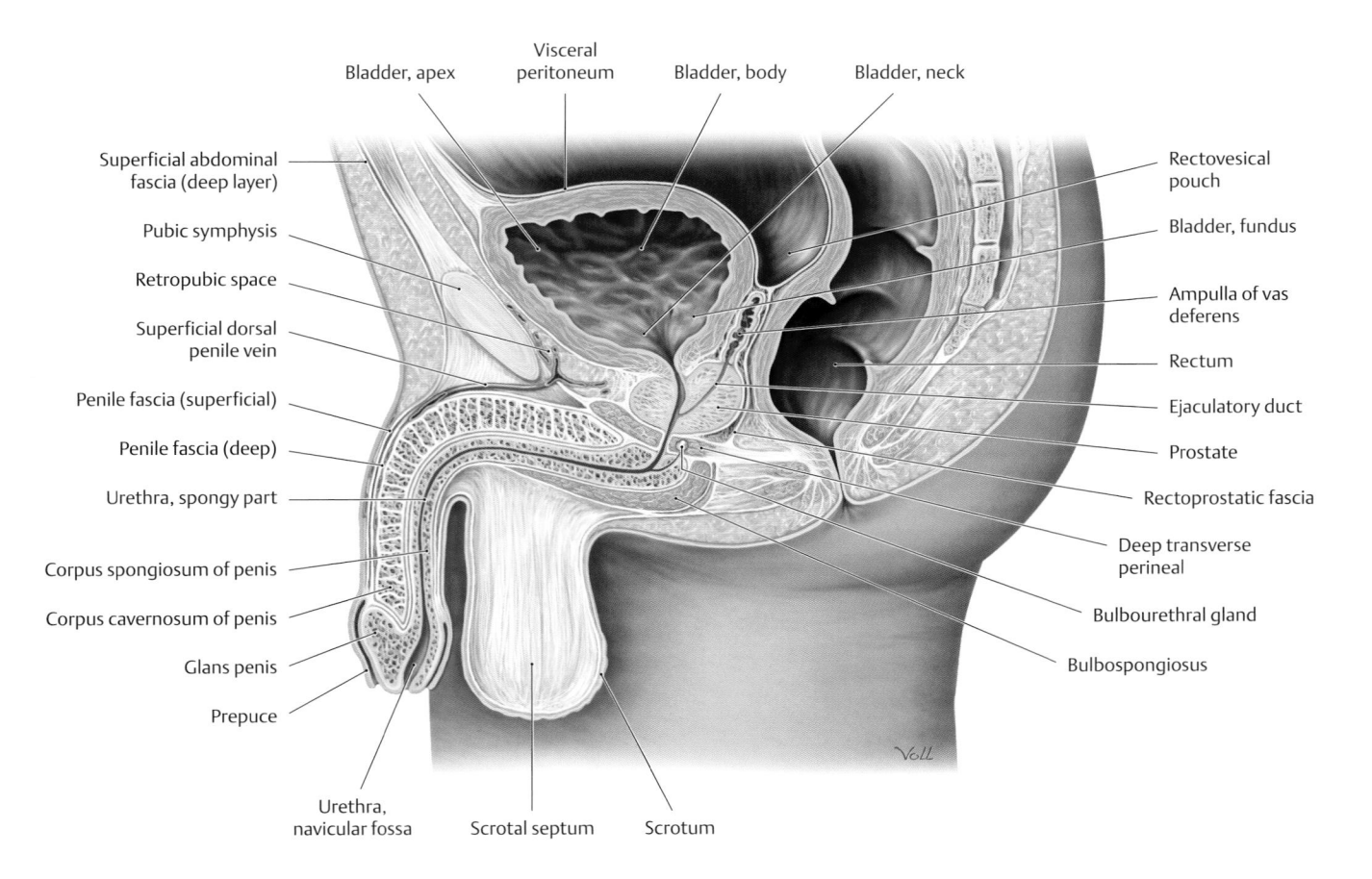

Visceral peritoneum
Bladder, apex
Bladder, body
Bladder, neck
Superficial abdominal fascia (deep layer)
Pubic symphysis
Retropubic space
Superficial dorsal penile vein
Penile fascia (superficial)
Penile fascia (deep)
Urethra, spongy part
Corpus spongiosum of penis
Corpus cavernosum of penis
Glans penis
Prepuce
Rectovesical pouch
Bladder, fundus
Ampulla of vas deferens
Rectum
Ejaculatory duct
Prostate
Rectoprostatic fascia
Deep transverse perineal
Bulbourethral gland
Bulbospongiosus
Urethra, navicular fossa
Scrotal septum
Scrotum

B The prostate in situ

Sagittal section through a male pelvis, viewed from the left side, with the bladder and rectum opened. This drawing is a composite from many planes to demonstrate the peritoneal relationships and the attachment of the seminal vesicle to the prostate and urethra. The paramedian ampulla of the vas deferens has been straightened somewhat and projected into the sectional plane with the ejaculatory duct and left bulbo- urethral gland. The prostate is located at the bladder outlet and encircles the urethra (see **C**). It borders posteriorly on the anterior wall of the rectum, separated from it by connective-tissue fascia. The prostate has no contact with the peritoneum and lies entirely in the pelvic extraperitoneal space. By contrast, the tips of the seminal vesicles are frequently covered by visceral peritoneum.

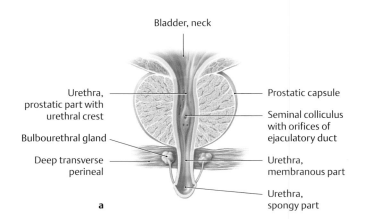

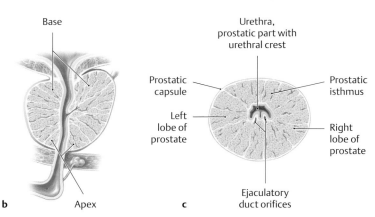

C Relationship of the prostate to the urethra

a Coronal section (anterior view), **b** sagittal section (left lateral view), and **c** transverse section (superior view) through the prostate and urethra.

The prostate is a chestnut-sized gland consisting of two lateral lobes (right and left) that are joined posteriorly by the median lobe and anteriorly by the prostatic isthmus. The entire gland is surrounded by a firm connective-tissue capsule (prostatic capsule). The prostate is a derivative of the urethral epithelium, appearing initially as a poste-

rior epithelial bud that later grows to encircle the urethra (prostatic part). Histologically, the prostate is composed of 30–50 tubuloalveolar glands that open into the prostatic part of the urethra via approximately 20 excretory ducts. The prostatic secretion makes up approximately 30 % of the volume of the ejaculate. It contains compounds that are important for active sperm motility. The secretion is colorless, watery, and slightly acidic (pH 6.4). It also contains a protein (prostate-specific antigen, PSA) whose serum levels are frequently elevated in patients with a prostatic malignancy.

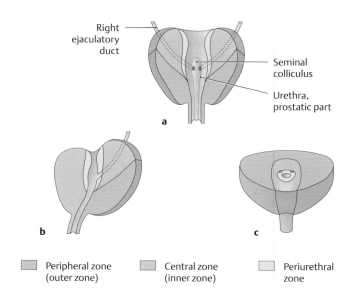

	Peripheral zone (outer zone)		Central zone (inner zone)		Periurethral zone

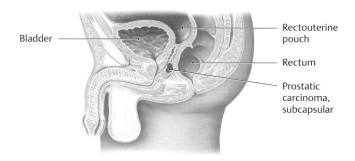

E Typical site of occurrence of prostatic carcinoma

Sagittal section through a male pelvis, viewed from the left side. Prostatic carcinoma is one of the most common malignant tumors in older males. It often grows at a subcapsular location in the peripheral zone of the prostate. Unlike BPH, which begins in the *central* part of the gland, prostatic carcinoma thus does *not* cause urinary outflow obstruction in its early stages. Being in the peripheral zone, however, the tumor is palpable as a firm mass through the anterior wall of the rectum. A digitally guided biopsy needle can be passed into the prostate through the rectal wall to obtain a tissue biopsy for histological examination.

D Clinical and histological division of the prostate into zones

Schematic representation of the prostate viewed in three sections: **a** coronal (anterior view), **b** sagittal (left lateral view), and **c** transverse (anterosuperior view). The ejaculatory duct is also shown for clarity. To aid in describing the location of certain disease processes, the prostate is divided **clinically** into three zones:

- Periurethral zone (the smallest zone)
- Central zone (inner zone, approximately 25 % of prostatic weight)
- Peripheral zone (outer zone, approximately 70 % of prostatic weight)

Histologically, it is not uncommon to add a transitional zone from aglandular to very glandular tissue (lateral to the proximal urethral segment) and an anterior aglandular zone. These zones show different predilections for disease: *Benign prostatic enlargement* (benign prostatic hyperplasia, BPH) most commonly involves the periurethral zone or transitional zone of the prostate, causing obstruction of urinary outflow. *Prostatic carcinoma*, on the other hand, tends to develop in the peripheral zone (see **E**).

F Normal values for the male accessory sex glands

Prostate		Seminal vesicle	
Sagittal diameter	ca. 2–3 cm	Length	
Width	ca. 4 cm	– Coiled	ca. 3–5 cm
Thickness	ca. 1–2 cm	– Uncoiled	ca. 15 cm
Glands	ca. 40 lobules	Secretion	pH 7,4; fructose-rich
Duct system	ca. 20 ducts		
Secretion	pH 6,4; enzyme-rich	**Bulbourethral gland**	
		Size	Pea-sized
Weight	ca. 20 g	Duct length	ca. 4 cm

2.41 Male Genitalia: Scrotum, Testis, and Epididymis

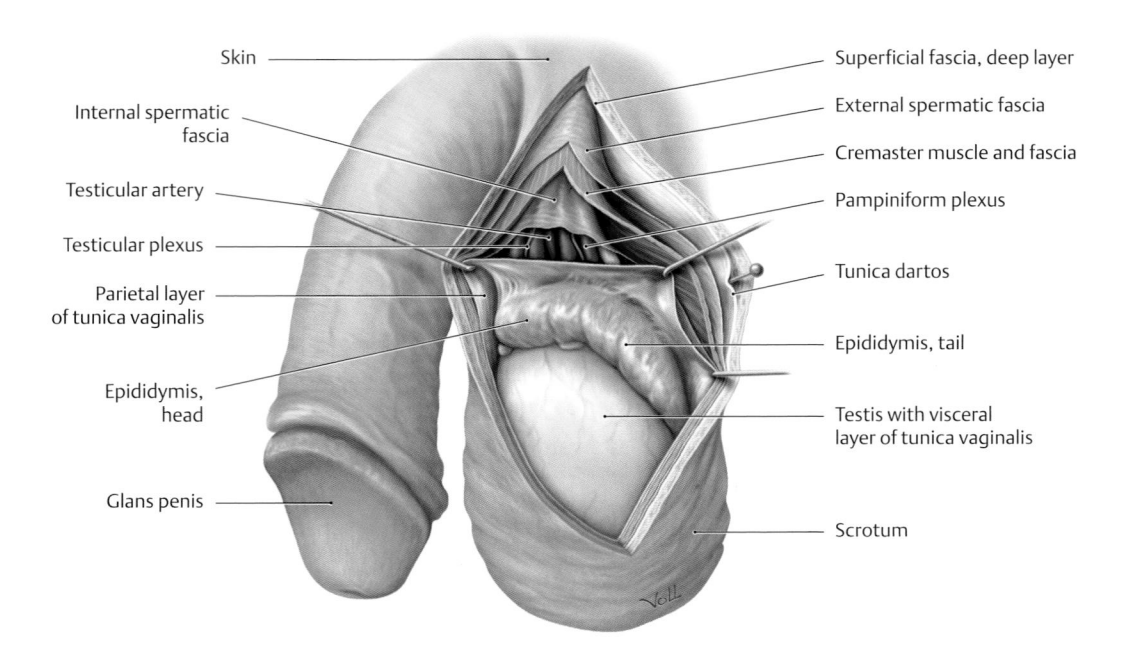

Skin
Internal spermatic fascia
Testicular artery
Testicular plexus
Parietal layer of tunica vaginalis
Epididymis, head
Glans penis

Superficial fascia, deep layer
External spermatic fascia
Cremaster muscle and fascia
Pampiniform plexus
Tunica dartos
Epididymis, tail
Testis with visceral layer of tunica vaginalis
Scrotum

A The scrotum and coverings of the testis in situ
Left lateral view with the scrotum opened in layers. The testis is a paired organ having the approximate size and shape of a plum (see **D**). It is divided by fibrous septa into approximately 350 lobules. The layers of the scrotum and coverings of the testis are formed by the layers of the anterior abdominal wall during the developmental descent of the testis (see **E**). As the testis descends, it carries with it a finger-shaped process of peritoneum (vaginal process) through the inguinal canal; normally this process becomes obliterated and separated from the peritoneal cavity at the internal (deep) inguinal ring. Thus the peritoneum forms a closed sac within the scrotum (tunica vaginalis) composed of a visceral layer and a parietal layer. An abnormal collection of serous fluid in the space between the two peritoneal layers (hydrocele) may exert pressure on the testis, causing clinical complaints. Occasionally, however, the peritoneal process remains patent and gives rise to a congenital indirect inguinal hernia.

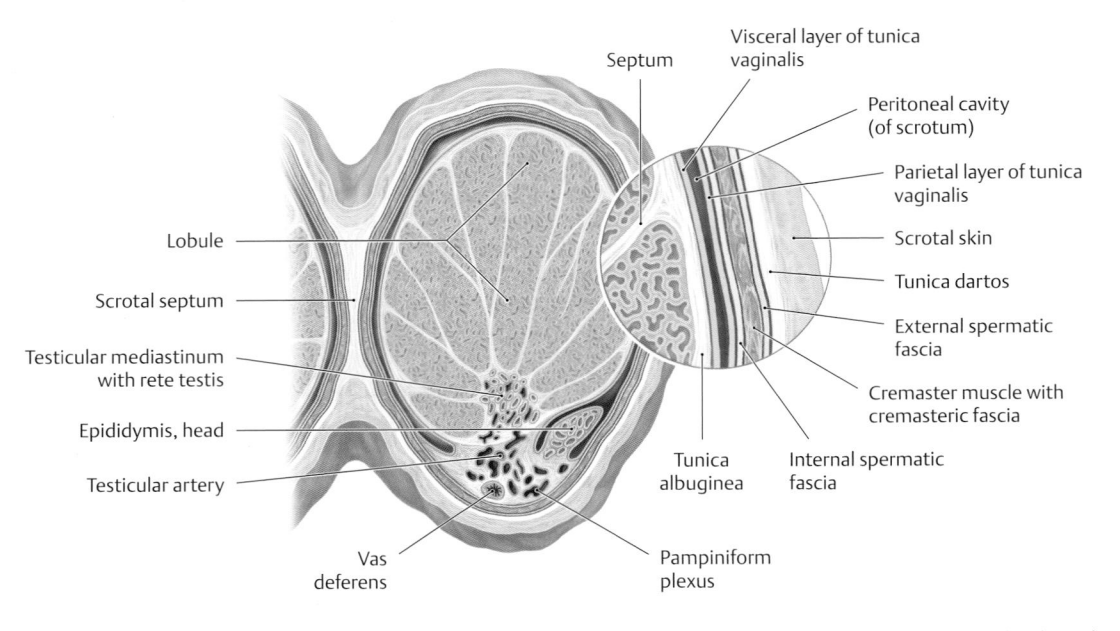

Septum
Visceral layer of tunica vaginalis
Peritoneal cavity (of scrotum)
Parietal layer of tunica vaginalis
Scrotal skin
Tunica dartos
External spermatic fascia
Cremaster muscle with cremasteric fascia
Internal spermatic fascia
Lobule
Scrotal septum
Testicular mediastinum with rete testis
Epididymis, head
Testicular artery
Vas deferens
Tunica albuginea
Pampiniform plexus

B Scrotum and coverings of the testis in cross-section
Transverse section through the right testis, viewed from above. The magnified view shows the various layers that make up the coverings of the testis. The testis is surrounded by a firm fibrous capsule, the tunica albuginea. Fine connective-tissue septa radiate inward from the tunica albuginea to the testicular mediastinum, subdividing the testis into approximately 350–370 lobules that contain the seminiferous tubules (see **C**). The seminiferous tubules are the sites where the spermatocytes develop (spermatogenesis). Groups of cells embedded in the interstitial connective tissue produce testosterone.

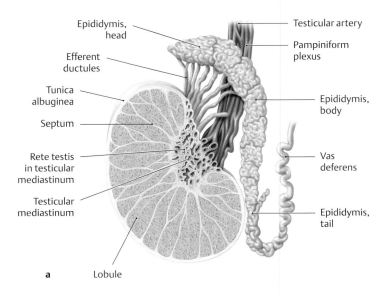

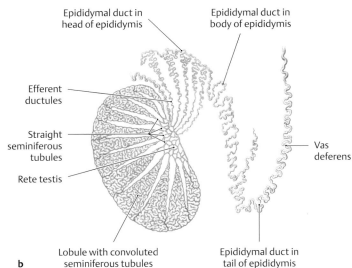

a Lobule

b Lobule with convoluted seminiferous tubules / Epididymal duct in tail of epididymis

C Structure of the testis and epididymis

Left lateral view of the left testis and epididymis. The testis has been sectioned in the sagittal plane, and the epididymis has been elevated from the testis. The wedge-shaped lobules of the testis contain the **seminiferous tubules** (convoluted seminiferous tubules, approximately 3 cm long coiled, 20 cm long uncoiled), where the sperm develop. The tissue between the convoluted seminiferous tubules contains the interstitial (Leydig) cells, which produce androgens, principally testosterone. The convoluted tubules continue into the *straight* seminiferous tubules, which continue into the rete testis, a network of anastomosing epithelium-lined channels. The rete testis is connected to approximately 12 efferent ductules, which open into the epididymis. Attached to the posterior aspect of the testis, the **epididymis** is the organ of storage and maturation for the spermatozoa. The head of the epididymis consists mostly of the efferent ductules, while its body and tail consist of the highly convoluted epididymal duct (approximately 6 m long when unraveled). In the head of the epididymis, the efferent ductules open into the epididymal duct, which is continuous at its caudal end with the vas deferens.

Note: The testis and epididymis lie inside the scrotum and *outside* the abdominal cavity because the temperature within the body cavity is too high for normal spermatogenesis. Thus, failure of the testis to descend normally into the scrotum (i.e., an inguinal testis) is frequently associated with infertility.

The formation and maturation of spermatocytes in the testis, the migration of spermatozoa in the epididymis, and their final storage in the caudal part of the epididymal duct takes approximately 80 days.

D Normal values for the testis and epididymis

Testis		Epididymis	
Weight	ca. 20 g	Length of epididymal duct	
Length	ca. 4 cm	– Uncoiled	ca. 6 m
Width	ca. 2 cm	– Coiled	ca. 6 cm
350–370 testicular lobules			
Approximately 12 efferent ductules			

E Coverings of the testis and layers of the abdominal wall

The inguinal canal is an evagination of the abdominal wall. As a result, the anatomical layers of the abdominal wall have their counterparts in the layers of the scrotum and testicular coverings.

Layers of the abdominal wall	Coverings of the testis
Abdominal skin	Scrotal skin
Superficial fascia	Tunica dartos
External oblique muscle	External spermatic fascia
Internal oblique muscle	Cremaster muscle* and its fascia
Transversus abdominis	(No counterpart)
Transversalis fascia	Internal spermatic fascia
Peritoneum	Tunica vaginalis

Note: the cremaster, like the internal oblique, is striated and receives somatic motor innervation, but is usually not under voluntary control.

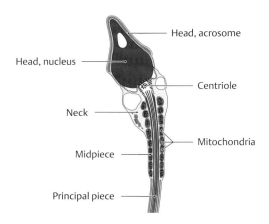

F Ultrastructure of a mature spermatozoon

It takes approximately 80 days for a spermatic stem cell (spermatogonium) to develop into a mature spermatozoon. The spermatogonia are formed in the convoluted seminiferous tubules, while final maturation takes place in the epididymis. The ultrastructural features of the spermatozoon, which is approximately 60 μm long (with tail), include the following:

- The *head* with the acrosome and nucleus
- The *tail* (flagellum), which contains the axonema (axial filament) and consists of several parts:
  - Neck
  - Midpiece
  - Principal piece
  - End piece (not shown here)

259

2.42 Male Genitalia: Seminiferous Structures and Ejaculate

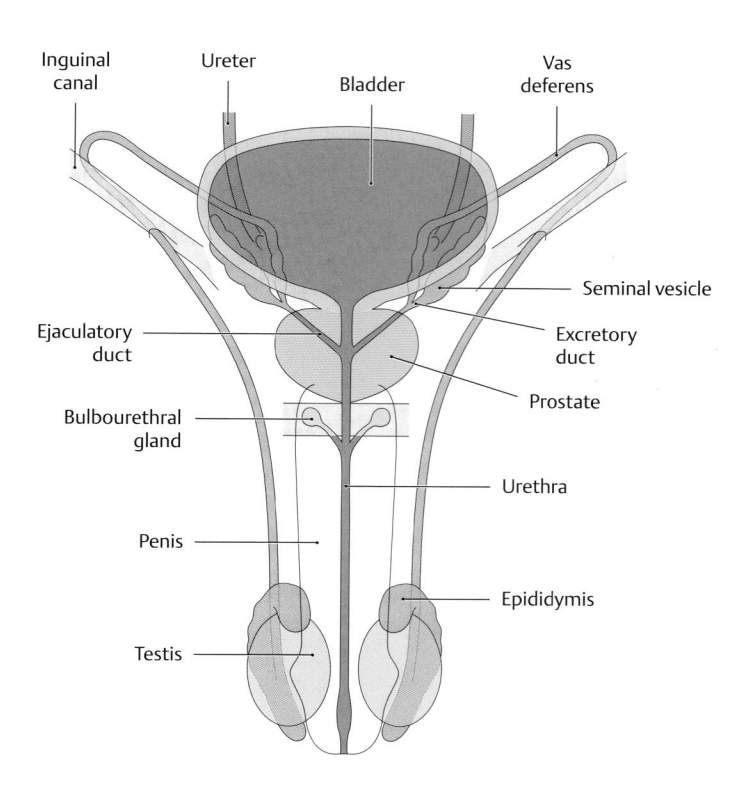

Inguinal canal · Ureter · Bladder · Vas deferens · Seminal vesicle · Ejaculatory duct · Excretory duct · Prostate · Bulbourethral gland · Urethra · Penis · Epididymis · Testis

A Overview of the seminiferous structures

Anterior view of the male reproductive tract. The bladder is also shown to aid orientation.

Note: The male urethra serves as a common urinary and genital passage.

The vas deferens and the duct of the seminal vesicle join to form the ejaculatory duct, which opens into the urethra (see **C**).

C Site of spermatogenesis and pathway of sperm transport

The seminiferous structures in the strict sense consist of the efferent ductules, epididymal duct, and vas deferens.

Testis	• Convoluted seminiferous tubules (spermatogenesis) • Straight seminiferous tubules • Rete testis • Efferent ductules
Epididymis: • Head	• Efferent ductules (open into epididymal duct)
• Body • Tail	• Epididymal duct • Epididymal duct (opens into vas deferens)
Inguinal canal and pelvic cavity	• Vas deferens
Prostate	• Ejaculatory duct (union of vas deferens and duct of seminal vesicle)
Pelvic floor and pelvis (corpus spongiosum)	• Urethra

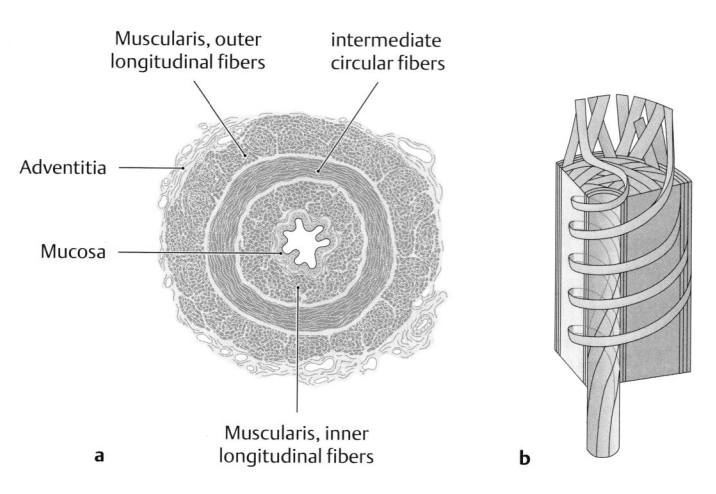

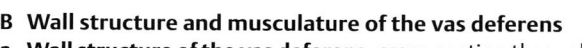

Muscularis, outer longitudinal fibers · intermediate circular fibers · Adventitia · Mucosa · Muscularis, inner longitudinal fibers

a   **b**

B Wall structure and musculature of the vas deferens

a Wall structure of the vas deferens, cross-section through the lumen. The vas deferens (ductus deferens) is approximately 40 cm long and 3 mm in diameter. It arises in continuity with the epididymal duct at the caudal end of the epididymis. Its function is to transport the sperm suspension rapidly toward the urethra during ejaculation. It is equipped for this task with powerful smooth muscle fibers that appear to be arranged in three layers (longitudinal, circular, and longitudinal; see **b**). Facing the lumen of the vas deferens is a simple columnar epithelium. Close to the epididymis the epithelium becomes pseudo stratified, and many cells bear stereocilia (nonmotile cellular projections).

b Musculature of the vas deferens, three-dimensional representation of the muscle fiber pattern (after Rauber and Kopsch). The smooth muscle of the vas deferens appears to have a three-layered arrangement when viewed in cross-section. Actually, however, the muscle fibers are arranged in a continuous pattern that spirals around the duct lumen in turns of varying obliquity. The smooth-muscle fibers of the vas deferens have an extremely rich sympathetic innervation, as ejaculation is triggered by the sympathetic nervous system.

D The ejaculate (normal values and terminology)

The ejaculate consists of spermatozoa and seminal fluid, which comes mainly from the seminal vesicles (approximately 70%) and prostate (approximately 30%).

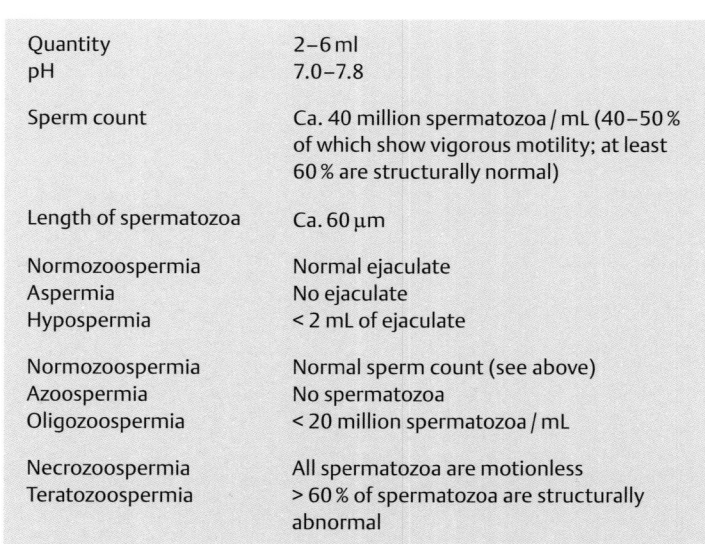

Quantity	2–6 ml
pH	7.0–7.8
Sperm count	Ca. 40 million spermatozoa / mL (40–50% of which show vigorous motility; at least 60% are structurally normal)
Length of spermatozoa	Ca. 60 μm
Normozoospermia Aspermia Hypospermia	Normal ejaculate No ejaculate < 2 mL of ejaculate
Normozoospermia Azoospermia Oligozoospermia	Normal sperm count (see above) No spermatozoa < 20 million spermatozoa / mL
Necrozoospermia Teratozoospermia	All spermatozoa are motionless > 60% of spermatozoa are structurally abnormal

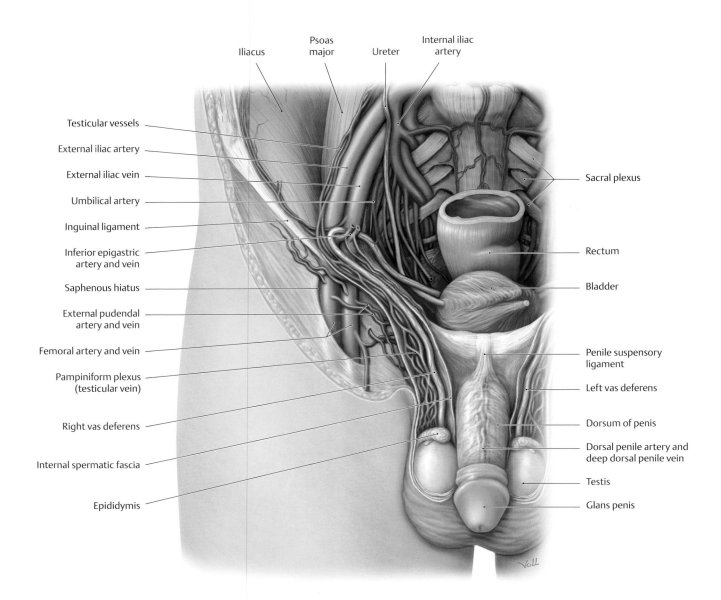

Iliacus · Psoas major · Ureter · Internal iliac artery

Testicular vessels

External iliac artery

External iliac vein

Umbilical artery

Inguinal ligament

Inferior epigastric artery and vein

Saphenous hiatus

External pudendal artery and vein

Femoral artery and vein

Pampiniform plexus (testicular vein)

Right vas deferens

Internal spermatic fascia

Epididymis

Sacral plexus

Rectum

Bladder

Penile suspensory ligament

Left vas deferens

Dorsum of penis

Dorsal penile artery and deep dorsal penile vein

Testis

Glans penis

E The spermatic cord in situ

Anterior view. The inguinal canal has been opened on both sides, and the coverings of the spermatic cord have been opened anteriorly to show the course of the vas deferens. The inguinal canal is markedly larger in the male than in the female due to the presence of the spermatic cord. This larger canal and the larger inguinal ring predispose the male to the herniation of abdominal viscera through the inguinal canal (inguinal hernia).

Note: The vas deferens passes lateral to the inferior epigastric artery and vein. This relationship should be noted in operations on the inguinal ring to avoid vascular injury.

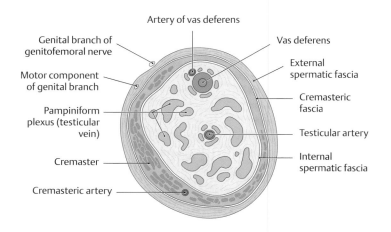

Genital branch of genitofemoral nerve

Motor component of genital branch

Pampiniform plexus (testicular vein)

Cremaster

Cremasteric artery

Artery of vas deferens

Vas deferens

External spermatic fascia

Cremasteric fascia

Testicular artery

Internal spermatic fascia

F Contents of the spermatic cord

Transverse section through the spermatic cord to display the wall layers of the cord and the arrangement of its contents. Even a normally developed venous network (pampiniform plexus) may be affected by abnormal varicose dilation about the testis (varicocele, due for example to a venous outflow obstruction) and may raise the temperature of the testis, leading to decreased fertility.

Note: The pampiniform plexus drains into the testicular vein. The right testicular vein opens into the inferior vena cava, while the left testicular vein runs close to the inferior pole of the kidney and enters the renal vein at almost a 90° angle. Thus, it is more common for varicoceles to develop on the left side than on the right side in response to a condition that obstructs testicular venous flow (mass on the lower renal pole, vein entering at a hemodynamically unfavorable angle).

3.1 Arteries of the Abdomen and Pelvis

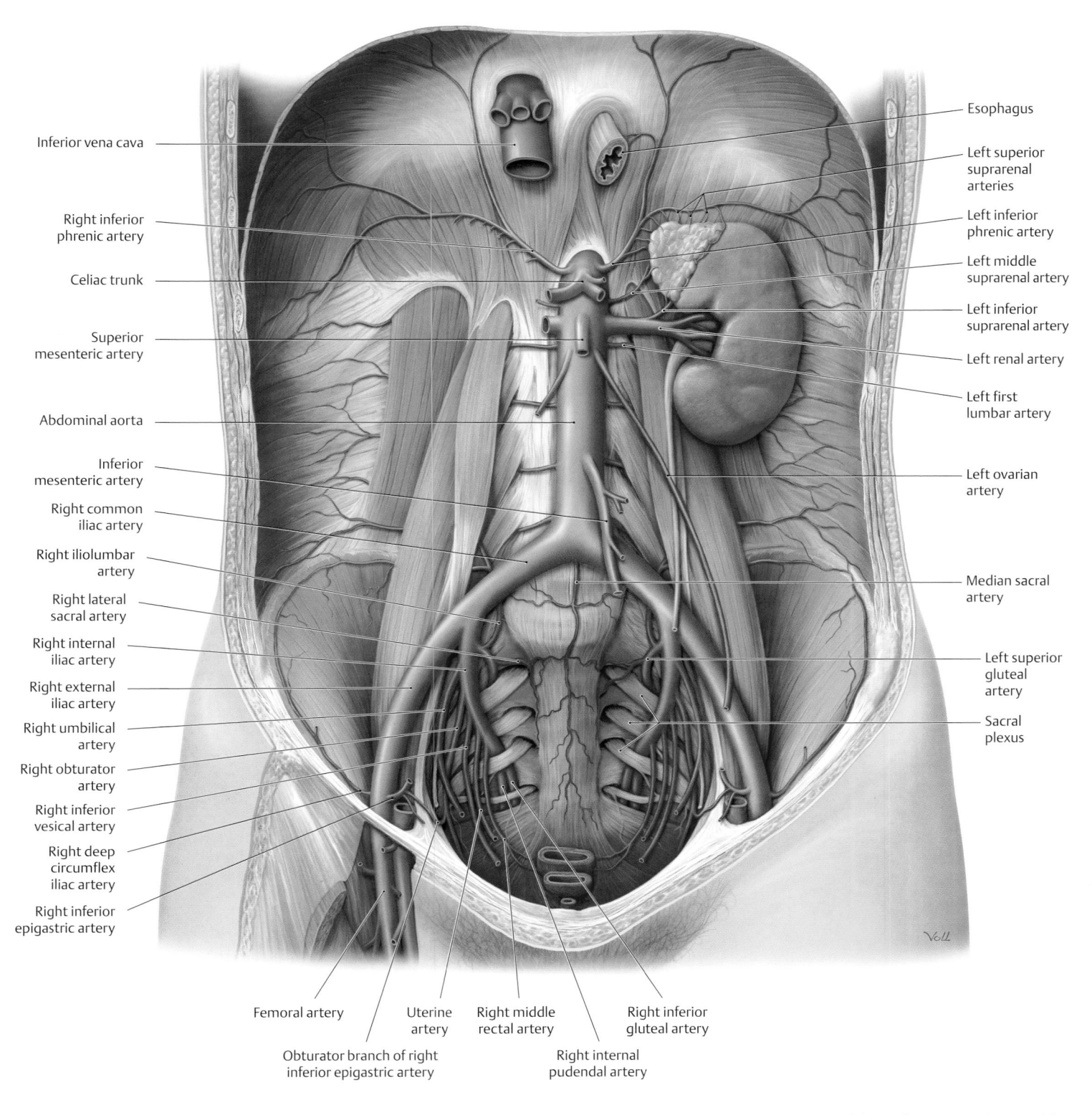

Inferior vena cava

Right inferior
phrenic artery

Celiac trunk

Superior
mesenteric artery

Abdominal aorta

Inferior
mesenteric artery

Right common
iliac artery

Right iliolumbar
artery

Right lateral
sacral artery

Right internal
iliac artery

Right external
iliac artery

Right umbilical
artery

Right obturator
artery

Right inferior
vesical artery

Right deep
circumflex
iliac artery

Right inferior
epigastric artery

Esophagus

Left superior
suprarenal
arteries

Left inferior
phrenic artery

Left middle
suprarenal artery

Left inferior
suprarenal artery

Left renal artery

Left first
lumbar artery

Left ovarian
artery

Median sacral
artery

Left superior
gluteal
artery

Sacral
plexus

Femoral artery   Uterine   Right middle   Right inferior
artery   rectal artery   gluteal artery

Obturator branch of right   Right internal
inferior epigastric artery   pudendal artery

A Overview of the abdominal aorta and pelvic arteries (abdominal organs removed)
Anterior view (female pelvis). The esophagus has been pulled slightly inferiorly, and the peritoneum has been completely removed.
The abdominal aorta is the distal continuation of the thoracic aorta. It descends slightly to the left of the midline to approximately the level of

the L 4 vertebra, as shown in **B** (or possibly to the L 5 vertebra in older individuals). There it divides into the paired common iliac arteries (aortic bifurcation). The common iliac arteries divide further into the internal and external iliac arteries. The abdominal aorta (see **C**) and its major branches give origin to various "subbranches" that supply the abdomen and pelvis (see **D**).

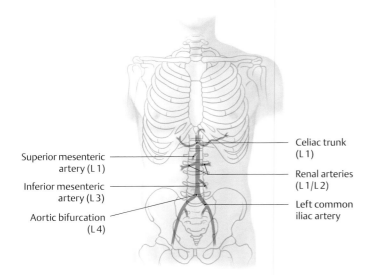

Superior mesenteric
artery (L 1)

Inferior mesenteric
artery (L 3)

Aortic bifurcation
(L 4)

Celiac trunk
(L 1)

Renal arteries
(L 1/L 2)

Left common
iliac artery

**B Projection of the abdominal aorta and its major branches onto
the vertebral column and pelvis**
Anterior view of the five major arterial trunks. The major branches of
the abdominal aorta can be identified in imaging studies based on their
relationship to the vertebrae.

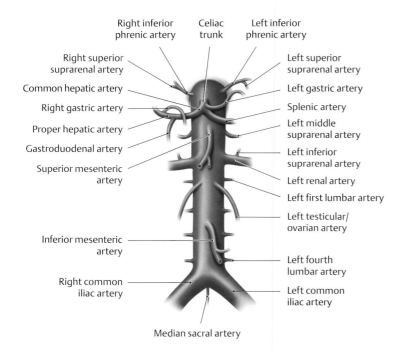

Right inferior
phrenic artery

Celiac
trunk

Left inferior
phrenic artery

Right superior
suprarenal artery

Common hepatic artery

Right gastric artery

Proper hepatic artery

Gastroduodenal artery

Superior mesenteric
artery

Inferior mesenteric
artery

Right common
iliac artery

Left superior
suprarenal artery

Left gastric artery

Splenic artery

Left middle
suprarenal artery

Left inferior
suprarenal artery

Left renal artery

Left first lumbar artery

Left testicular/
ovarian artery

Left fourth
lumbar artery

Left common
iliac artery

Median sacral artery

C Sequence of branches from the abdominal aorta

D Functional groups of arteries that supply the abdomen and pelvis
The branches of the abdominal aorta and pelvic arteries can be divided
into five broad functional groups (→ = give rise to)

Paired branches (and one unpaired branch) that supply the diaphragm, kidneys, suprarenal glands, posterior abdominal wall, spinal cord, and gonads (see **C**)

- Right and left inferior phrenic arteries
    - → Right and left superior suprarenal arteries
- Right and left middle suprarenal arteries
- Right and left renal arteries
    - → Right and left inferior suprarenal arteries
- Right and left testicular (ovarian) arteries
- Right and left lumbar arteries (first through fourth)
- Median sacral artery (with lowest lumbar arteries)

One unpaired trunk that supplies the liver, gallbladder, pancreas, spleen, stomach, and duodenum (see **C** and p. 265)

- Celiac trunk with
  - Left gastric artery → Esophageal branches
  - Splenic artery → Left gastro-omental artery
    - → Pancreatic branches
    - → Great pancreatic artery
    - → Dorsal pancreatic artery
    - → Posterior gastric artery
  - Common hepatic artery → Proper hepatic artery
    - → Cystic artery
    - → Right gastric artery
    - → Gastroduodenal artery
      - → Supraduodenal branch (inconstant branch of gastroduodenal artery)
      - → Right gastro-omental artery
      - → Duodenal branches
      - → Retroduodenal arteries
      - → Anterior and posterior superior pancreaticoduodenal arteries

One unpaired trunk that supplies the small intestine and large intestine as far as the left colic flexure (see **C**, p. 269)

- Superior mesenteric artery
    - → Inferior pancreaticoduodenal artery
    - → Jejunal arteries
    - → Ileal arteries
    - → Ileocolic artery
    - → Right colic artery
    - → Middle colic artery

One unpaired trunk that supplies the large intestine from the left colic flexure (see **C**, p. 271)

- Inferior mesenteric artery → Left colic artery
    - → Sigmoid arteries
    - → Superior rectal artery

One indirect (see below) paired trunk that supplies the pelvis (see **A**)

- Internal iliac artery (from the common iliac artery, not directly from the aorta, hence an "indirect paired trunk") with branches that supply:
    - → Umbilical artery
      - → Superior vesical artery
    - → Inferior vesical artery
    - → Uterine artery (or artery of vas deferens)
    - → Middle rectal artery
    - → Internal pudendal artery

The pelvic walls (parietal branches)
- → Iliolumbar artery
- → Lateral sacral artery
- → Obturator artery
- → Superior and inferior gluteal arteries

3.2 Branches of the Celiac Trunk: Arteries Supplying the Stomach, Liver, and Gallbladder

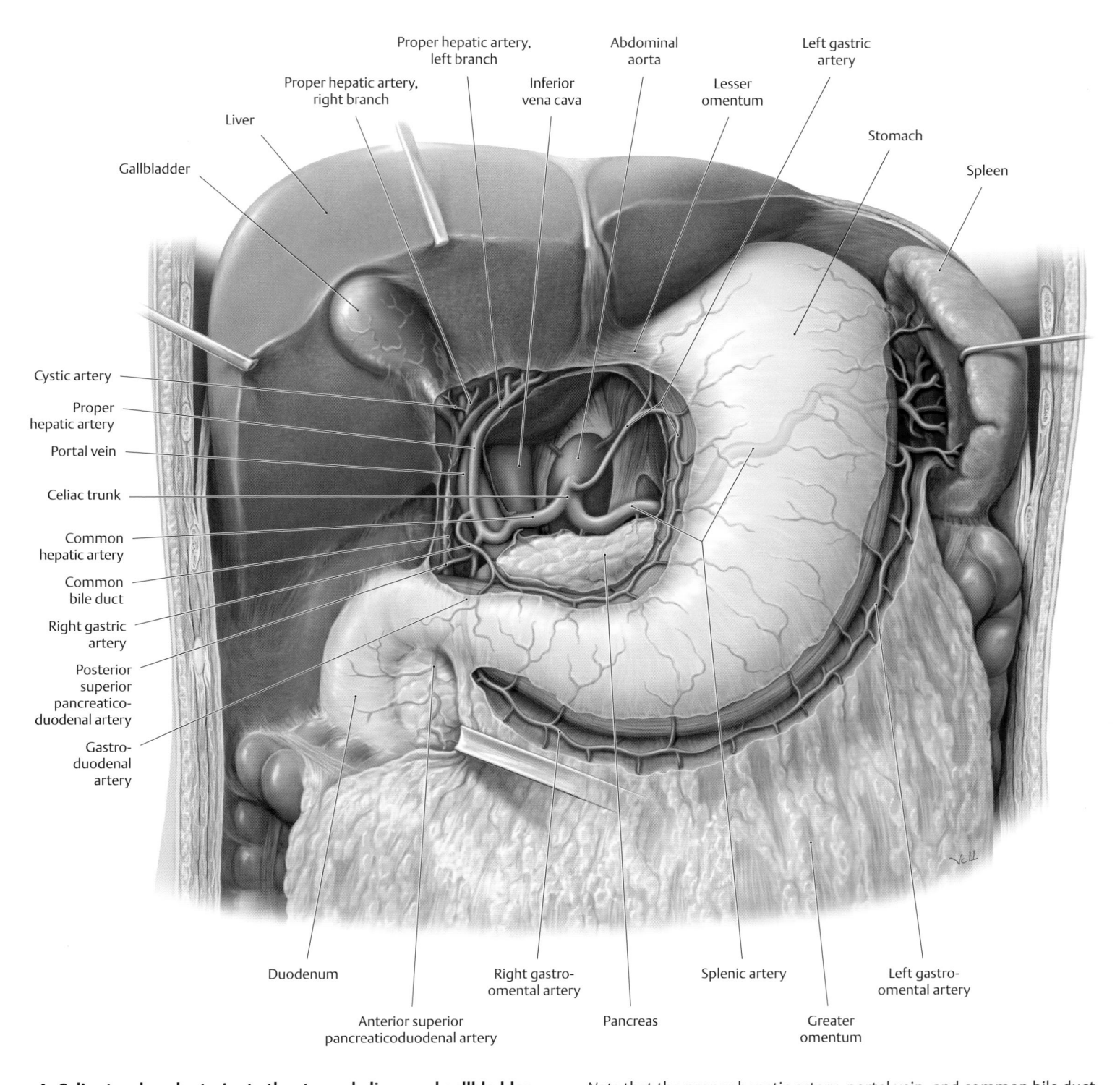

A Celiac trunk and arteries to the stomach, liver, and gallbladder
Anterior view. The lesser omentum (see p. 183) has been opened to display the celiac trunk. The greater omentum (see pp. 156 and 183) has been incised to demonstrate the gastro-omental arteries.
The celiac trunk is the first anterior visceral branch of the abdominal aorta. It is only about 1 cm long. In 25% of cases it divides into three arterial branches in a tripod-like configuration, as illustrated here. The principal variants of the celiac trunk are shown in **C**.

Note that the proper hepatic artery, portal vein, and common bile duct reach the liver by passing through the hepatoduodenal ligament, which is part of the lesser omentum. These vessels must be protected in surgical operations on the gallbladder and bile duct.

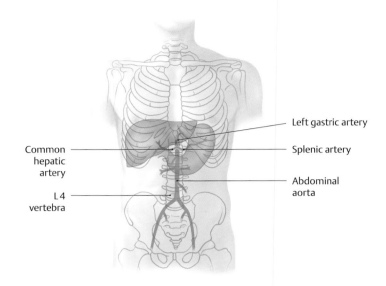

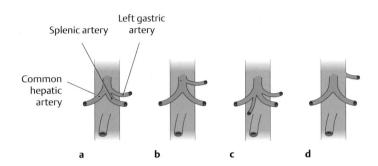

B Projection of the celiac trunk onto the vertebral column (T 12) and its relationship to the liver and stomach

C Variants of the celiac trunk (after Lippert and Pabst)
a The common hepatic artery, left gastric artery, and splenic artery have a common origin (approximately 25 % of cases).
b The celiac trunk divides into the left gastric artery and hepatosplenic artery (approximately 50 % of cases).
c The celiac trunk gives off a fourth branch to the pancreas (approximately 10 % of cases).
d The left gastric artery branches directly from the abdominal aorta (approximately 5 % of cases). All other variants have an incidence less than 5 %.

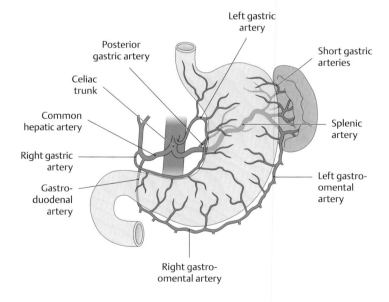

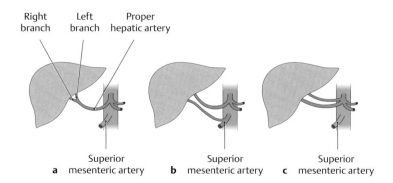

D Arteries of the stomach
Note that the *posterior wall* of the stomach is supplied by the posterior gastric artery, which arises from the splenic artery in 60 % of cases. Variants of the gastric arteries do occur, but for simplicity they are not illustrated here.

E Variants in the arterial supply to the liver (after Lippert and Pabst)
a Typical division of the proper hepatic artery into a right and left branch (approximately 75 % of cases).
b The right branch arises from the superior mesenteric artery (approximately 10 %).
c Both branches arise separately from the celiac trunk (less than 5 %).

3.3 Branches of the Celiac Trunk: Arteries Supplying the Pancreas, Duodenum, and Spleen

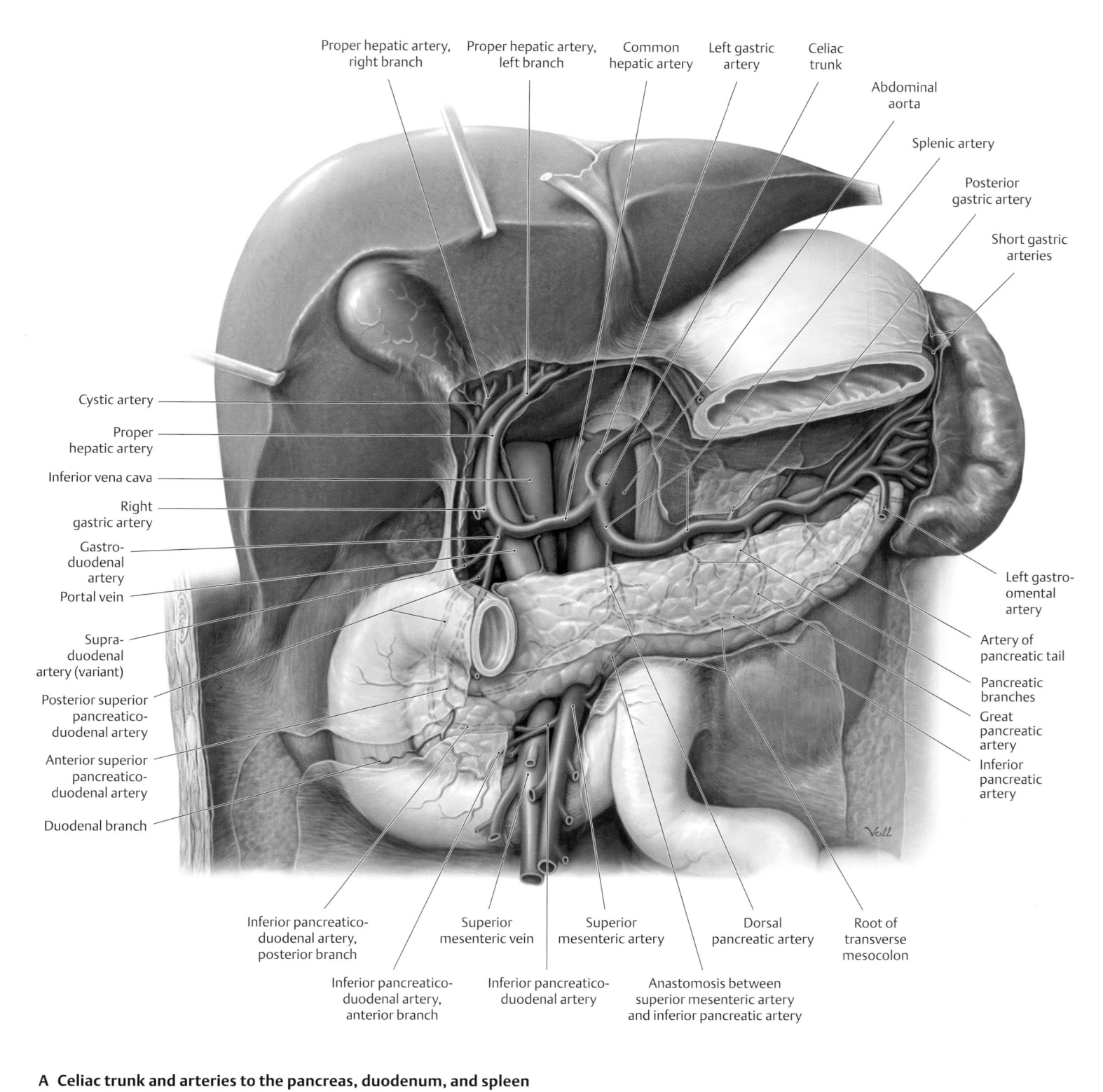

Proper hepatic artery, right branch

Proper hepatic artery, left branch

Common hepatic artery

Left gastric artery

Celiac trunk

Abdominal aorta

Splenic artery

Posterior gastric artery

Short gastric arteries

Cystic artery

Proper hepatic artery

Inferior vena cava

Right gastric artery

Gastro-duodenal artery

Portal vein

Supra-duodenal artery (variant)

Posterior superior pancreatico-duodenal artery

Anterior superior pancreatico-duodenal artery

Duodenal branch

Left gastro-omental artery

Artery of pancreatic tail

Pancreatic branches

Great pancreatic artery

Inferior pancreatic artery

Inferior pancreatico-duodenal artery, posterior branch

Superior mesenteric vein

Superior mesenteric artery

Dorsal pancreatic artery

Root of transverse mesocolon

Inferior pancreatico-duodenal artery, anterior branch

Inferior pancreatico-duodenal artery

Anastomosis between superior mesenteric artery and inferior pancreatic artery

A Celiac trunk and arteries to the pancreas, duodenum, and spleen
Anterior view with the body of the stomach and the lesser omentum removed. The root of the transverse mesocolon extends anterior to the duodenum, pancreas, and the superior mesenteric artery and vein. As a result, tumors of the head of the pancreas may impinge upon the superior mesenteric artery or vein and restrict their blood flow (see **C**).

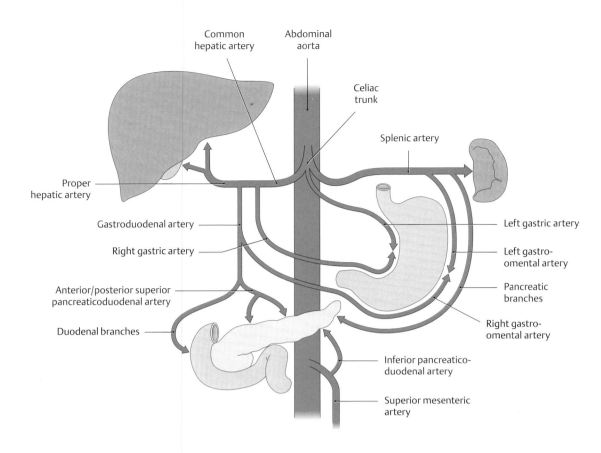

B Schematic overview of the distribution of the celiac trunk
Note: The pancreas is additionally supplied by branches from the superior mesenteric artery.

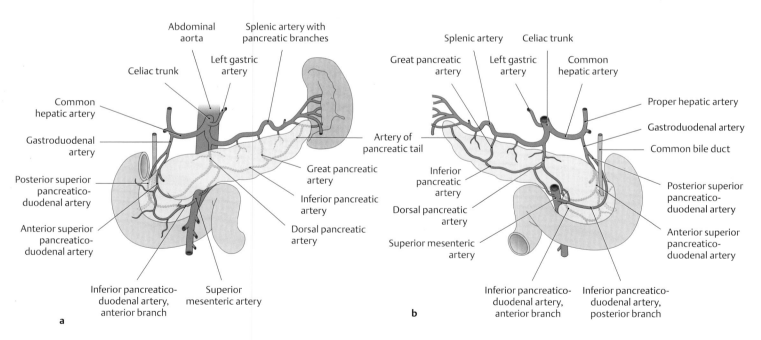

a

b

C Arterial supply to the pancreas

a Anterior view, **b** posterior view. In **b**, the abdominal aorta has been removed to show the origins of the celiac trunk and superior mesenteric artery.

Note that the pancreas is supplied by branches from the celiac trunk as well as branches from the superior mesenteric artery. The superior and inferior arteries that supply the pancreas are arranged in an anastomosing system called the "pancreatic arcade." The largest of the anastomoses between the splenic artery and inferior pancreatic artery is called the great pancreatic artery.

3.4 Branches of the Superior Mesenteric Artery: Arteries Supplying the Pancreas, Small Intestine, and Large Intestine

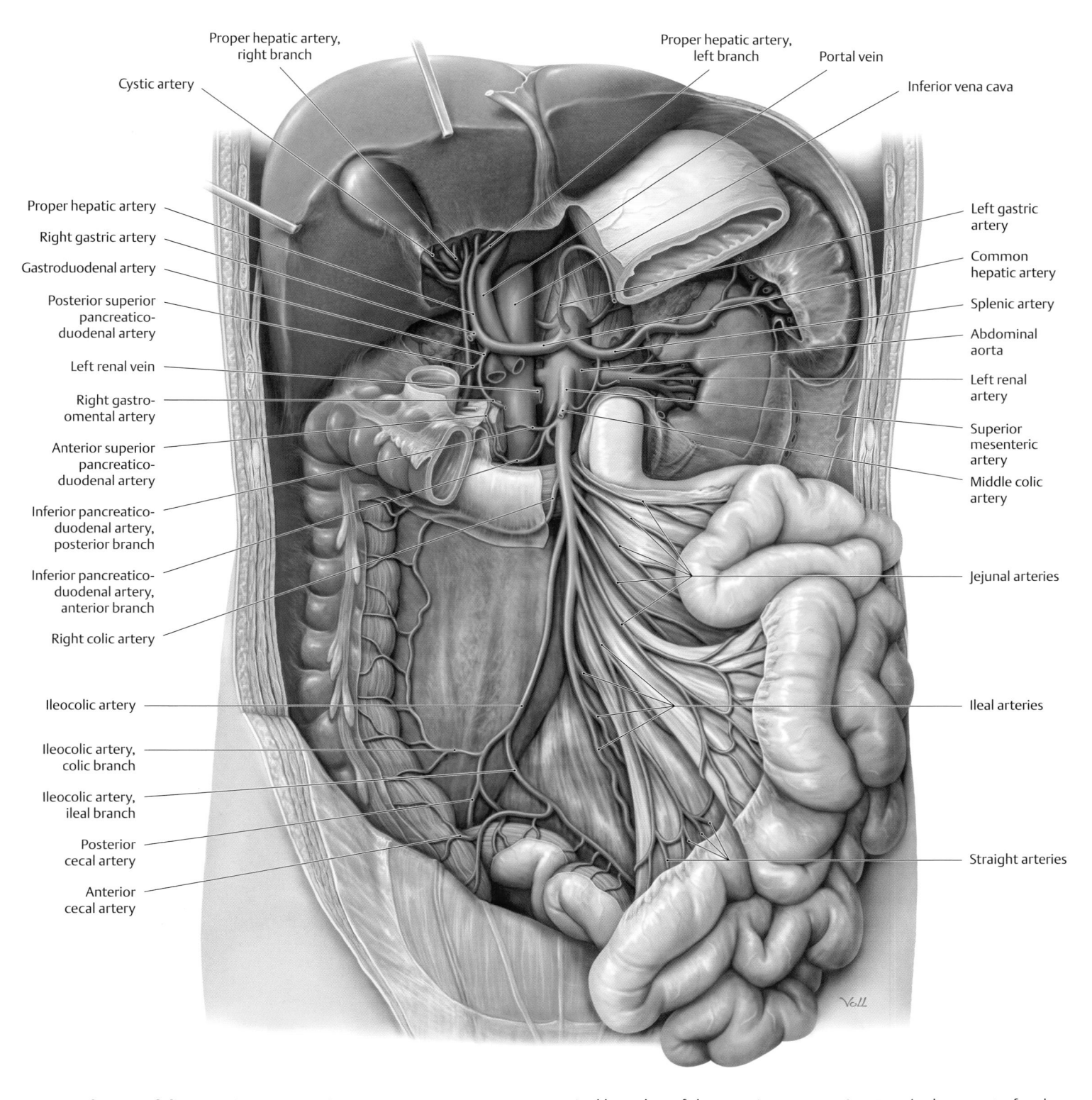

Proper hepatic artery, right branch

Cystic artery

Proper hepatic artery, left branch

Portal vein

Inferior vena cava

Proper hepatic artery

Right gastric artery

Gastroduodenal artery

Posterior superior pancreatico-duodenal artery

Left renal vein

Right gastro-omental artery

Anterior superior pancreatico-duodenal artery

Inferior pancreatico-duodenal artery, posterior branch

Inferior pancreatico-duodenal artery, anterior branch

Right colic artery

Ileocolic artery

Ileocolic artery, colic branch

Ileocolic artery, ileal branch

Posterior cecal artery

Anterior cecal artery

Left gastric artery

Common hepatic artery

Splenic artery

Abdominal aorta

Left renal artery

Superior mesenteric artery

Middle colic artery

Jejunal arteries

Ileal arteries

Straight arteries

Voll

A Distribution of the superior mesenteric artery

Anterior view. For clarity, the stomach and peritoneum have been partially removed or windowed, leaving intact most of the retroperitoneal connective tissue below the transverse colon.

The superior mesenteric artery arises from the front of the abdominal aorta at the level of the first lumbar (L 1) vertebra. It passes anteriorly and inferiorly, distributing most its numerous branches to the right side. Thus, it is clearly accessible to inspection and dissection only when the loops of small intestine are reflected to the left side, as illustrated here. This view also displays the series of arcades formed by the intes-

tinal branches of the superior mesenteric artery (only one set of arches is present along the jejunum, but the arches increase distally and form multiple sets along the ileum). Straight arteries (vasa recta) extend from the arcades to the associated bowel segments. The superior mesenteric artery and its numerous branches supply the small intestine, portions of the pancreas (see p. 267), and a considerable part of the large intestine (see **C**), almost as far as the left colic flexure (not visible here). The trunk of the superior mesenteric artery passes over the duodenum and left renal vein (see **D**).

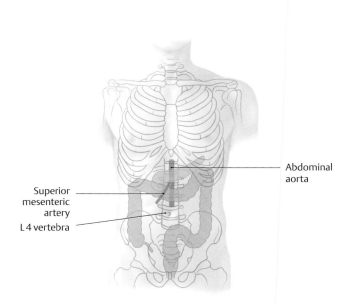

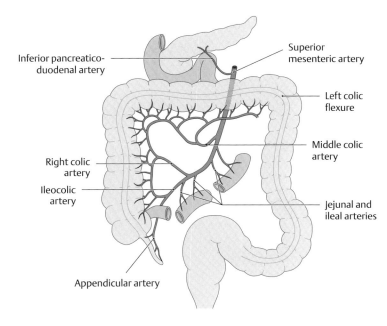

B Projection of the superior mesenteric artery onto the vertebral column and its relationship to the large intestine and pancreas

The superior mesenteric artery arises at the level of the first lumbar vertebra.

C Sequence of branches from the superior mesenteric artery
(see also **E**)

Relationship of the superior mesenteric artery to specific organs. The territory of the superior mesenteric artery ends just proximal to the left colic flexure, at which point the supply by the *inferior* mesenteric artery begins (see pp. 270 and 271). It is common for multiple anastomoses to exist between the two mesenteric systems (see **E** and **F**, p. 271).

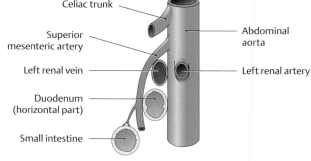

D Relationship of the superior mesenteric artery to the duodenum and left renal vein

Left lateral view.

Note: The superior mesenteric artery descends in front of the duodenum and left renal vein. The left renal vein lies within the aorticomesenteric angle, where it may become entrapped and compressed (see p. 272).

E Branches of the superior mesenteric artery, listed in the sequence of the organs they supply

- Inferior pancreaticoduodenal artery
- Jejunal and ileal arteries (approximately 14–20)
- Ileocolic artery with anterior and posterior cecal arteries and appendicular artery
- Right colic artery
- Middle colic artery

The arteries to the small and large intestine form numerous arcades from which small straight arteries (vasa recta) pass through the mesentery to supply the various parts of the intestine.

3.5 Branches of the Inferior Mesenteric Artery: Arteries Supplying the Large Intestine

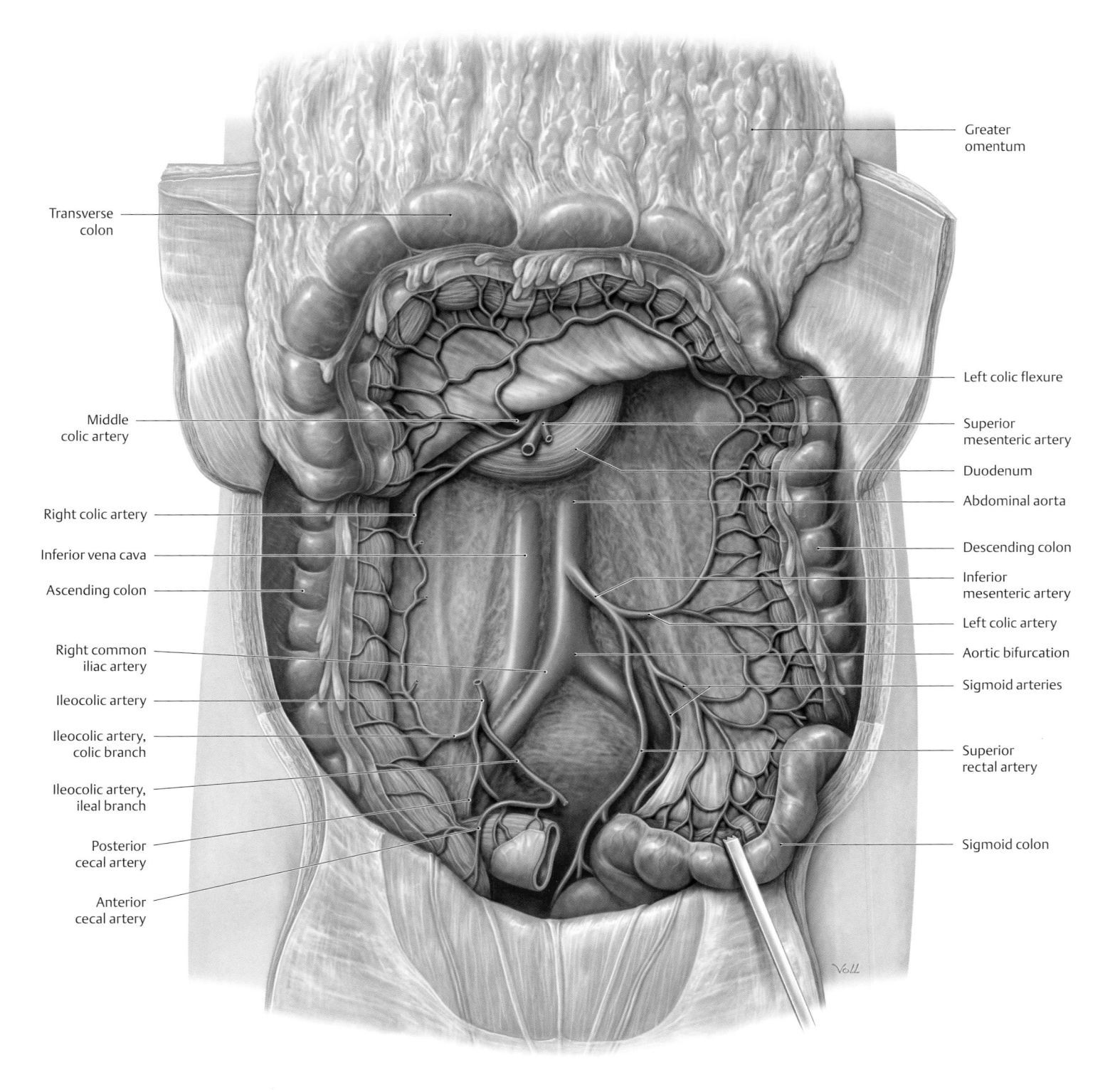

Greater
omentum

Transverse
colon

Left colic flexure

Middle
colic artery

Superior
mesenteric artery

Duodenum

Right colic artery

Abdominal aorta

Inferior vena cava

Descending colon

Ascending colon

Inferior
mesenteric artery

Left colic artery

Right common
iliac artery

Aortic bifurcation

Ileocolic artery

Sigmoid arteries

Ileocolic artery,
colic branch

Superior
rectal artery

Ileocolic artery,
ileal branch

Posterior
cecal artery

Sigmoid colon

Anterior
cecal artery

A Arterial supply to the large intestine from the superior and inferior mesenteric arteries

Anterior view. The jejunum and most of the ileum have been removed, and the transverse colon (see p. 193) has been reflected superiorly. The peritoneum has been windowed or removed at several sites, leaving part of the retroperitoneal connective tissue in place.

The inferior mesenteric artery arises from the abdominal aorta at the 3 level (see **B**) and descends toward the left side. Thus, it is clearly accessible to inspection and dissection only when the loops of small intestine are reflected to the right side (bowel loops have been removed here). This view also displays the numerous sets of arcades formed by the branches of the inferior mesenteric artery. This artery supplies the distal portions of the large intestine, starting approximately at the left colic flexure.

Note: The rectum is supplied by three arteries (see **D**), only one of which, the superior rectal artery, is visible in this dissection.

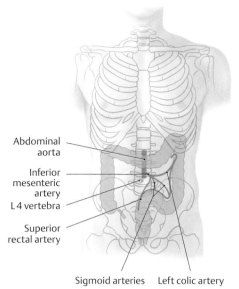

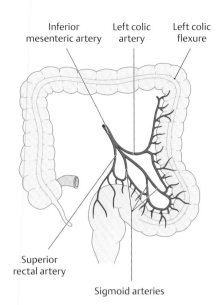

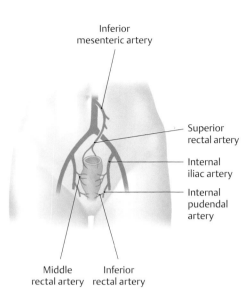

B Projection of the inferior mesenteric artery onto the vertebral column and its relationship to the large intestine

The inferior mesenteric artery branches from the abdominal aorta at the level of the L 3 vertebrae.

C Sequence of branches from the inferior mesenteric artery (see also **D**, p. 263)

Left colic artery, sigmoid arteries (two or three), superior rectal artery.

Note that the left colic flexure marks the approximate boundary between the blood supply by the superior and inferior mesenteric arteries.

D Contribution of the inferior mesenteric artery to the rectal blood supply

The rectum is supplied by three different arteries or branches (see p. 288):

- The inferior mesenteric artery (or its branch, the superior rectal artery)
- The middle rectal artery (directly)
- The internal pudendal artery (or its branch, the inferior rectal artery)

The inferior mesenteric artery supplies most of the rectum from above, while the other two arteries supply the smaller, lower portions of the rectum.

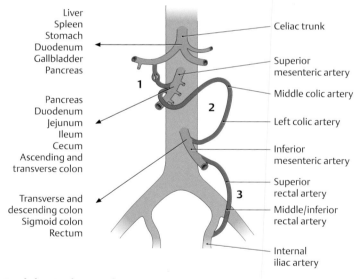

E Abdominal arterial anastomoses

1 Between the celiac trunk and superior mesenteric artery via the pancreaticoduodenal arteries
2 Between the superior and inferior mesenteric arteries (middle and left colic arteries; Riolan and Drummond anastomoses, see **F**);
3 Between the inferior mesenteric artery and internal iliac artery (superior rectal artery and middle or inferior rectal artery)

These anastomoses are important in that they can function as collaterals, delivering blood to intestinal areas that have been deprived of their normal blood supply.

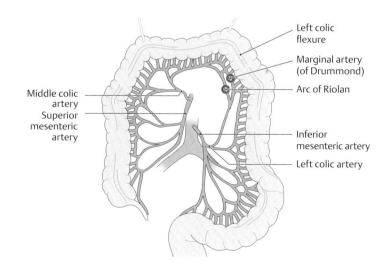

F Anastomoses between the middle and left colic arteries

The anastomoses between these two vessels are located near the left colic flexure and should be noted during operations in this region (vascular ligations). One of these vessels can compensate for decreased blood flow in the other.

3.6 Tributaries of the Inferior Vena Cava

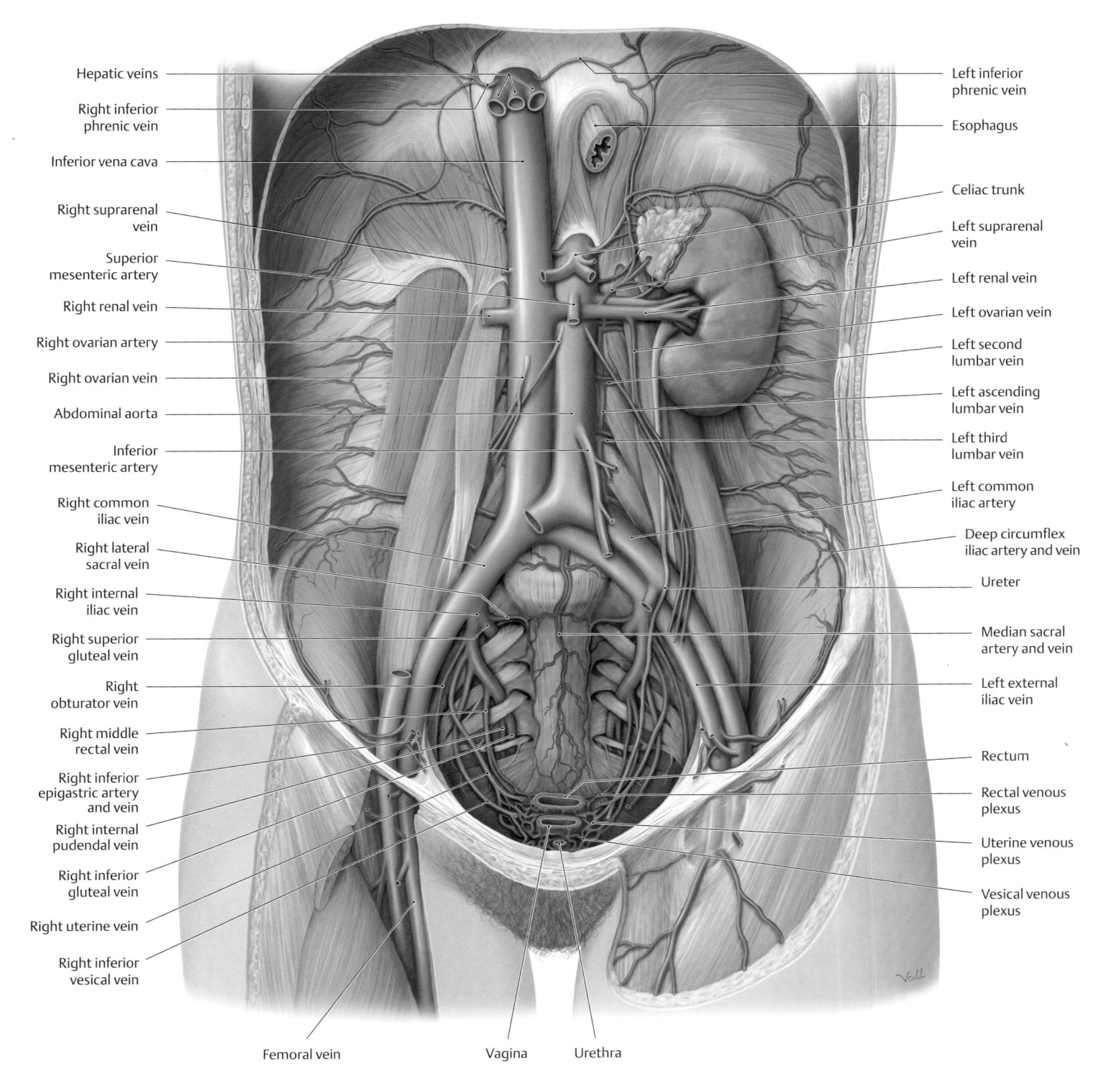

Hepatic veins

Right inferior phrenic vein

Inferior vena cava

Right suprarenal vein

Superior mesenteric artery

Right renal vein

Right ovarian artery

Right ovarian vein

Abdominal aorta

Inferior mesenteric artery

Right common iliac vein

Right lateral sacral vein

Right internal iliac vein

Right superior gluteal vein

Right obturator vein

Right middle rectal vein

Right inferior epigastric artery and vein

Right internal pudendal vein

Right inferior gluteal vein

Right uterine vein

Right inferior vesical vein

Left inferior phrenic vein

Esophagus

Celiac trunk

Left suprarenal vein

Left renal vein

Left ovarian vein

Left second lumbar vein

Left ascending lumbar vein

Left third lumbar vein

Left common iliac artery

Deep circumflex iliac artery and vein

Ureter

Median sacral artery and vein

Left external iliac vein

Rectum

Rectal venous plexus

Uterine venous plexus

Vesical venous plexus

Femoral vein   Vagina   Urethra

A Tributaries of the inferior vena cava in the posterior abdomen and pelvis

Anterior view of an opened female abdomen. All organs but the left kidney and suprarenal gland have been removed, and the esophagus has been pulled slightly inferiorly.

The inferior vena cava receives numerous tributaries that return venous blood from the abdomen and pelvis (and, of course, from the lower limbs), analogous to the distribution of the paired abdominal aortic branches in this region. The inferior vena cava is formed by the union of the two common iliac veins at the approximate level of the L 5 vertebra (see **C**), behind and slightly inferior to the aortic bifurcation.

Note the special location of the left renal vein and its risk of compression by the superior mesenteric artery (see p. 269): The left renal vein passes in front of the abdominal aorta but behind the superior mesenteric artery. Veins in the male pelvis are described on p. 286.

The veins in the pelvis have numerous variants. For example, the tributaries of the internal iliac vein are frequently multiple (unlike those shown above) but unite to form a single trunk before entering the iliac vein (see also p. 287).

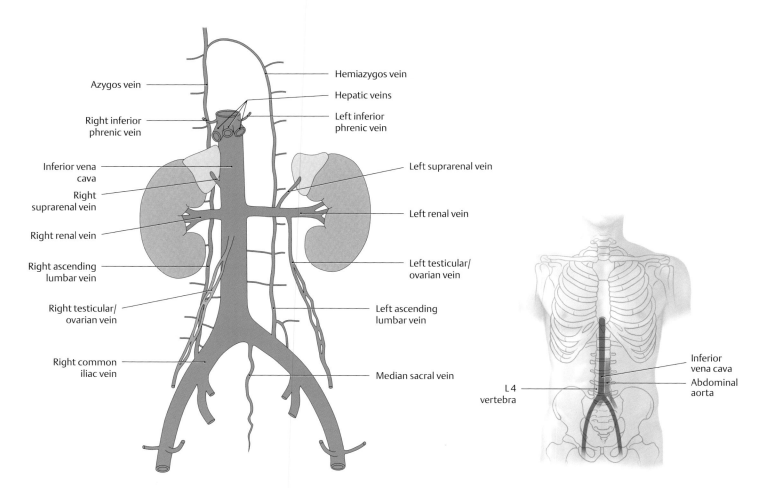

B Tributaries of the inferior vena cava
The difference in the venous drainage of the right and left kidneys is displayed more clearly here than in **A**. The continuity of the right ascending lumbar vein with the azygos vein is also shown.

Direct tributaries return venous blood directly to the inferior vena cava without passing through an intervening capillary bed. Direct tributaries drain the following organs:

- The diaphragm, abdominal wall, kidneys, suprarenal glands, testes / ovaries, and liver
- For the *pelvis* (via the common iliac vein) from: the pelvic wall and floor, uterus, fallopian tubes, bladder, ureters, accessory sex glands, lower rectum, and lower limb

Indirect tributaries return blood that has passed through the capillary bed of the liver via the hepatic portal system (see p. 274). The following organs have indirect tributaries:

- The spleen
- The organs of the digestive tract: pancreas, duodenum, jejunum, ileum, cecum, colon, and upper rectum

Note: Venous blood from the inferior vena cava may drain through the ascending lumbar veins into the azygos or hemiazygos vein and thence to the superior vena cava. Thus a connection between the two venae cavae exists on the posterior wall of the abdomen and thorax: a cavocaval or intercaval anastomosis. The location and significance of cavocaval anastomoses are discussed on p. 292. Frequently an anastomosis exists between the suprarenal vein and inferior phrenic vein (not shown here, see **A**) on the left side of the body.

C Projection of the inferior vena cava onto the vertebral column
The inferior vena cava ascends on the right side of the abdominal aorta and pierces the diaphragm at the vena caval hiatus located at the T 8 level. The common iliac veins unite at the L 5 level to form the inferior vena cava (see also **A**).

D Direct tributaries of the inferior vena cava

- Right and left inferior phrenic veins
- Hepatic veins
- Right suprarenal vein
- Right and left renal veins at the L 1/ L 2 level (the left testicular / ovarian vein and left suprarenal vein terminate in the left renal vein)
- Lumbar veins
- Right testicular / ovarian vein
- Common iliac veins (L 5 level)
- Median sacral vein (often terminates in the left common iliac vein)

3.7 Tributaries of the Portal Vein

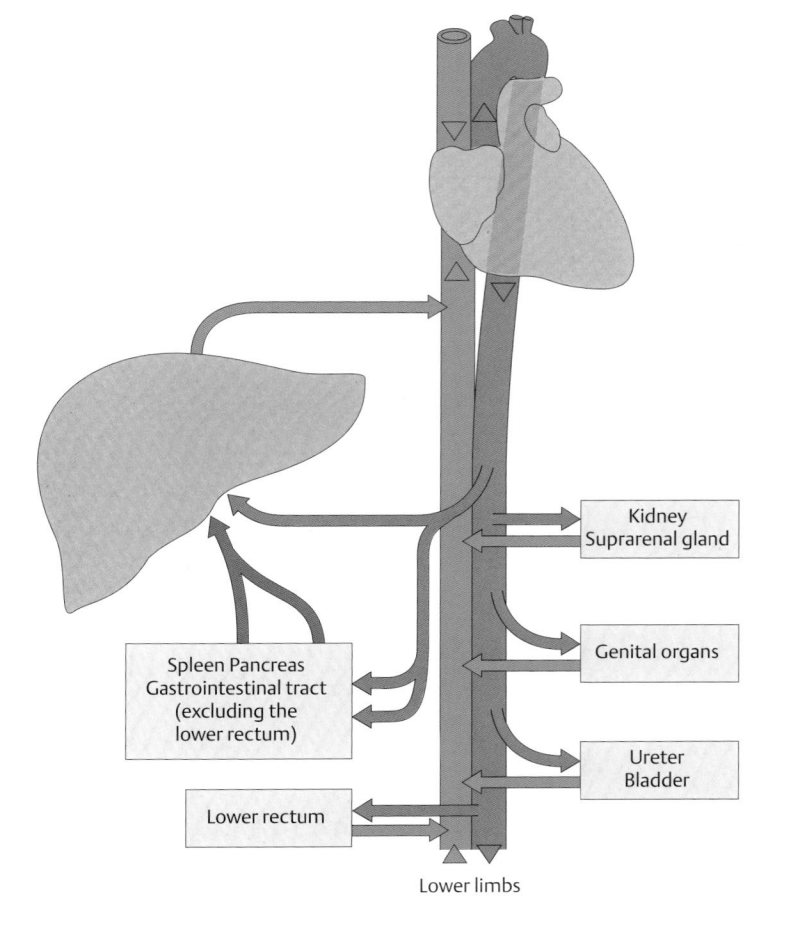

A The portal venous system in the abdomen

The arterial blood supply and venous drainage of the abdominal and pelvic organs differ in their functional organization: While they derive their arterial blood supply entirely from the abdominal aorta or one of its major branches, *venous drainage* is accomplished by one of *two different venous systems*:

1. Organ veins that drain directly or indirectly (via the iliac veins) into the inferior vena cava, which then returns the blood to the right heart (see also p. 272)
2. Organ veins that first drain directly or indirectly (via the mesenteric veins or splenic vein) *into the portal vein* — and thus to the liver — before the blood enters the inferior vena cava and returns to the right heart.

The *first pathway* serves the urinary organs, suprarenal glands, genital organs, and the walls of the abdomen and pelvis. The *second pathway* serves the organs of the digestive system (hollow organs of the gastrointestinal tract, pancreas, gallbladder) and the spleen (see **D**). Only the lower portions of the rectum are exempt from this pathway and drain directly through the iliac veins to the inferior vena cava. This (re)routing of venous blood through the hepatic portal system ensures that the organs of the digestive tract deliver their nutrient-rich blood to the liver for metabolic processing before it is returned to the heart. It also provides a route by which elements of degenerated red blood cells can be conveyed from the spleen to the liver. Thus, the portal vein functions to deliver blood to the liver to support metabolism. This contrasts with the proper hepatic artery, which supplies the liver with oxygen and other nutrients. Anastomoses may develop between the portal venous system and vena caval system (portacaral anastomosis) and function as collateral pathways in certain diseases (see p. 293).

B Projection of the portal vein and its two major tributaries onto the vertebral column

The portal vein of the liver is formed by the union of the *superior* mesenteric vein and splenic vein to the right of the midline at the L 1 level. The *inferior* mesenteric vein typically opens into the splenic vein, also conveying its blood to the portal vein via this route.
Note the relationship of the portal vein to the liver, stomach, and pancreas.

C Tributaries of the portal vein

- **Superior mesenteric vein** (see p. 278) with its tributaries:
  - Pancreaticoduodenal veins
  - Pancreatic veins
  - Right gastro-omental vein
  - Jejunal veins
  - Ileal veins
  - Ileocolic vein
  - Right colic vein
  - Middle colic vein
- **Inferior mesenteric vein** (see p. 279) with its tributaries:
  - Left colic vein
  - Sigmoid veins
  - Superior rectal vein
- **Splenic vein** (see p. 277) with its tributaries:
  - Left gastro-omental vein
  - Pancreatic veins
  - Short gastric veins
- **Direct tributaries** (see pp. 276–279)
  - Cystic vein
  - Left gastric vein with esophageal veins
  - Right gastric vein
  - Posterior superior pancreaticoduodenal vein
  - Prepyloric vein
  - Paraumbilical veins

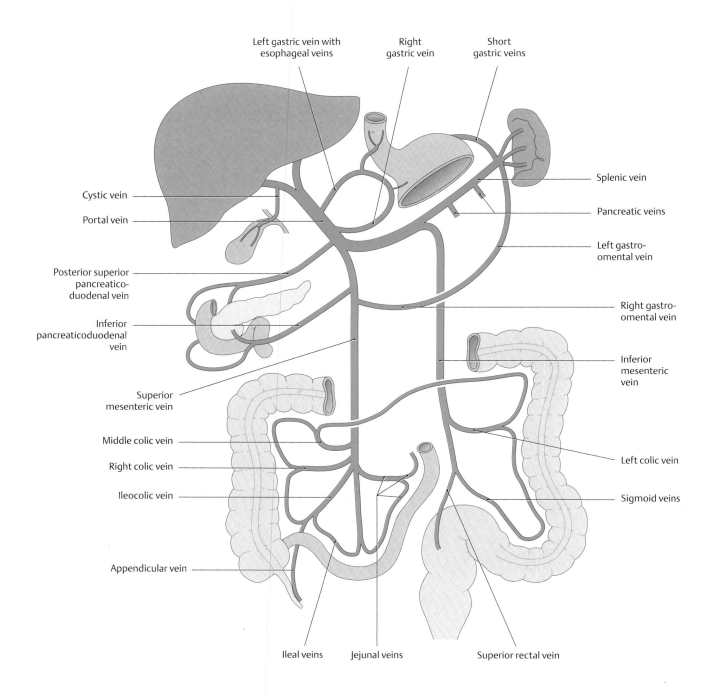

Left gastric vein with esophageal veins

Right gastric vein

Short gastric veins

Cystic vein

Portal vein

Splenic vein

Pancreatic veins

Left gastro-omental vein

Posterior superior pancreatico-duodenal vein

Inferior pancreaticoduodenal vein

Right gastro-omental vein

Inferior mesenteric vein

Superior mesenteric vein

Middle colic vein

Right colic vein

Ileocolic vein

Left colic vein

Sigmoid veins

Appendicular vein

Ileal veins

Jejunal veins

Superior rectal vein

D Distribution of the portal vein (see also **C**)

The portal vein of the liver is a short vessel (total length 6–12 cm) with a large caliber. On entering the liver, it divides into two main branches, one for each of the hepatic lobes. The region drained of the portal vein corresponds to the region supplied by the celiac trunk and the superior and inferior mesenteric arteries. The portal vein receives venous blood from the hollow organs of the gastrointestinal tract (excluding the lower rectum) and from the pancreas, gallbladder, and spleen. Some of this blood flows directly to the portal vein through the corresponding organ veins, and the rest reaches the portal vein indirectly by way of the mesenteric veins or splenic vein.

3.8 Portal Vein: Venous Drainage of the Stomach, Duodenum, Pancreas, and Spleen

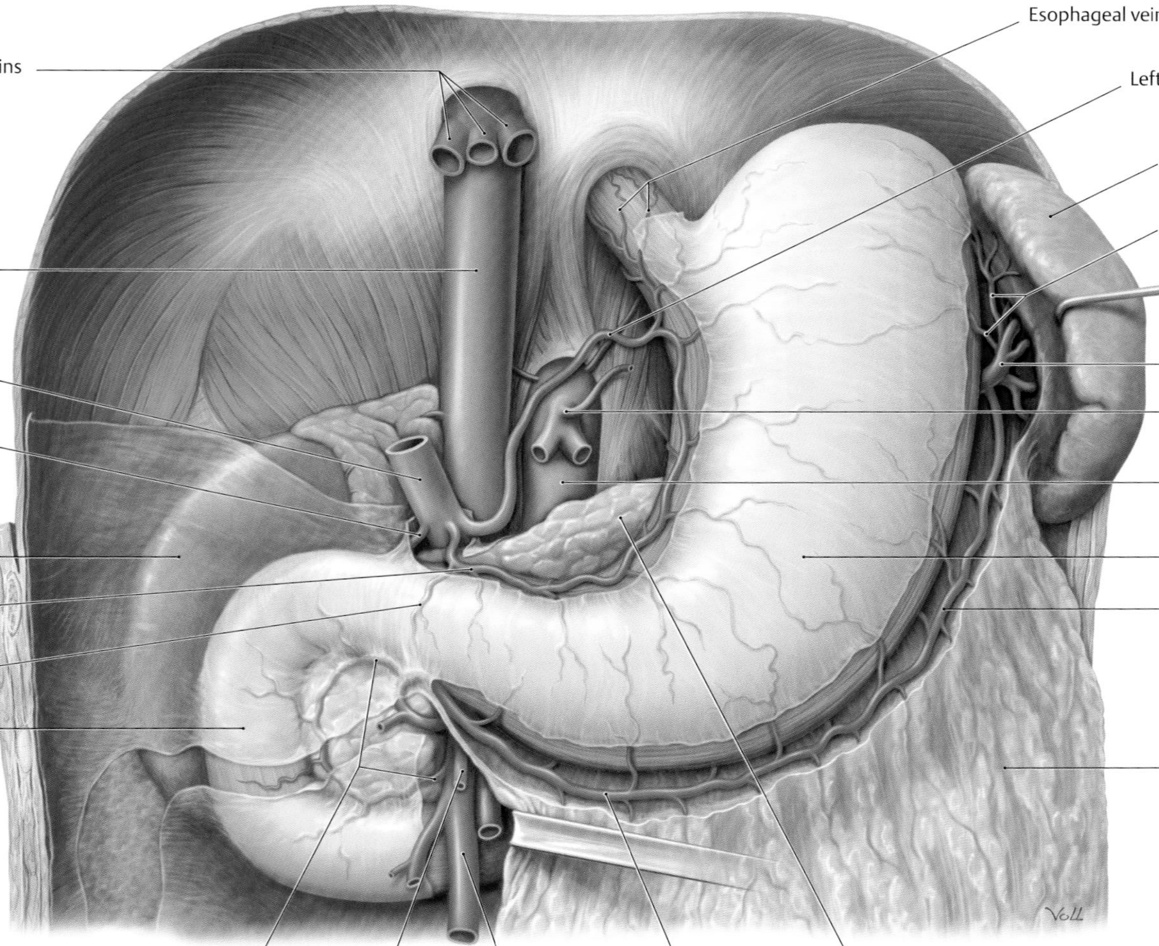

Hepatic veins

Esophageal veins

Left gastric vein

Spleen

Short gastric veins

Inferior vena cava

Portal vein

Posterior superior pancreatico-duodenal vein

Splenic vein

Celiac trunk

Abdominal aorta

Right kidney

Stomach

Right gastric vein

Left gastro-omental vein

Prepyloric vein

Duodenum

Greater omentum

Pancreatico-duodenal vein

Middle colic vein

Superior mesenteric vein

Right gastro-omental vein

Pancreas

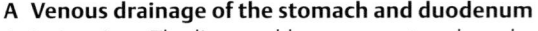

A Venous drainage of the stomach and duodenum

Anterior view. The liver and lesser omentum have been removed, and the greater omentum has been opened and retracted to the left. The stomach has been pulled slightly inferiorly, and the peritoneum has been removed or windowed at several sites to display the termination of the hepatic veins in the inferior vena cava and the communication of the gastric veins with the portal venous system.

Blood from the *lesser curvature of the stomach* generally flows directly into the portal vein, while blood from the *greater curvature* reaches the portal vein by way of the splenic vein and superior mesenteric vein. The lower portions of the duodenum drain chiefly to the superior mesenteric vein, while the upper portions usually drain directly to the portal vein. Variants are common, however.

Note how the esophageal veins drain into the portal vein by way of the left gastric veins. This is important in the portacaval collateral circulation (see **B** and p. 293).

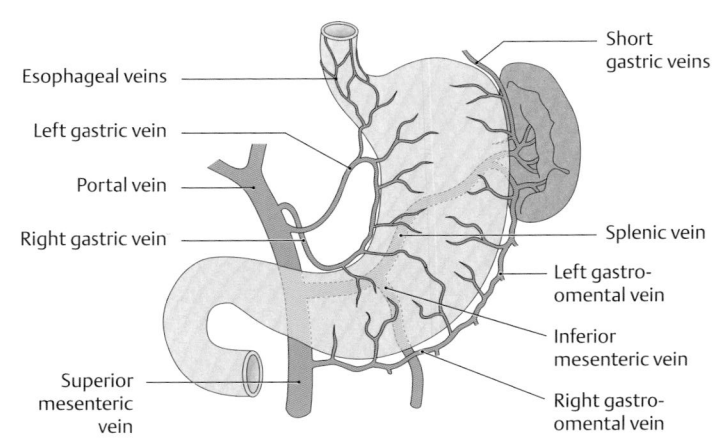

Esophageal veins

Left gastric vein

Portal vein

Right gastric vein

Superior mesenteric vein

Short gastric veins

Splenic vein

Left gastro-omental vein

Inferior mesenteric vein

Right gastro-omental vein

B Junction of the inferior mesenteric vein and splenic vein

Anterior view. This view, with the stomach translucent, demonstrates the site where the inferior mesenteric vein typically opens into the splenic vein behind the stomach.

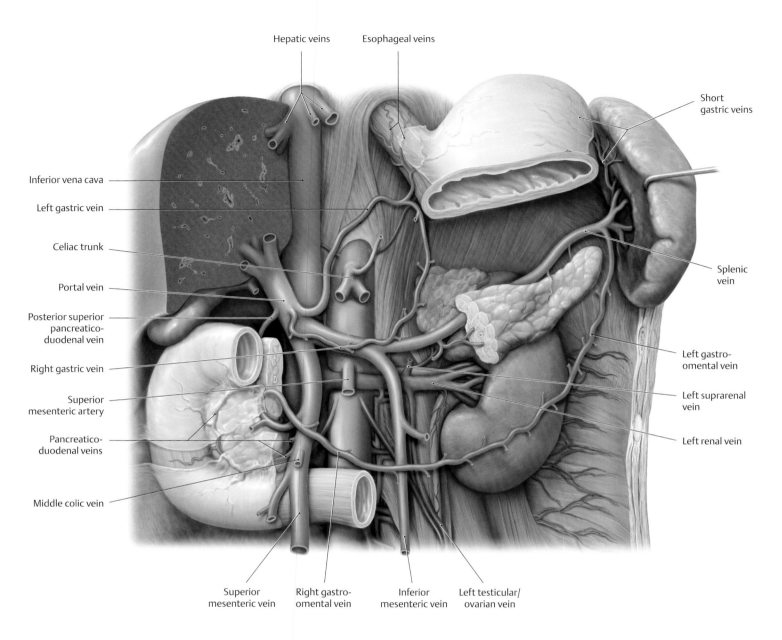

Hepatic veins   Esophageal veins

Short gastric veins

Inferior vena cava

Left gastric vein

Celiac trunk

Portal vein

Posterior superior pancreatico-duodenal vein

Right gastric vein

Superior mesenteric artery

Pancreatico-duodenal veins

Middle colic vein

Splenic vein

Left gastro-omental vein

Left suprarenal vein

Left renal vein

Superior mesenteric vein   Right gastro-omental vein   Inferior mesenteric vein   Left testicular/ovarian vein

C Venous drainage of the pancreas and spleen

Anterior view. The stomach has been partially removed and pulled slightly inferiorly for better exposure, and most of the peritoneum has been removed.

This dissection clearly shows how the portal vein is formed by the junction of the superior mesenteric vein and splenic vein near the liver. In 70% of cases the splenic vein receives the inferior mesenteric vein, as shown here, before uniting with the superior mesenteric vein (see also **B**).

Venous blood from the spleen is carried by the splenic vein *directly* to the portal vein, while blood from the *pancreas* takes various routes: Most

of the pancreatic veins (mainly from the tail and body of the pancreas) open into the splenic vein. A few (mainly from the head of the pancreas) open into the superior mesenteric vein or drain directly into the portal vein.

Note the venous arcade along the pancreas (which is richly vascularized) and the close relationship of the head of the pancreas to the portal vein tributaries. Because of this, a tumor in the head of the pancreas may impinge upon the portal vein tributaries (especially the superior mesenteric vein), leading to venous obstruction and ascites (accumulation of intra-abdominal fluid).

3.9 Superior and Inferior Mesenteric Vein: Venous Drainage of the Small and Large Intestine

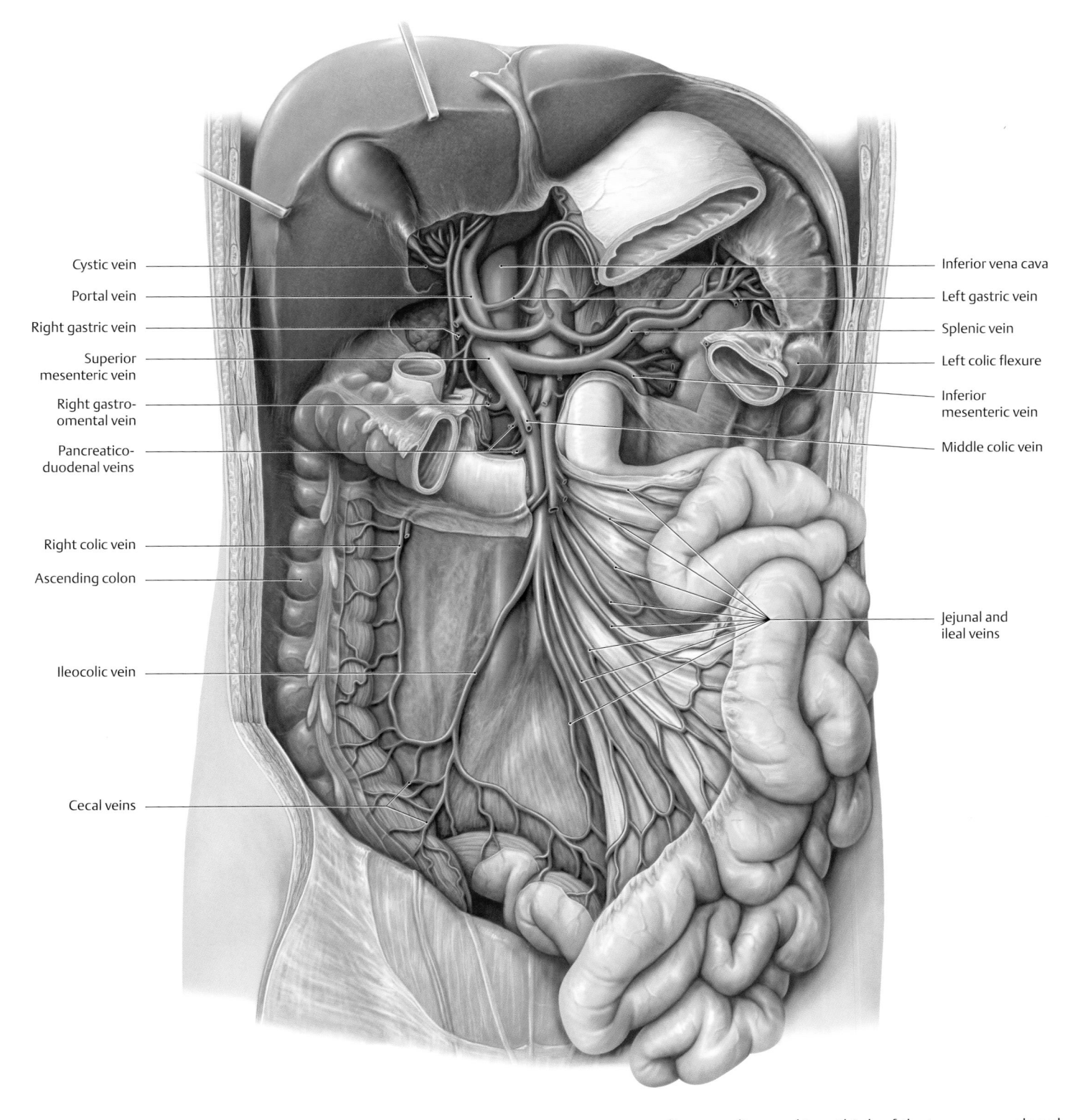

Cystic vein
Portal vein
Right gastric vein
Superior mesenteric vein
Right gastro-omental vein
Pancreatico-duodenal veins
Right colic vein
Ascending colon
Ileocolic vein
Cecal veins

Inferior vena cava
Left gastric vein
Splenic vein
Left colic flexure
Inferior mesenteric vein
Middle colic vein
Jejunal and ileal veins

A Tributaries of the superior mesenteric vein

Anterior view. Most of the stomach has been removed, and the peritoneum has been removed or windowed at multiple sites, leaving some of the retroperitoneal connective tissue in place. The mesentery and transverse colon have been partially removed, and the loops of small intestine have been displaced to the left.

The superior mesenteric vein unites with the splenic vein at the L 1 level to form the portal vein (see **B**, p. 274).

The *small intestine* drains *exclusively* into branches of the *superior* mesenteric vein. The superior mesenteric vein also collects blood from the cecum, appendix, ascending, and two-thirds of the transverse colon almost to the left colic flexure. From that point the colon is drained by the *inferior* mesenteric vein. As with the mesenteric arteries, multiple anastomoses are present between these two large veins. The superior mesenteric vein drains a much larger territory than the inferior mesenteric. Thus, the venous drainage of the small and large intestine follows the pattern of their arterial supply.

Note: The ascending colon, which is secondarily retroperitoneal, may also be drained by veins in the retroperitoneum (lumbar veins) that empty into the inferior vena cava. This is another example of a portacaval collateral pathway (see p. 293).

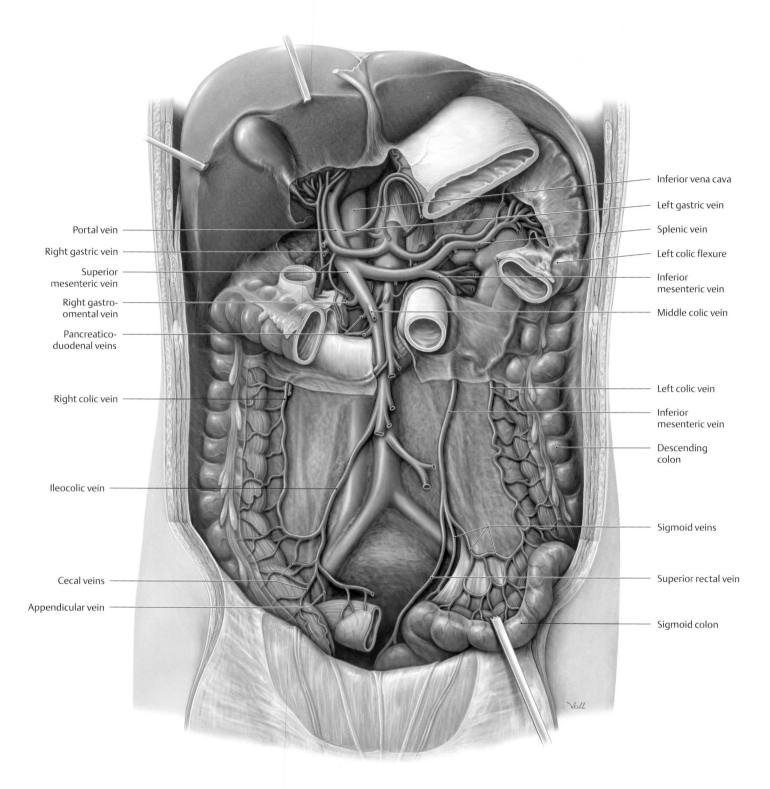

Inferior vena cava

Left gastric vein

Splenic vein

Left colic flexure

Inferior mesenteric vein

Middle colic vein

Left colic vein

Inferior mesenteric vein

Descending colon

Sigmoid veins

Superior rectal vein

Sigmoid colon

Portal vein

Right gastric vein

Superior mesenteric vein

Right gastro- omental vein

Pancreatico- duodenal veins

Right colic vein

Ileocolic vein

Cecal veins

Appendicular vein

B Tributaries of the inferior mesenteric vein

Anterior view. Most of the stomach, pancreas, and small intestine have been removed. The peritoneum has been removed or windowed at several sites, leaving some of the retroperitoneal connective tissue in place.

The inferior mesenteric vein is formed by the union of the left colic vein, sigmoid veins, and superior rectal vein. Unlike the *superior* mesenteric vein, the inferior mesenteric vein runs separate from the artery and generally opens into the splenic vein behind the stomach and pancreas (see p. 277). Thus the *inferior* mesenteric vein returns blood *only from the large intestine*. The boundary between the territories of the superior and inferior mesenteric veins is usually located in the transverse colon near the left colic flexure, although multiple anastomoses exist between the two mesenteric veins.

The descending colon, which is secondarily retroperitoneal, may also be drained by veins in the retroperitoneum (lumbar veins), again establishing a portosystemic collateral pathway.

Note: Blood from the *upper rectum* drains through the *superior* rectal vein to the inferior mesenteric vein before entering the *portal vein*. The *lower rectum* (not shown here) is drained by the middle and inferior rectal veins, which drain into the *inferior vena cava* by way of the iliac veins. A portacaval anastomosis may also be present in this region. This explains why malignant tumors of the upper rectum metastasize to the liver, while malignant tumors of the lower rectum tend to metastasize to the lung.

3.10 Arteries and Veins of the Kidneys and Suprarenal Glands: Overview

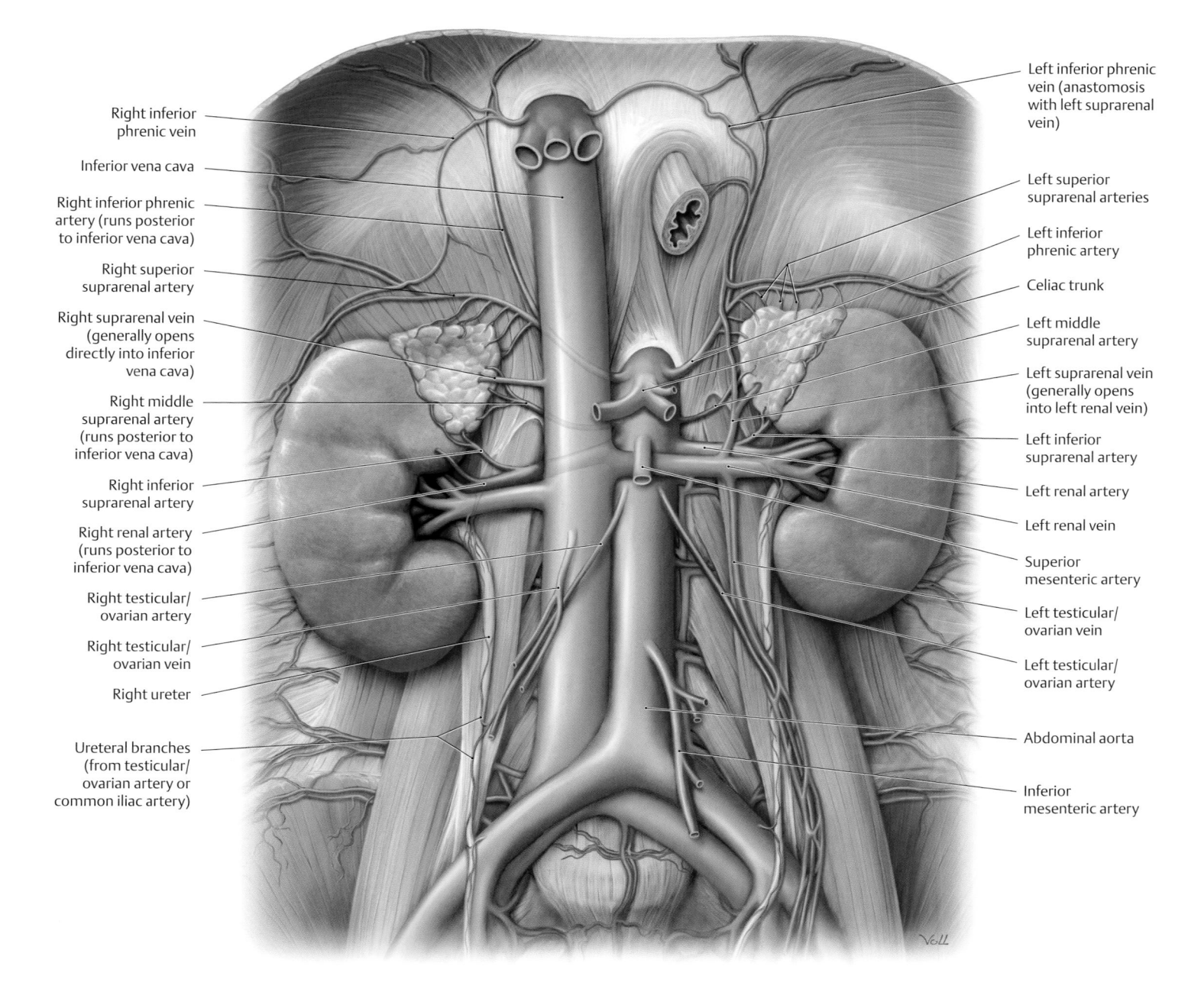

Right inferior phrenic vein

Inferior vena cava

Right inferior phrenic artery (runs posterior to inferior vena cava)

Right superior suprarenal artery

Right suprarenal vein (generally opens directly into inferior vena cava)

Right middle suprarenal artery (runs posterior to inferior vena cava)

Right inferior suprarenal artery

Right renal artery (runs posterior to inferior vena cava)

Right testicular/ ovarian artery

Right testicular/ ovarian vein

Right ureter

Ureteral branches (from testicular/ ovarian artery or common iliac artery)

Left inferior phrenic vein (anastomosis with left suprarenal vein)

Left superior suprarenal arteries

Left inferior phrenic artery

Celiac trunk

Left middle suprarenal artery

Left suprarenal vein (generally opens into left renal vein)

Left inferior suprarenal artery

Left renal artery

Left renal vein

Superior mesenteric artery

Left testicular/ ovarian vein

Left testicular/ ovarian artery

Abdominal aorta

Inferior mesenteric artery

A Overview of the arteries and veins of the kidneys and suprarenal glands

Anterior view. The esophagus has been pulled slightly inferiorly, and the right kidney and suprarenal gland have been pulled away from the inferior vena cava to show the vascular anatomy of the suprarenal gland. The other abdominal organs have been removed.

Renal artery: The renal arteries branch from the sides of the abdominal aorta at the level of the L 1/L 2 vertebrae (see **C**). The *right* renal artery runs *posterior* to the inferior vena cava (shown transparent in the drawing), and the *left* renal artery runs *posterior* to the left renal vein. Each renal artery divides into an anterior and posterior branch. The renal artery gives off the inferior suprarenal arteries to the suprarenal gland; capsular (perirenal) branches to tissues surrounding the kidney and to the renal capsule (fibrous capsule and perirenal fat capsule, removed here for clarity); and ureteral branches to supply the proximal ureter and distal renal pelvis. Possible variants are illustrated in **E**, p. 283.

Suprarenal arteries: Superior, middle and inferior suprarenal arteries (from the inferior phrenic artery, abdominal aorta, and renal artery, see above).

Renal vein: The renal vein on each side is generally formed by the union of two or three venous branches (variants are shown in **F**, p. 283). While the *left renal vein* receives the left suprarenal vein and left testicular or ovarian vein, the *right renal vein* opens directly into the inferior vena cava without receiving these tributaries (see also **D**). The renal vein also receives capsular branches from the renal fibrous capsule in addition to small branches from the renal pelvis and proximal ureter (not shown here).

Suprarenal veins:

Note: The three main arteries of the suprarenal glands (see above) are generally accompanied *by only one vein* (rarely two), the *suprarenal vein*. While the *left* suprarenal vein opens into the left renal vein, frequently anastomosing with the left inferior phrenic vein (as shown here), the *right* suprarenal vein empties directly into the inferior vena cava (see also **D**).

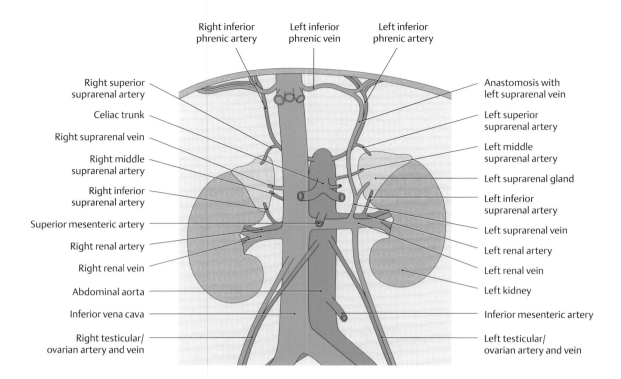

B Arteries and veins of the kidneys and suprarenal glands
Anterior view. The right kidney and suprarenal gland have been slightly retracted from the inferior vena cava to display their blood vessels more clearly.
It is evident in this diagram and in **A** that the suprarenal glands have a more complex vascular anatomy than the kidneys: More than 50 small branches may pass from the arterial trunks of the suprarenal glands (superior, middle and inferior suprarenal arteries) into the glands.
Note that the three main arteries of the suprarenal glands are generally accompanied by only one vein, the suprarenal vein. This vessel opens *directly* into the inferior vena cava on the *right* side and into the renal vein on the *left* side (see **D**).

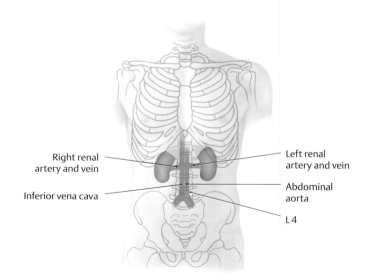

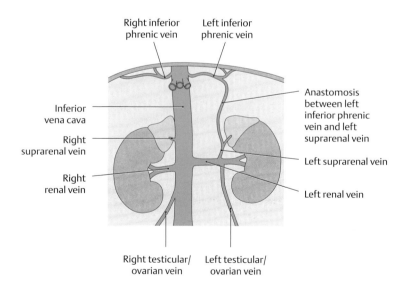

C Projection of the renal arteries and veins onto the vertebral column
The renal artery arises from the abdominal aorta at the L 1/ L 2 level.
Note: The renal veins lie anterior to the arteries.

D Tributaries of the left renal vein
The renal vein has more tributaries on the left side than on the right. The *left* renal vein receives the left suprarenal vein (often anastomosing with the left inferior phrenic vein, see **A**) and the left testicular / ovarian vein, whereas the corresponding veins on the *right* side open *directly* into the inferior vena cava. Because of this arrangement, varicose dilations of the veins in the spermatic cord (varicoceles) are more common on the left side than on the right.

3.11 Arteries and Veins of the Kidneys and Suprarenal Glands: Topographical Anatomy and Variants

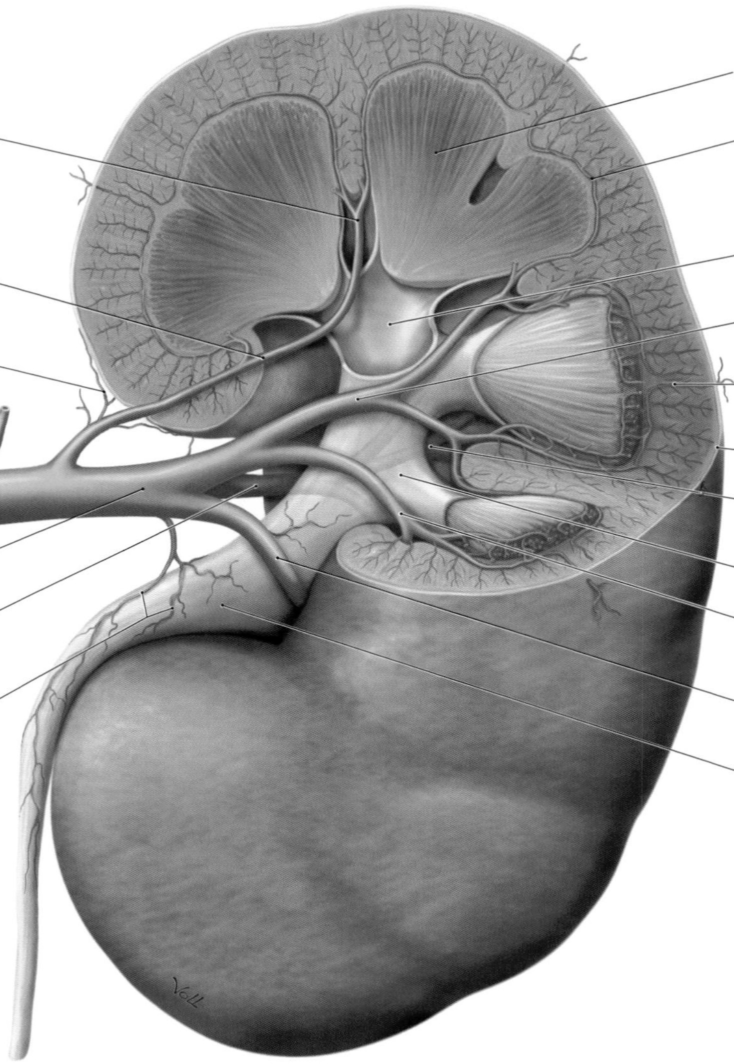

Interlobar artery
(between the
medullary pyramids)

Superior segmental artery

Capsular branches

Inferior suprarenal artery

Left renal artery
(main trunk)

Anterior branch
of renal artery

Posterior branch
of renal artery

Ureteral branches
(here from left
renal artery)

Pyramid

Arcuate artery
(at base of medullary
pyramids)

Major calix

Anterior superior
segmental artery

Interlobular artery

Fibrous capsule

Branch of posterior
segmental artery

Renal pelvis

Anterior inferior
segmental artery

Inferior segmental artery

Left ureter
(origin from
renal pelvis)

A Division of the renal artery into segmental arteries
Anterior view of the left kidney.
The main trunk of the renal artery divides into an anterior and posterior branch. The anterior branch divides further into four segmental arteries:

- Superior segmental artery
- Anterior superior segmental artery
- Anterior inferior segmental artery
- Inferior segmental artery

The posterior branch gives rise to only one segmental vessel, the posterior segmental artery.

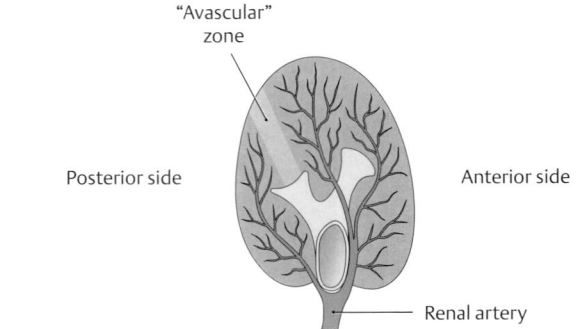

"Avascular"
zone

Posterior side

Anterior side

Renal artery

B "Avascular" zone in the kidney
Inferior view of the right kidney.
Between the posterior segment and anterior segments is a relatively avascular zone of the kidney, which otherwise is *very heavily vascularized*. This zone provides an important line of access for intrarenal surgery.

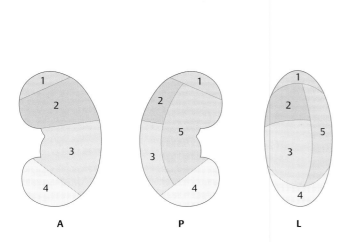

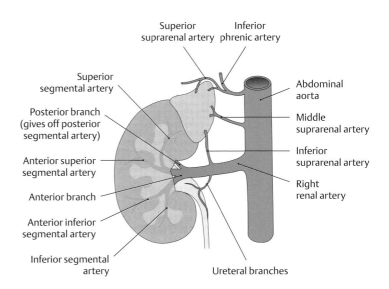

A   **P**   **L**

C Vascular segmentation of the kidney

Left kidney viewed from the anterior (A), posterior (P) and lateral (L) sides.

The renal artery and its branches divide the kidney into five segments:

1 Superior segment
2 Anterior superior segment
3 Anterior inferior segment
4 Inferior segment
5 Posterior segment

D Relationship of the renal arterial branches to the renal segments

Anterior view of the right kidney, demonstrating the origins of the renal artery, middle suprarenal artery, and inferior phrenic artery from the abdominal aorta.

Note the division of the renal artery into an anterior branch (anterior segments, superior and inferior segment) and a posterior branch (for the posterior segment, see also **A**). The upper part of the ureter is supplied by ureteral branches from the renal artery.

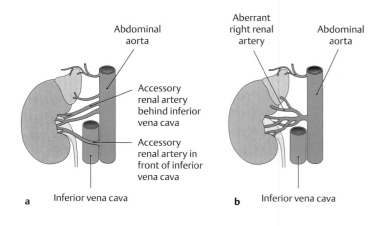

E Variants of the renal arteries

Anterior view of the right kidney.

a Two accessory renal arteries (one crossing in front of the inferior vena cava): Accessory renal arteries are extra arteries that pass from the abdominal aorta to the renal hilum. As a common variant with accessory renal arteries, the inferior suprarenal artery does not arise from the renal artery.

b An *aberrant* renal artery is one that does not enter the kidney at the renal hilum.

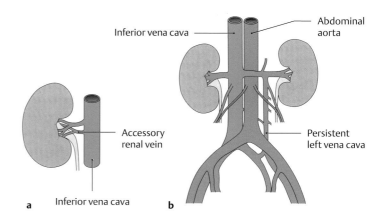

F Variants of the renal veins

Anterior view.

a Accessory (supernumerary) renal veins.

b A left vena cava (persistent lower part of the supracardinal vein) ascends to the level of the left renal vein and opens into it.

283

3.12 Divisions and Topographical Anatomy of the Internal Iliac Artery

Abdominal aorta

Right common iliac artery

Right internal iliac artery

Right external iliac artery

Umbilical artery, patent part

Internal iliac artery, anterior trunk

Obturator nerve

Obturator artery

Inferior epigastric artery

Obturator branch of inferior epigastric artery

L 5 vertebra

Median sacral artery

Iliolumbar artery

Internal iliac artery, posterior trunk

Lateral sacral artery

Superior gluteal artery

Inferior gluteal artery

Sacral plexus

Inferior vesical artery

Middle rectal artery

Coccygeus

Obturator internus

Internal pudendal artery

Pudendal nerve

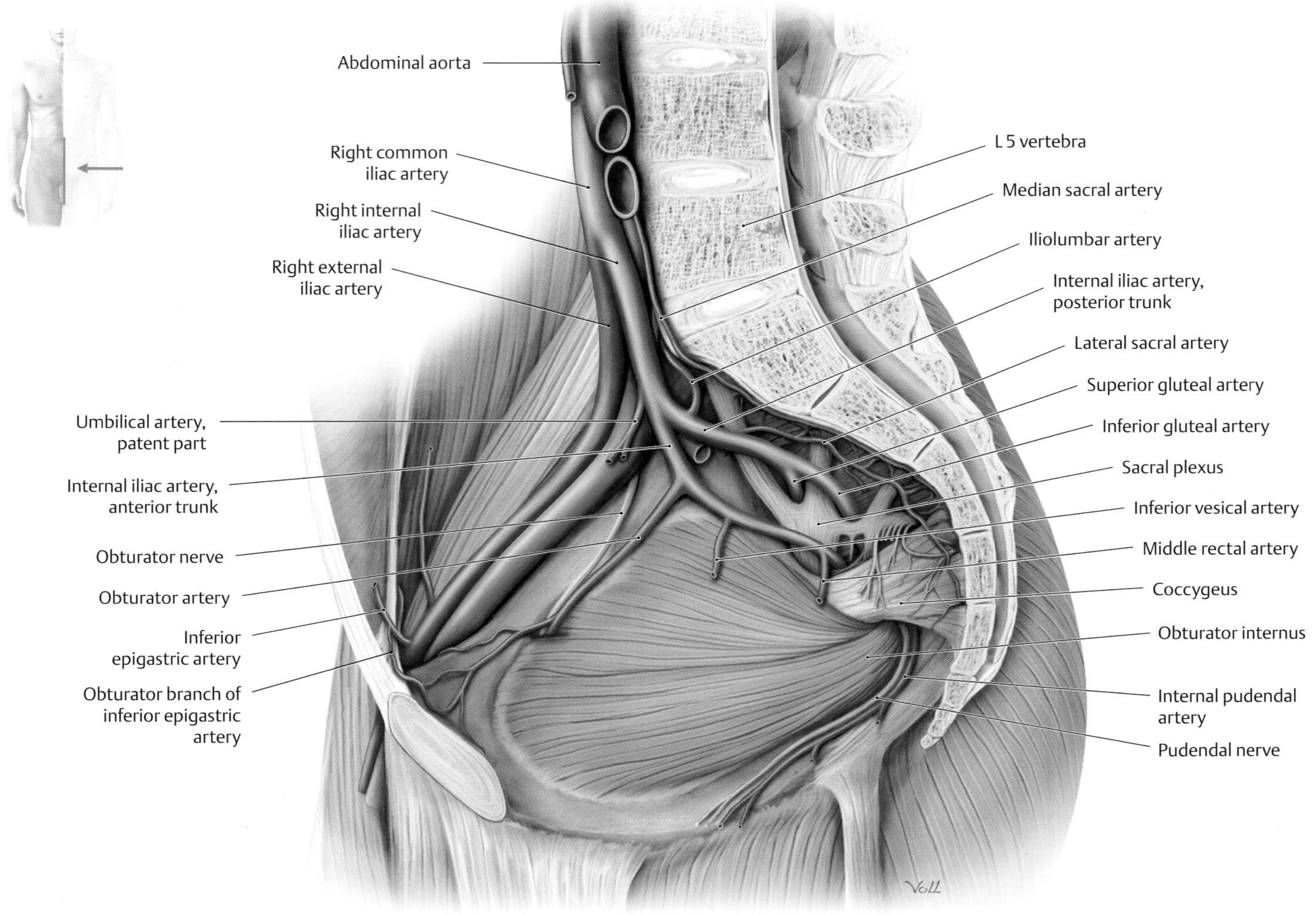

A Branches of the right internal iliac artery in the male pelvis
Left lateral view with the pelvic organs removed. This illustration is an idealized composite of a series of saggital sections that include the midline and more lateral structures.

The internal iliac artery arises from the common iliac artery. In 60% of cases it divides anterior to the piriformis (see **C**) into an anterior and posterior trunk. The anterior trunk gives off visceral branches and also parietal branches to the pelvic wall, while the posterior trunk gives off branches only to the pelvic wall. The sequence of the branches is shown in **D**.

Note the relationship of the internal iliac artery and its branches to the sacral plexus. Several branches of the internal iliac artery "disappear" behind this nerve plexus. The relationship of the internal iliac artery to the bony pelvic wall and pelvic apertures is shown in **C**.

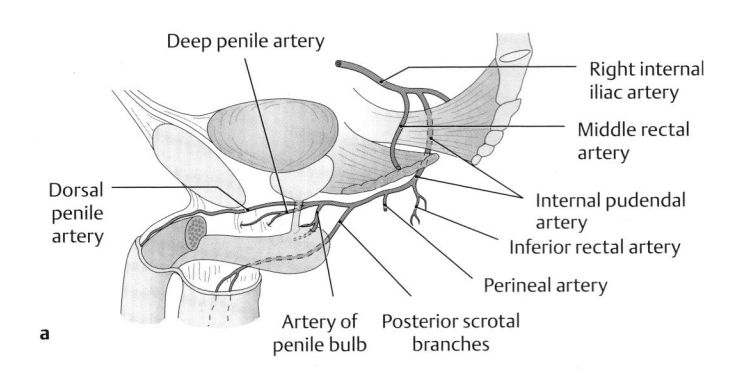

Deep penile artery

Right internal iliac artery

Middle rectal artery

Internal pudendal artery

Inferior rectal artery

Perineal artery

Dorsal penile artery

Artery of penile bulb

Posterior scrotal branches

a

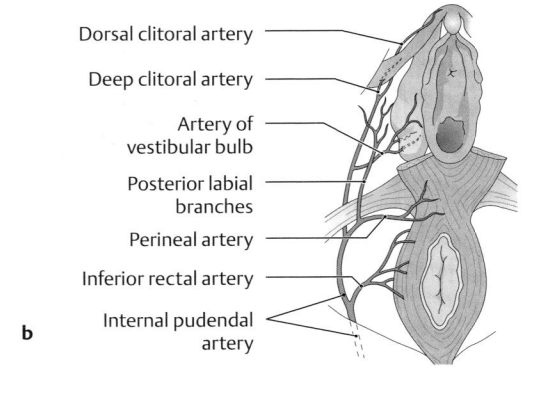

Dorsal clitoral artery

Deep clitoral artery

Artery of vestibular bulb

Posterior labial branches

Perineal artery

Inferior rectal artery

Internal pudendal artery

b

B Course and branches of the right internal pudendal artery on the pelvic floor
The internal pudendal artery is only partially visible in **A**. This diagram illustrates its further course.

a Course of the artery in the male (same perspective as in **A**).
b Course of the artery in the female. The course of the internal pudendal artery is analogous to its course in the male pelvis. An inferior view is shown to supplement the lateral view in **a**, and because this view is important in surgical procedures on the female pelvic floor.

C Sequence of branches of the right internal iliac artery and their projection onto the male pelvis

Compared with **A**, this diagram additionally shows the superior vesical artery, which arises from the umbilical artery (in **A** the umbilical artery was transected above the origin of the superior vesical artery). This drawing also shows the relationship of the vessels to the greater sciatic foramen, while **A** emphasized their relationship to the sacral plexus. The sequence of internal iliac branches in the female pelvis is shown in **E**, p. 287.

D Sequence of branches of the internal iliac artery

Each internal iliac artery supplies the walls and organs of the pelvis with five parietal branches and five or six visceral branches (→ = "gives off").

Parietal branches (pelvic walls)	
Iliolumbar artery to the lateral pelvic wall	→ *Lumbar branch* → *Spinal branch* → *Iliac branch*
Lateral sacral artery to the posterior pelvic wall	→ *Spinal branches*
Obturator artery to the medial thigh and lateral pelvic wall	→ *Pubic branch* → *Acetabular branch* → *Anterior branch* → *Posterior branch*
Superior gluteal artery to the gluteal region	→ *Superficial branch* → *Deep branch*
Inferior gluteal artery to the gluteal region	→ *Accompanying artery of sciatic nerve*

Visceral branches (pelvic organs)	
Umbilical artery patent part gives off:	→ *Artery of vas deferens* → *Superior vesical artery (to the bladder)*
Inferior vesical artery to the bladder fundus	→ *Prostatic branches*
Uterine artery to the uterus, fallopian tubes, vagina, and ovaries	→ *Helicine branches* → *Vaginal branches* → *Ovarian branch* → *Tubal branch*
Vaginal artery May arise as a separate branch from the internal iliac artery (as shown here) or, more commonly, from the inferior vesical artery or uterine artery ("vaginal azygos artery")	
Middle rectal artery to the rectal ampulla and levator ani	→ *Vaginal branches (f)* → *Prostatic branches (m)*
Internal pudendal artery (included with the visceral branches because it gives off the inferior rectal artery)	→ *Inferior rectal artery (to the terminal rectum, etc.)* → *Perineal artery* → *Posterior scrotal branches (m), posterior labial branches (f)* → *Urethral artery* → *Artery of vestibular bulb (f), artery of penile bulb (m)* → *Dorsal clitoral artery (f), dorsal penile artery (m)* → *Deep clitoral artery (f), deep penile artery (m)* → *Perforator arteries of penis*

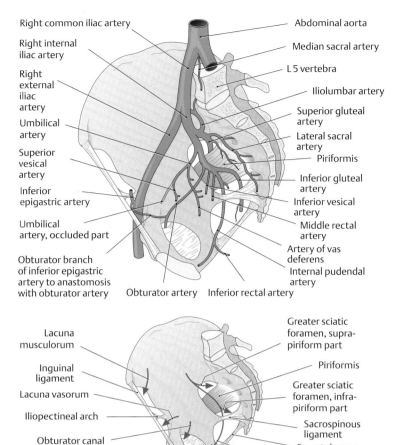

E Arterial pathways in the pelvic wall

View of a right hemipelvis showing the pelvic apertures that transmit the arteries and corresponding veins. There are a total of six pathways, whose landmarks are the piriformis, sacrospinous ligament, sacrotuberous ligament, inguinal ligament, and obturator membrane (see also **F**).

F Neurovascular tracts on the pelvic wall

There are six major neurovascular tracts on the pelvic walls, four of which (*) contain branches from the internal iliac artery.

Tract	Neurovascular structures transmitted
Posterior Greater sciatic foramen, suprapiriform part* (above the piriformis)	Superior gluteal artery and vein, superior gluteal nerve
Greater sciatic foramen, infrapiriform part* (below the piriformis)	Inferior gluteal artery and vein, inferior gluteal nerve, sciatic nerve, internal pudendal artery and vein, pudendal nerve, posterior femoral cutaneous nerve
On pelvic floor Pudendal canal*	Internal pudendal artery and vein, pudendal nerve
Lateral Obturator canal*	Obturator artery and vein, obturator nerve
Anterior Lacuna musculorum (posterior to inguinal ligament, lateral to iliopectineal arch)	Femoral nerve, lateral femoral cutaneous nerve
Lacuna vasorum (posterior to inguinal ligament, medial to iliopectineal arch)	Femoral artery and vein, lymphatic vessels (the femoral artery is a branch of the external iliac artery), femoral branch of genitofemoral nerve

3.13 Arteries and Veins of the Pelvic Organs

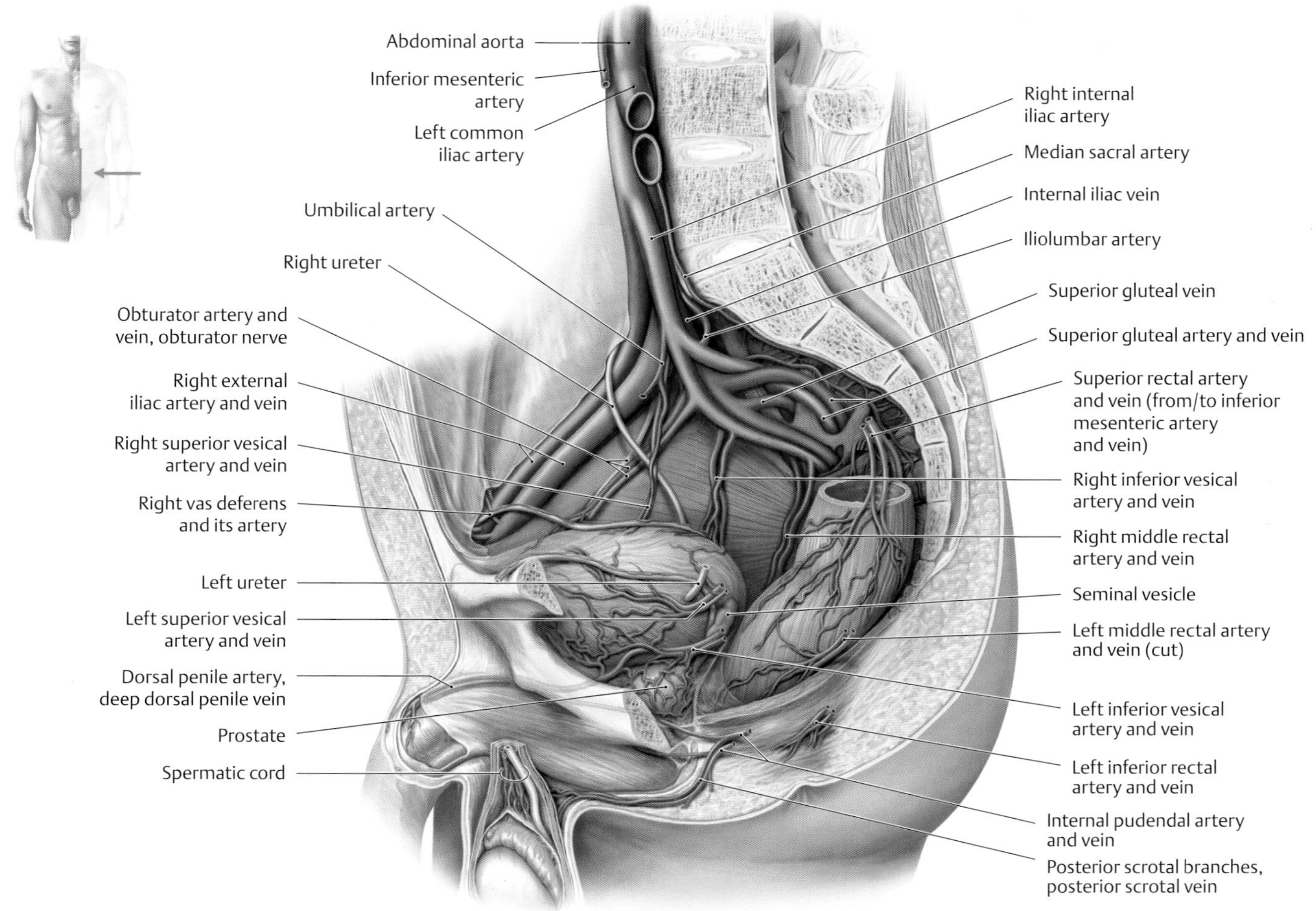

Abdominal aorta

Inferior mesenteric artery

Left common iliac artery

Umbilical artery

Right ureter

Obturator artery and vein, obturator nerve

Right external iliac artery and vein

Right superior vesical artery and vein

Right vas deferens and its artery

Left ureter

Left superior vesical artery and vein

Dorsal penile artery, deep dorsal penile vein

Prostate

Spermatic cord

Right internal iliac artery

Median sacral artery

Internal iliac vein

Iliolumbar artery

Superior gluteal vein

Superior gluteal artery and vein

Superior rectal artery and vein (from/to inferior mesenteric artery and vein)

Right inferior vesical artery and vein

Right middle rectal artery and vein

Seminal vesicle

Left middle rectal artery and vein (cut)

Left inferior vesical artery and vein

Left inferior rectal artery and vein

Internal pudendal artery and vein

Posterior scrotal branches, posterior scrotal vein

A Arterial supply and venous drainage of the pelvic organs in the male (overview)

Right hemipelvis (compiled from multiple sagittal sections) viewed from the left side, idealized. The pelvic organs derive their **arterial supply** from the visceral branches of the internal iliac artery (see p. 285). Their **venous drainage** is by corresponding veins (often running parallel to the arteries), which drain to the internal iliac vein. The veins, unlike the arteries, are frequently multiple on each side of the pelvis and are often expanded near the organs to form large plexuses. The main differences in the arterial supply and venous drainage of the pelvic organs in the male and female are based on the copious blood supply to the uterus and vagina in the female (see p. 290): The uterus and vagina are supplied by *their own* major vessels. In the male, however, the accessory sex glands are supplied by smaller branches arising from the vessels of nearby organs (bladder, rectum).

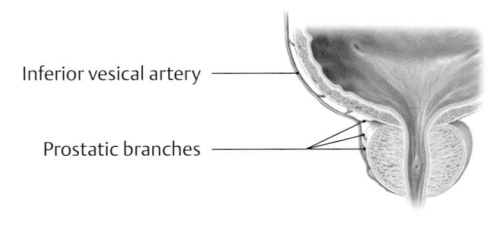

Inferior vesical artery

Prostatic branches

B Arterial supply of the prostate

Coronal section, anterior view. Most prostatic branches arise from the inferior vesical artery, and a smaller number arise from the middle rectal artery (not shown here). The prostatic branches ramify into a great many branchlets outside the organ capsule of the prostate.

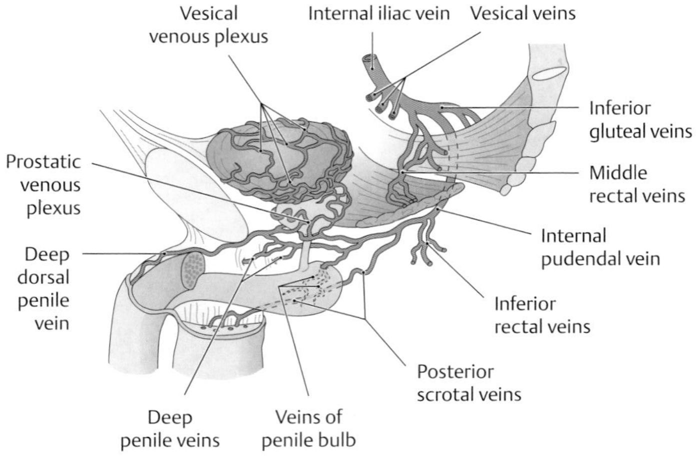

Vesical venous plexus

Internal iliac vein

Vesical veins

Prostatic venous plexus

Deep dorsal penile vein

Inferior gluteal veins

Middle rectal veins

Internal pudendal vein

Inferior rectal veins

Posterior scrotal veins

Deep penile veins

Veins of penile bulb

C Venous drainage of the bladder and male genitalia

Large venous plexuses around the bladder (vesical venous plexus) and prostate (prostatic venous plexus) drain through the vesical veins to the internal iliac vein. An anastomotic connection between the prostatic venous plexus and vertebral venous plexus (not shown here, aids venous drainage of the vertebral column and spinal canal) creates a route by which tumor cells from a prostatic carcinoma may metastasize to the spine (which may first come to clinical attention as back pain).

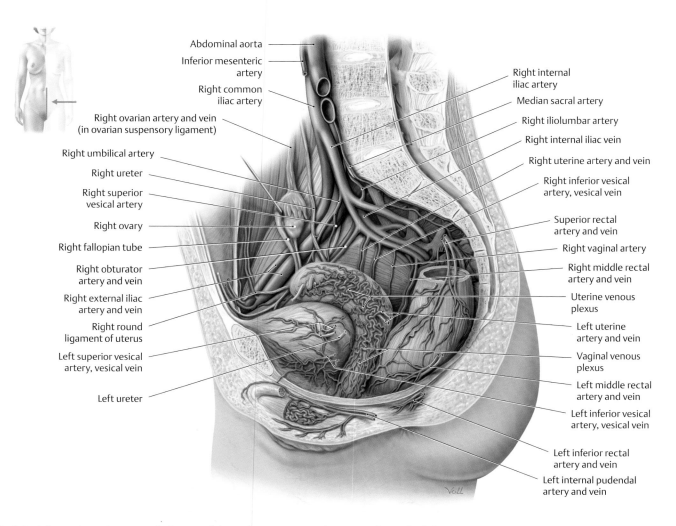

Abdominal aorta
Inferior mesenteric artery
Right common iliac artery
Right ovarian artery and vein (in ovarian suspensory ligament)
Right umbilical artery
Right ureter
Right superior vesical artery
Right ovary
Right fallopian tube
Right obturator artery and vein
Right external iliac artery and vein
Right round ligament of uterus
Left superior vesical artery, vesical vein
Left ureter

Right internal iliac artery
Median sacral artery
Right iliolumbar artery
Right internal iliac vein
Right uterine artery and vein
Right inferior vesical artery, vesical vein
Superior rectal artery and vein
Right vaginal artery
Right middle rectal artery and vein
Uterine venous plexus
Left uterine artery and vein
Vaginal venous plexus
Left middle rectal artery and vein
Left inferior vesical artery, vesical vein
Left inferior rectal artery and vein
Left internal pudendal artery and vein

D Arterial supply and venous drainage of the pelvic organs in the female (overview)

Right hemipelvis (compiled from multiple sagittal sections) viewed from the left side, idealized. The supply of the internal genital organs, which represent a significant fraction of the total vascular demand in the female pelvis, is described on p. 290.

Right common iliac artery
Abdominal aorta
Iliolumbar artery
Right internal iliac artery
Umbilical artery, patent part
Obturator artery
Right external iliac artery
Superior vesical artery
Inferior vesical artery

Superior gluteal artery
Lateral sacral artery
Uterine artery
Internal pudendal artery
Inferior gluteal artery
Vaginal artery (here arising separately from the internal iliac artery)
Middle rectal artery
Vaginal branch of uterine artery

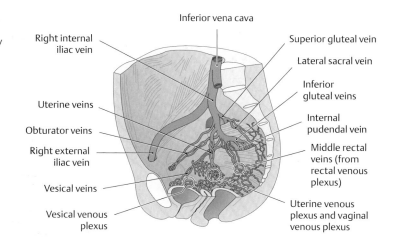

Right internal iliac vein
Uterine veins
Obturator veins
Right external iliac vein
Vesical veins
Vesical venous plexus

Inferior vena cava
Superior gluteal vein
Lateral sacral vein
Inferior gluteal veins
Internal pudendal vein
Middle rectal veins (from rectal venous plexus)
Uterine venous plexus and vaginal venous plexus

E Sequence of branches of the internal iliac artery in the female pelvis

Left lateral view. The vessels to the uterus and vagina mark the principal difference from the vasculature of the male pelvis (see also **E**, p. 285). The **uterus** receives a large vessel, the uterine artery, which usually arises separately from the internal iliac artery (the analogous vessel in the male, the artery of the vas deferens, usually branches from the umbilical artery). The uterine artery *may* also arise from the middle rectal artery, which is larger in those cases. The arterial supply to the **vagina** is also subject to variation. The vagina may be supplied by a separate vaginal artery branching from the internal iliac artery or by a vaginal branch arising from either the uterine artery or the inferior vesical artery.

F Venous drainage of the organs of the female pelvis

Left lateral view showing the right internal iliac vein. The female pelvic organs are generally drained by four plexuses (see also **E**, p. 291):

- Vesical venous plexus (vesical veins)
- Vaginal venous plexus (vesical veins)
- Uterine venous plexus (uterine vein)
- Rectal venous plexus (rectal veins)

The middle and inferior rectal veins drain to the internal iliac vein. The superior rectal vein drains into the inferior mesenteric vein. (The superior and inferior rectal veins are not shown here.)

287

3.14 Arteries and Veins of the Rectum

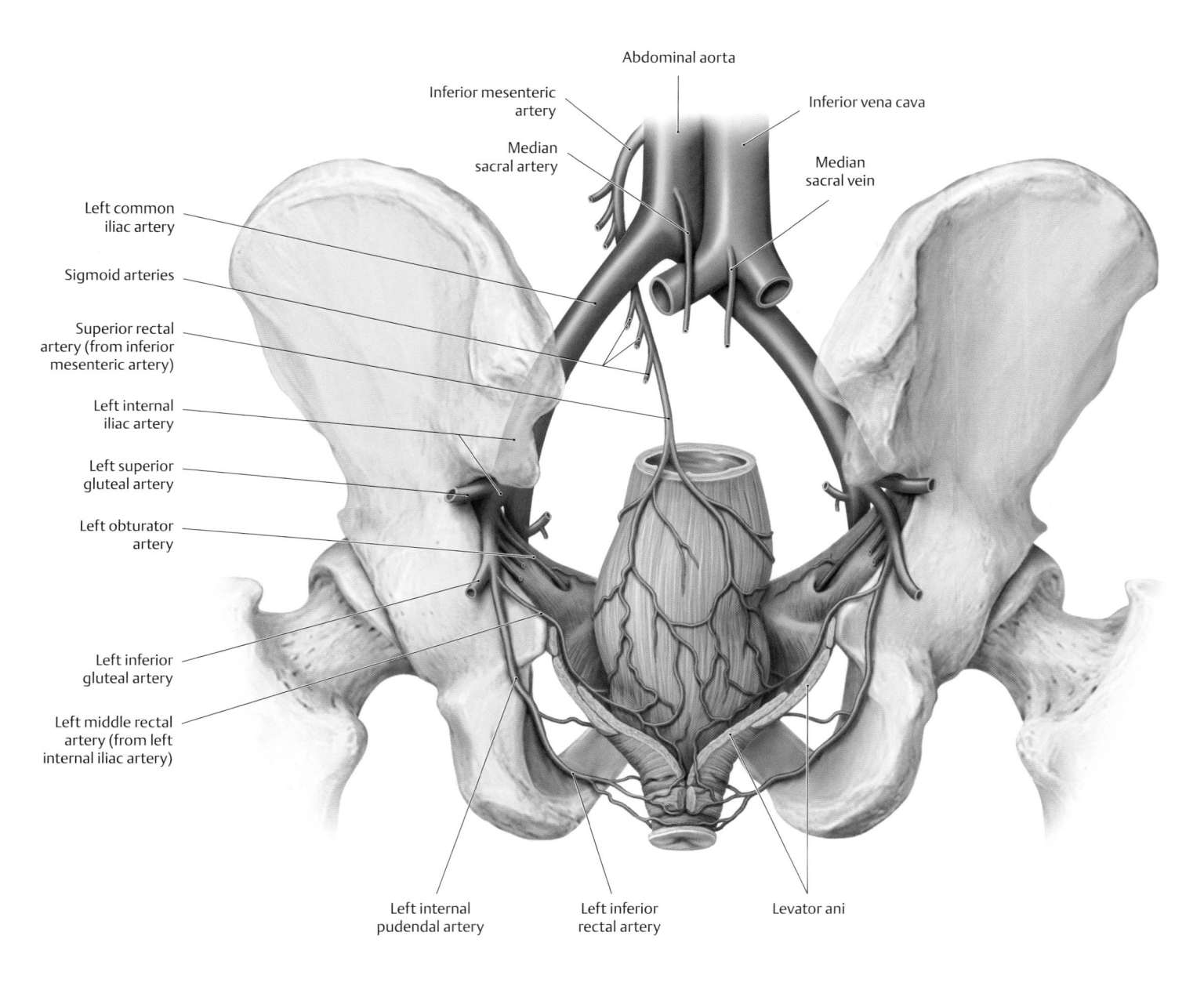

A Arterial supply of the rectum

Posterior view. For clarity, portions of the ilium are shown translucent. *Note:* The unpaired *superior* rectal artery (from the unpaired inferior mesenteric artery) divides into two branches on reaching the rectum. By contrast, the *middle* rectal arteries (from the internal iliac artery) and inferior rectal arteries (from the internal pudendal artery) are paired owing to their origin from paired parent vessels. In the female, it is not unusual for the middle rectal artery to arise from the uterine artery. The *inferior* rectal artery leaves the internal pudendal artery in the pudendal canal (*Alcock's canal*). The superior rectal artery approaches the rectum from above and posteriorly, also coming in contact with the peritoneal covering of the rectum (for clarity, not shown here). The middle and inferior rectal arteries approach the rectum from the sides, the levator ani forming a well-defined partition between them: The middle rectal arteries pass to the rectum above that muscle, the inferior rectal arteries below it. Because the levator ani forms an essential part of the "pelvic diaphragm" (see p. 168), the course of the middle and inferior rectal arteries is also described as *supradiaphragmatic* and *infradiaphragmatic*, respectively. The rectal arteries frequently accompany the rectal veins for a considerable distance.

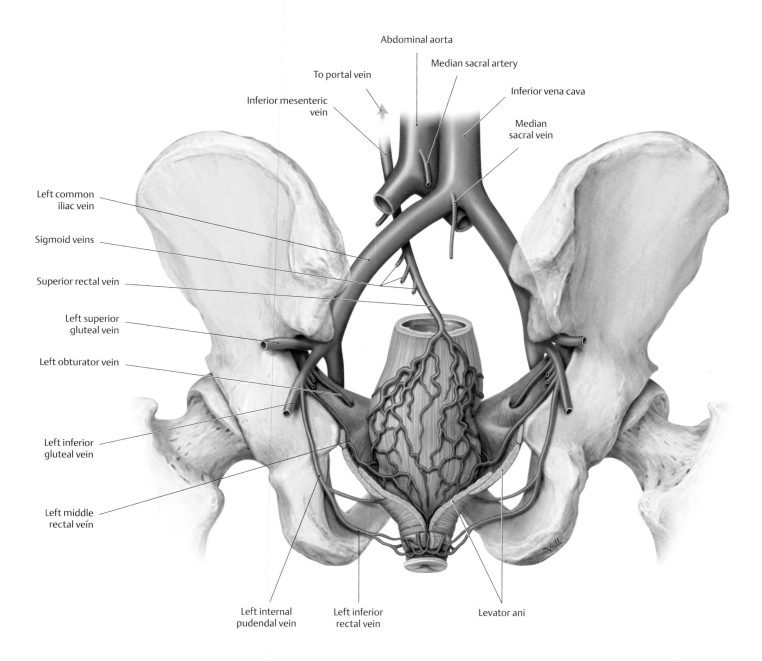

Abdominal aorta

Median sacral artery

To portal vein

Inferior mesenteric vein

Inferior vena cava

Median sacral vein

Left common iliac vein

Sigmoid veins

Superior rectal vein

Left superior gluteal vein

Left obturator vein

Left inferior gluteal vein

Left middle rectal vein

Left internal pudendal vein

Left inferior rectal vein

Levator ani

B Venous drainage of the rectum

Posterior view. Portions of the ilium are shown translucent for clarity.
Note: The unpaired *superior* rectal vein (to the unpaired inferior mesenteric vein) divides into two branches on reaching the rectum. By contrast, the *middle* rectal veins (to the internal iliac vein) and *inferior* rectal veins (to the internal pudendal vein) are paired owing to their termination in paired venous trunks.

Because the rectal veins accompany the corresponding arteries for some distance, their course is analogous to that previously described for the arteries (see **A**): The superior rectal vein follows an abdominal route, while the middle and inferior rectal veins take supra- and infradiaphragmatic routes. The superior rectal vein drains to the hepatic portal system by way of the inferior mesenteric vein (see pp. 275 and 279).
Note: Tumors in the region drained by the *superior* rectal vein can metastasize through the portal venous system to the capillary bed of the liver (hepatic metastases), whereas tumors in the region drained by the *middle* and *inferior* rectal veins metastasize through the inferior vena cava to the capillary bed of the lung (pulmonary metastases). Note also the importance of these veins as portacaval collaterals (see p. 293).

3.15 Arteries and Veins of the Female Genitalia and Urinary Organs

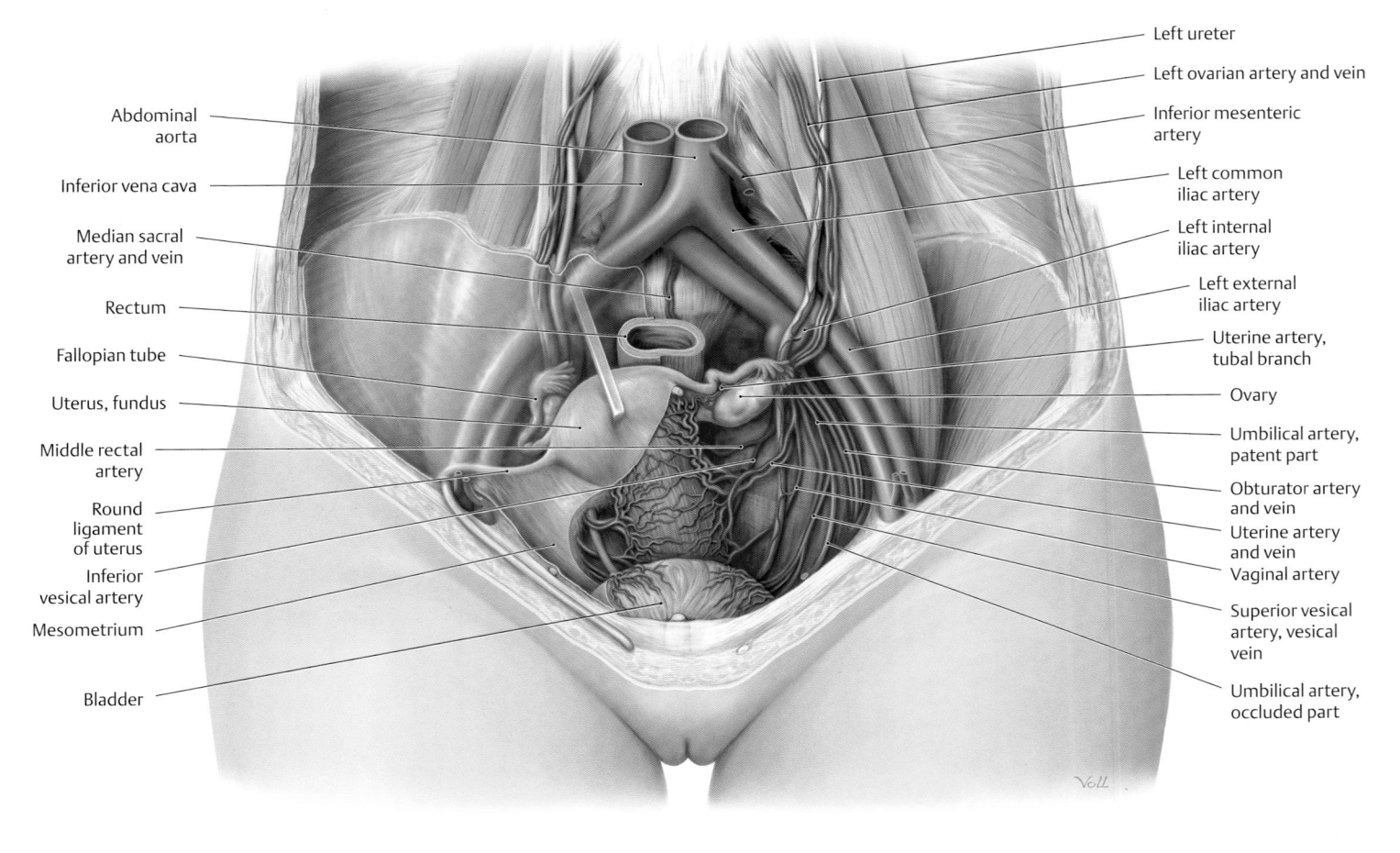

Left ureter

Left ovarian artery and vein

Inferior mesenteric artery

Left common iliac artery

Left internal iliac artery

Left external iliac artery

Uterine artery, tubal branch

Ovary

Umbilical artery, patent part

Obturator artery and vein

Uterine artery and vein

Vaginal artery

Superior vesical artery, vesical vein

Umbilical artery, occluded part

Abdominal aorta

Inferior vena cava

Median sacral artery and vein

Rectum

Fallopian tube

Uterus, fundus

Middle rectal artery

Round ligament of uterus

Inferior vesical artery

Mesometrium

Bladder

A Vascular supply of the female internal genitalia

Anterior view. All of the peritoneum has been removed on the left side, and most has been removed on the right side. The uterus has been straightened and tilted to the right.

The (internal) female genital organs are supplied by two large **arteries** that arise from different trunks. The *ovary* is supplied mainly by the ovarian artery (usually arising from the abdominal aorta, see variants in **B**), and the *uterus* is supplied by the uterine artery, a visceral branch of the internal iliac artery. The fallopian tube receives one tubal branch from the uterine artery and one from the ovarian artery. The ovary is additionally supplied by an ovarian branch of the uterine artery. The uterine artery passes to the uterus in the base of the broad ligament (see

p. 246). The ureter crosses just inferior to the artery, and this relationship should be noted in operations on the uterus (see **G**). The uterine artery enters the uterus at the junction of the body of the uterus and the cervix. At that point it often gives off a vaginal branch to the vagina and then runs a very tortuous course to the uterine fundus. This tortuosity provides redundant vessel length that allows the artery to stretch when the uterus enlarges during pregnancy. The **venous drainage** of the uterus is to the uterine plexus, which is drained on each side by the uterine vein. The uterine vein empties into the internal iliac vein, running a course analogous to that of the uterine artery. The right ovarian vein drains blood from the right ovary directly into the inferior vena cava, while blood from the left ovary drains to the left renal vein before reaching the vena cava.

Abdominal aorta

Right renal artery

Left renal artery

b

a

Right ovarian/ testicular artery

Left ovarian/ testicular artery

c

B Variants in the origin of the ovarian and testicular arteries
(after Lippert and Pabst)
a Typical case: The ovarian or testicular arteries arise from the abdominal aorta (approximately 70 % of cases).
b Accessory vessels are present (approximately 15 %).
c The arteries arise from the renal artery (approximately 15 %).

C Range of variation in the location of the ovarian arteries
(after von Lanz and Wachsmuth)
Anterior view showing the relationship of the arteries to the ureters.

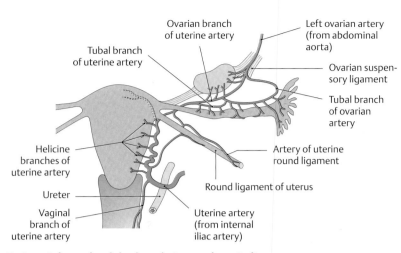

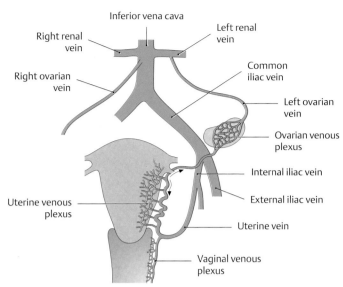

D Arterial supply of the female internal genitalia

Anterior view.

Note: Two arteries supply the ovary in the "ovarian arcade": the ovarian artery from the abdominal aorta (courses in the ovarian suspensory ligament) and the ovarian branch of the uterine artery (runs along the fallopian tube). Attention must be given to both vessels during adnexal surgery. With a tumor or cyst of the ovary, "ovarian torsion" may occur, causing a dangerous reduction in the ovarian blood supply. Reason: The plum-sized ovary is suspended on a vascular cord, the suspensory ligament (consisting of the ovarian artery and vein and surrounding peritoneum, not shown here). An ovarian cyst or tumor leads to *eccentric* enlargement of the ovary. When the human body spins or rotates (e.g., during sports), the affected ovary may become twisted about the axis of this vascular pedicle, strangulating the vessels and constricting or totally occluding the ovarian blood supply.

E Venous drainage of the female internal genitalia

Anterior view. The uterine vein (often multiple on both sides, but shown here as a single vessel for clarity) collects venous blood from the uterine plexus and also drains a portion of the vaginal plexus. The ovarian venous plexus creates an anastomosis between the ovarian vein and uterine vein (it is drained by both veins).

Note the different modes of termination of the left and right ovarian veins.

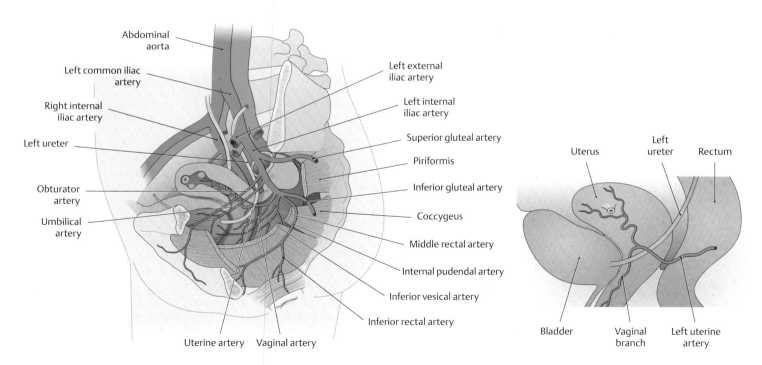

F Arterial supply of the uterus, vagina, and bladder

View into the pelvis from the left side. The uterine broad ligament has been cut open to display the branches of the left internal iliac artery.

Note: The serpentine course of the uterine artery along the uterine body is particularly well demonstrated in this lateral view (see also **A**). The origins of the uterine artery and vaginal artery are subject to considerable variation.

G Relationship of the uterine artery and ureter

Left lateral view of the left uterine artery and left ureter. The ureter crosses inferior to the uterine artery in the base of the broad ligament (see also **A**) and is therefore susceptible to injury in operations on the uterus.

291

3.16 Venous Anastomoses in the Abdomen and Pelvis

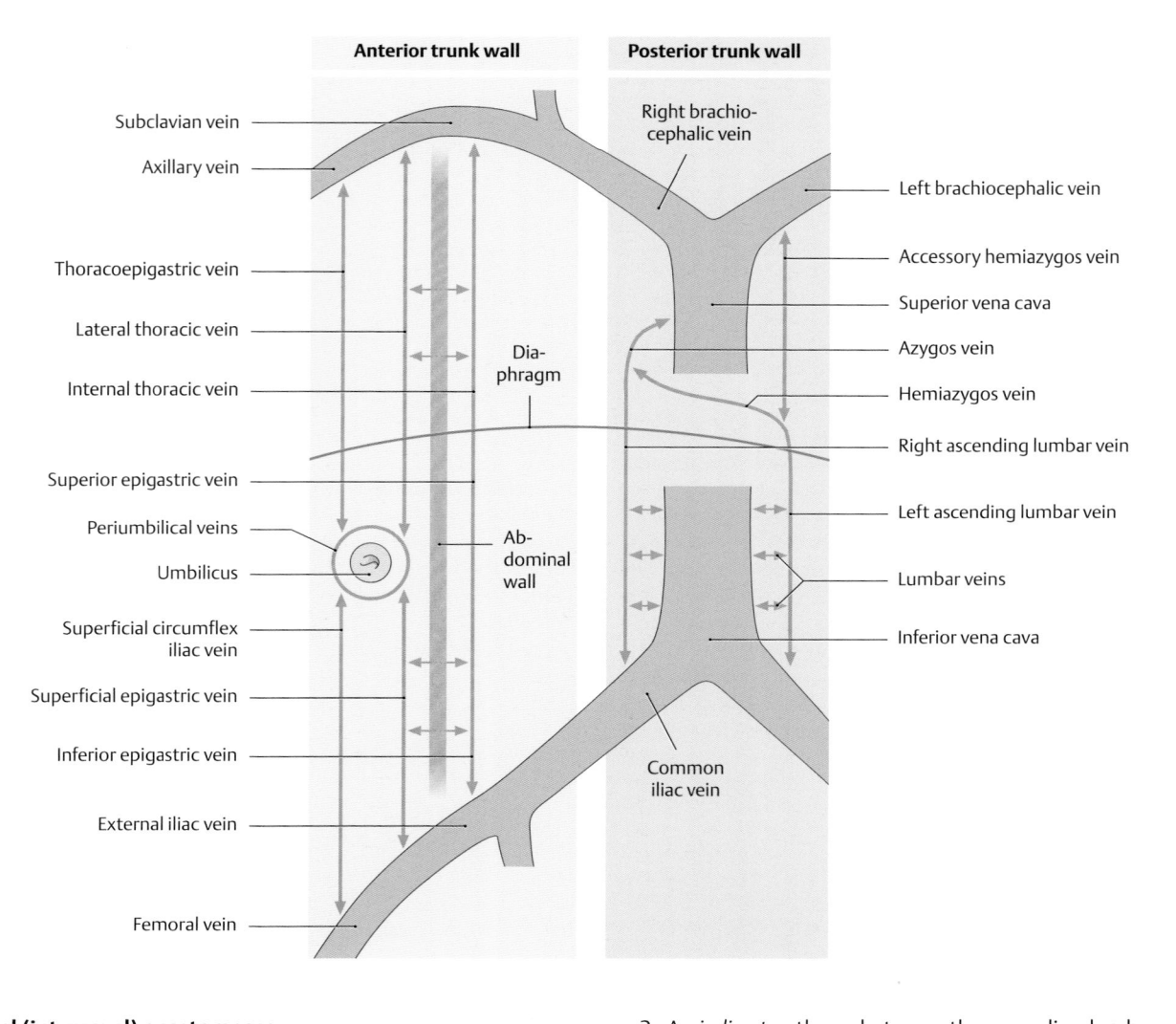

A Cavocaval (intercaval) anastomoses

Large venous anastomoses are present between the inferior and superior vena cava on the anterior and posterior trunk walls. Known as *cavocaval* or *intercaval anastomoses*, they provide collateral pathways for returning venous blood to the *superior* vena cava and right heart in patients with outflow obstructions affecting the *inferior* vena cava in the abdomen or the common iliac veins in the pelvis. Veins of the chest wall form the cranial portion of this collateral network. The veins of the *anterior* abdominal wall provide both a *superficial* pathway (anterior to the rectus abdominis) and a *deep* pathway (posterior to the rectus abdominis). (In the chest, these pathways lie outside or inside the thoracic skeleton.)

Note: On the *anterior* trunk wall, the paraumbilical veins (see **B**) establish a collateral pathway between the portal vein and drainage to the venae cavae. This portosystemic (portacaval) pathway is important in patients with obstructed portal venous flow and may affect the superficial and deep anterior pathways.

- Anastomoses on the *posterior wall* of the abdomen. They utilize the connection between the ascending lumbar vein and the azygos / hemiazygos vein. Two pathways are available:

  1. A *direct* pathway between the ascending lumbar vein and azygos / hemiazygos vein:
     Inferior vena cava → (possibly via the common iliac vein) ascending lumbar vein → azygos / hemiazygos vein → **superior vena cava**.

  2. An *indirect* pathway between the ascending lumbar vein and azygos / hemiazygos vein by way of horizontal trunk wall veins (intercostal and lumbar veins, mediated by venous plexuses on the spinal column; for clarity, not shown here):
     Inferior vena cava → (possibly via the common iliac vein) ascending lumbar vein → lumbar veins → vertebral venous plexus → posterior intercostal veins → azygos / hemiazygos vein → **superior vena cava**.

- Anastomoses on the *anterior* wall of the abdomen. They utilize superficial and deep cutaneous veins, which may exchange blood between them. Two pathways are available:

  1. Deep pathway (posterior to the rectus abdominis):
     Inferior vena cava → common iliac vein → external iliac vein → inferior epigastric vein → superior epigastric vein → internal thoracic vein → subclavian vein → brachiocephalic vein → **superior vena cava**.

  2. Superficial pathway (anterior to the rectus abdominis):
     Inferior vena cava → common iliac vein → external iliac vein → femoral vein → superficial epigastric vein / superficial circumflex iliac vein → thoracoepigastric vein / lateral thoracic vein → axillary vein → subclavian vein → brachiocephalic vein → **superior vena cava**.

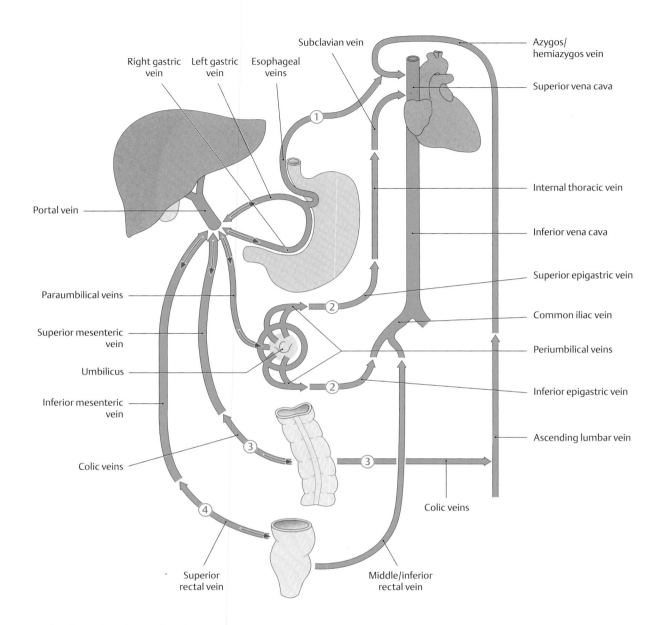

Right gastric vein | Left gastric vein | Esophageal veins | Subclavian vein | Azygos/hemiazygos vein

Superior vena cava

Portal vein

Internal thoracic vein

Inferior vena cava

Paraumbilical veins

Superior epigastric vein

Superior mesenteric vein

Common iliac vein

Umbilicus

Periumbilical veins

Inferior mesenteric vein

Inferior epigastric vein

Ascending lumbar vein

Colic veins

Colic veins

Superior rectal vein

Middle/inferior rectal vein

B Schematic of collateral pathways for the portal vein (portosystemic collaterals)

Venous collateral pathways are also available between the portal venous system and the inferior and superior venae cavae. These *portosystemic* collaterals are physiological pathways that can develop in response to (1) overlapping venous territories in organs (venous plexuses in the esophagus, colon, rectum) or (2) the persistence of patent blood vessels that are normally obliterated after birth (umbilical vein, paraumbilical veins). These collateral pathways become clinically significant when the portal system is compromised (as in hepatic cirrhosis, for example). As venous pressure increases, the portal vein can divert blood away from the liver and return it to the supplying vessels. Thus, veins that are normally *afferent* vessels for the liver undergo a *flow reversal* (see red arrows) and transport blood back through the inferior or superior vena cava and and back to the heart. Portosystemic shunts can be life-saving, but nevertheless cause significant additional problems, because some of the vessels in the shunt pathways (in the esophagus and rectum, specifically) are barely capable of handling the significant redirected blood flow, with consequent rise of pressure in the system, and are thus liable to rupture. The following four **collateral pathways** are of key importance:

① Through veins of the stomach and distal esophagus (dilation of these veins may lead to esophageal varices, with risk of life-threatening hemorrhage):

Portal vein ← gastric veins ← *esophageal veins* → azygos/hemiazygos vein → **superior vena cava.**

② Through veins of the anterior abdominal wall:
Portal vein ← umbilical vein (patent part) ← *paraumbilical veins* → superior epigastric vein → internal thoracic vein → subclavian vein → **superior vena cava** or
Portal vein ← umbilical vein (patent part) → *paraumbilical veins* → inferior epigastric vein → external iliac vein → **inferior vena cava.**
Drainage from paraumbilical veins into the superficial veins (rare) of the anterior abdominal wall (thoracoepigastric vein, lateral thoracic vein, superficial epigastric vein, see **A**) leads to dilation of these tortuous veins (Medusa head, caput medusae).

③ Through veins of the posterior abdominal wall:
Portal vein ← superior and inferior mesenteric vein ← *colic veins* → ascending lumbar veins → azygos/hemiazygos vein → **superior vena cava**. The ascending lumbar veins may also divert blood to the inferior vena cava.

④ Through the rectal venous plexus (with dilation):
Portal vein ← inferior mesenteric vein ← superior rectal vein ← *middle/inferior rectal veins* → internal iliac vein → **inferior vena cava.**

4.1 Overview of Lymphatic Trunks and Lymph Node Groups in the Abdomen and Pelvis

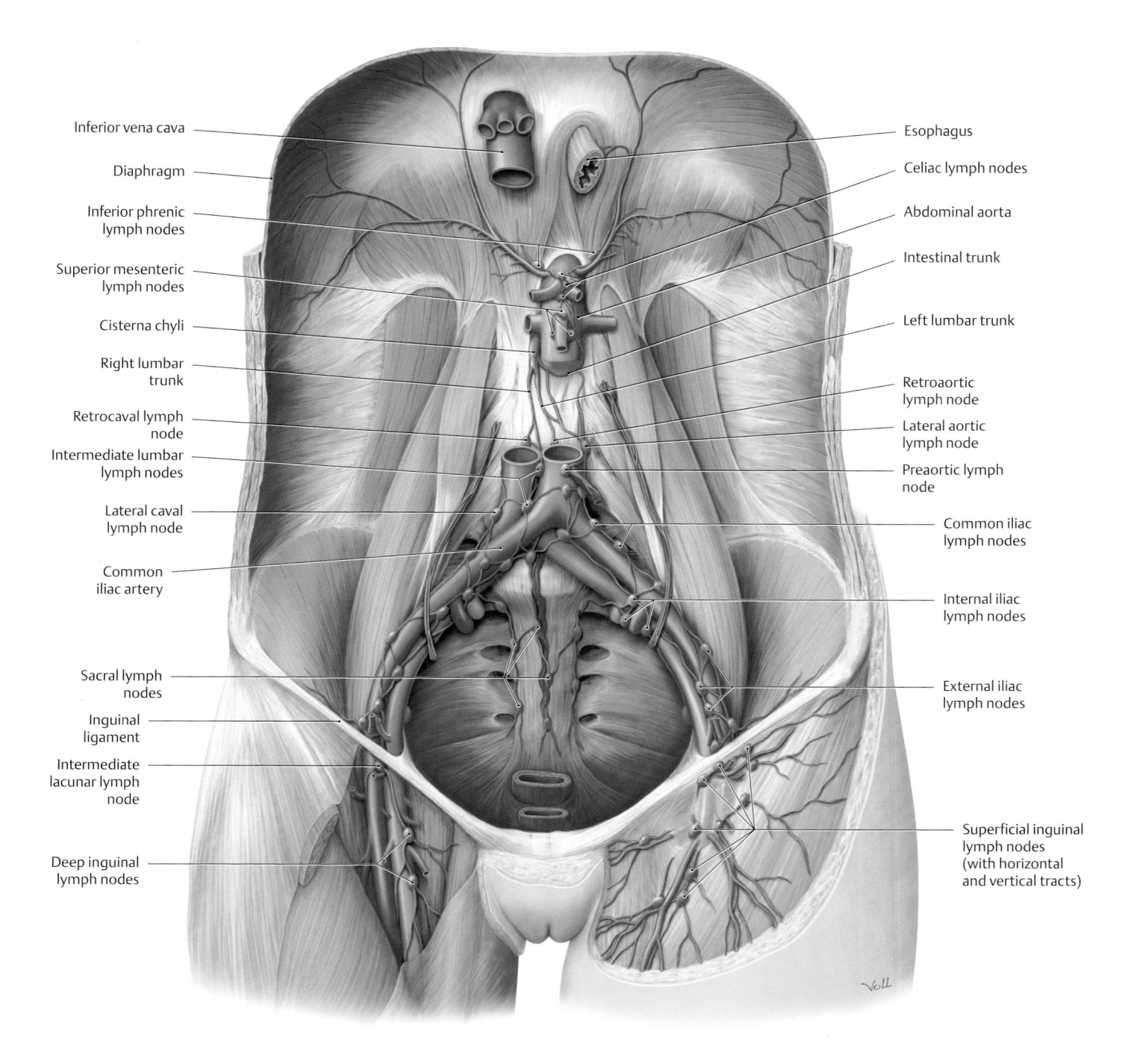

A Overview of parietal lymph nodes in the abdomen and pelvis

Anterior view of an opened female abdomen. All visceral structures have been removed except for major vessels, and the lymphatic vessels are shown larger for clarity. Size disparities between the lymph nodes (1 mm to over 1 cm) and actual numbers (several hundred) are ignored. Regional lymph nodes (see **C**) may be arranged so densely that individual groups can scarcely be identified. Lymph nodes in the abdomen and pelvis are classified by their location as *parietal* or *visceral*. Parietal lymph nodes are located *near the trunk wall* (often distributed along blood vessels), while visceral lymph nodes are located *near organs* in the connective tissue of the extraperitoneal space or in the mesentery attached to an organ. A large percentage of parietal lymph nodes are located on the posterior wall of the abdomen and pelvis: they are clustered around the large vessels that course on the posterior abdominal

and pelvic walls, such as the abdominal aorta and inferior vena cava in the abdomen and the iliac arteries and veins and their branches in the pelvis. Only a few lymph nodes are located on the anterior wall, such as the inguinal lymph nodes and the nodes around the external iliac artery (iliac lymph nodes). The lymph nodes and lymphatic vessels are arranged in an intricate network in the abdomen and pelvis, as they generally are elsewhere in the body. As a result, lymphatic drainage tends to follow multiple regional patterns of flow rather than a single well-defined pathway (see p. 296). Potential drainage routes are particularly numerous for the organs of the pelvis, where several organs may share lymphatic pathways. For example, certain lymph nodes are utilized (with varying degrees of preference) by the bladder, genital organs, and rectum.

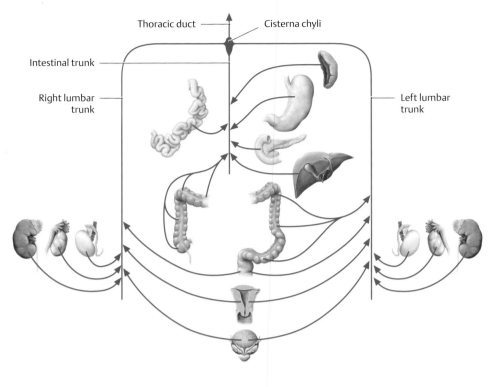

Thoracic duct — Cisterna chyli

Intestinal trunk

Right lumbar trunk

Left lumbar trunk

B Lymphatic trunks in the abdomen and pelvis

Lymph from the abdominal and pelvic organs drains to the lumbar and intestinal trunks (see p. 296) after first passing through one or more lymph node groups (see **C**). An expansion, the cisterna chyli, is frequently present at the union of these trunks. Lymph from the cisterna chyli drains through the thoracic duct to the junction of the left subclavian and internal jugular veins. The thoracic duct is the principal lymphatic trunk that returns lymph to the venous system.

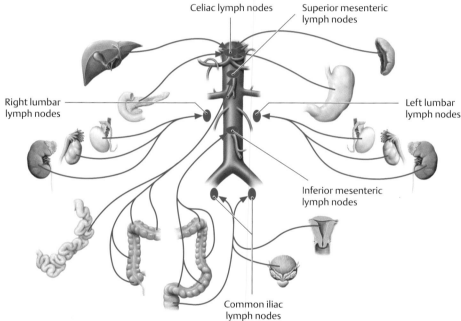

Celiac lymph nodes

Superior mesenteric lymph nodes

Right lumbar lymph nodes

Left lumbar lymph nodes

Inferior mesenteric lymph nodes

Common iliac lymph nodes

C Lymph node groups in the abdomen and pelvis

Before lymph from the organs of the abdomen and pelvis enters the lymphatic trunks, it is filtered by **lymph nodes** that collect the lymph from a particular organ (or region). After leaving the regional nodes, the lymph drains to **collecting lymph nodes**. These are the nodes that collect lymph from several lymph node groups and carry it to the lymphatic trunks. In the abdomen and pelvis, these are the lumbar and intestinal trunks.

Note: One lymph node may function as a *regional lymph node* for *various* organs, but at the same time it may collect lymph from several regional nodes, functioning also as a *collecting lymph node*. This principle is illustrated in the abdomen and pelvis by the lumbar lymph nodes: They function as regional lymph nodes for the kidneys, suprarenal glands, gonads, and adnexa (see pp. 302–305) and as collecting lymph nodes for the iliac nodes.

D Lymph node groups and tributary regions

Lymph node groups and collecting lymph nodes	Location (see C)	Organs or organ segments that drain to these lymph node groups (tributary regions)
Celiac lymph nodes	Around the celiac trunk	Distal third of esophagus, stomach, greater omentum, duodenum (superior and descending parts), pancreas, spleen, liver, and gallbladder
Superior mesenteric lymph nodes	At the origin of the superior mesenteric artery	Second through fourth parts of duodenum, jejunum and ileum, cecum with vermiform appendix, ascending colon, transverse colon (proximal two-thirds)
Inferior mesenteric lymph nodes	At the origin of the inferior mesenteric artery	Transverse colon (distal third), descending colon, sigmoid colon, rectum (proximal part)
Lumbar lymph nodes (right, intermediate, left)	Around the abdominal aorta and inferior vena cava	Diaphragm (abdominal side), kidneys, suprarenal glands, testis and epididymis, ovary, fallopian tube, uterine fundus, ureters, retroperitoneum
Iliac lymph nodes	Around the iliac vessels	Rectum (anal end), bladder and urethra, uterus (body and cervix), vas deferens, seminal vesicle, prostate, external genitalia (via inguinal lymph nodes)

4.2 Overview of the Lymphatic Drainage of Abdominal and Pelvic Organs

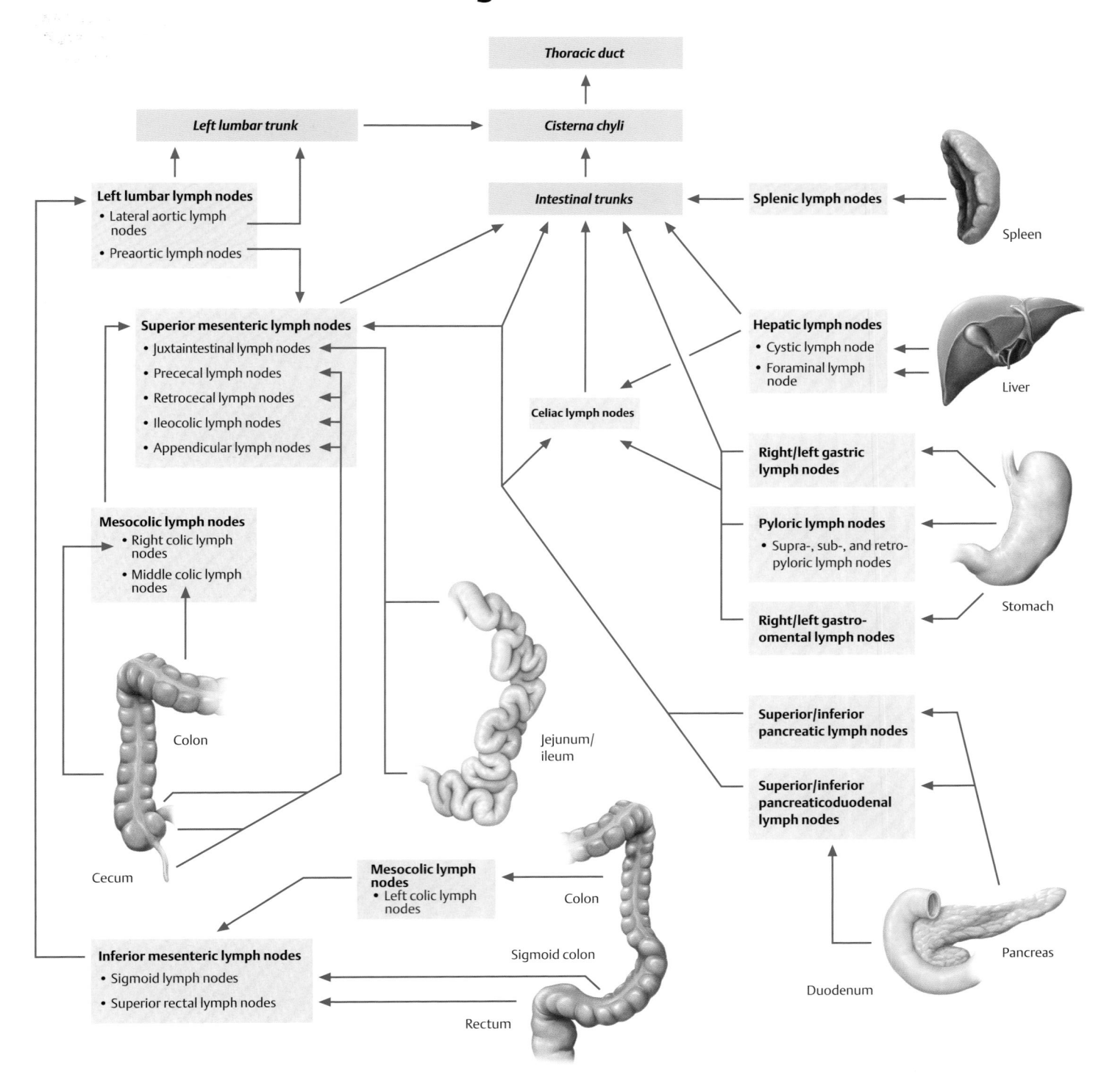

A Principal lymphatic pathways draining the digestive organs and spleen

Lymph from the spleen and most of the digestive organs drains directly from regional lymph nodes or through intervening collecting lymph nodes to the *intestinal trunks*. Exceptions are the descending colon, sigmoid colon, and the upper part of the rectum, which are drained by the *left lumbar trunk*. The organs and visceral lymph nodes in the above schematic are served mainly by three large collecting stations (individual lymph nodes are covered later in the chapter):

• Celiac lymph nodes: collect lymph from the stomach, duodenum, pancreas, spleen, and liver. Topographically and at dissection, they are often indistinguishable from the regional lymph nodes of nearby upper abdominal organs.
• Superior mesenteric lymph nodes: collect lymph from the jejunum, ileum, ascending colon, and transverse colon.
• Inferior mesenteric lymph nodes: collect lymph from the descending colon, sigmoid colon, and rectum.

These collecting lymph nodes drain *principally* through the intestinal trunks to the cisterna chyli. There is also an *accessory* drainage route to the cisterna chyli by way of the left lumbar lymph nodes.
The lymphatic drainage of the rectum is described on p. 301.

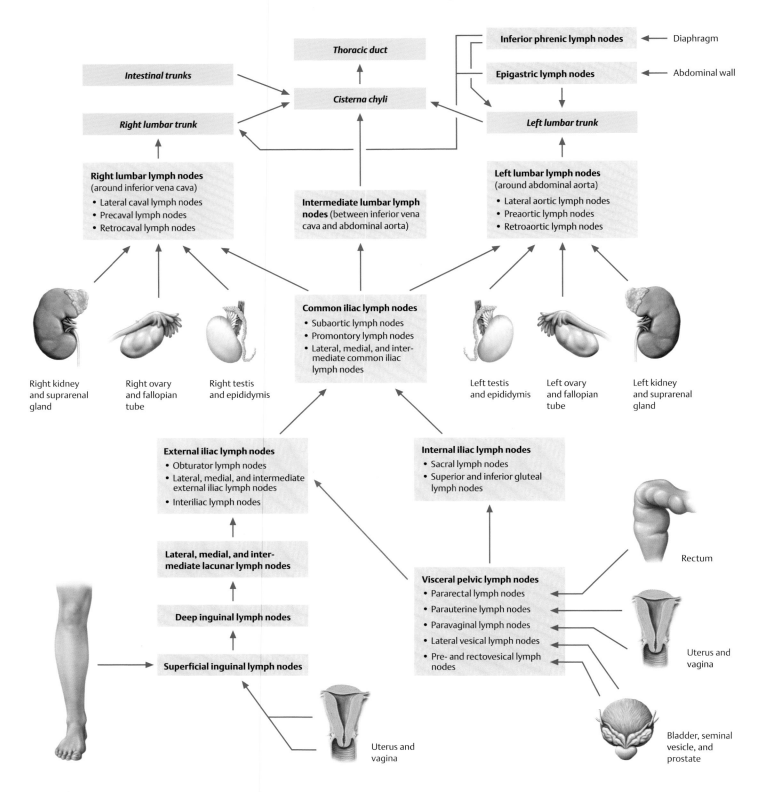

B Principal lymphatic pathways draining the organs of the retroperitoneum and pelvis (and lower limb)

Lymph from these organs drains principally to the right and left lumbar trunks. The following are important lymph node groups for the organs of the retroperitoneum and pelvis (and lower limb):

- Common iliac lymph nodes: collect lymph from the pelvic organs and lower limb.
- Right and left lumbar lymph nodes: collecting lymph nodes for the common iliac nodes, also regional lymph nodes for the organs of the retroperitoneum *and* the gonads, although the latter are located in the pelvis or scrotum. As the gonads undergo their developmental descent, they maintain their lymphatic connection to the lumbar lymph nodes (analogous to their blood supply, see p. 290). As a result, when tumors of the testis (or ovary), for example, undergo lymphogenous spread, they tend to metastasize directly to the abdomen rather than to the pelvis.

Both the iliac lymph nodes and the lumbar lymph nodes are classified as *parietal* nodes, a category that includes the phrenic and epigastric nodes. Lymph nodes such as the pararectal and parauterine lymph nodes are classified as *visceral* nodes.

4.3 Lymphatic Drainage of the Stomach, Spleen, Pancreas, Duodenum, and Liver

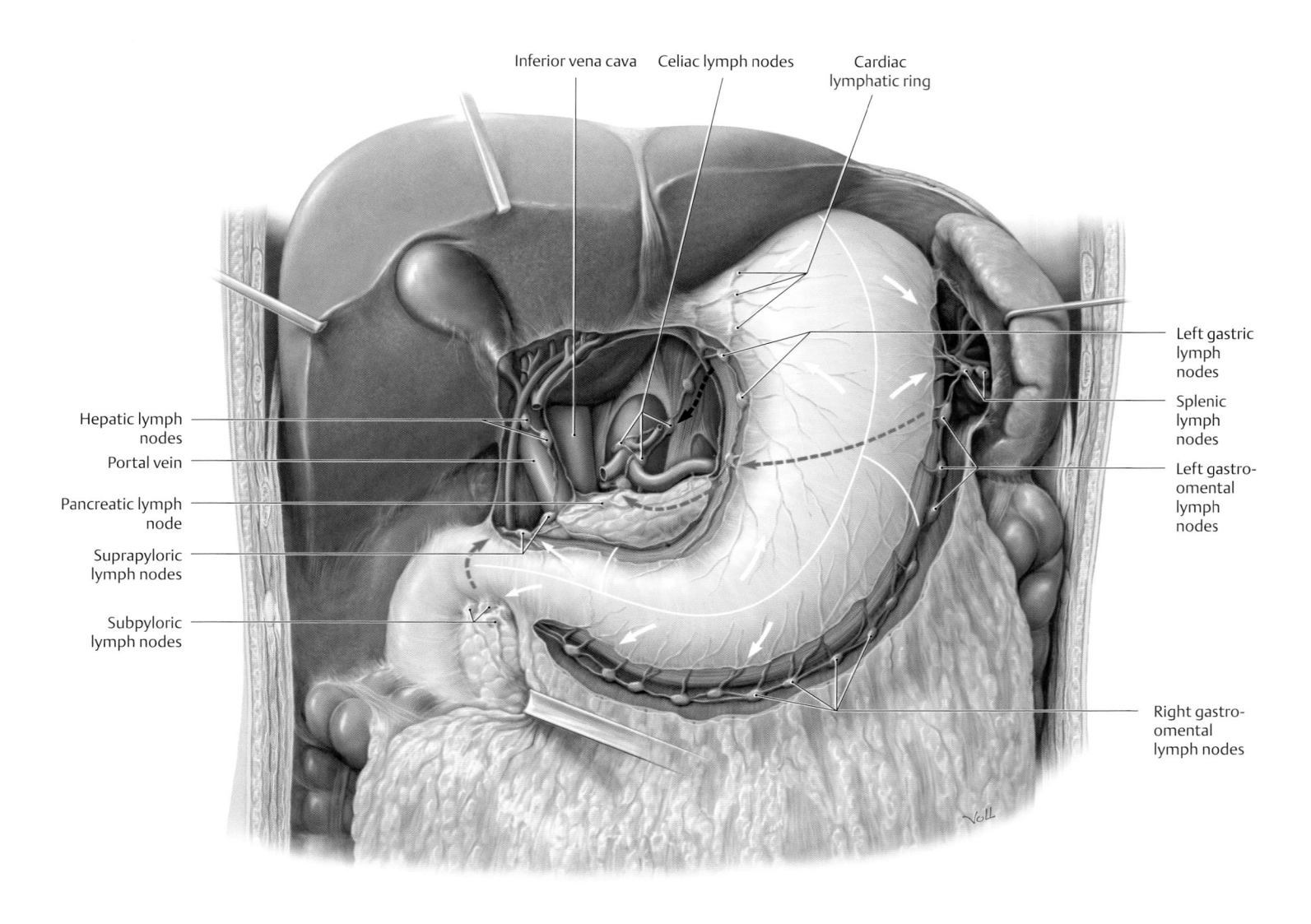

Inferior vena cava   Celiac lymph nodes   Cardiac lymphatic ring

Left gastric lymph nodes

Splenic lymph nodes

Left gastro-omental lymph nodes

Hepatic lymph nodes

Portal vein

Pancreatic lymph node

Suprapyloric lymph nodes

Subpyloric lymph nodes

Right gastro-omental lymph nodes

A Lymphatic drainage of the stomach

Anterior view. The lesser omentum has been removed, the greater omentum has been partially opened along the greater curvature of the stomach, and the liver has been retracted slightly superiorly. The following lymphatic pathways are important in this region:

- Drainage toward the **greater and lesser curvatures of the stomach**. Initial drainage is to the regional lymph nodes: the right and left gastric lymph nodes (toward the lesser curvature) or the right and

left gastro-omental lymph nodes (toward the greater curvature, see white lines and arrows). These regional lymph nodes convey lymph either directly or indirectly to the celiac lymph nodes (indirectly by way of the pyloric and splenic nodes). From there the lymph drains to the intestinal trunk.

- Drainage from the **fundus and cardia**: initially to the inconstant (not always present) lymphatic ring of the gastric cardia, then to the intestinal trunk.

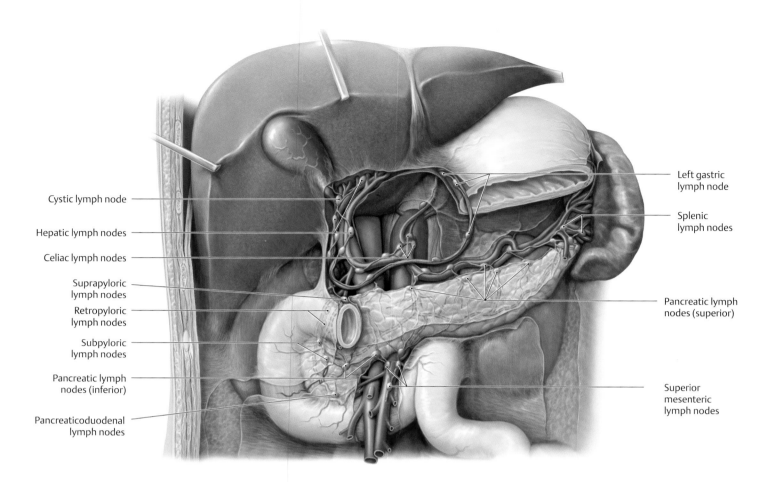

Cystic lymph node

Hepatic lymph nodes

Celiac lymph nodes

Suprapyloric
lymph nodes

Retropyloric
lymph nodes

Subpyloric
lymph nodes

Pancreatic lymph
nodes (inferior)

Pancreaticoduodenal
lymph nodes

Left gastric
lymph node

Splenic
lymph nodes

Pancreatic lymph
nodes (superior)

Superior
mesenteric
lymph nodes

B Lymphatic drainage of the spleen, pancreas, and duodenum

Anterior view. Most of the stomach has been removed, the colon has been detached, and the liver has been retracted upward. The following lymph nodes and groups of nodes are important in this region:

- **Spleen:** drains initially to the *splenic lymph nodes*, then directly or indirectly to the *intestinal trunk* (the indirect route may be through the superior pancreatic lymph nodes *alone* or through the superior pancreatic nodes and the celiac nodes).
- **Pancreas:** drains initially to the *superior and inferior pancreatic lymph nodes*, then directly or indirectly (via the celiac nodes) to the intestinal trunk; *or* drains initially to the *superior and inferior pancreaticoduo-*

denal lymph nodes (mainly on the posterior side of the pancreas), then directly or indirectly via the superior mesenteric nodes to the intestinal trunk.

- **Duodenum:** The *upper portion* of the duodenum drains initially to the *pyloric lymph nodes* (see **C**), then to the superior pancreaticoduodenal lymph nodes and from there to the hepatic lymph nodes, or directly to the celiac nodes in some cases, before entering the intestinal trunk. The *lower portion* of the duodenum first drains to the *superior and inferior pancreaticoduodenal lymph nodes*, then directly to the intestinal trunk.

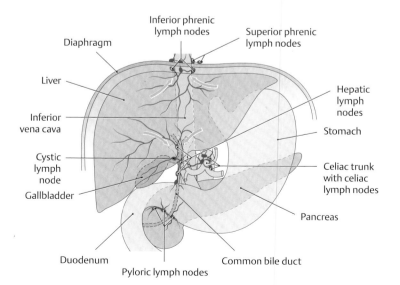

Diaphragm

Liver

Inferior
vena cava

Cystic
lymph
node

Gallbladder

Inferior phrenic
lymph nodes

Superior phrenic
lymph nodes

Hepatic
lymph
nodes

Stomach

Celiac trunk
with celiac
lymph nodes

Pancreas

Duodenum

Pyloric lymph nodes

Common bile duct

C Lymphatic pathways for the liver and biliary tract

Anterior view. The following lymphatic pathways are important in this region:

Liver and intrahepatic bile ducts (three drainage pathways):

- Most lymph drains inferiorly through the hepatic lymph nodes to the celiac lymph nodes and then to the intestinal trunk and cisterna chyli, or it may drain directly from the hepatic lymph nodes to the intestinal trunk and cisterna chyli.
- A small amount of lymph drains cranially through the inferior phrenic lymph nodes to the lumbar trunk.
- In some cases lymph drains through the diaphragm (partly through the vena caval hiatus and partly through muscular openings in the diaphragm) to the superior phrenic lymph nodes and then to the bronchomediastinal trunk.

Gallbladder: Lymph from the gallbladder drains initially to the cystic lymph node, then follows the pathway described above.

Common bile duct: Lymph from the bile duct drains through the pyloric lymph nodes (supra-, sub-, and retropyloric nodes) and the foraminal lymph node to the celiac nodes, then to the intestinal trunk.

299

4.4 Lymphatic Drainage of the Small and Large Intestine

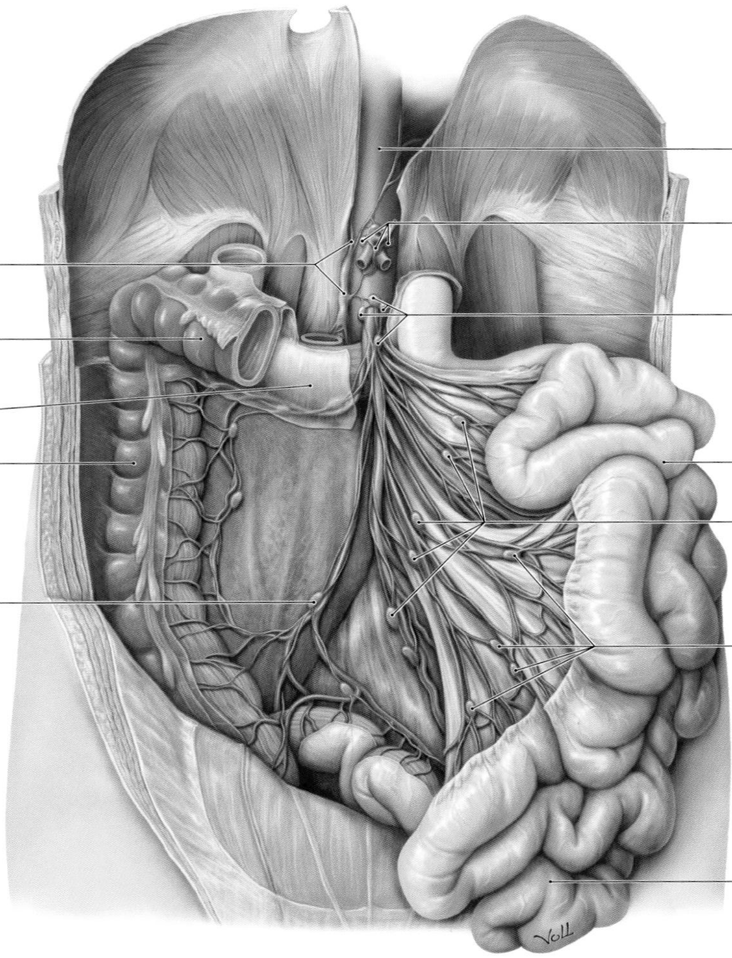

Abdominal aorta

Celiac lymph nodes

Superior mesenteric lymph nodes

Thoracic duct with cisterna chyli

Transverse colon

Duodenum

Ascending colon

Jejunum

Intermediate mesenteric lymph nodes

Ileocolic lymph nodes

Juxtaintestinal lymph nodes

Ileum

A Lymph nodes and lymphatic drainage of the jejunum and ileum
Anterior view. The stomach, liver, pancreas, and most of the colon have been removed. The lymph nodes of the small intestine are the largest group of lymph nodes in the human body, numbering approximately 100 150 nodes of greatly varying size. For clarity, the above drawing shows only a few lymph nodes that are representative of larger groups. Lymph from both the jejunum and ileum drains initially to regional lymph nodes (juxtaintestinal lymph nodes), then to the superior mesenteric lymph nodes, and finally to the intestinal trunk. The lymph nodes and vessels in the *mesentery* basically follow the distribution of the arteries and veins.

They are called "intermediate" because they are situated *between* visceral and collecting lymph nodes (the superior and inferior mesenteric lymph nodes). In patients with a malignant tumor, it is desirable to remove as many lymph nodes as possible along a drainage pathway to ensure the removal of any micrometastases (metastases not grossly visible) that may be present in the nodes. In the case of the duodenum, this means that the resection should include not only the affected part of the duodenum but also the attached portion of the mesentery and the (intermediate) lymph nodes that it contains. Occasionally even the superior and inferior mesenteric lymph nodes are also removed.

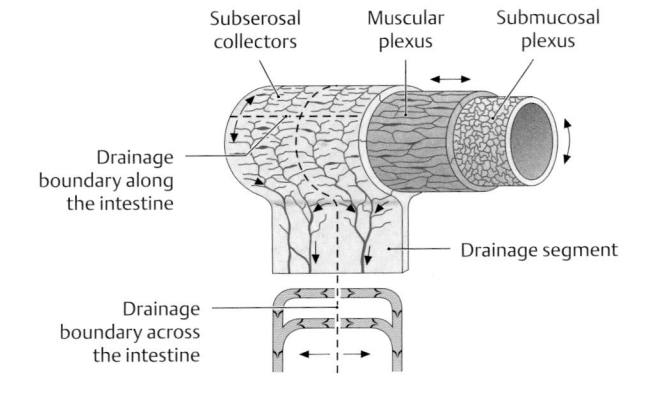

Subserosal collectors

Muscular plexus

Submucosal plexus

Drainage boundary along the intestine

Drainage segment

Drainage boundary across the intestine

B Lymphatic drainage of the intestine by segments
(after Földi and Kubik)
Lymph is collected in several plexuses (networks of lymphatic vessels and lymph collectors) in the intestinal wall. The lymphatics accompany the mesenteric arteries and veins through the mesentery, and in principle they drain the intestinal segment that is supplied by those vessels. Valves in the subserous collectors determine the direction of flow and define the boundaries of the individual drainage segments in the intestinal wall. Because of these segmental boundaries, it is rare for a tumor to spread extensively along the intestine by the lymphatic route.
Arrows: principal direction of lymphatic drainage.

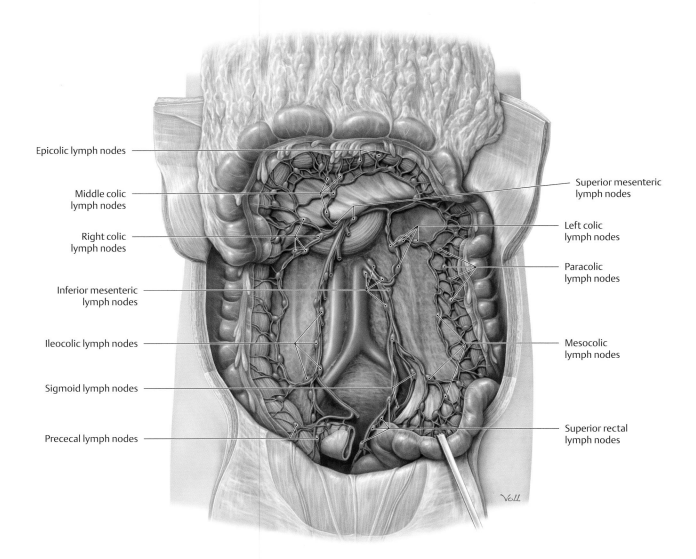

Epicolic lymph nodes

Middle colic lymph nodes

Right colic lymph nodes

Inferior mesenteric lymph nodes

Ileocolic lymph nodes

Sigmoid lymph nodes

Prececal lymph nodes

Superior mesenteric lymph nodes

Left colic lymph nodes

Paracolic lymph nodes

Mesocolic lymph nodes

Superior rectal lymph nodes

C Lymphatic drainage of the large intestine
(modified from Földi and Kubik)

Anterior view. The transverse colon and greater omentum have been reflected superiorly. The following lymphatic pathways are important in this region:

- **Ascending colon, cecum, and transverse colon:** Lymph from these structures drains initially to the *right and middle colic lymph nodes*, then to the *superior mesenteric lymph nodes*, and finally to the *intestinal trunk*.
- **Descending colon:** Lymph from the descending colon drains initially to regional lymph nodes, the *left colic lymph nodes*, then to the *inferior mesenteric lymph nodes*, and then drains via the *left lumbar lymph nodes* (not visible here) into the *left lumbar trunk* (not visible here).
- **Sigmoid colon:** Lymph from the sigmoid colon drains initially to the sigmoid lymph nodes, then follows the pathway described for the descending colon (above).

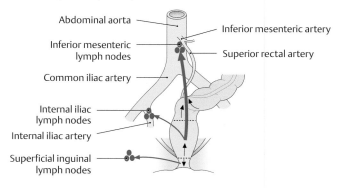

Abdominal aorta

Inferior mesenteric lymph nodes

Common iliac artery

Internal iliac lymph nodes

Internal iliac artery

Superficial inguinal lymph nodes

Inferior mesenteric artery

Superior rectal artery

- **Upper rectum** (see also **D**): Lymph from the upper rectum drains initially to the *superior rectal lymph nodes*, then follows the pathway described for the sigmoid colon (above).

Thus, a malignant tumor undergoing lymphogenous spread must negotiate several lymph node groups (all of which should be removed in tumor resections) before the malignant cells can reach the intestinal trunk and thoracic duct and finally enter the bloodstream. This long route of lymphogenous spread improves the prospects for a cure.

The lymph nodes of the large intestine can be classified *clinically* and *functionally* into more groups than by anatomical criteria alone: lymph nodes of the intestinal wall (epicolic group), lymph nodes near the intestine (paracolic group), lymph nodes at the origins of the three large intestinal arteries (central group), and lymph nodes at the origins of the mesenteric arteries (collecting lymph nodes). In standard anatomical nomenclature, the epicolic nodes are not distinguished as a seperate group, and the paracolic and central groups are considered collectively as mesocolic lymph nodes.

D Lymphatic drainage of the rectum

Anterior view. The rectum has three levels and three principal directions of lymphatic drainage (direct or indirect via the pararectal lymph nodes on the rectal wall):

- Upper level: through superior rectal lymph nodes (not shown here) to inferior mesenteric lymph nodes (→ intestinal trunk and left lumbar trunk).
- Middle level: internal iliac lymph nodes (→ right and left lumbar trunks).
- Lower level:
  - Columnar zone: to internal iliac lymph nodes.
  - Cutaneous zone: through superficial inguinal lymph nodes to external iliac lymph nodes (→ lumbar trunks).

301

4.5 Lymphatic Drainage of the Kidneys, Suprarenal Glands, Ureter, and Bladder

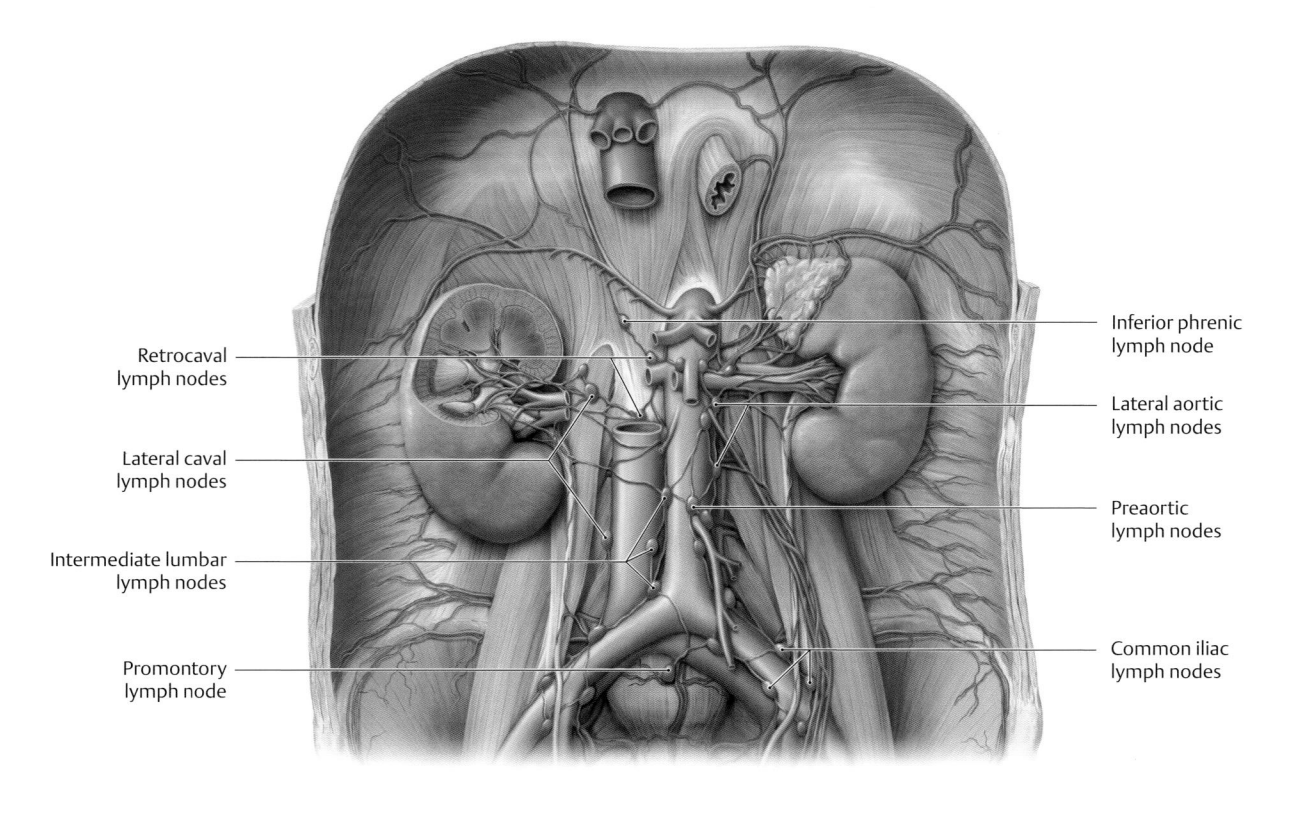

A Lymphatic drainage of the kidney, suprarenal gland, and ureter
(abdominal part; the pelvic part is shown in **C**)
Anterior view. The following lymphatic pathways are important in this region (see also p. 297):

- **Right kidney and suprarenal gland:** drain to the *right lumbar lymph nodes* (= lateral caval, precaval and retrocavcaval lymph nodes, see **B**), then to the *right lumbar trunk*.

- **Left kidney and suprarenal gland:** drain to the *left lumbar lymph nodes* (lateral aortic, preaortic and retroaortic lymph nodes, see **B**), then to the *left lumbar trunk*.
- **Ureter (abdominal part):** follows the pathway for the right and left kidneys and suprarenal glands (see also **C**).

The lumbar lymph nodes additionally function as collecting lymph nodes for the common iliac nodes.

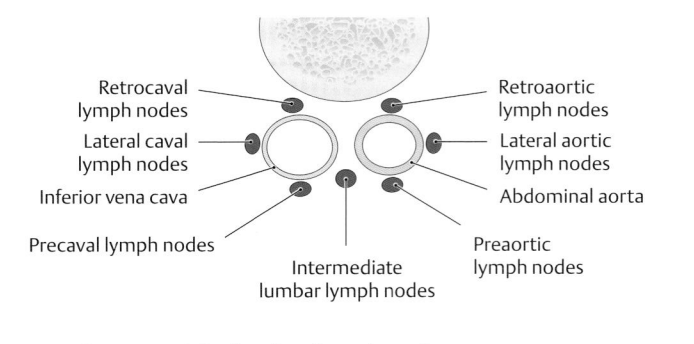

B Classification of the lumbar lymph nodes
Transverse section, viewed from above. The lumbar lymph nodes are distributed around the abdominal aorta and inferior vena cava. They are divided into three groups based on their relationship to these vessels:

- Left lumbar lymph nodes (around the aorta)
- Intermediate lumbar lymph nodes (between the aorta and inferior vena cava)
- Right lymph nodes (around the inferior vena cava)

These groups are further divided into subgroups (see legend of **A**).

C Lymph nodes of the ureter
Anterior view of the right ureter.
The lymphatic drainage of the ureter is roughly divided into two levels:

- Abdominal part of the ureter: lumbar lymph nodes
  - Right: lateral caval lymph nodes (= right lumbar lymph nodes)
  - Left: lateral aortic lymph nodes (= left lumbar lymph nodes)
- Pelvic part of the ureter: external and internal iliac lymph nodes

Both pathways empty into the lumbar trunks.

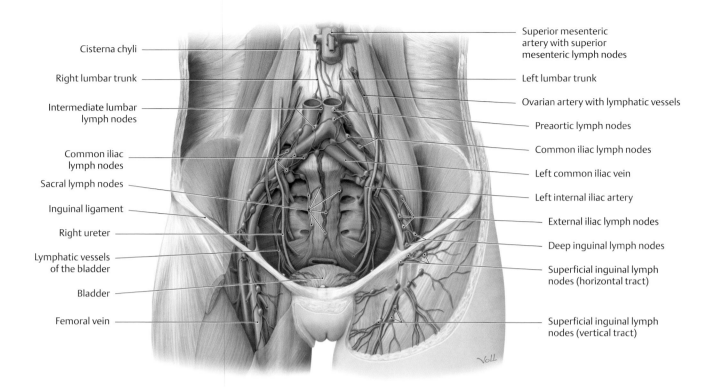

D Overview of the pelvic lymph nodes and the lymphatic drainage of the bladder

Anterior view of an opened female abdomen and pelvis. All organs have been removed except for the bladder and a small rectal stump, and the peritoneum has been removed. The bladder is distended, making it visible above the pubic symphysis. This drawing clearly shows the numerous parietal lymph nodes that are distributed around the iliac vessels in the pelvis (see **E**). Lymph from the bladder usually drains first to groups of visceral lymph nodes: the lateral vesical lymph nodes and the pre- and retrovesical lymph nodes (known collectively as the paravesical nodes). These nodes are embedded in the pelvic connective tissue surrounding the bladder and lie so deep within the pelvis that they are not visible here. Lymph from these visceral nodes drains directly or indirectly along two major pathways, reaching lymph nodes lateral to the abdominal aorta and inferior vena cava (lumbar lymph nodes) and finally entering the lumbar trunks. These pathways are illustrated in **F**.

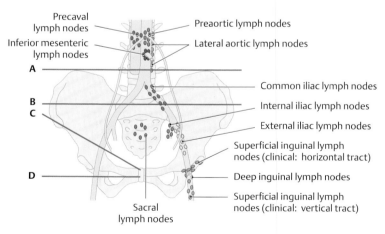

E Overview of the pelvic lymph nodes

The pelvic lymph nodes are distributed along major blood vessels and in front of the sacrum. The blood vessels are not visualized by lymphography (contrast radiography of the lymph nodes), however, and so the location of the pelvic lymph nodes must be determined by other means. One method is to use four reference lines based on skeletal landmarks:

A Iliolumbar line: horizontal line tangent to the superior borders of the iliac crests
B Iliosacral line: horizontal line through the center of the sacroiliac joint
C Inguinal line: line along the inguinal ligament
D Obturator line: horizontal line through the center of the obturator foramen

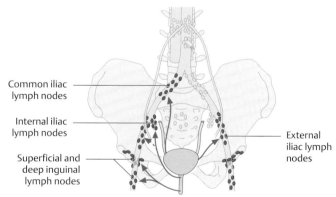

F Lymphatic drainage of the bladder and urethra

The **bladder** is drained by two principal pathways:

- Cranially along the visceral iliac vessels (see **D**),
- To the internal and external iliac lymph nodes (mainly at the base of the bladder)

Portions of the bladder near the internal urethral orifice are drained by the superficial and deep inguinal lymph nodes. The **urethra** drains chiefly to the deep and superficial inguinal lymph nodes (the latter mainly draining areas near the external urethral orifice). The proximal portions of the urethra are drained by the iliac lymph nodes, particularly the internal iliac nodes.

Note: The penis, like the urethra, is drained by the superficial and deep inguinal lymph nodes.

4.6 Lymphatic Drainage of the Male and Female Genitalia

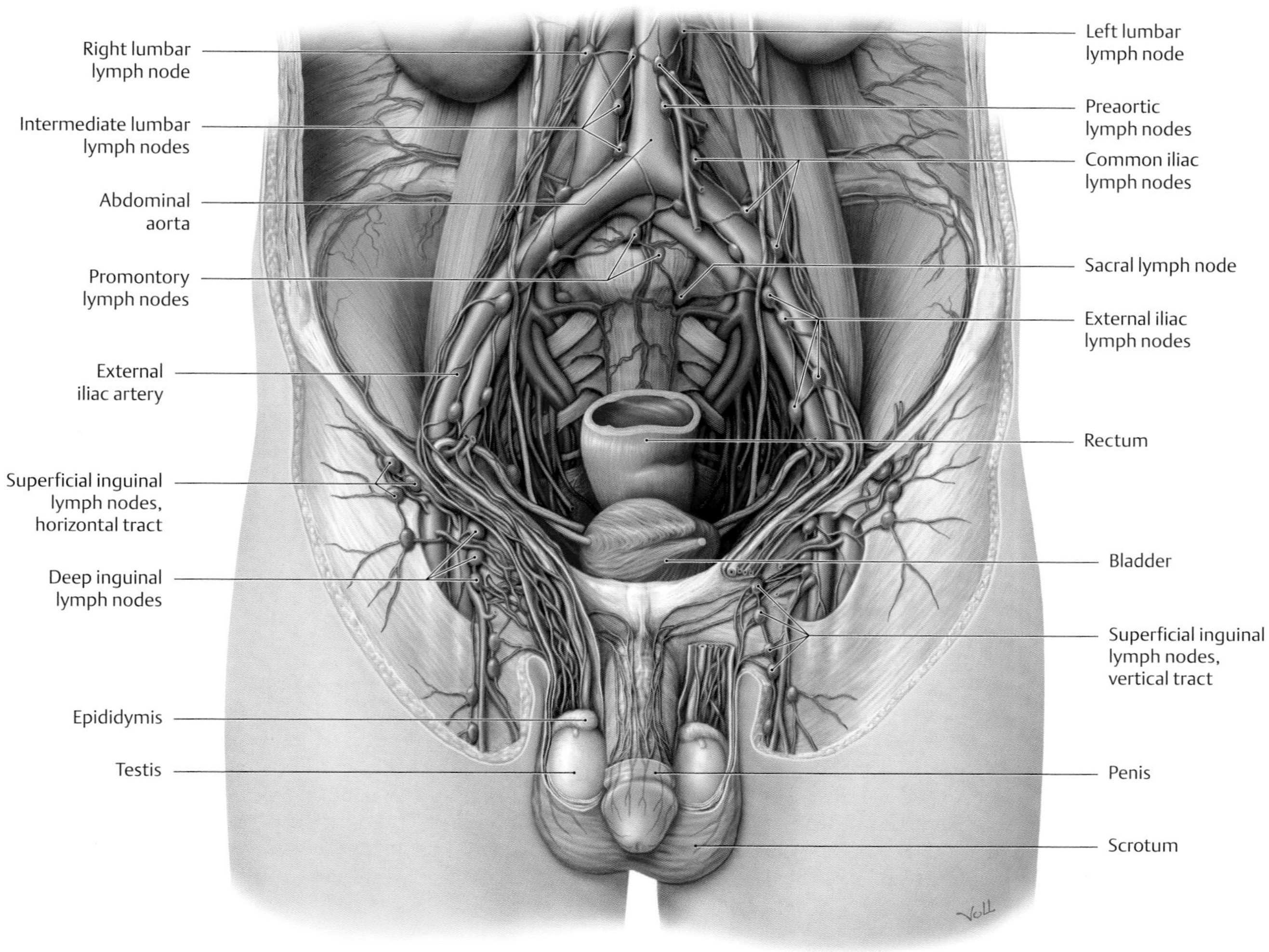

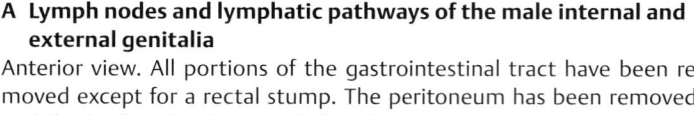

Right lumbar lymph node

Intermediate lumbar lymph nodes

Abdominal aorta

Promontory lymph nodes

External iliac artery

Superficial inguinal lymph nodes, horizontal tract

Deep inguinal lymph nodes

Epididymis

Testis

Left lumbar lymph node

Preaortic lymph nodes

Common iliac lymph nodes

Sacral lymph node

External iliac lymph nodes

Rectum

Bladder

Superficial inguinal lymph nodes, vertical tract

Penis

Scrotum

A Lymph nodes and lymphatic pathways of the male internal and external genitalia

Anterior view. All portions of the gastrointestinal tract have been removed except for a rectal stump. The peritoneum has been removed, and the bladder has been pulled slightly to the left. The *external genitalia* consist of the penis and scrotum, while the testis and epididymis (despite their location) are included with the *internal genitalia* because of their embryonic origin, along with the prostate and seminal vesicles. (The lymphatic drainage of the prostate, testis, and epididymis is described in **B**.)

Note: The lumbar lymph nodes that drain the *testis and epididymis* are located farther from these organs than most "visceral lymph nodes." As with the ovary, this results in a long drainage pathway from the testis and epididymis to the lumbar nodes. Metastases from a testicular malignancy are most frequently encountered in the lumbar lymph nodes. The *external genitalia* are drained by the superficial and deep inguinal lymph nodes. The lymphatic vessels on the dorsum of the penis are connected by anastomoses that allow for bilateral lymphatic drainage. Because of this bilateral arrangement, a malignant tumor on the *right* side of the penis may metastasize to the right *and* left inguinal lymph nodes.

B Lymphatic drainage of the testis, epididymis, and accessory sex glands

All lymph from the male genitalia is ultimately channeled by various groups of parietal lymph nodes to lumbar nodes distributed around the abdominal aorta and inferior vena cava (see pp. 297 and 302). The following specific drainage pathways are available:

Testis and epididymis: long, direct drainage pathway along the testicular vessels to the right and left lumbar lymph nodes

Vas deferens: to the iliac lymph nodes (the external more than the internal)

Seminal vesicle: internal and external iliac lymph nodes (same pathway as the vas deferens)

Prostate (multiple pathways): external iliac lymph nodes; along the vesicular vessels to the internal iliac lymph nodes; sacral lymph nodes (and on to the lumbar nodes)

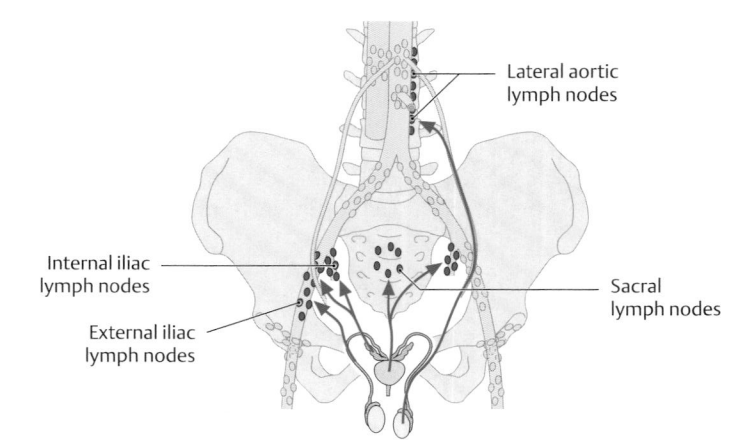

Lateral aortic lymph nodes

Internal iliac lymph nodes

External iliac lymph nodes

Sacral lymph nodes

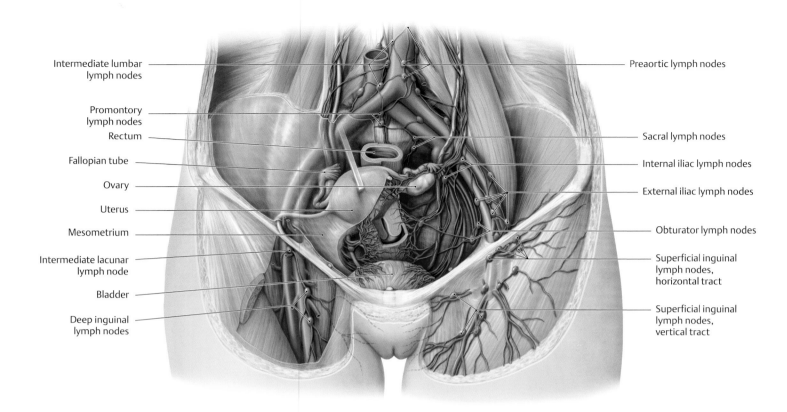

C Lymph nodes and lymphatic pathways of the female internal and external genitalia

Anterior view. The uterus is retracted to the right. The broad ligament (see p. 246) has been removed on the left side and partially opened on the right side to display the numerous lymphatic vessels that traverse the ligament. For clarity, the drawing shows only isolated lymph nodes within certain groups of nodes. *Lymph from the internal genitalia* in the female pelvis drains principally to the iliac and lumbar lymph nodes, while *lymph from the external genitalia* drains mainly to the inguinal

lymph nodes. The inguinal lymph nodes are divided by clinical criteria into a horizontal tract and vertical tract. It is believed that the *external genitalia* are drained mainly by the vertical tract.

Note: The ovary, though located in the pelvis, drains to the lumbar lymph nodes. A large portion of the lymphatic vessels of the uterus course within the broad ligament. Consequently the lymphogenous spread of malignant uterine tumors takes place along that ligament, proceeding laterally toward the pelvic wall.

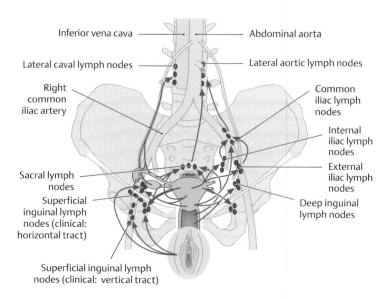

D Lymphatic drainage of the female genitalia

All of the genitalia are drained by various groups of parietal lymph nodes, which ultimately drain to lumbar nodes distributed around the abdominal aorta and inferior vena cava (see pp. 297 and 302).

External genitalia (and lowest portions of the vagina): superficial and deep inguinal lymph nodes, plus an accessory route (not shown) directly to the iliac lymph nodes.

Internal genitalia:

• Ovary, uterine fundus, and (mainly distal) portions of the fallopian tube: long drainage pathway to the lumbar lymph nodes around the abdominal aorta and inferior vena cava

• Uterine fundus and body and (mainly proximal) portions of the fallopian tube: sacral lymph nodes, internal and external iliac lymph nodes

• Uterus (cervix) and middle and upper portions of vagina: deep inguinal lymph nodes

Note: Small visceral lymph nodes for the uterus and vagina (parauterine and paravaginal lymph nodes, not shown here) are embedded in regional pelvic connective tissue close to the organs they serve.

5.1 Organization of the Sympathetic and Parasympathetic Nervous Systems

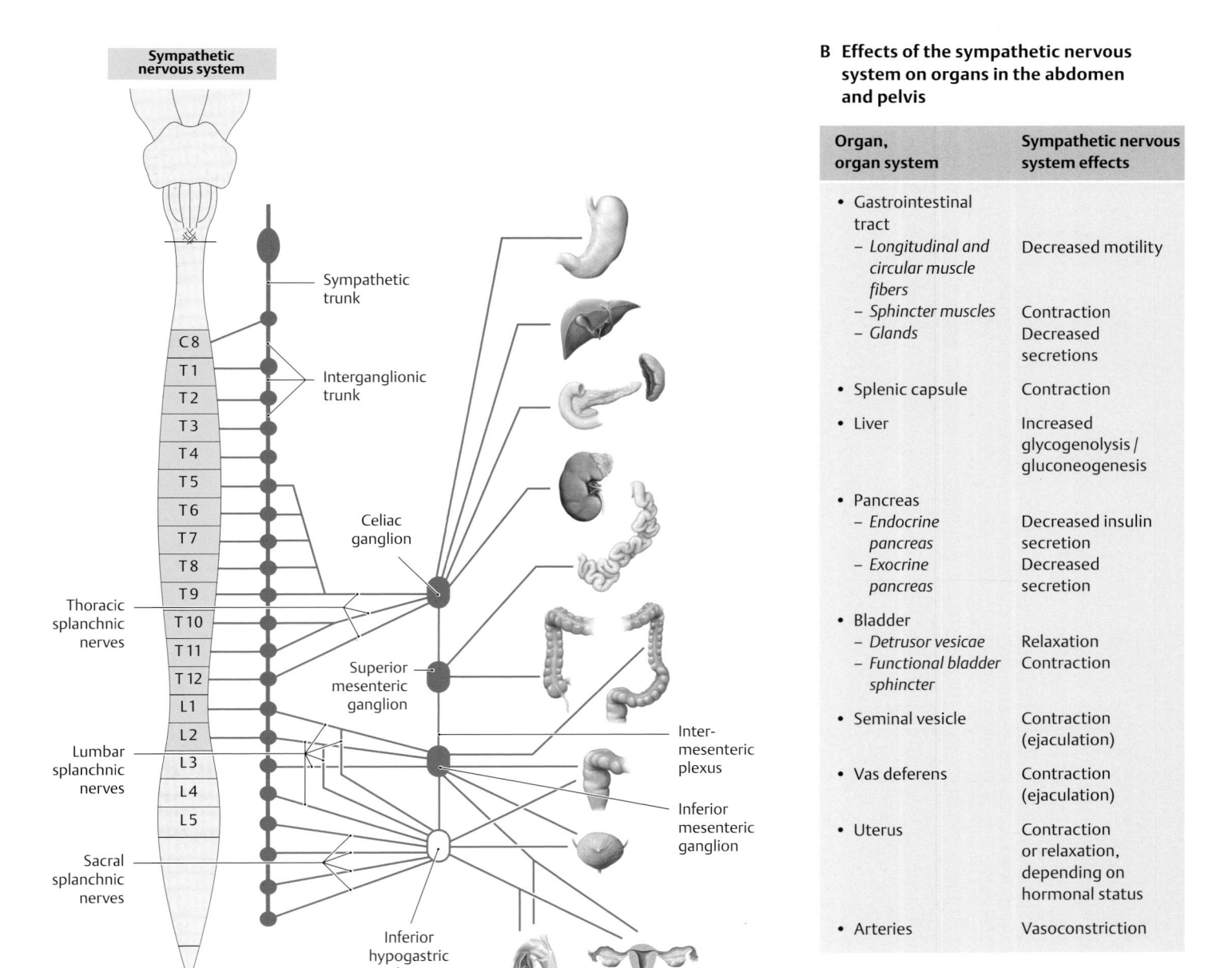

Sympathetic nervous system

- Sympathetic trunk
- C8
- T1
- T2 — Interganglionic trunk
- T3
- T4
- T5
- T6
- T7 — Celiac ganglion
- T8
- T9
- Thoracic splanchnic nerves — T10
- T11
- T12 — Superior mesenteric ganglion
- L1
- L2
- Lumbar splanchnic nerves — L3
- L4
- L5
- Sacral splanchnic nerves
- Inferior hypogastric plexus

- Inter-mesenteric plexus
- Inferior mesenteric ganglion

B Effects of the sympathetic nervous system on organs in the abdomen and pelvis

Organ, organ system	Sympathetic nervous system effects
• Gastrointestinal tract	
– *Longitudinal and circular muscle fibers*	Decreased motility
– *Sphincter muscles*	Contraction
– *Glands*	Decreased secretions
• Splenic capsule	Contraction
• Liver	Increased glycogenolysis / gluconeogenesis
• Pancreas	
– *Endocrine pancreas*	Decreased insulin secretion
– *Exocrine pancreas*	Decreased secretion
• Bladder	
– *Detrusor vesicae*	Relaxation
– *Functional bladder sphincter*	Contraction
• Seminal vesicle	Contraction (ejaculation)
• Vas deferens	Contraction (ejaculation)
• Uterus	Contraction or relaxation, depending on hormonal status
• Arteries	Vasoconstriction

A Organization of the sympathetic nervous system in the abdomen and pelvis

The first, or presynaptic, neurons of the sympathetic system that supply the **organs of the abdomen** are located in the lateral horns of spinal cord segments T 5 –T 12. Their presynaptic axons pass *without synapsing* through the ganglia of the sympathetic trunk and form the thoracic splanchnic nerves (= greater and lesser thoracic splanchnic nerves, and occasionally a least thoracic splanchnic nerve from T 12). The *synapse with the second , or postsysnaptic, neuron* is located in the celiac ganglion, the superior (or inferior) mesenteric ganglion, or the aorticorenal ganglion (see p. 308).

The first, or presynaptic, neurons of the sympathetic system that supply the **organs of the pelvis** are located in the lateral horns of spinal cord segments L 1 and L 2. Their presynaptic axons pass through the lumbar ganglia of the sympathetic trunk and form the lumbar splanchnic nerves. The *synapse with the second, or postsynaptic, neuron* may be located in the lumbar ganglia, inferior mesenteric ganglion, or inferior hy-

pogastric plexus. Beyond that point the postsynaptic fibers of the postsynaptic neuron generally pass to the target organ with its artery, usually accompanied by parasympathetic fibers of the autonomic nervous system.

Note: The peripheral ganglia of the sympathetic nervous system are distributed along the sides of the vertebral column (paravertebral). Peripheral ganglia in the abdomen and pelvis are also placed anterior to the vertebral column (prevertebral) and sacrum.

The paravertebral ganglia are interconnected by interganglionic connections to form the sympathetic trunk — two long pathways extending along each side of the vertebral column. The ganglia are named for the corresponding levels of the spine (thoracic ganglia, lumbar ganglia, etc.) and are variable in number. The prevertebral ganglia are located at the origins of the major arteries from the abdominal aorta and are named accordingly (celiac ganglion, superior and inferior mesenteric ganglia, etc.).

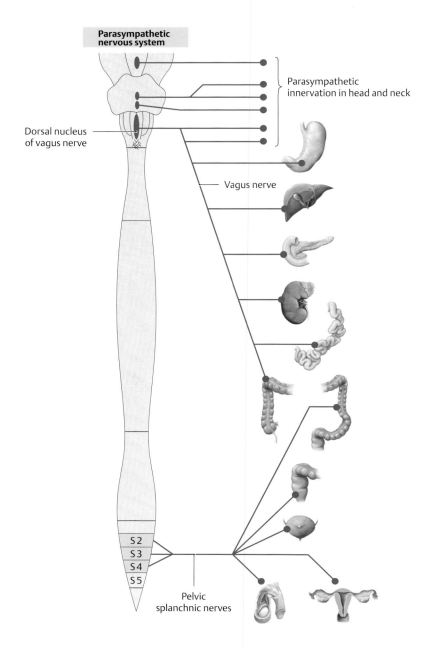

Parasympathetic nervous system

Parasympathetic innervation in head and neck

Dorsal nucleus of vagus nerve

Vagus nerve

S2
S3
S4
S5

Pelvic splanchnic nerves

D Effects of the parasympathetic nervous system on organs in the abdomen and pelvis

Organ, organ system	Parasympathetic nervous system effects
• Gastrointestinal tract	
– *Longitudinal and circular muscle fibers*	Increased motility
– *Sphincter muscles*	Relaxation
– *Glands*	Increased secretions
• Splenic capsule	–
• Liver	–
• Pancreas	
– *Endocrine pancreas*	–
– *Exocrine pancreas*	Increased secretion
• Bladder	
– *Detrusor vesicae*	Contraction
– *Functional bladder sphincter*	–
• Seminal vesicle	–
• Vas deferens	–
• Uterus	–
• Arteries	Vasodilation of the arteries in the penis or clitoris (erection)

C Organization of the parasympathetic nervous system in the abdomen and pelvis

Contrasting with the thoracolumbar organization of the sympathetic nervous system, the parasympathetic nervous system in the abdomen and pelvis consists of *two topographically distinct systems*: a cranial part and a sacral part. This system also differs from the sympathetic nervous system in that the synapse of the first, or presynaptic, neuron with the second or postsynaptic neuron is located in the intramural ganglia of the organ walls.

- **Cranial part of the parasympathetic nervous system in the abdomen and pelvis:** The presynaptic neuron is located in the dorsal nucleus of the vagus nerve (i.e., the nucleus of cranial nerve X in the medulla oblongata). The axons (presynaptic nerve fibers) course with the vagus nerve to visceral or intramural ganglia, where they synapse with the postsynaptic neuron. The *distribution* of the cranial part includes the stomach, liver, gallbladder, pancreas, duodenum, kidney, suprarenal gland, small intestine, and the large intestine from the ascending colon to near the left colic flexure.

- **Sacral part of the parasympathetic nervous system in the abdomen and pelvis:** Its origin is located in the lateral horns of spinal cord segments S2 – S4 (sacral intermediolateral nucleus). The axons (synaptic nerve fibers) run a very short distance with spinal nerves S2 – S4, then separate from them and course as the pelvic splanchnic nerves to ganglion cells in the inferior hypogastric plexus or organ wall, where they synapse with the postsynaptic neuron. The *distribution* of the sacral part of the parasympathetic nervous system in the abdomen and pelvis includes left colic flexure, the descending and sigmoid colon, rectum, anus, bladder, urethra, and the internal and external genitalia.

5.2 Autonomic Ganglia and Plexuses

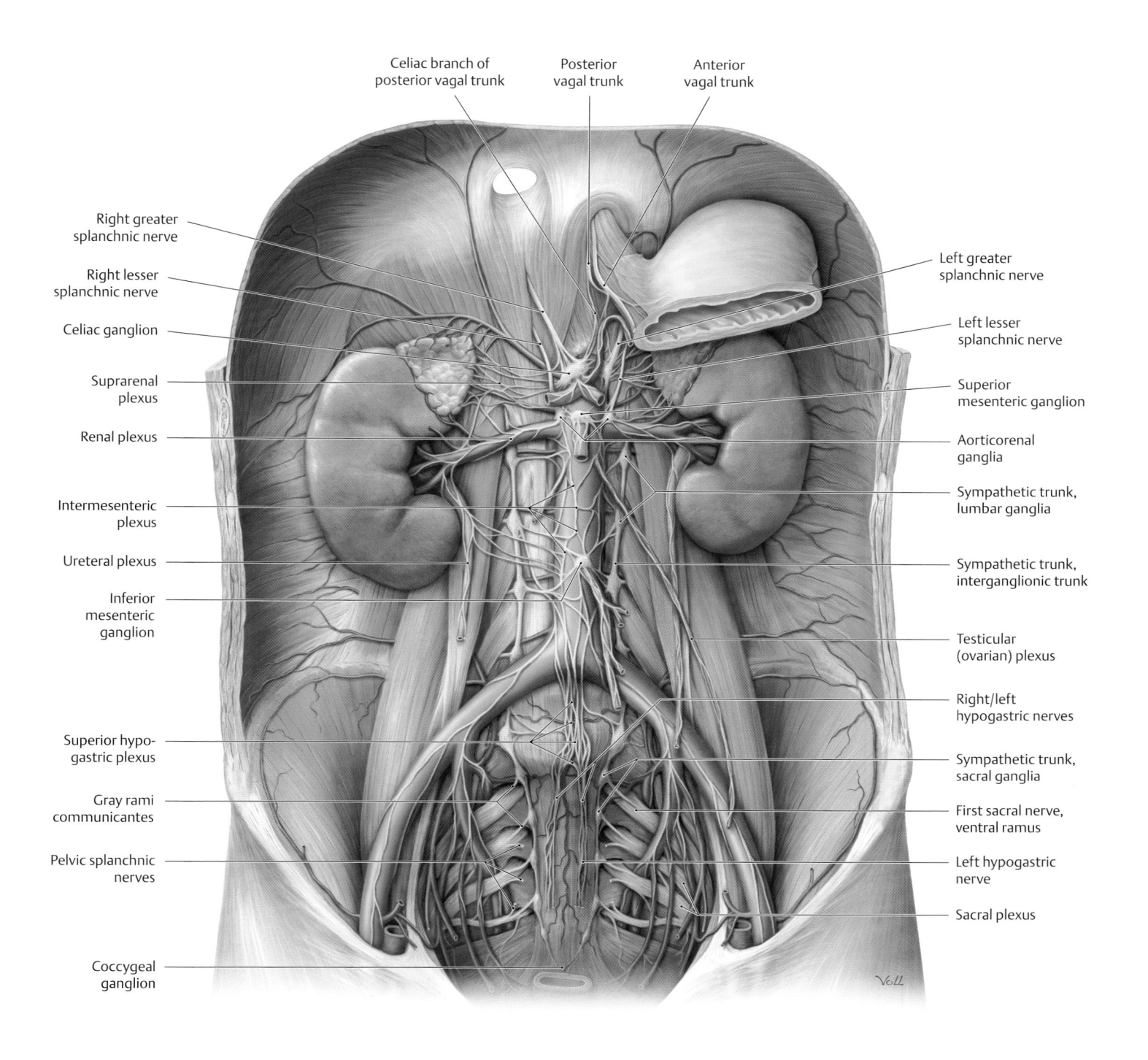

Celiac branch of posterior vagal trunk

Posterior vagal trunk

Anterior vagal trunk

Right greater splanchnic nerve

Right lesser splanchnic nerve

Celiac ganglion

Suprarenal plexus

Renal plexus

Intermesenteric plexus

Ureteral plexus

Inferior mesenteric ganglion

Superior hypo-gastric plexus

Gray rami communicantes

Pelvic splanchnic nerves

Coccygeal ganglion

Left greater splanchnic nerve

Left lesser splanchnic nerve

Superior mesenteric ganglion

Aorticorenal ganglia

Sympathetic trunk, lumbar ganglia

Sympathetic trunk, interganglionic trunk

Testicular (ovarian) plexus

Right/left hypogastric nerves

Sympathetic trunk, sacral ganglia

First sacral nerve, ventral ramus

Left hypogastric nerve

Sacral plexus

A Overview of autonomic ganglia and plexuses in the abdomen and pelvis

Anterior view of an opened male abdomen and pelvis with all of the peritoneum removed. Almost all of the stomach has been removed, and the gastric stump and esophagus have been pulled slightly inferior. The pelvic organs have been removed except for a rectal stump. The autonomic nervous system forms extensive *plexuses* and a number of *ganglia* around the abdominal aorta and within the pelvis, the ganglia marking the sites where the first presynaptic neuron synapses with the second postsynaptic neuron. All of the autonomic plexuses in front of and alongside the abdominal aorta are collectively termed the *abdominal aortic plexus*. This structure also includes the individual plexuses located

at the origins of the paired and unpaired branches of the abdominal aorta (see **B**). As a general rule, sympathetic and parasympathetic nerve fibers come together in the plexuses on their way to the target organ. *Note:* The left and right vagus nerves are organized around the esophagus to form the anterior and posterior vagal trunks. Both trunks contain fibers from both vagus nerves, the *anterior* vagal trunk containing more fibers from the left vagus nerve, the *posterior* trunk containing more fibers from the right vagus nerve. While the anterior vagal trunk generally terminates at the stomach, the posterior vagal trunk goes on to supply the entire small intestine and the large intestine approximately to the junction of the middle and distal thirds of the transverse colon.

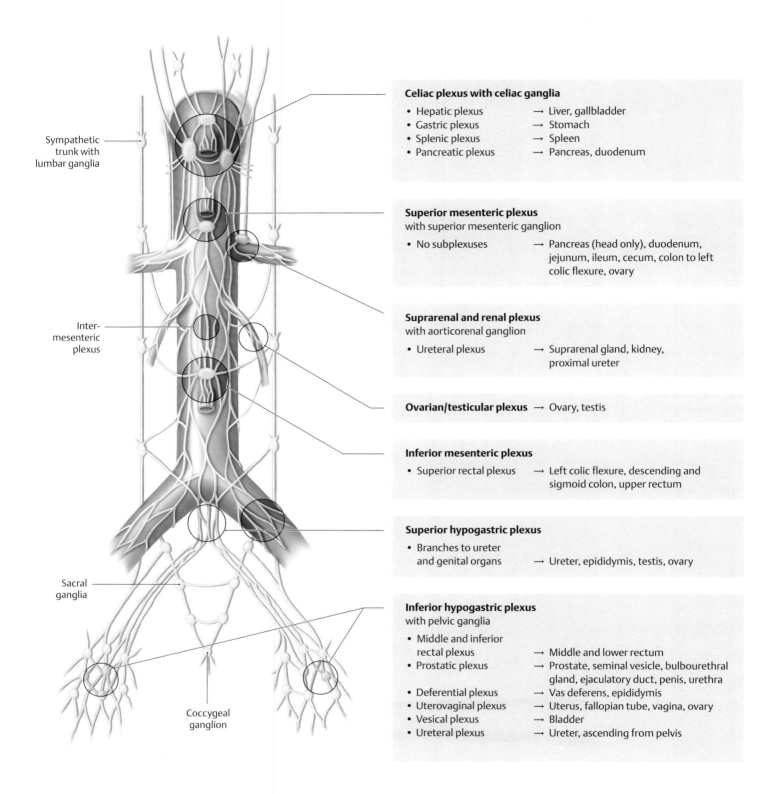

Sympathetic trunk with lumbar ganglia

Inter-mesenteric plexus

Sacral ganglia

Coccygeal ganglion

Celiac plexus with celiac ganglia

- Hepatic plexus   → Liver, gallbladder
- Gastric plexus   → Stomach
- Splenic plexus   → Spleen
- Pancreatic plexus   → Pancreas, duodenum

Superior mesenteric plexus
with superior mesenteric ganglion

- No subplexuses   → Pancreas (head only), duodenum, jejunum, ileum, cecum, colon to left colic flexure, ovary

Suprarenal and renal plexus
with aorticorenal ganglion

- Ureteral plexus   → Suprarenal gland, kidney, proximal ureter

Ovarian/testicular plexus → Ovary, testis

Inferior mesenteric plexus

- Superior rectal plexus   → Left colic flexure, descending and sigmoid colon, upper rectum

Superior hypogastric plexus

- Branches to ureter and genital organs   → Ureter, epididymis, testis, ovary

Inferior hypogastric plexus
with pelvic ganglia

- Middle and inferior rectal plexus   → Middle and lower rectum
- Prostatic plexus   → Prostate, seminal vesicle, bulbourethral gland, ejaculatory duct, penis, urethra
- Deferential plexus   → Vas deferens, epididymis
- Uterovaginal plexus   → Uterus, fallopian tube, vagina, ovary
- Vesical plexus   → Bladder
- Ureteral plexus   → Ureter, ascending from pelvis

B Organization of autonomic ganglia and plexuses in the abdomen and pelvis

The ganglia and plexuses of the autonomic nervous system are named for the arteries that they accompany or around which they are distributed (e.g., the celiac ganglion and mesenteric plexus). In the *sympathetic* system, the presynaptic neuron synapses with the postsynaptic neuron in ganglia *distant* from the organs (or ganglion cells in a plexus distant from the organs); in the *parasympathetic* system, this synapse occurs in ganglia *near* the organs (or ganglion cells in a plexus near the

organs). Thus, the parasympathetic ganglia are usually located on the target organ or in its wall, where they receive branches from the vagal trunks or pelvic splanchnic nerves.

Note: Even plexuses may contain aggregations of ganglion cells, sometimes very small. An example is the renal plexus, which contains the renal ganglia (too small to be shown in the drawing).

The autonomic plexuses contain efferent (visceromotor) fibers as well as numerous afferent (viscerosensory) fibers for both their sympathetic and parasympathetic components.

5.3 Autonomic Innervation of the Liver, Gallbladder, Stomach, Duodenum, Pancreas, and Spleen

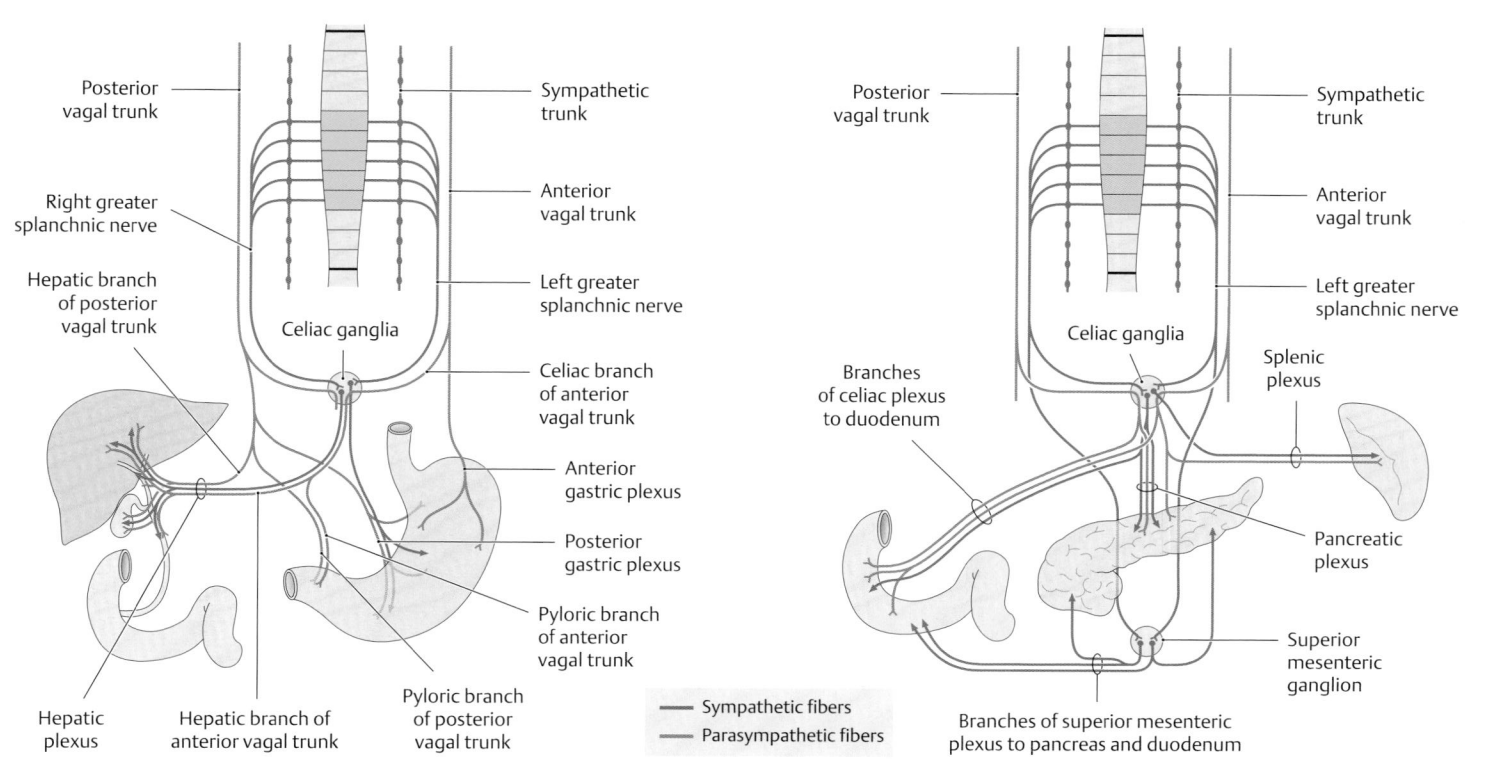

A Autonomic innervation of the liver, gallbladder, and stomach

These organs receive their **sympathetic supply** from the celiac ganglia. The *postsynaptic* fibers course with the branches of the celiac trunk, while the *presynaptic* fibers form the splanchnic nerves (mainly the greater splanchnic nerve) and synapse with the postsynaptic neuron in the ganglion. They receive their **parasympathetic supply** from the vagal trunks (presynaptic fibers). The *anterior* vagal trunk (preponderance of left vagus nerve fibers) terminates at the stomach, while the *posterior* vagal trunk goes on to supply large portions of the intestine. The anterior and posterior gastric plexuses are distributed to the anterior and posterior walls of the stomach. The synapse with the postsynaptic parasympathetic neuron occurs in small ganglia located directly on the stomach wall.

Sympathetic and parasympathetic fibers pass along the proper hepatic artery to the porta hepatis as the hepatic plexus. After dividing at the liver, this plexus also distributes fibers to the gallbladder and the intra- and extrahepatic bile ducts.

B Autonomic innervation of the pancreas, duodenum, and spleen

These organs receive their **sympathetic supply** from the celiac ganglia and superior mesenteric ganglion. The *postsynaptic* fibers pass along the branches of the celiac trunk and superior mesenteric artery. The *presynaptic* fibers form the greater and lesser splanchnic nerves. They receive their **parasympathetic supply** from the vagal trunks (mainly the posterior trunk).

Sympathetic and parasympathetic fibers course with the splenic artery to the spleen as the *splenic plexus*, and they course with branches of the splenic artery and superior mesenteric artery to the pancreas as the *pancreatic plexus*. The fibers to the duodenum reach that organ via the gastroduodenal artery, pancreaticoduodenal artery, and duodenal branches as part of the *superior mesenteric plexus*. The synapse with the second parasympathetic neuron occurs in small ganglia located near the organs.

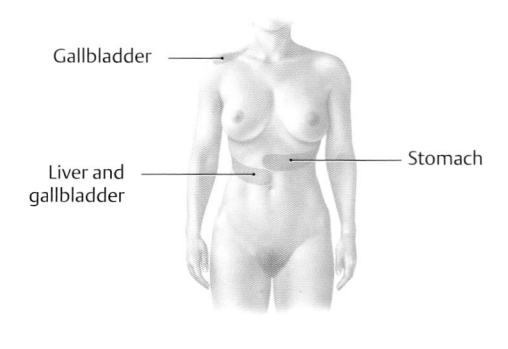

C Referred pain from the liver, gallbladder, and stomach

The Head zones (see p. 146) of the liver, gallbladder, and stomach extend from the right and left hypochondriac regions to the epigastric region. Gallbladder pain may also radiate to the right shoulder. (There are no Head zones associated with the duodenum and spleen.)

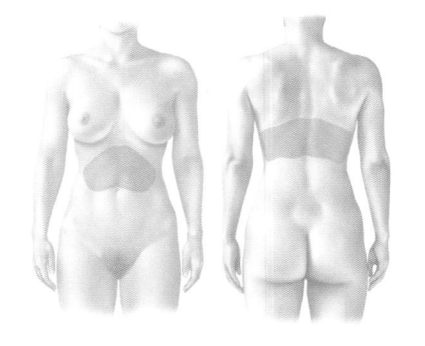

D Referred pain from of the pancreas

The Head zone of the pancreas girdles the abdomen. Pain due to pancreatic disease may be perceived not just in the upper abdomen but also in the back. The anterior Head zone overlaps with the zones of the liver and stomach.

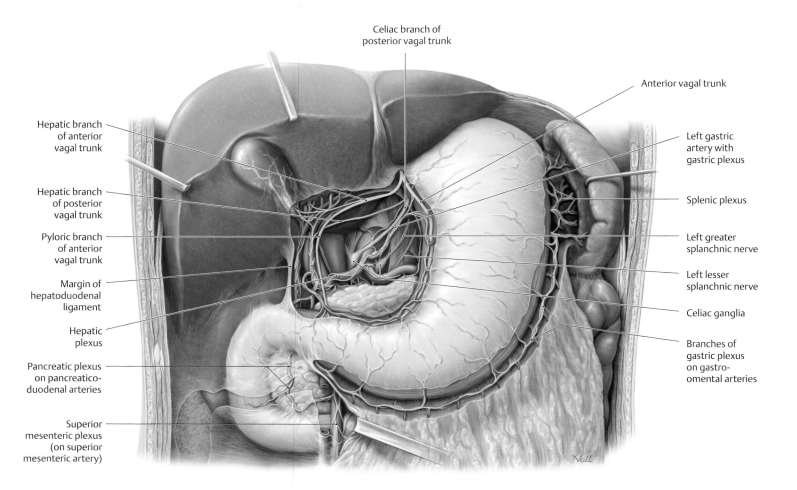

Celiac branch of
posterior vagal trunk

Anterior vagal trunk

Hepatic branch
of anterior
vagal trunk

Hepatic branch
of posterior
vagal trunk

Pyloric branch
of anterior
vagal trunk

Margin of
hepatoduodenal
ligament

Hepatic
plexus

Pancreatic plexus
on pancreatico-
duodenal arteries

Superior
mesenteric plexus
(on superior
mesenteric artery)

Left gastric
artery with
gastric plexus

Splenic plexus

Left greater
splanchnic nerve

Left lesser
splanchnic nerve

Celiac ganglia

Branches of
gastric plexus
on gastro-
omental arteries

E Innervation of the liver, gallbladder, stomach, duodenum, pancreas, and spleen

Anterior view. The lesser omentum has been broadly removed, and the greater omentum has been opened. The ascending colon and part of the transverse colon have been removed. The retroperitoneal fat and connective tissue has been partially removed to improve the exposure. The visceral plexuses arising from the celiac ganglion mainly accompany the arteries as they pass to their target organs.

Note: The pylorus is generally supplied by separate pyloric branches that arise from the vagal trunks (parasympathetic supply) and often run initially with the hepatic branches. Because of this arrangement, the function of the pylorus is not impaired when the vagal trunks are divided

distal to the origin of the pyloric branches, as it is by a *selective proximal vagotomy* (see **F**). Thus it is possible to reduce acid production by the parietal cells in the body and fundus of the stomach without affecting necessary gastrin production in the antrum and pylorus or compromising the motor function of the pylorus.

The **liver and bile ducts** receive their autonomic supply from *parasympathetic* hepatic branches that join the *sympathetic* fibers in the hepatic plexus. The *hepatic plexus* accompanies the proper hepatic artery to the liver and gives off branches that supply the gallbladder and biliary tract. The **spleen and pancreas** receive autonomic fibers from the splenic and pancreatic plexuses. The **duodenum** derives part of its supply from the superior mesenteric ganglion and superior mesenteric plexus.

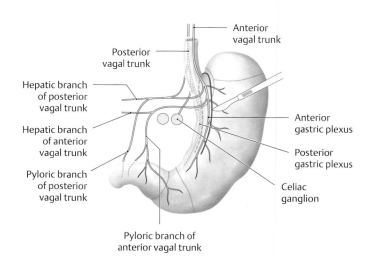

Anterior
vagal trunk

Posterior
vagal trunk

Hepatic branch
of posterior
vagal trunk

Hepatic branch
of anterior
vagal trunk

Pyloric branch
of posterior
vagal trunk

Anterior
gastric plexus

Posterior
gastric plexus

Celiac
ganglion

Pyloric branch of
anterior vagal trunk

F Selective proximal vagotomy

Impulses from the vagus nerve stimulate the production of HCl (hydrochloric adic). Thus, a selective proximal vagotomy may be considered for the treatment of gastric hyperacidity that is *refractory to medical treatment*. This is an operation in which the vagus fibers that stimulate the acid-producing parietal cells (mainly in the gastric body and fundus) are transected on the stomach wall, at a site which is past the origin of the pyloric branches from the vagal trunks. The pyloric branches are left intact, ensuring the maintenance of normal pyloric function.

5.4 Autonomic Innervation of the Intestine: Distribution of the Superior Mesenteric Plexus

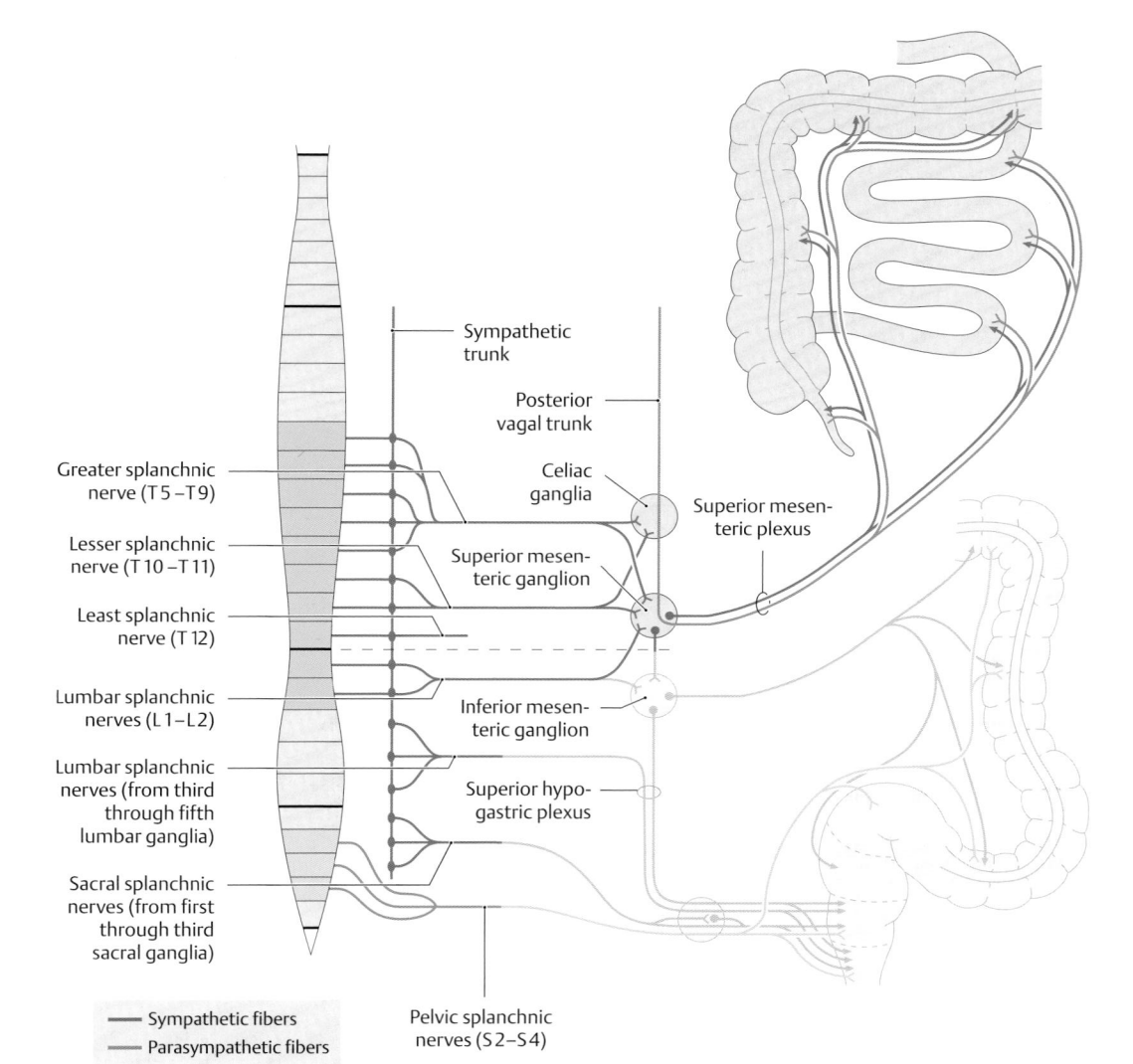

Greater splanchnic nerve (T 5 –T 9)

Lesser splanchnic nerve (T 10 –T 11)

Least splanchnic nerve (T 12)

Lumbar splanchnic nerves (L 1–L 2)

Lumbar splanchnic nerves (from third through fifth lumbar ganglia)

Sacral splanchnic nerves (from first through third sacral ganglia)

Sympathetic trunk

Posterior vagal trunk

Celiac ganglia

Superior mesenteric ganglion

Inferior mesenteric ganglion

Superior hypo-gastric plexus

Superior mesenteric plexus

—— Sympathetic fibers
—— Parasympathetic fibers

Pelvic splanchnic nerves (S 2–S 4)

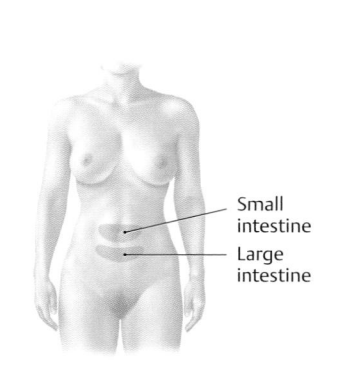

Small intestine

Large intestine

B Referred pain from the small and large intestine
In many cases the pain associated with intestinal diseases is not localized precisely to the bowel. Frequently the pain is projected to the color-shaded areas on the abdominal wall.

A Autonomic distribution of the superior mesenteric plexus
While a clear distinction is drawn between the small and large intestine topographically and histologically, autonomic innervation is based on the supply of a particular intestinal segment by a particular plexus, regardless of whether that segment is part of the small or large intestine. The main distinction to be made is whether the intestinal segment is supplied by the *superior* or *inferior* mesenteric plexus. This principle is illustrated in the above diagram (see also p. 314):

Sympathetic innervation:
• The *jejunum, ileum, cecum, ascending colon*, and the *proximal two-thirds of the transverse colon* are supplied by postsynaptic branches of the *superior* mesenteric ganglion via the superior mesenteric plexus, which is distributed to the various intestinal segments along the branches of the superior mesenteric artery.
• Similarly, the *distal third of the transverse colon*, the *descending colon, sigmoid colon*, and *upper rectum* are innervated by postsynaptic branches of the *inferior* mesenteric ganglion and the associated plexus, which is distributed along the branches of the inferior mesenteric artery (see p. 315).
• The *middle and lower rectum* are supplied by the lumbar and sacral splanchnic nerves via the inferior hypogastric plexus (the supply to the three levels of the rectum is shown on p. 314).

The superior mesenteric ganglion, then, provides **sympathetic** innervation to the entire small intestine and part of the large intestine, supplying by far the greater portion of the entire bowel.

The **parasympathetic innervation** of the small and large intestine is analogous to their sympathetic innervation.
• The *small intestine, cecum, ascending colon*, and *proximal two-thirds of the transverse colon* are supplied by the *vagal trunk* and its branches.
• The remaining *colon* and *rectum* are innervated by the *pelvic splanchnic nerves* from segments S2–S4 (see p. 314). Some of these nerves have their synapses in ganglion cells within the inferior hypogastric plexus and some in ganglion cells on the organ wall.

Thus, the vagal trunk (i.e., elements of the cranial part of the parasympathetic nervous system) provides **parasympathetic** innervation to the entire small intestine and part of the large intestine, supplying the greater portion of the entire bowel. A site on the transverse colon called the *Cannon-Böhm point* marks the boundary between the proximal and distal territories of the autonomic nervous system.

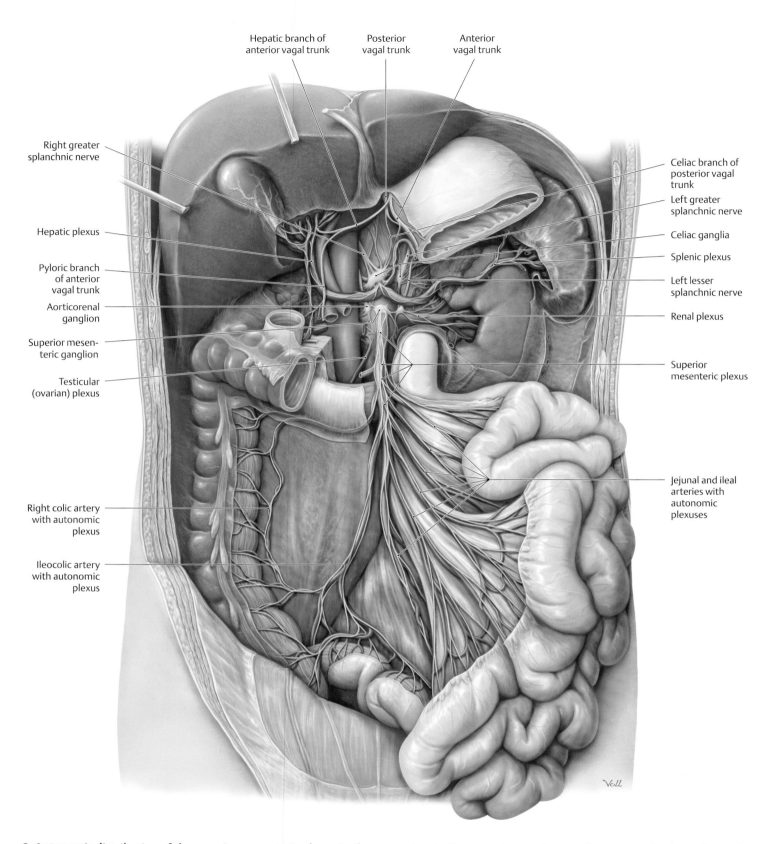

Hepatic branch of anterior vagal trunk

Posterior vagal trunk

Anterior vagal trunk

Right greater splanchnic nerve

Hepatic plexus

Pyloric branch of anterior vagal trunk

Aorticorenal ganglion

Superior mesenteric ganglion

Testicular (ovarian) plexus

Right colic artery with autonomic plexus

Ileocolic artery with autonomic plexus

Celiac branch of posterior vagal trunk

Left greater splanchnic nerve

Celiac ganglia

Splenic plexus

Left lesser splanchnic nerve

Renal plexus

Superior mesenteric plexus

Jejunal and ileal arteries with autonomic plexuses

Voll

C Autonomic distribution of the superior mesenteric plexus to the intestine

Anterior view. The liver has been retracted superiorly, and the stomach and pancreas have been partially removed. Most of the distal part of the transverse colon has been removed, and all loops of small intestine have been reflected toward the left side.

The postsynaptic branches of the superior mesenteric ganglion (**sympathetic supply**) pass along the branches of the superior mesenteric artery in the mesentery as the superior mesenteric plexus, being distributed to the jejunum, ileum, cecum (and vermiform appendix), and the colon as far as the junction of the middle and distal thirds of the transverse colon. Past that point the bowel receives its sympathetic innervation from the inferior mesenteric ganglion (not visible here). **Parasympathetic innervation** from the jejunum to the distal third of the transverse colon is supplied by the vagal trunk and its branches. The innervation of the remaining colon and rectum is described on p. 314.

5.5 Autonomic Innervation of the Intestine: Distribution of the Inferior Mesenteric Plexus and Inferior Hypogastric Plexus

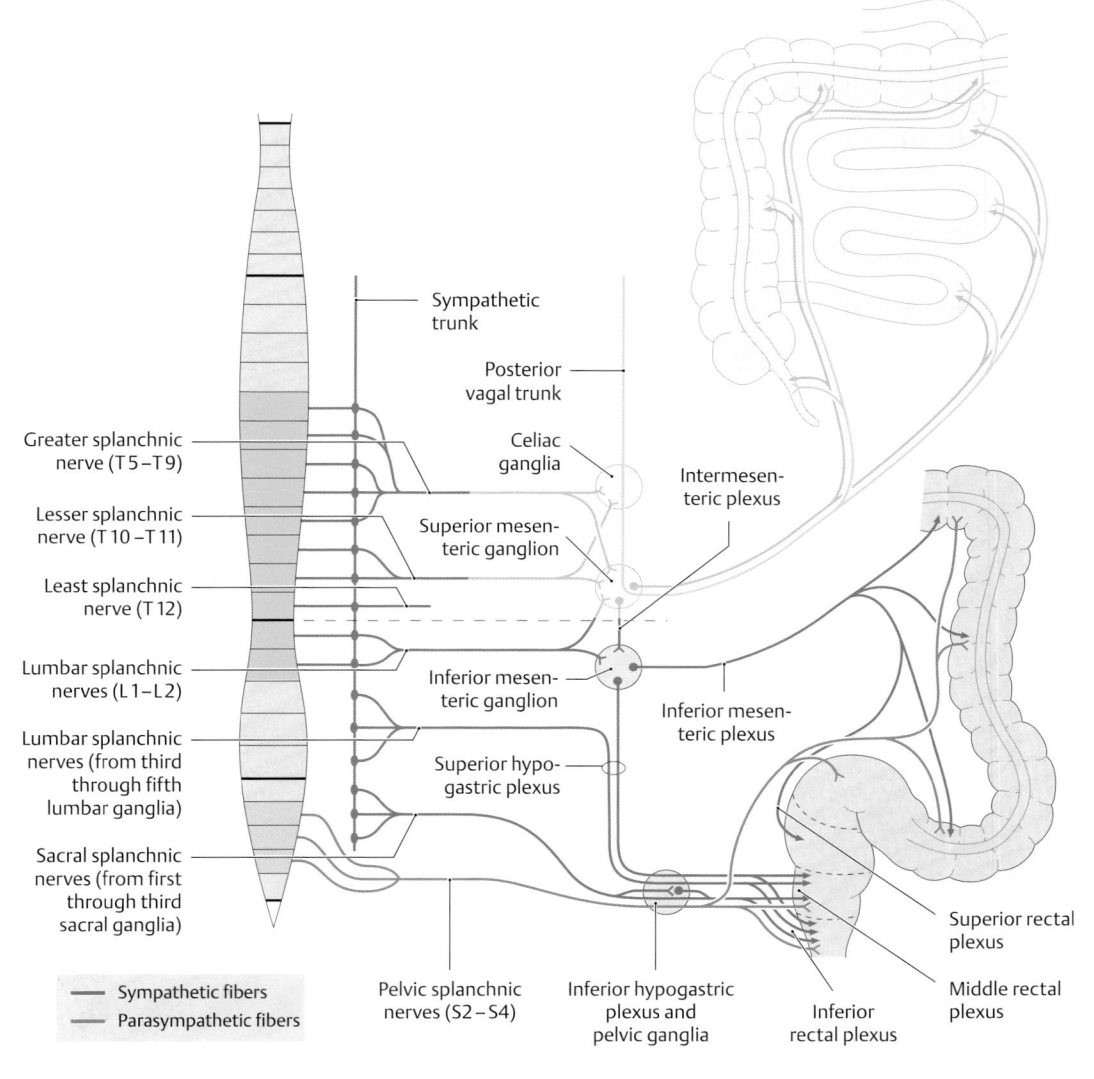

Sympathetic trunk

Posterior vagal trunk

Greater splanchnic nerve (T5–T9)

Celiac ganglia

Intermesenteric plexus

Lesser splanchnic nerve (T10–T11)

Superior mesenteric ganglion

Least splanchnic nerve (T12)

Lumbar splanchnic nerves (L1–L2)

Inferior mesenteric ganglion

Inferior mesenteric plexus

Lumbar splanchnic nerves (from third through fifth lumbar ganglia)

Superior hypogastric plexus

Sacral splanchnic nerves (from first through third sacral ganglia)

Superior rectal plexus

—— Sympathetic fibers
—— Parasympathetic fibers

Pelvic splanchnic nerves (S2–S4)

Inferior hypogastric plexus and pelvic ganglia

Inferior rectal plexus

Middle rectal plexus

A Autonomic distribution of the inferior mesenteric plexus and inferior hypogastric plexus

Note: The autonomic innervation of the bowel is not divided anatomically between the small and large intestine. It is best understood in terms of the particular bowel segment that is supplied by a particular plexus (superior or inferior mesenteric plexus, inferior hypogastric

plexus). Because this unit is concerned mainly with the distribution of the inferior mesenteric plexus and inferior hypogastric plexus (see also **C**), the regions supplied by these plexuses are highlighted in the above diagram. Further details on the innervation pattern are given on p. 309.

Muscularis externa, longitudinal layer

Muscularis externa, circular layer

Submucosa

Serosa

Mucosa

Subserosal plexus

Submucosal plexus

Myenteric plexus

B Organization of the enteric plexus

The enteric plexus is the portion of the autonomic nervous system that specifically serves *all the organs of the gastrointestinal tract*. Located within the wall of the digestive tube (intramural nervous system), it is subject to both sympathetic and parasympathetic influences. Congenital absence of the enteric plexus leads to severe disturbances of gastrointestinal transit (e.g., Hirschsprung disease). The enteric plexus has basically the same organization throughout the gastrointestinal tract, although there is an area in the wall of the lower rectum that is devoid of ganglion cells (see p. 201). Three subsystems are distinguished in the enteric plexus:

- Submucosal plexus (Meissner plexus)
- Myenteric plexus (Auerbach plexus)
- Subserosal plexus

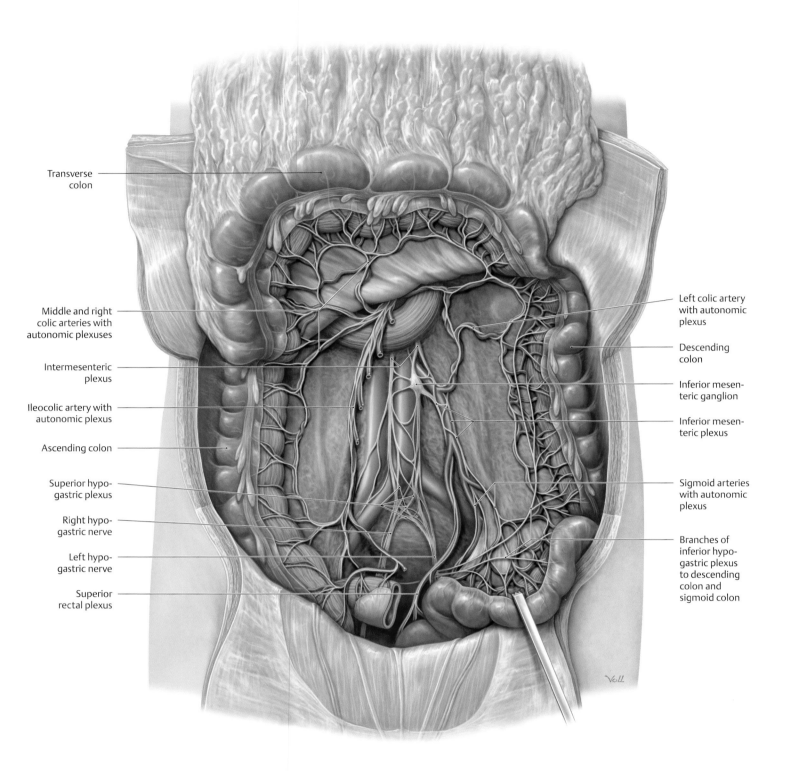

Transverse colon

Middle and right colic arteries with autonomic plexuses

Intermesenteric plexus

Ileocolic artery with autonomic plexus

Ascending colon

Superior hypo-gastric plexus

Right hypo-gastric nerve

Left hypo-gastric nerve

Superior rectal plexus

Left colic artery with autonomic plexus

Descending colon

Inferior mesen-teric ganglion

Inferior mesen-teric plexus

Sigmoid arteries with autonomic plexus

Branches of inferior hypo-gastric plexus to descending colon and sigmoid colon

C Autonomic distribution of the inferior mesenteric plexus and inferior hypogastric plexus to the bowel

Anterior view. The jejunum and ileum have been removed, leaving a short ileal stump on the cecum. The transverse colon has been reflected superiorly, and the sigmoid colon has been retracted inferiorly.

Sympathetic innervation:

- The *cecum, vermiform appendix, ascending colon*, and *proximal two-thirds of the transverse colon* (plus all of the small intestine, not visible here) are supplied by postsynaptic branches of the superior mesenteric ganglion.
- The *distal third of the transverse colon, descending colon, sigmoid colon*, and *upper rectum* are supplied by postsynaptic branches of the

inferior mesenteric ganglion, which follow the branches of the inferior mesenteric artery as the inferior mesenteric plexus.

- The *middle and lower rectum** are supplied by the lumbar and sacral splanchnic nerves via the inferior hypogastric plexus (which follows the visceral branches of the internal iliac artery).

Parasympathetic innervation is also divided at the junction of the middle and distal thirds of the transverse colon:

- The *proximal* portion is innervated by the vagal trunk and its branches (i.e., the *cranial* part of the parasympathetic nervous system).
- The *distal* portion is innervated by the pelvic splanchnic nerves of segments S2 – S4 and parts of the inferior hypogastric plexus (i.e., the *sacral* part of the parasympathetic nervous system; see also p. 312).

* Rectal innervation is described more fully on pp. 316 and 318.

315

5.6 Autonomic Innervation of the Urinary Organs and Suprarenal Glands

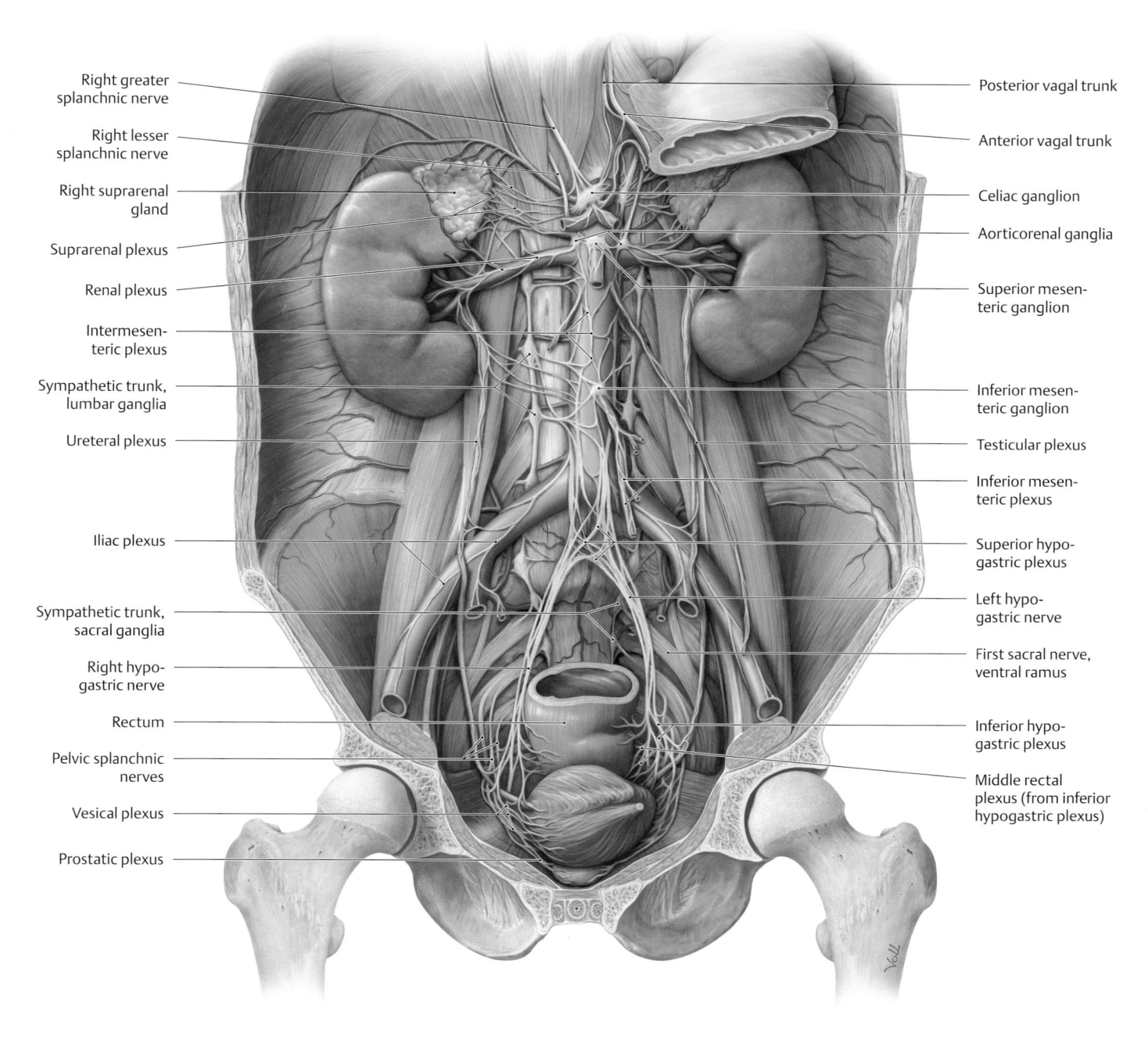

Right greater splanchnic nerve
Right lesser splanchnic nerve
Right suprarenal gland
Suprarenal plexus
Renal plexus
Intermesenteric plexus
Sympathetic trunk, lumbar ganglia
Ureteral plexus
Iliac plexus
Sympathetic trunk, sacral ganglia
Right hypogastric nerve
Rectum
Pelvic splanchnic nerves
Vesical plexus
Prostatic plexus

Posterior vagal trunk
Anterior vagal trunk
Celiac ganglion
Aorticorenal ganglia
Superior mesenteric ganglion
Inferior mesenteric ganglion
Testicular plexus
Inferior mesenteric plexus
Superior hypogastric plexus
Left hypogastric nerve
First sacral nerve, ventral ramus
Inferior hypogastric plexus
Middle rectal plexus (from inferior hypogastric plexus)

A Overview of the autonomic innervation of the urinary organs and suprarenal glands

Anterior view into an opened male abdomen and pelvis. The stomach has been largely removed and pulled slightly inferior with the esophagus for better exposure. The right kidney has been displaced slightly laterally, and the bladder has been straightened and retracted to the left. The pelvis has been sectioned in a coronal plane passing approximately through the center of the acetabula. The autonomic innervation of the urinary organs and suprarenal glands varies according to the location of the specific organ:

- The **kidneys in the retroperitoneum** and portions of the upper urinary tract **(proximal ureters)** receive *sympathetic* fibers initially from the lesser, least, and lumbar splanchnic nerves (see **B**), which synapse with the postsynaptic neuron in the aorticorenal or renal ganglia. The *parasympathetic* fibers originate from the posterior vagal trunk and partly from the pelvic splanchnic nerves (the plexuses are described in **B**).

- The **suprarenal cortex and medulla in the retroperitoneum** receive *sympathetic* fibers from the greater and lesser splanchnic nerves. They receive *parasympathetic* fibers from the posterior vagal trunk, which pass with the renal plexus to the suprarenal glands as the suprarenal plexus. The *sympathetic* autonomic innervation of the suprarenal medulla is exceptional in that the suprarenal medulla is supplied only by presynaptic sympathetic fibers from the suprarenal plexus. These axons directly innervate the suprarenal medullary cells (see p. 220). At present, there is no convincing evidence that the suprarenal medulla receives *parasympathetic* innervation.

- The **bladder, most of the abdominal part** and **pelvic part of the ureter** (and the **urethra**, not shown here) **in the pelvis** (see **D**) receive *sympathetic* fibers from the lumbar and sacral splanchnic nerves, and they receive *parasympathetic* fibers from the pelvic splanchnic nerves (S2–S4). The plexuses are shown in **D**, and the autonomic innervation of the **rectum** is described on p. 312.

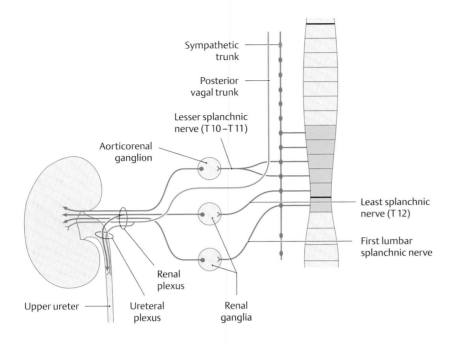

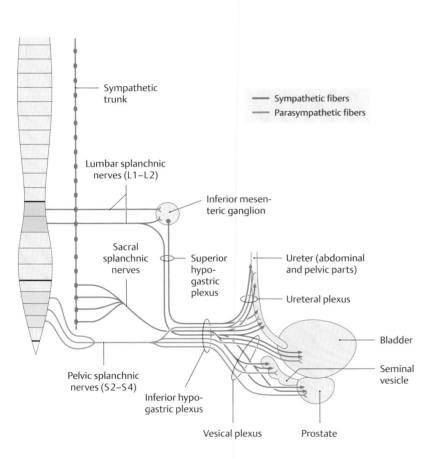

B Autonomic innervation of the kidney and upper ureter

The sympathetic fibers from the aorticorenal ganglia and renal ganglia combine with the parasympathetic fibers from the posterior vagal trunk to form the *renal plexus*, which passes to the kidney. Branches from that plexus form the *ureteral plexus*, which supplies the abdominal (upper) part of the ureter. Presynaptic sympathetic fibers form the thoracic splanchnic nerves (not shown here).

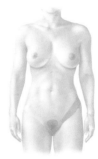

C Referred pain from the left kidney and bladder

Pain associated with diseases of the kidney and bladder (inflammation, calculi) may be perceived in these skin areas. Occasionally the pain radiates into the groin ("loin to groin pain").

D Autonomic innervation of the bladder and the abdominal and pelvic parts of the ureter

Sympathetic fibers from the lumbar and sacral splanchnic nerves pass with the parasympathetic fibers from the pelvic splanchnic nerves to the inferior hypogastric plexus. Branches from that plexus are distributed to form additional plexuses, including the vesical and ureteral plexuses that supply the bladder and ureter (its abdominal and pelvic parts). For the *parasympathetic* fibers, the synapse with the postsynaptic neuron is located entirely in the inferior hypogastric plexus (or organ wall).

The *sympathetic* fibers synapse partly in the inferior mesenteric ganglion and partly in the inferior hypogastric plexus (see the fibers that continue from the superior hypogastric plexus to the inferior hypogastric plexus).

Note: With a complete transection of the spinal cord, the effect of higher CNS centers on the central parasympathetic neurons of S2 – S4 (= pelvic splanchnic nerves) is abolished. Because the pelvic splanchnic nerves initiate and control micturition, a complete cord lesion also causes problems of bladder control.

5.7   Autonomic Innervation of the Male Genitalia

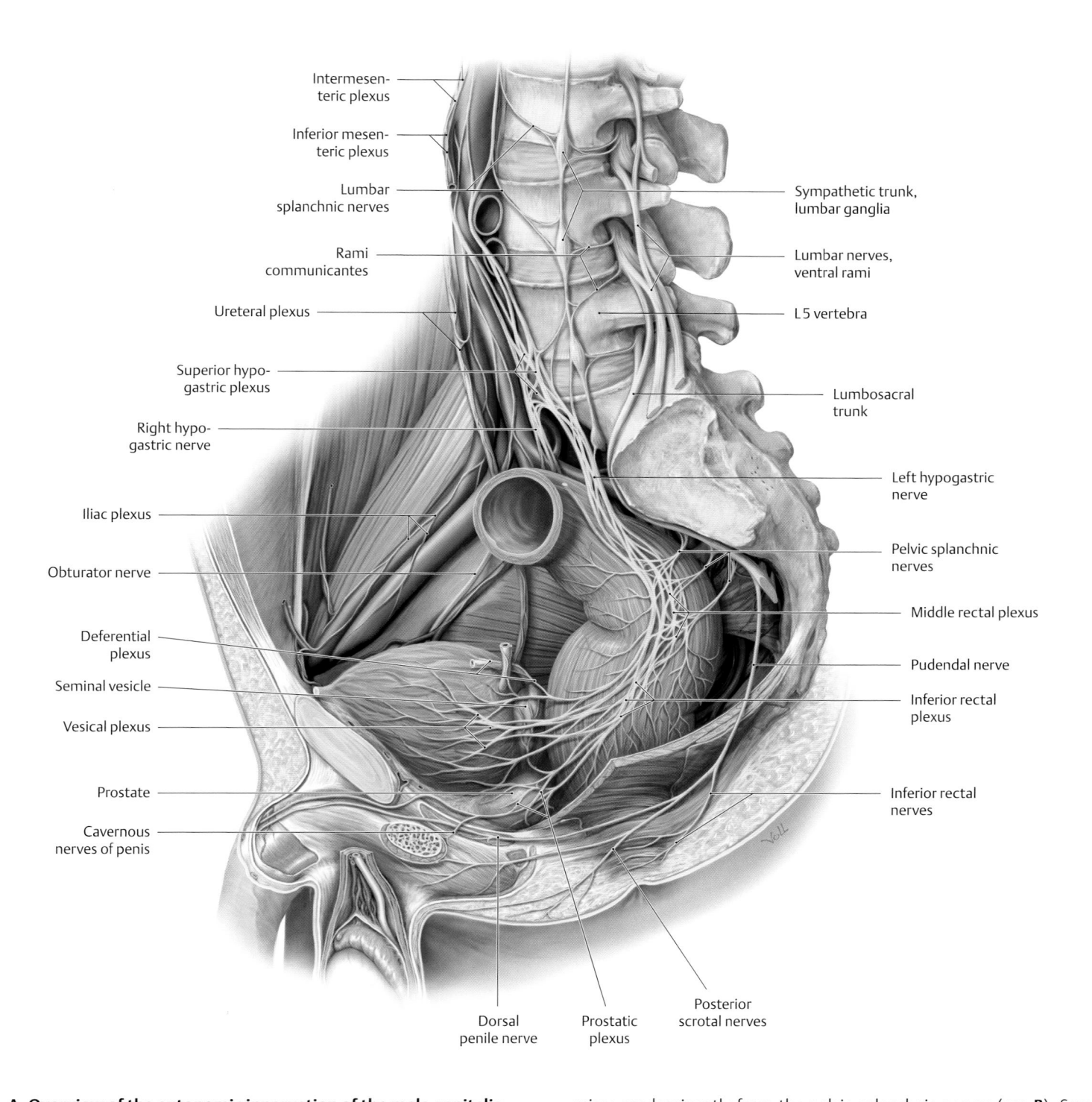

Intermesen-
teric plexus

Inferior mesen-
teric plexus

Lumbar
splanchnic nerves

Rami
communicantes

Ureteral plexus

Superior hypo-
gastric plexus

Right hypo-
gastric nerve

Iliac plexus

Obturator nerve

Deferential
plexus

Seminal vesicle

Vesical plexus

Prostate

Cavernous
nerves of penis

Sympathetic trunk,
lumbar ganglia

Lumbar nerves,
ventral rami

L5 vertebra

Lumbosacral
trunk

Left hypogastric
nerve

Pelvic splanchnic
nerves

Middle rectal plexus

Pudendal nerve

Inferior rectal
plexus

Inferior rectal
nerves

Posterior
scrotal nerves

Dorsal
penile nerve

Prostatic
plexus

A Overview of the autonomic innervation of the male genitalia
Opened male pelvis viewed from the left side. This drawing is a composite from many planes of section to show the three-dimensional relationships more clearly. The *sympathetic* fibers that supply the testis and epididymis form the lesser, least and lumbar splanchnic nerves. Those that supply the accessory sex glands (prostate, seminal vesicle, and bulbourethral glands), penis, and vas deferens arise from the lumbar and sacral splanchnic nerves. The *parasympathetic* supply to the male genitalia is much more modest than the sympathetic supply; it

arises predominantly from the pelvic splanchnic nerves (see **B**). Sympathetic and parasympathetic fibers join to form the *inferior hypogastric plexus*, which also receives the hypogastric nerves (arise from the division of the superior hypogastric plexus). The paired inferior hypogastric plexuses, which give origin to the plexuses that supply the urinary organs (see p. 309), then divide into multiple plexuses that innervate the genital organs (see **C**). The innervation of the rectum is described on pp. 312 and 314.

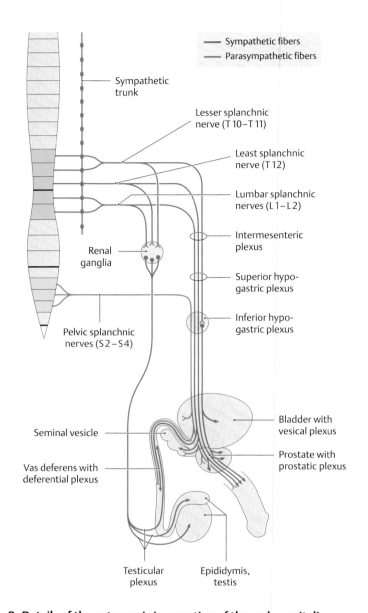

Sympathetic fibers
Parasympathetic fibers

Sympathetic trunk

Lesser splanchnic nerve (T 10–T 11)

Least splanchnic nerve (T 12)

Lumbar splanchnic nerves (L 1–L 2)

Intermesenteric plexus

Renal ganglia

Superior hypogastric plexus

Inferior hypogastric plexus

Pelvic splanchnic nerves (S 2–S 4)

Seminal vesicle

Bladder with vesical plexus

Vas deferens with deferential plexus

Prostate with prostatic plexus

Testicular plexus

Epididymis, testis

C Autonomic innervation of the male genitalia

First neuron	Peripheral course (sympathetic and parasympathetic)	Target organ	Effect
Sympathetic:			
T 10–T 12 (lesser and least splanchnic nerves)	Via renal ganglia to testicular plexus	• Testis • Epididymis	• Vasoconstriction
L 1–L 2 (lumbar and sacral splanchnic nerves)	Via superior hypogastric plexus and inferior hypogastric plexus to prostatic plexus and to:	• Prostate	• Stimulate secretions
		• Bulbourethral glands and seminal vesicle	
	Deferential plexus	• Penis (partly) • Vas deferens	• Ejaculation • Contraction
Parasympathetic:			
S 2–S 4 (pelvic splanchnic nerves)	Via inferior hypogastric plexus to prostatic plexus, continuing to the cavernous nerves of the penis	• Penis, erectile tissues	• Erection

B Details of the autonomic innervation of the male genitalia

- The **accessory sex glands (prostate, seminal vesicle, and bulbourethral glands)** receive their autonomic innervation from the prostatic plexus, which branches from the inferior hypogastric plexus (also believed to carry pain fibers).
- The **penis** also receives its autonomic innervation from branches of the prostatic plexus and from the cavernous nerves of the penis (see **A**). In both cases the synapse with the postsynaptic neuron occurs in the ganglion cells of the inferior hypogastric plexus.
- The **vas deferens** is supplied mainly by the deferential plexus, which also branches from the inferior hypogastric plexus and to a lesser degree from the testicular plexus that runs along the testicular artery.
- The **testis**, because of its developmental descent, receives most of its autonomic innervation from the testicular plexus (sympathetic fibers along the testicular artery, which synapse in the renal ganglia). The testicular plexus also gives off fibers to the epididymis. Both organs receive a smaller amount of autonomic innervation from the inferior hypogastric plexus (not included in **C**).

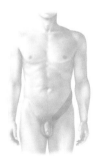

D Referred pain from the male gonads
The pain associated with diseases of the testis (e.g., inflammation) may be referred to this skin area. Gonadal pain, like intestinal pain, is not perceived at the anatomical location of the organ (referred pain [see p. 146]).

5.8 Autonomic Innervation of the Female Genitalia

Intermesen-
teric plexus

Inferior mesen-
teric plexus

Lumbar
splanchnic nerve

Rami
communicantes

Ureteral plexus

Superior hypo-
gastric plexus

Right hypo-
gastric nerve

Ovarian plexus

Obturator nerve

Right inferior
hypogastric
plexus

Vesical plexus

Right utero-
vaginal plexus

Sympathetic trunk,
lumbar ganglia

Lumbar nerves,
ventral rami

L 5 vertebra

Left hypo-
gastric nerve

First sacral nerve,
ventral ramus

Lumbosacral
trunk

Sacral plexus

Pelvic splanchnic
nerves

Pudendal nerve

Right middle
rectal plexus

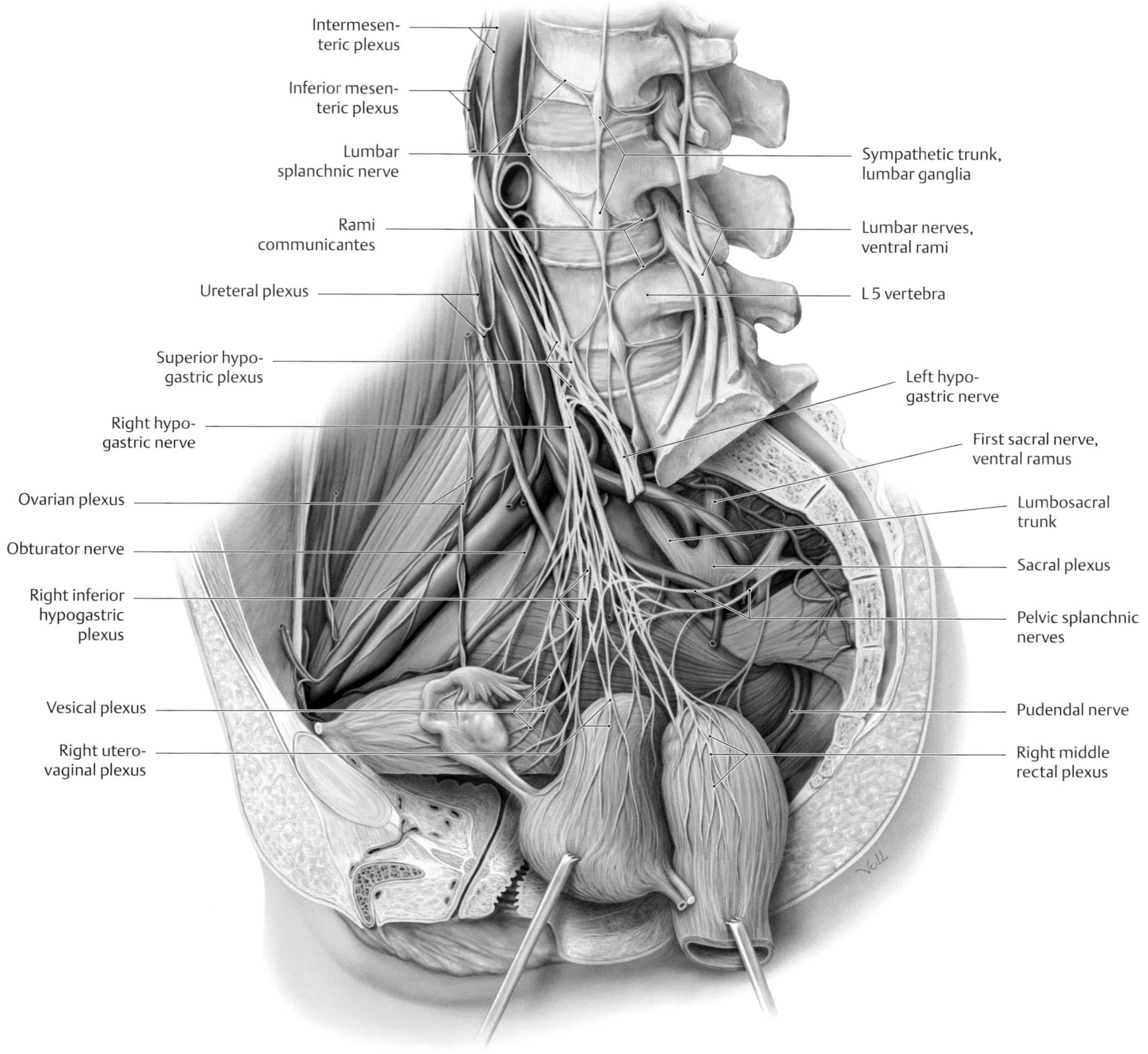

A Overview of the autonomic innervation of the female genitalia
An opened female pelvis viewed from the left side, with the rectum and
uterus reflected. This drawing was composited from multiple planes of
section to show the three-dimensional relationships more clearly. The
sympathetic fibers for the uterus, fallopian tubes, and ovaries arise predominantly from the lesser, least, and lumbar splanchnic nerves. The
parasympathetic fibers arise from the pelvic splanchnic nerves.
Note: The fibers that are distributed to the ovary synapse mainly in the
renal ganglia because as the ovary undergoes its developmental descent, it carries its autonomic supply from the abdomen with it. The fibers then continue on to the ovarian plexus, which also receives fibers
from the superior mesenteric plexus. This is analogous to the innervation of the testis via the renal ganglia and the superior and inferior mesenteric plexus and testicular plexus in the male.

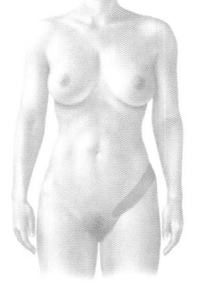

B Referred pain from the female gonads
The pain associated with ovarian diseases (e.g., inflammation) may
project to these skin areas and may not be perceived within the organ
itself (see p. 146).

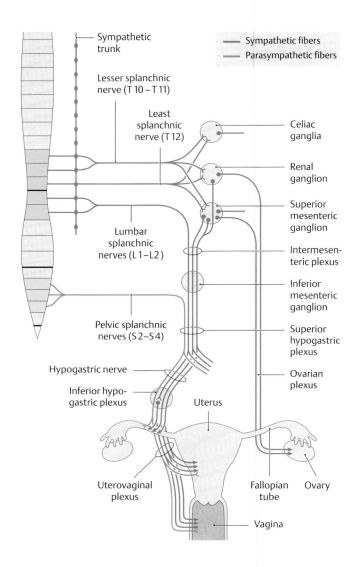

Sympathetic fibers
Parasympathetic fibers

D Autonomic innervation of the female genitalia

First neuron	Peripheral course (sympathetic and parasympathetic)	Target organ	Effect
Sympathetic:			
T 10–T 12 (lesser and least splanchnic nerves)	Via renal ganglia and superior mesenteric ganglion to ovarian plexus	• Ovary	• Vasoconstriction
L 1–L 2 (lumbar splanchnic nerves)	Via superior hypogastric plexus, hypogastric nerves, and inferior hypogastric plexus to uterovaginal plexus	• Uterus • Fallopian tube • Vagina	• Contraction (in uterus, depends on hormone status)
		• Vagina	• Vasoconstriction
Parasympathetic:			
S 2–S 4 (pelvic splanchnic nerves	Inferior hypogastric plexus to uterovaginal plexus, continuing to cavernous nerves of clitoris	• Uterus, fallopian tube	• Vasodilation
		• Vagina • Clitoris	• Transudation • Erection

C Autonomic innervation of the female genitalia

Because of the developmental descent of the **ovary**, its nerve supply extends a considerable distance along the ovarian artery in the ovarian suspensory ligament (the ovarian plexus, which arises from the abdominal aortic plexus via the renal ganglia — analogous to the innervation of the testis via the testicular plexus).

The **uterus, fallopian tube**, and **vagina** receive their autonomic innervation from the inferior hypogastric plexus. The *sympathetic* portion is derived from the lesser, least, and lumbar splanchnic nerves, which synapse partly in the mesenteric ganglia and partly in the ganglion cells of the inferior hypogastric plexus. The *parasympathetic* fibers are derived from the pelvic splanchnic nerves (S 2–S 4), which synapse in the inferior hypogastric plexus or in / on the organ wall. Branches from the inferior hypogastric plexus form the prominent uterovaginal plexus (of Frankenhauser) located on both sides of the uterus. The ovary may receive additional autonomic innervation along the fallopian tube from the inferior hypogastric plexus.

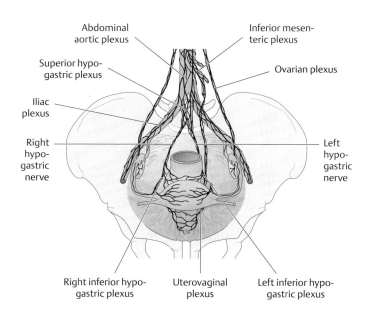

E Overview of the autonomic plexuses in the female pelvis
Anterior view.

Note the division of the of the superior hypogastric plexus into *two hypogastric nerves*, which are continuous with *both inferior hypogastric plexuses*. The latter then give off individual visceral plexuses to the rectum, uterus, vagina, and bladder (see p. 318 for the vesical plexus).

The ovary is supplied chiefly by the ovarian plexus, which runs along the ovarian artery in the ovarian suspensory ligament. Thus, the autonomic supply of the female pelvis corresponds to that in the male, although the plexuses in the female pelvis are more strongly developed due to the very rich nerve supply of the uterus.

321

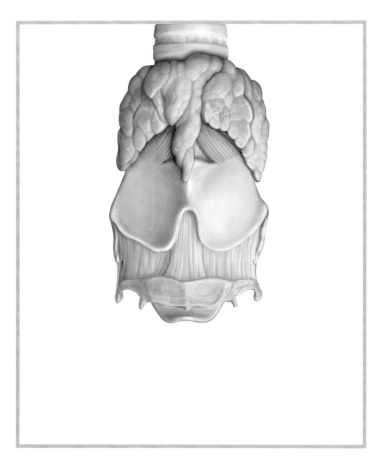

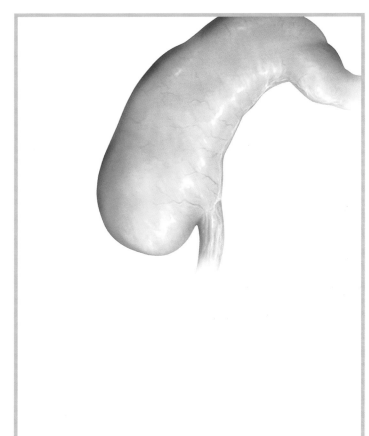

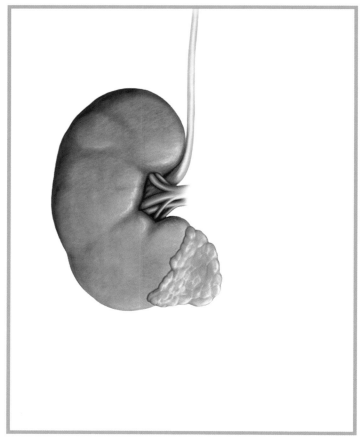

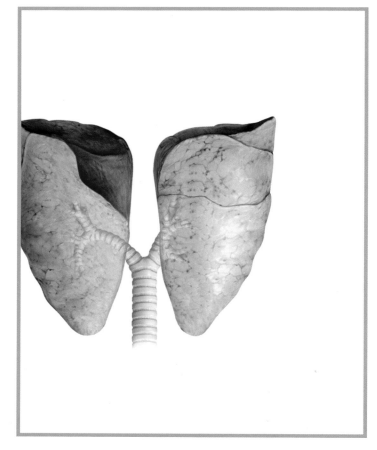

Neurovascular Supply to the Organs: A Schematic Approach

How to Use this Chapter

Each of the sections in this chapter reviews the neurovascular supply to an organ or group of organs in a schematized form. The following **subgroups** are distinguished in the diagrams:

- Arterial supply (red)
- Venous drainage (blue)
- Lymphatic drainage (green)
- Innervation (yellow)

The schematics can be used in various ways:

- *Reviewing* for a test: The student can quickly obtain a basic grasp of neurovascular structures and pathways.
- *Looking up* a specific structure: The diagrams make it easy to locate and identify a particular neurovascular supply.
- *Understanding* complex anatomy by appreciating the basic neurovascular supply to an organ in the diagrams and then referring back to the more complex anatomical relationships shown in earlier chapters.

Points to keep in mind when using the **schematics:**

- They reflect a simplified, idealized view.
- Topographical anatomy is ignored, and the structures are not drawn to scale.
- Organs that are in close proximity to each other but are supplied by different groups of neurovascular structures are shown in separate diagrams.
- By and large, variants are disregarded.
- In cases where the neurovascular supply is bilaterally symmetrical, only one side is shown.

1.1 Thymus

Arteries

Subclavian artery

↓

Internal thoracic artery → (Pericardiaco-phrenic artery)

↓ ↓

Thymic branches   Thymic branches

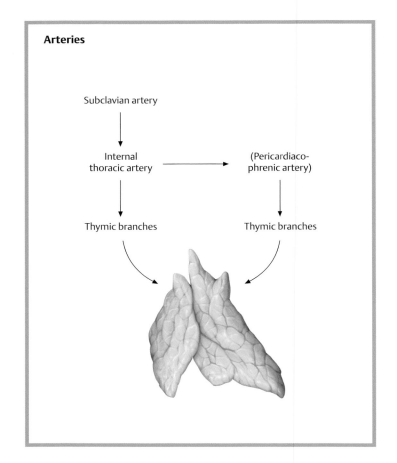

Veins

Superior vena cava

Right brachio-cephalic vein   Left brachio-cephalic vein

Thymic veins

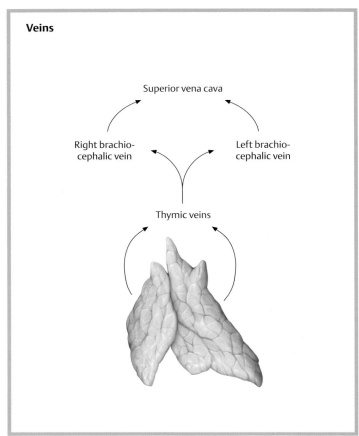

Lymph nodes

Junction of right subclavian and internal jugular veins   Junction of left subclavian and internal jugular veins

↑ ↑

Right broncho-mediastinal trunk   Left broncho-mediastinal trunk

Brachiocephalic lymph nodes

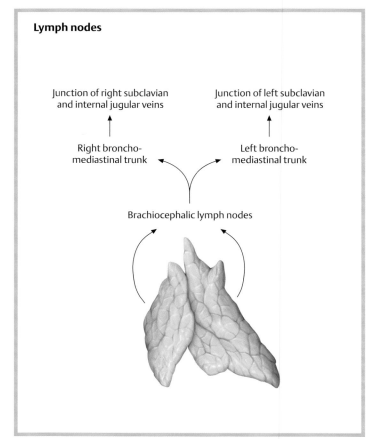

Innervation

Sympathetic	Parasympathetic

Sympathetic trunk   Vagus nerves

↓

Superior, inferior, middle cervical ganglia   Recurrent laryngeal nerves

↓

Cervical cardiac nerves   Cervical cardiac branches

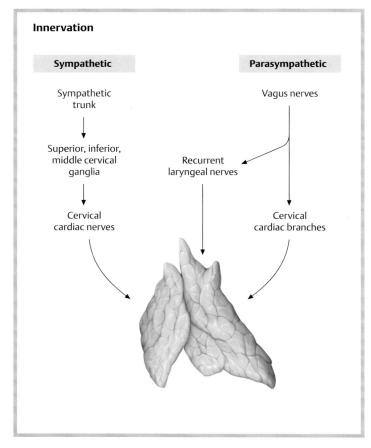

1.2 Larynx

Arteries

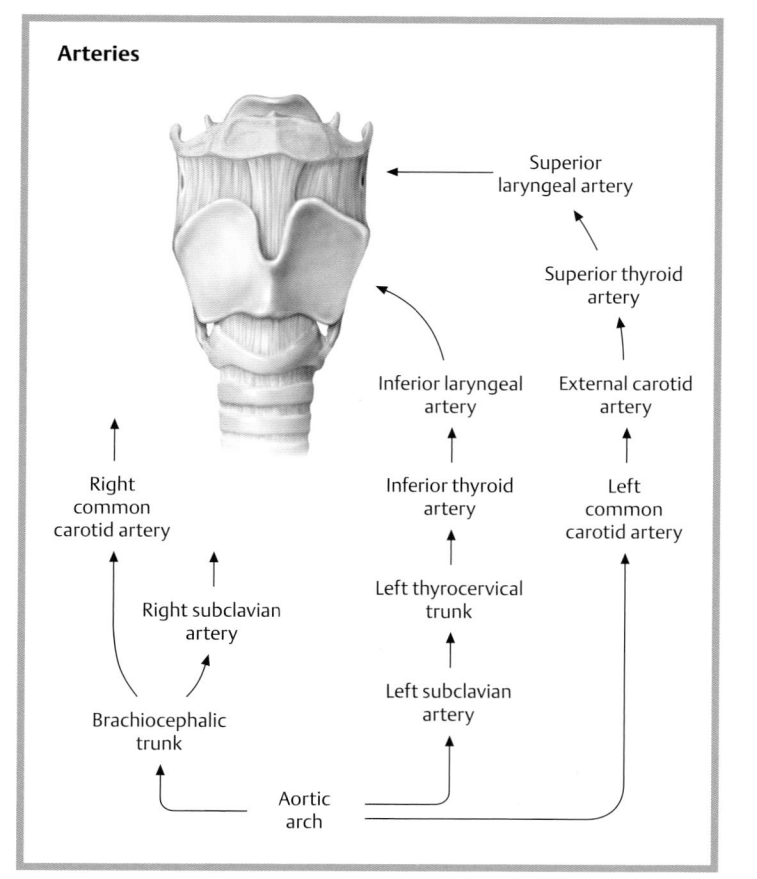

Superior laryngeal artery

Superior thyroid artery

Inferior laryngeal artery

External carotid artery

Right common carotid artery

Inferior thyroid artery

Left common carotid artery

Right subclavian artery

Left thyrocervical trunk

Brachiocephalic trunk

Left subclavian artery

Aortic arch

Veins

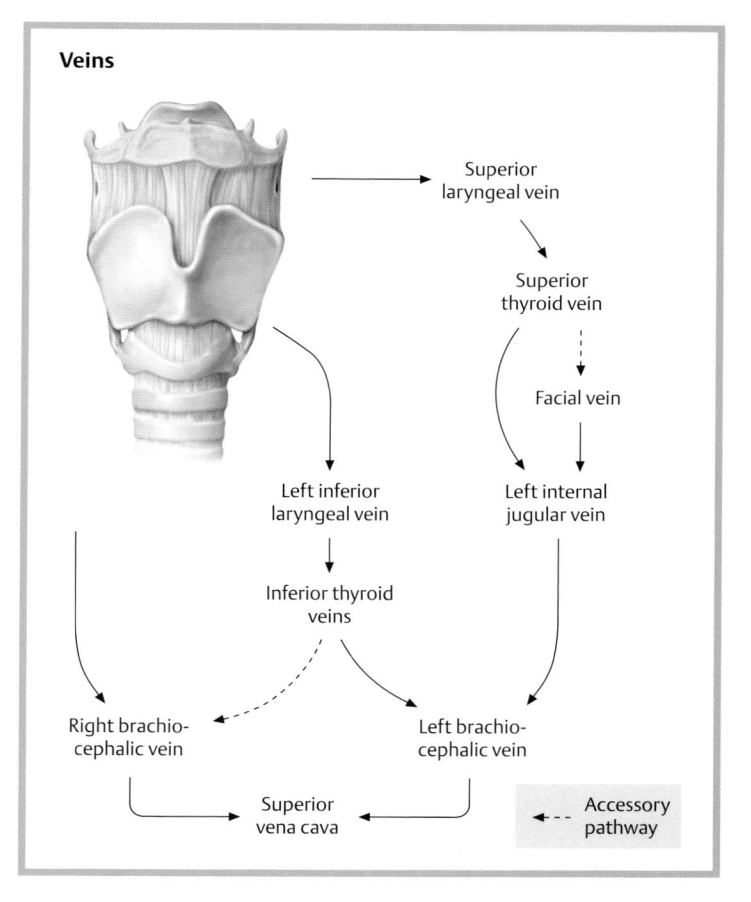

Superior laryngeal vein

Superior thyroid vein

Facial vein

Left inferior laryngeal vein

Left internal jugular vein

Inferior thyroid veins

Right brachio-cephalic vein

Left brachio-cephalic vein

Superior vena cava

◀--- Accessory pathway

Lymph nodes

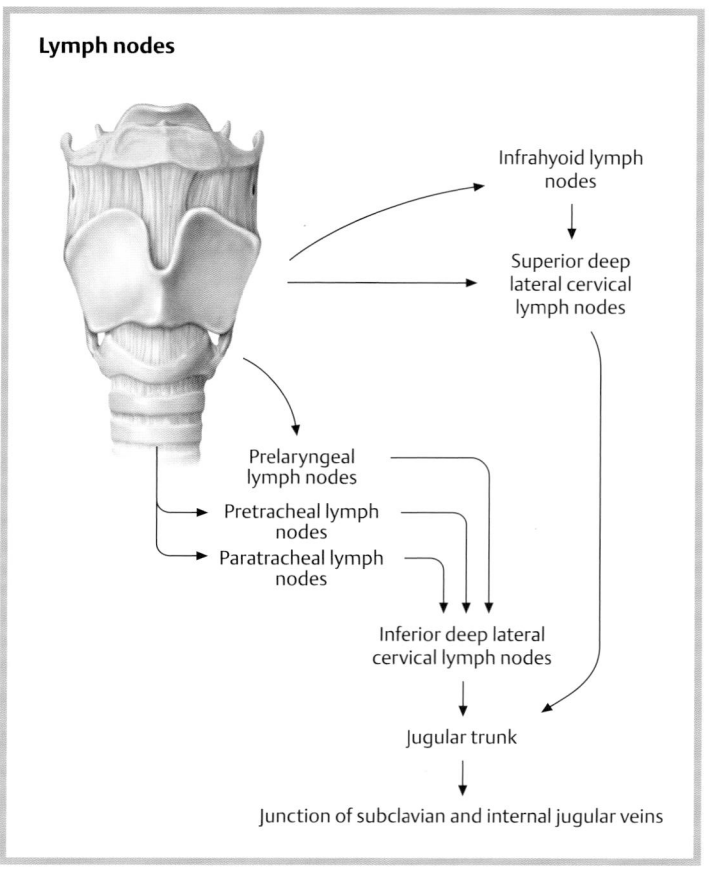

Infrahyoid lymph nodes

Superior deep lateral cervical lymph nodes

Prelaryngeal lymph nodes

Pretracheal lymph nodes

Paratracheal lymph nodes

Inferior deep lateral cervical lymph nodes

Jugular trunk

Junction of subclavian and internal jugular veins

Innervation

Sympathetic	Somatomotor	Parasympathetic
Sympathetic trunk	Nucleus ambiguus	Dorsal vagal nucleus
Carotid plexus		Vagus nerve
Laryngeal plexus		Superior laryngeal nerve

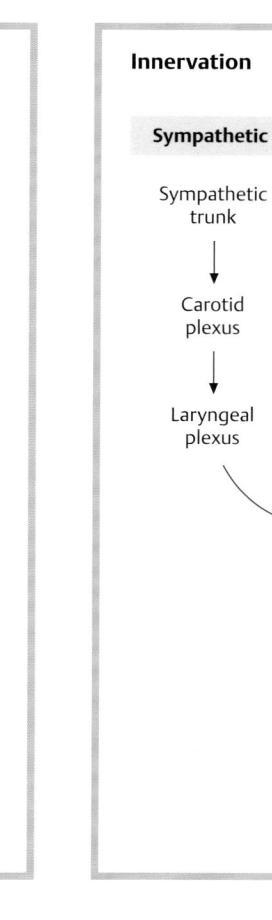

Recurrent laryngeal nerve

1.3 Thyroid Gland

Arteries

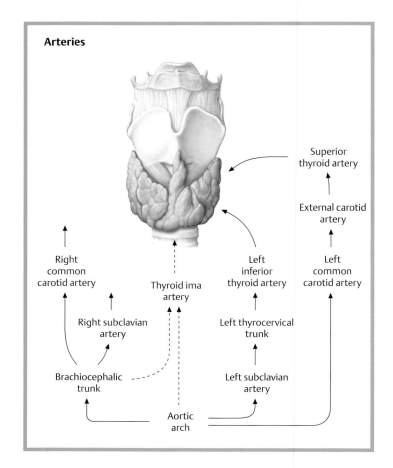

Superior thyroid artery

External carotid artery

Right common carotid artery

Thyroid ima artery

Left inferior thyroid artery

Left common carotid artery

Right subclavian artery

Left thyrocervical trunk

Brachiocephalic trunk

Left subclavian artery

Aortic arch

Veins

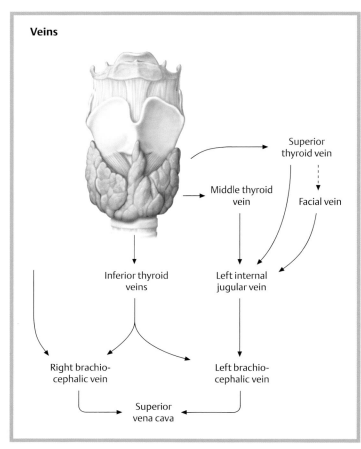

Superior thyroid vein

Middle thyroid vein

Facial vein

Inferior thyroid veins

Left internal jugular vein

Right brachio-cephalic vein

Left brachio-cephalic vein

Superior vena cava

Lymph nodes

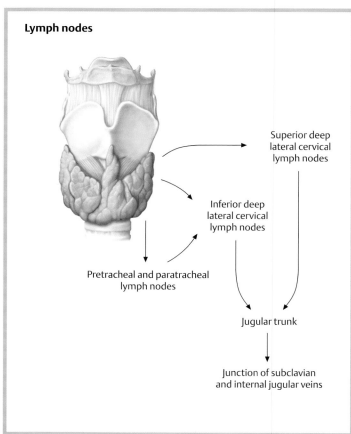

Superior deep lateral cervical lymph nodes

Inferior deep lateral cervical lymph nodes

Pretracheal and paratracheal lymph nodes

Jugular trunk

Junction of subclavian and internal jugular veins

Innervation

Sympathetic	Parasympathetic
Sympathetic trunk	Vagus nerve

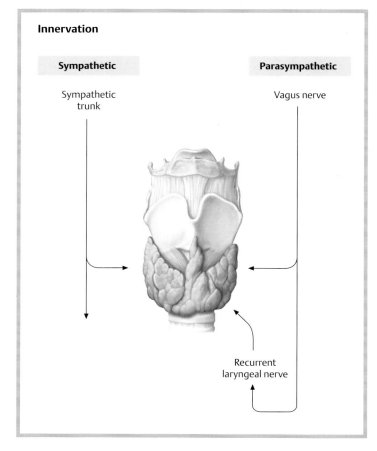

Recurrent laryngeal nerve

327

1.4 Pharynx*

Arteries

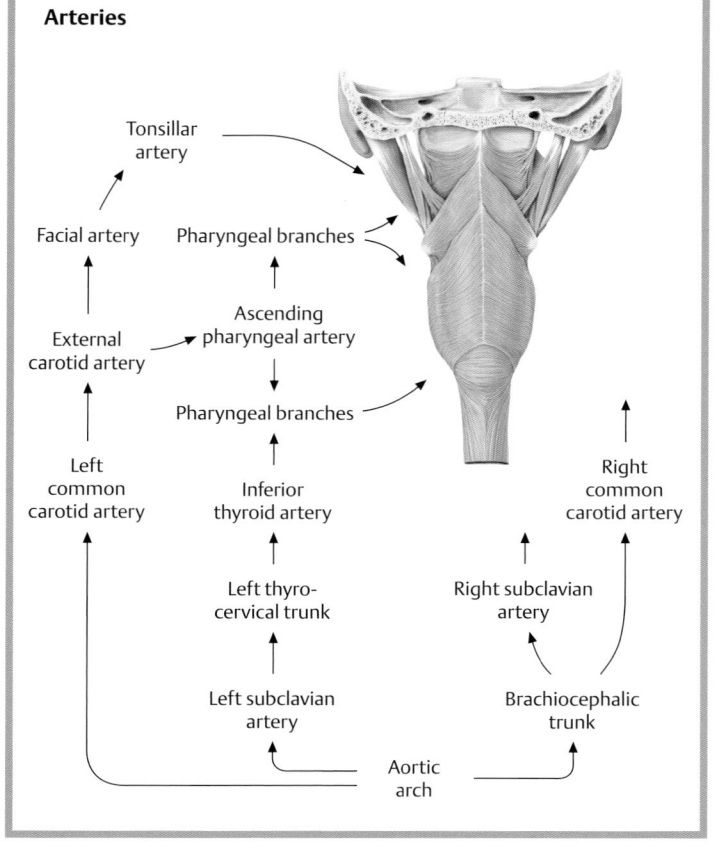

Tonsillar artery

Facial artery ← Pharyngeal branches

External carotid artery → Ascending pharyngeal artery

Ascending pharyngeal artery ↓ Pharyngeal branches

Pharyngeal branches ← Inferior thyroid artery

Left common carotid artery

Left thyro-cervical trunk

Left subclavian artery

Right common carotid artery

Right subclavian artery

Brachiocephalic trunk

Aortic arch

Veins

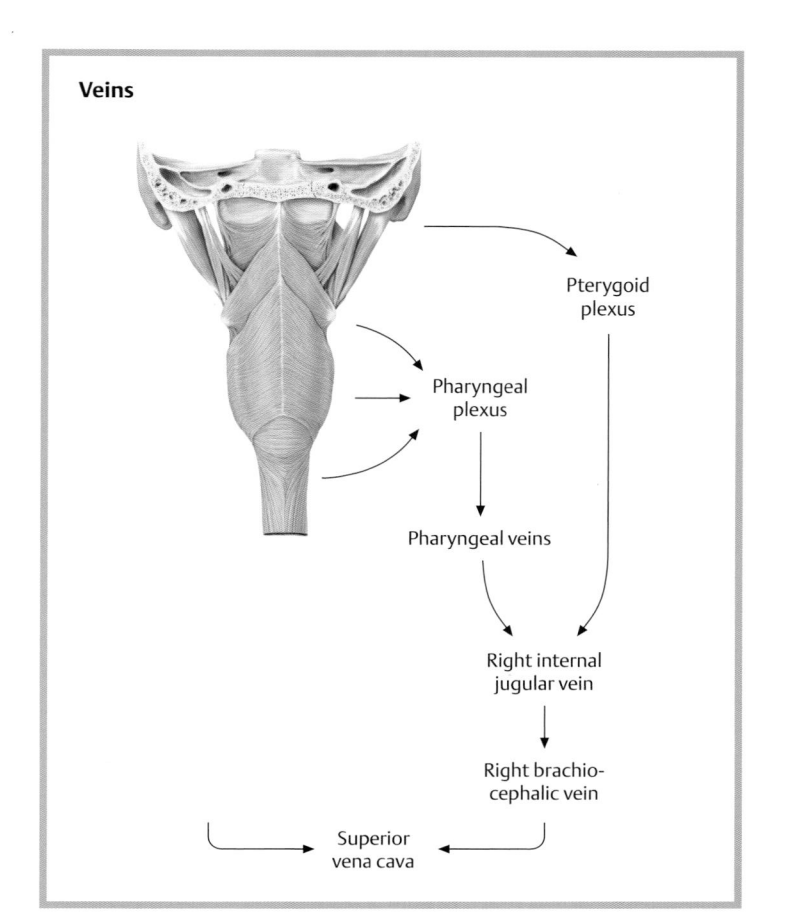

Pterygoid plexus

Pharyngeal plexus

Pharyngeal veins

Right internal jugular vein

Right brachio-cephalic vein

Superior vena cava

Lymph nodes

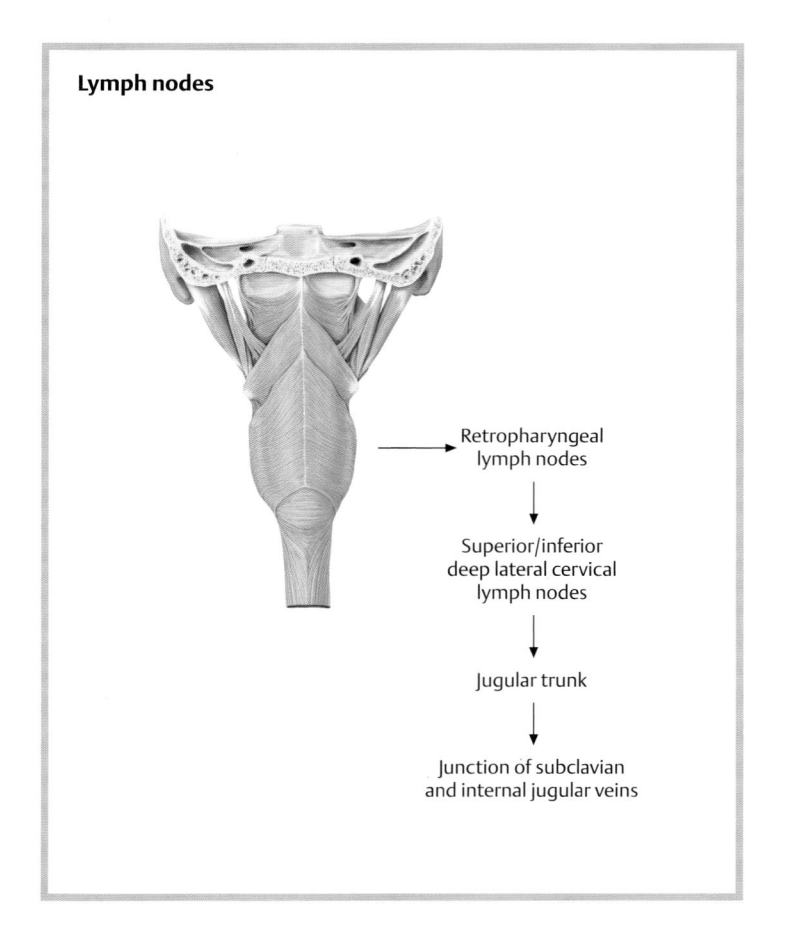

Retropharyngeal lymph nodes

↓

Superior/inferior deep lateral cervical lymph nodes

↓

Jugular trunk

↓

Junction of subclavian and internal jugular veins

Innervation

Sympathetic	Somatomotor	Parasympathetic
Sympathetic trunk	Nucleus ambiguus	Dorsal vagal nucleus
	Glossopharyngeal nerve	Vagus nerve
	Pharyngeal branches	Recurrent laryngeal nerve
	Pharyngeal plexus	

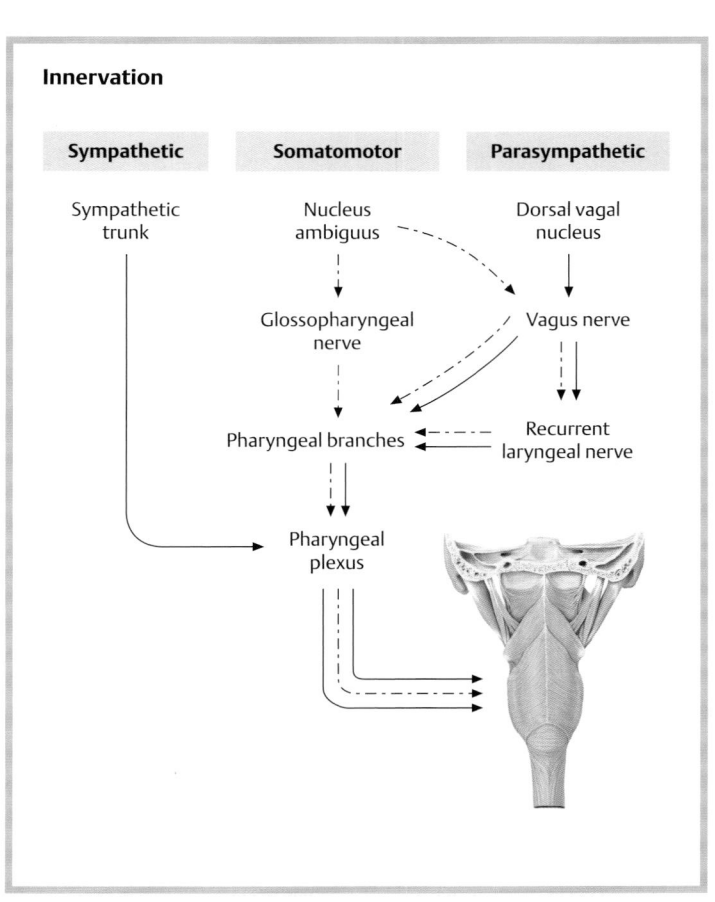

* Posterior view

1.5 Esophagus

Arteries

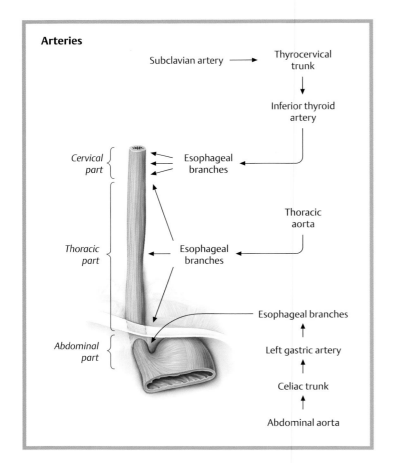

Subclavian artery → Thyrocervical trunk
↓
Inferior thyroid artery

Cervical part ← Esophageal branches

Thoracic aorta

Thoracic part ← Esophageal branches ←

Abdominal part

Esophageal branches
↑
Left gastric artery
↑
Celiac trunk
↑
Abdominal aorta

Veins

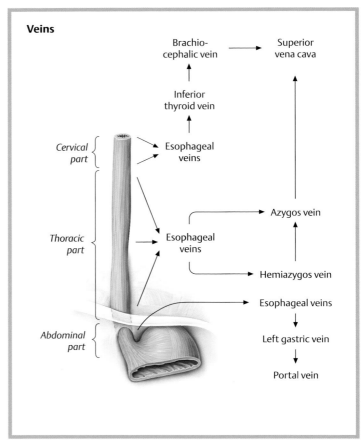

Brachio-cephalic vein → Superior vena cava

Inferior thyroid vein
↑

Cervical part → Esophageal veins

Thoracic part → Esophageal veins → Azygos vein

Hemiazygos vein

Abdominal part

Esophageal veins
↓
Left gastric vein
↓
Portal vein

Lymph nodes

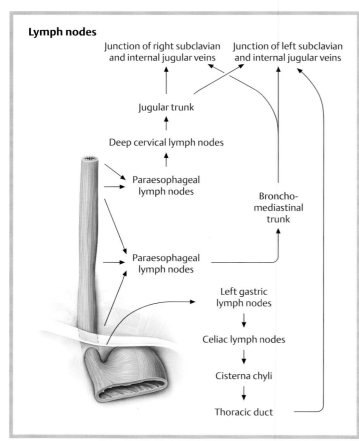

Junction of right subclavian and internal jugular veins   Junction of left subclavian and internal jugular veins
↑   ↑
Jugular trunk
↑
Deep cervical lymph nodes
↑
Paraesophageal lymph nodes

Broncho-mediastinal trunk

Paraesophageal lymph nodes

Left gastric lymph nodes
↓
Celiac lymph nodes
↓
Cisterna chyli
↓
Thoracic duct

Innervation

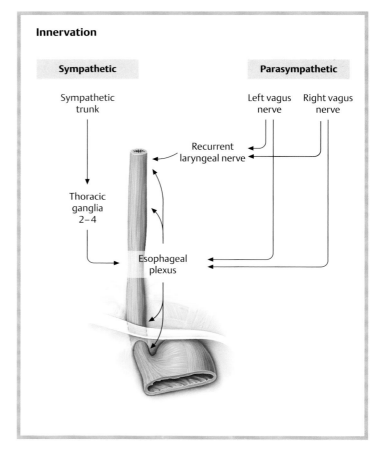

Sympathetic	**Parasympathetic**

Sympathetic trunk   Left vagus nerve   Right vagus nerve

Recurrent laryngeal nerve

Thoracic ganglia 2–4

Esophageal plexus

1.6 **Heart**

Arteries

Left
ventricle
↓
Ascending aorta

Right coronary
artery

Left coronary
artery

Posterior
interventricular
branch

Anterior
interventricular
branch

Circumflex
branch

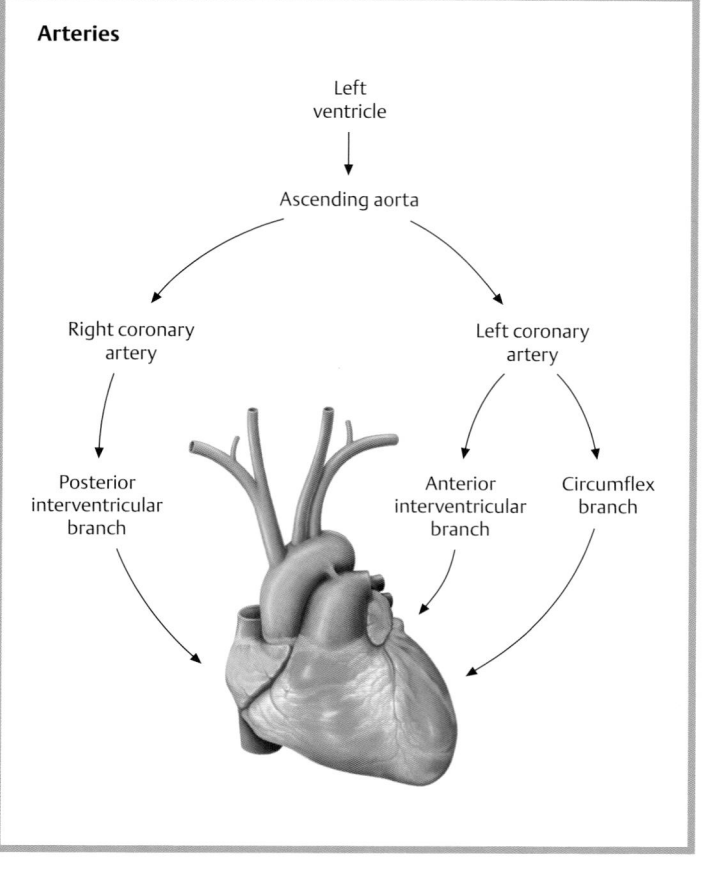

Veins

Right
atrium
↑
Coronary sinus

Middle
cardiac vein

Great
cardiac vein

Small
cardiac vein

Posterior
vein of left
ventricle

Anterior
vein of left
ventricle

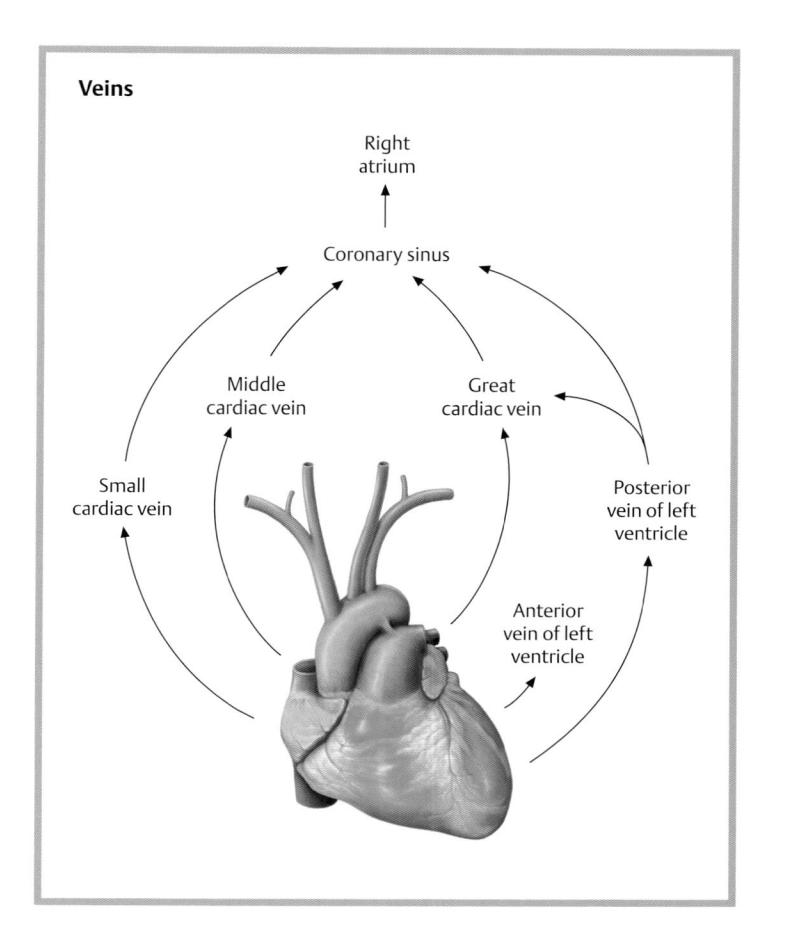

Lymph nodes

Bronchomediastinal
trunk
↑
Brachiocephalic lymph nodes,
tracheobronchial lymph nodes

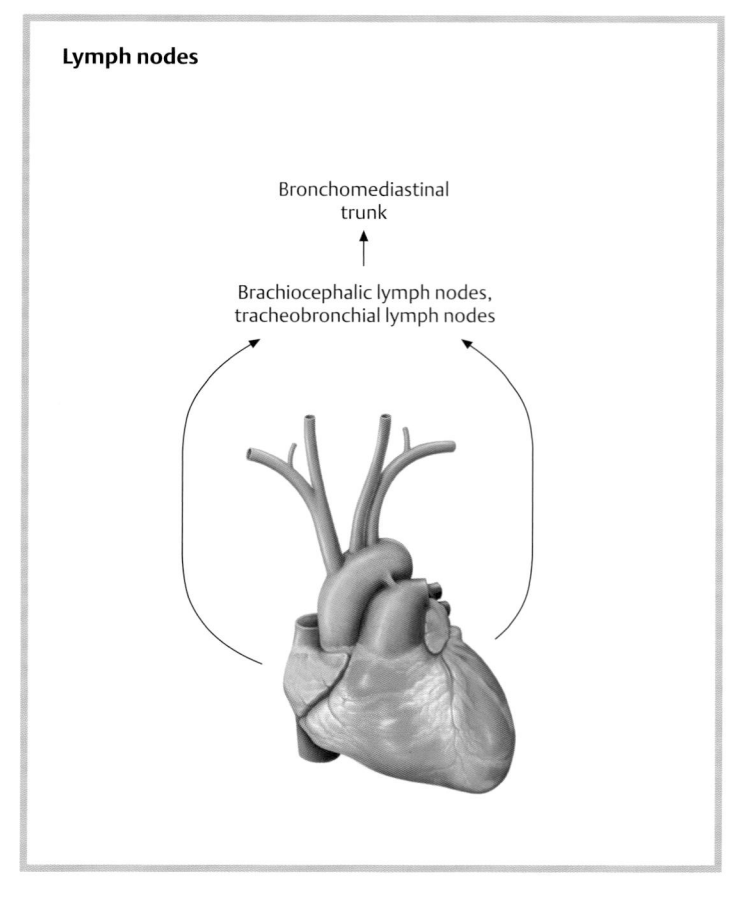

Innervation

Sympathetic	Parasympathetic

Sympathetic
trunk

Vagus nerves

Thoracic
ganglia
2–4 (5)

Cervical
ganglia

Cervical
cardiac nerves

Cervical
cardiac branches

Thoracic
cardiac branches

Thoracic
cardiac branches

Cardiac plexus

Myocardium

Coronary
arteries

Sinoatrial
node

Atrioventricular
node

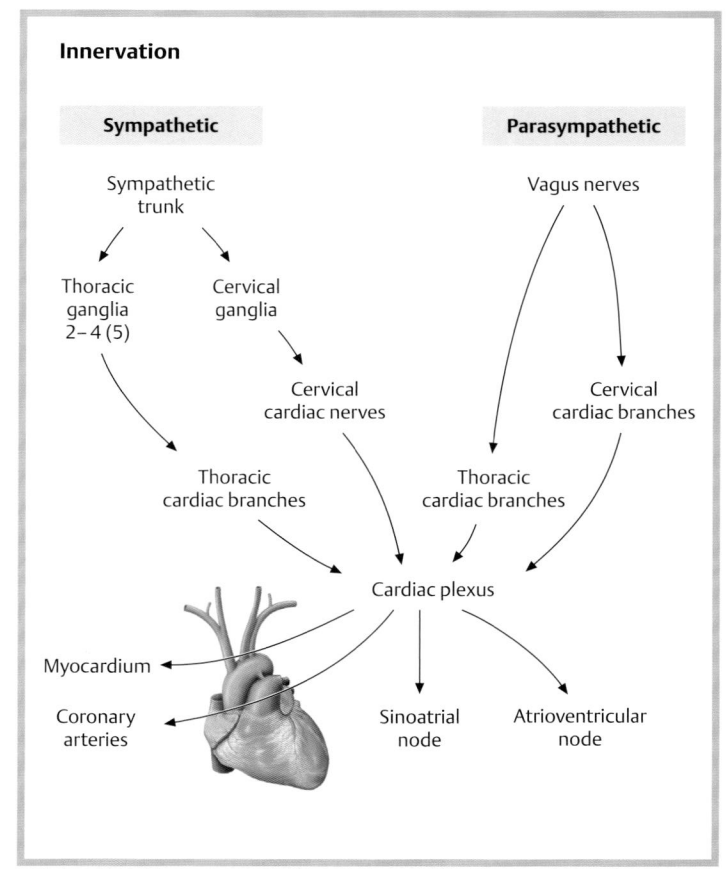

1.7 Pericardium

Arteries

Subclavian artery

↓

Internal
thoracic artery

↓

Pericardiaco-
phrenic artery

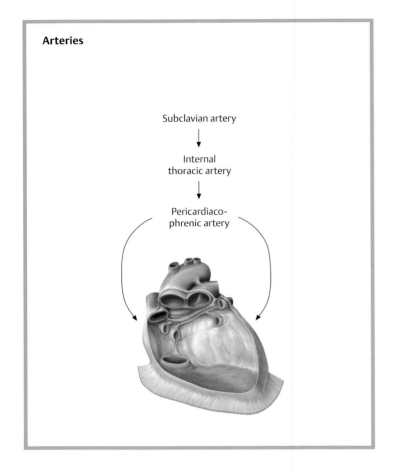

Veins

Superior vena cava

↑

Brachiocephalic
vein

↑

Internal
thoracic vein

↑

Pericardiaco-
phrenic vein

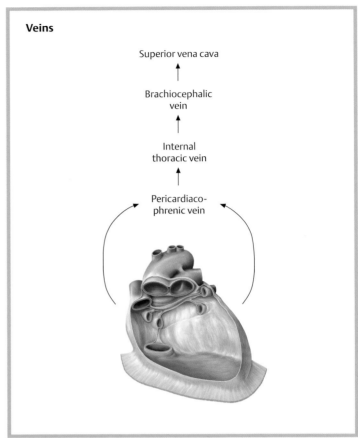

Lymph nodes

Bronchomediastinal
trunk

↑

Parasternal lymph nodes

↑

Prepericardial
lymph nodes

Lateral pericardial
lymph nodes

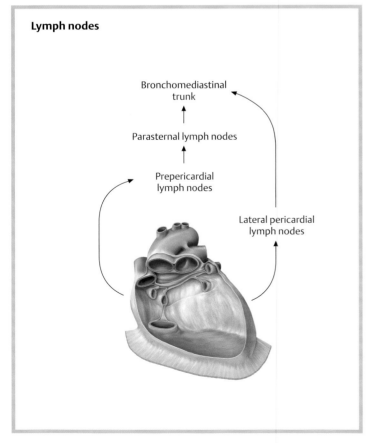

Innervation

Spinal cord
segments C(3)–4–(5)

↑

Cervical plexus

↑

Phrenic nerve

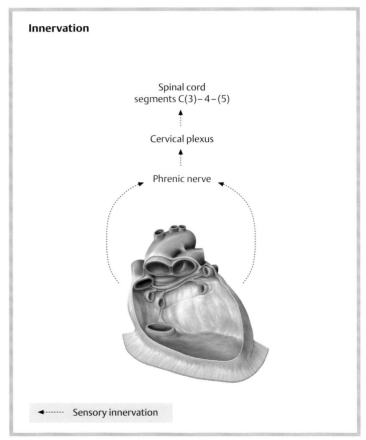

◄------ Sensory innervation

1.8 Lung and Trachea

Arteries

Pulmonary vessels

Right
ventricle

↓

Pulmonary
trunk

Right/left
pulmonary artery

Bronchial vessels

Left
ventricle

↓

Thoracic
aorta

↓

Bronchial branches

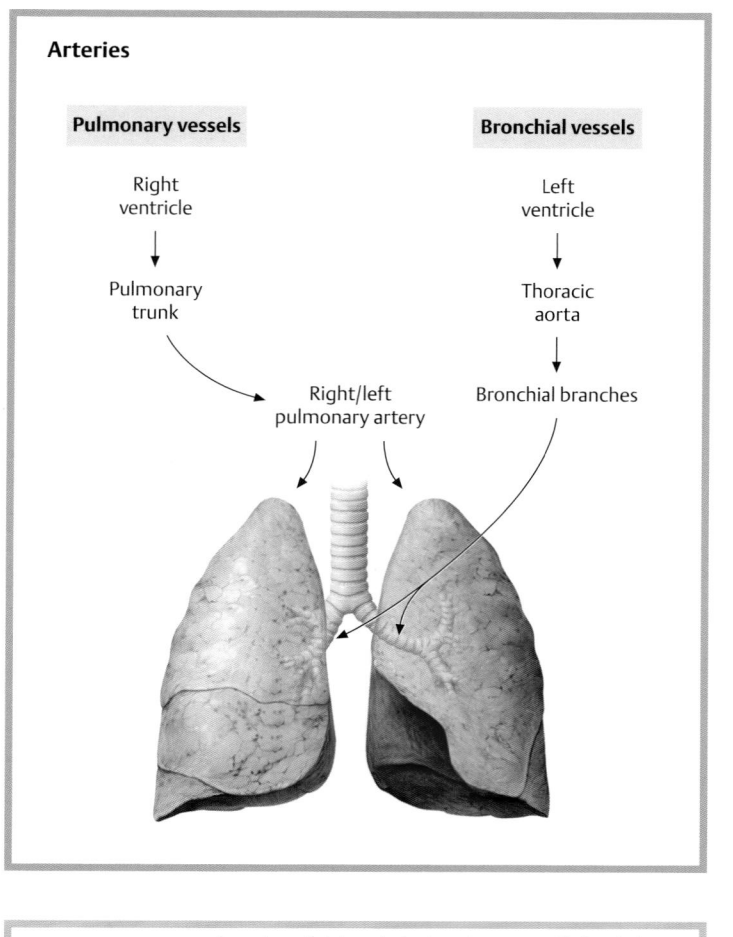

Veins

Pulmonary vessels

Left
atrium

↑

Pulmonary
trunk

Right/left
pulmonary veins

Bronchial vessels

Right
atrium

↑

Superior vena cava

↑

Azygos vein ←

(Accessory)
hemiazygos vein

↑

Bronchial veins

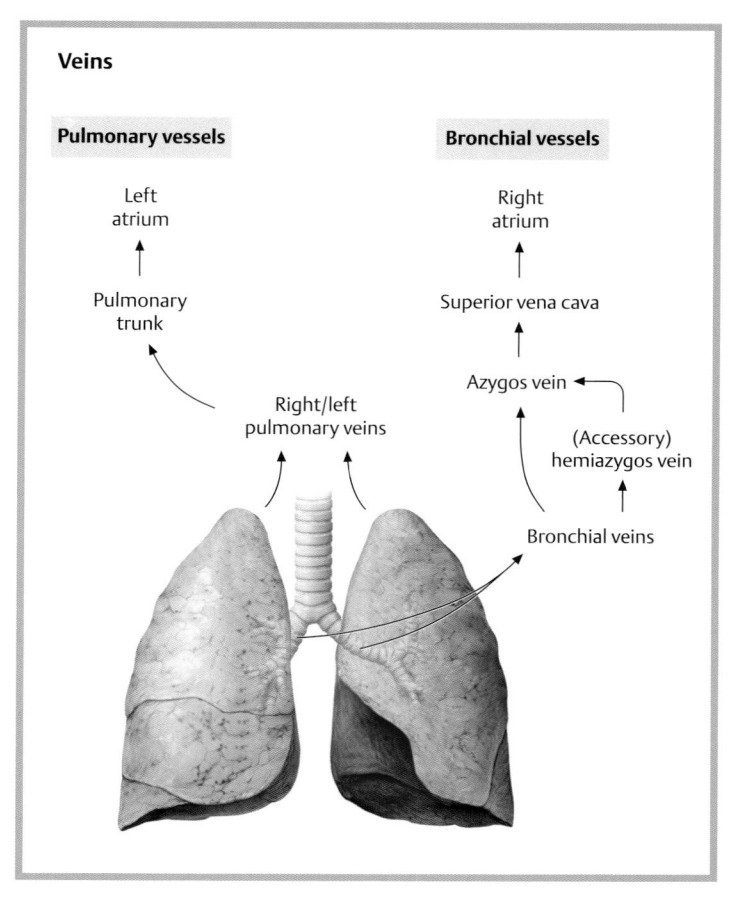

Lymph nodes

Junction of right subclavian
and internal jugular veins

Junction of left subclavian
and internal jugular veins

↑

Right/left bronchomediastinal trunk

↑ ↑

Paratracheal lymph nodes

↑ ↑

Superior/inferior tracheobronchial lymph nodes

Broncho-
pulmonary
lymph nodes

Intrapulmonary
lymph nodes

Superior phrenic lymph nodes

Inferior phrenic lymph nodes

↓

Lumbar trunk

↓

Cisterna chyli ⟶ Thoracic
duct

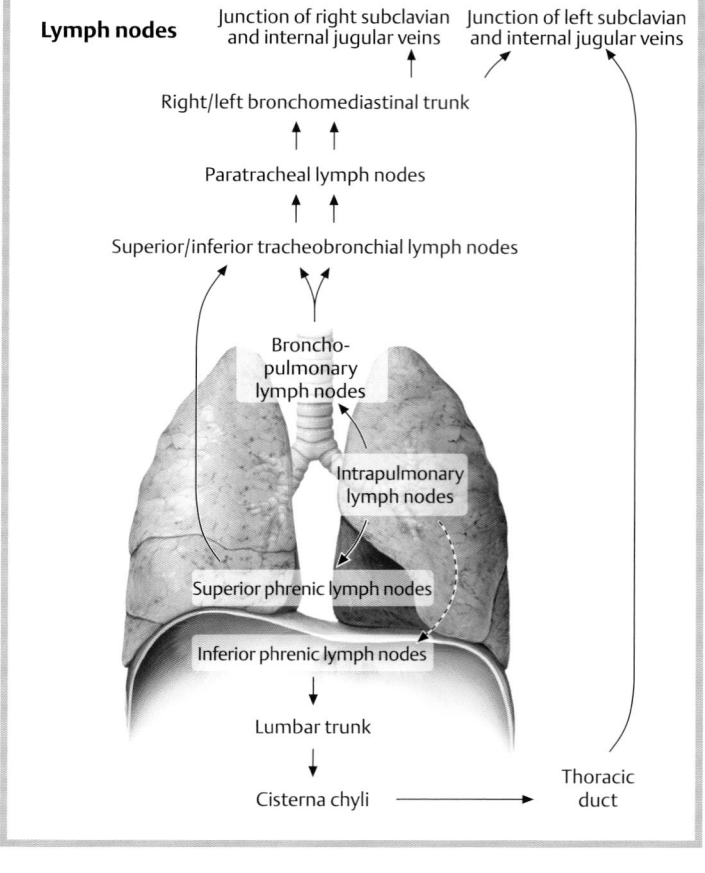

Innervation

Sympathetic

Sympathetic
trunk

↓

Thoracic
ganglia 3–4

Pulmonary branches

Parasympathetic

Left
vagus nerve

Right
vagus nerve

Recurrent
laryngeal nerve

Tracheal
branches

Bronchial branches

Pulmonary plexus

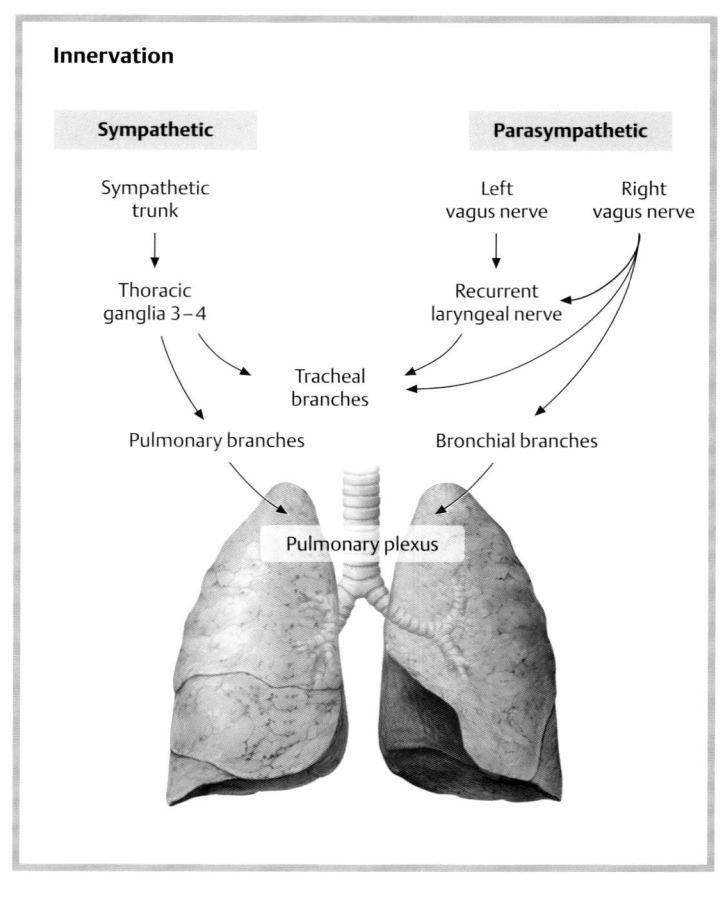

1.9 Diaphragm

Arteries

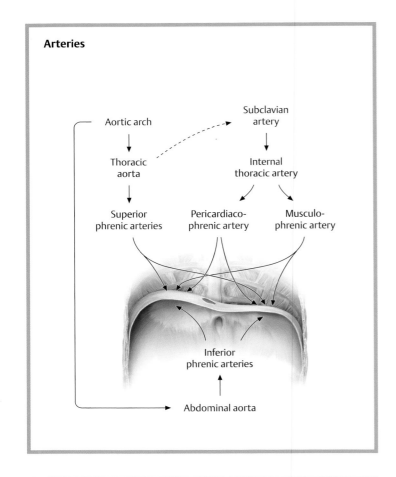

Aortic arch → Thoracic aorta

Subclavian artery → Internal thoracic artery

Thoracic aorta → Superior phrenic arteries

Internal thoracic artery → Pericardiaco-phrenic artery

Internal thoracic artery → Musculo-phrenic artery

Superior phrenic arteries, Pericardiaco-phrenic artery, Musculo-phrenic artery

Inferior phrenic arteries

Abdominal aorta

Veins

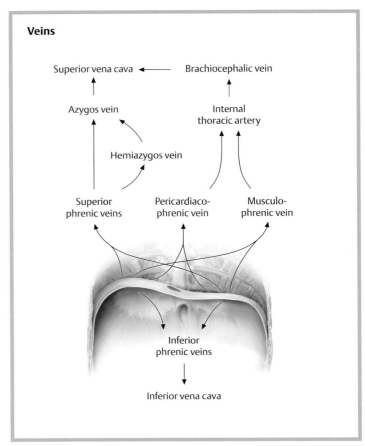

Superior vena cava ← Brachiocephalic vein

Azygos vein

Hemiazygos vein

Internal thoracic artery

Superior phrenic veins, Pericardiaco-phrenic vein, Musculo-phrenic vein

Inferior phrenic veins

Inferior vena cava

Lymph nodes

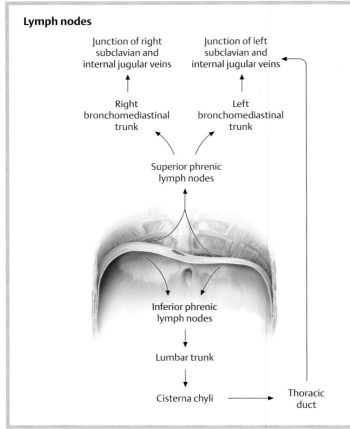

Junction of right subclavian and internal jugular veins

Junction of left subclavian and internal jugular veins

Right bronchomediastinal trunk

Left bronchomediastinal trunk

Superior phrenic lymph nodes

Inferior phrenic lymph nodes

Lumbar trunk

Cisterna chyli → Thoracic duct

Innervation

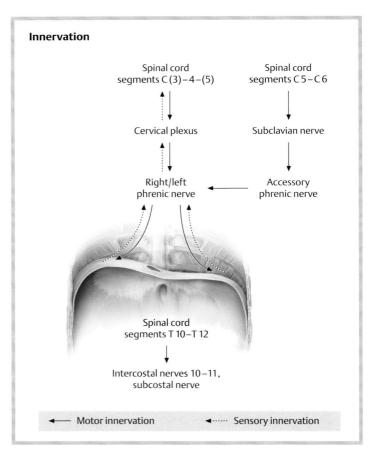

Spinal cord segments C (3)–4–(5)

Spinal cord segments C 5–C 6

Cervical plexus

Subclavian nerve

Right/left phrenic nerve ← Accessory phrenic nerve

Spinal cord segments T 10–T 12

Intercostal nerves 10–11, subcostal nerve

⟵ Motor innervation   ⟵······ Sensory innervation

1.10   Liver, Gallbladder, and Spleen

Arteries

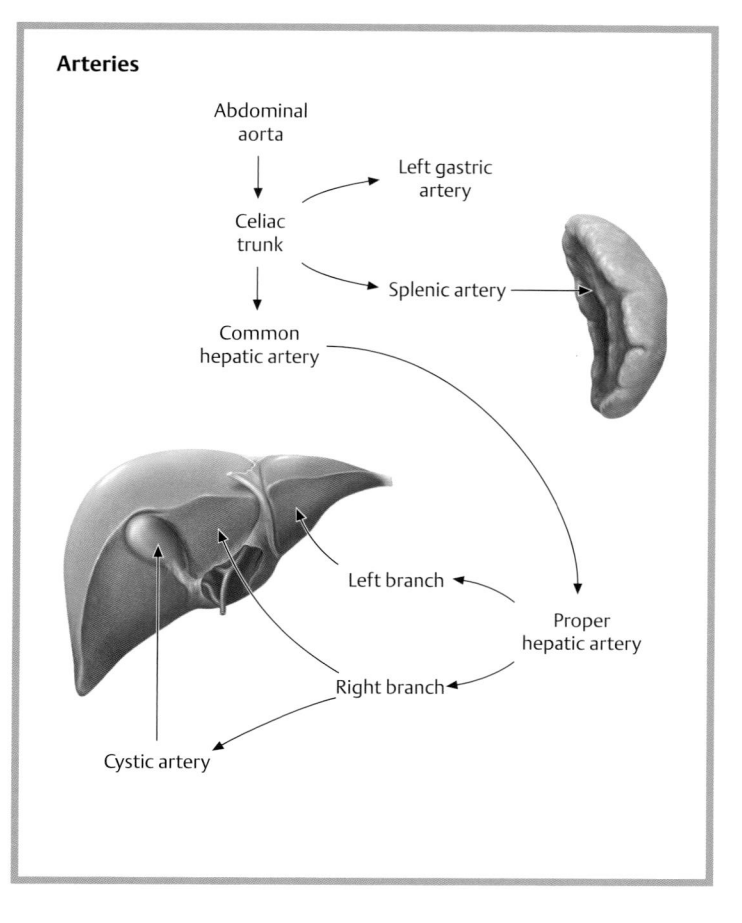

Abdominal aorta → Celiac trunk

Celiac trunk → Left gastric artery

Celiac trunk → Splenic artery

Splenic artery → (spleen)

Celiac trunk → Common hepatic artery

Common hepatic artery → Proper hepatic artery

Proper hepatic artery → Left branch

Proper hepatic artery → Right branch

Right branch → Cystic artery

Veins

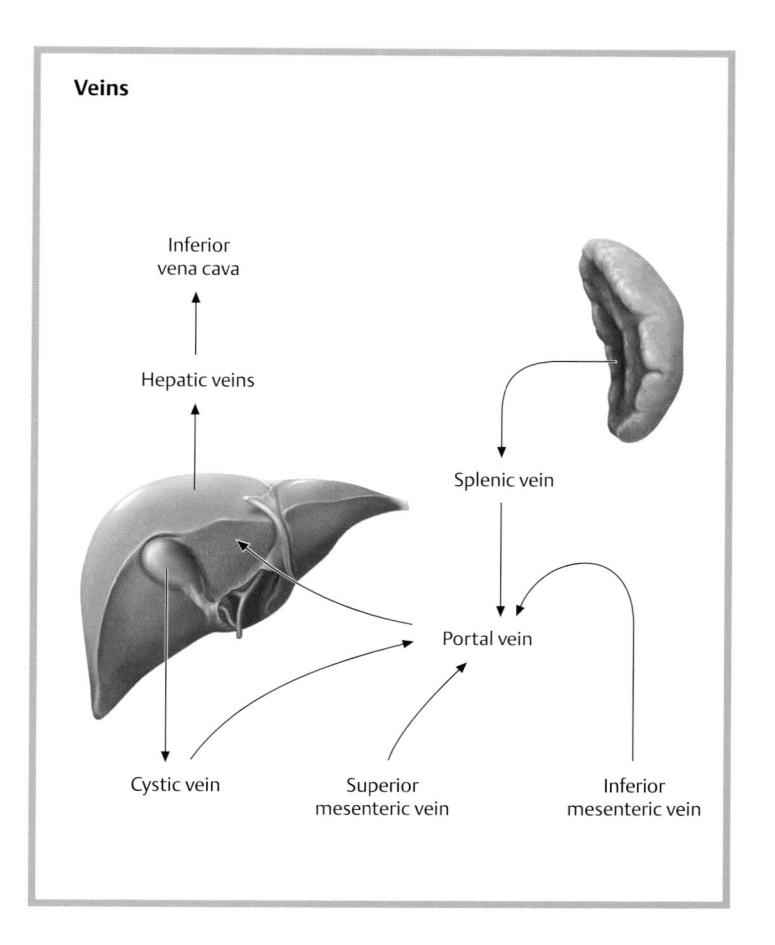

Hepatic veins → Inferior vena cava

(spleen) → Splenic vein

Splenic vein → Portal vein

Cystic vein → Portal vein

Superior mesenteric vein → Portal vein

Inferior mesenteric vein → Portal vein

Lymph nodes

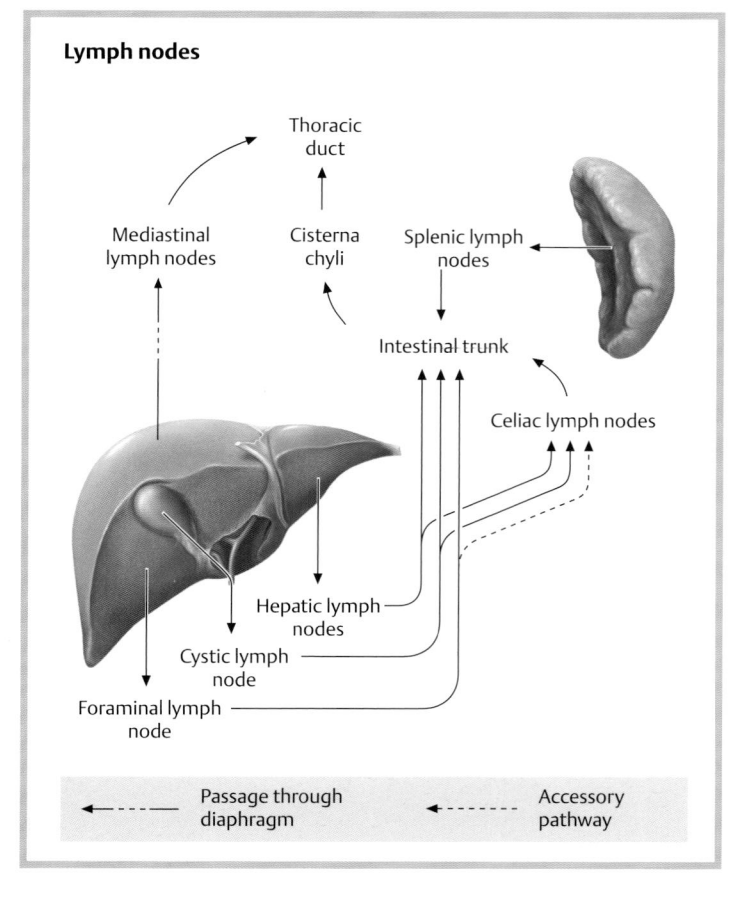

Mediastinal lymph nodes → Thoracic duct

Cisterna chyli → Thoracic duct

Intestinal trunk → Cisterna chyli

Splenic lymph nodes → Intestinal trunk

(spleen) → Splenic lymph nodes

Celiac lymph nodes

Hepatic lymph nodes

Cystic lymph node

Foraminal lymph node

◄- - - - - Passage through diaphragm   ◄- - - - - Accessory pathway

Innervation

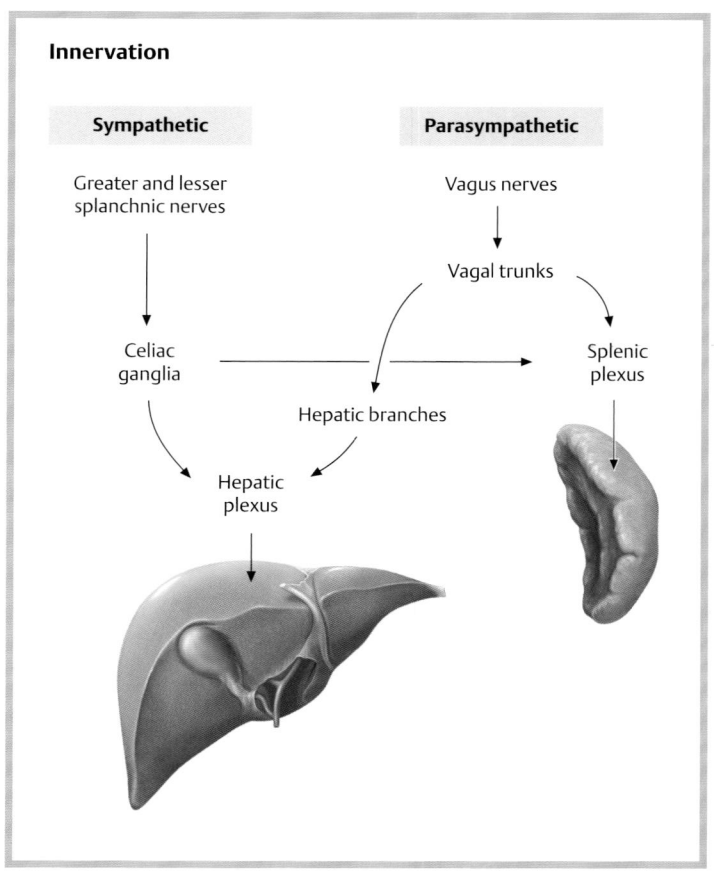

Sympathetic

Greater and lesser splanchnic nerves → Celiac ganglia

Parasympathetic

Vagus nerves → Vagal trunks

Vagal trunks → Splenic plexus

Vagal trunks → Hepatic branches

Celiac ganglia → Splenic plexus

Celiac ganglia → Hepatic plexus

Hepatic branches → Hepatic plexus

Hepatic plexus → (liver)

Splenic plexus → (spleen)

1.11 Stomach

Arteries

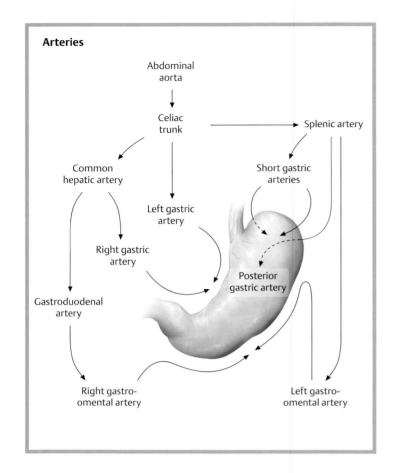

Abdominal aorta

Celiac trunk

Splenic artery

Common hepatic artery

Short gastric arteries

Left gastric artery

Right gastric artery

Posterior gastric artery

Gastroduodenal artery

Right gastro-omental artery

Left gastro-omental artery

Veins

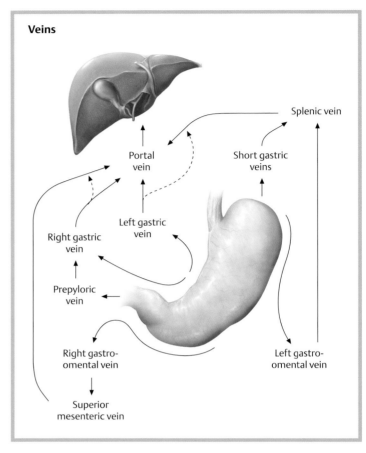

Splenic vein

Portal vein

Short gastric veins

Right gastric vein

Left gastric vein

Prepyloric vein

Right gastro-omental vein

Left gastro-omental vein

Superior mesenteric vein

Lymph nodes

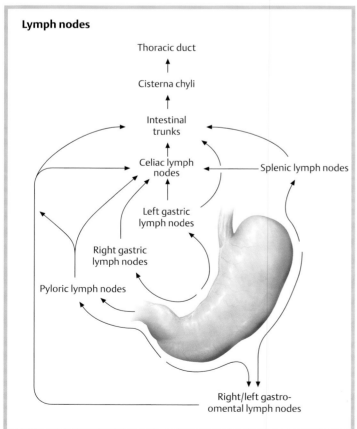

Thoracic duct

Cisterna chyli

Intestinal trunks

Celiac lymph nodes

Splenic lymph nodes

Left gastric lymph nodes

Right gastric lymph nodes

Pyloric lymph nodes

Right/left gastro-omental lymph nodes

Innervation

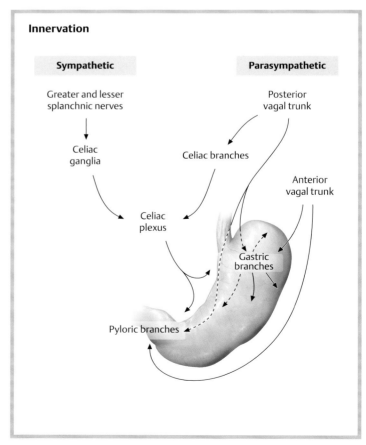

Sympathetic	**Parasympathetic**

Greater and lesser splanchnic nerves

Posterior vagal trunk

Celiac ganglia

Celiac branches

Anterior vagal trunk

Celiac plexus

Gastric branches

Pyloric branches

1.12 Duodenum and Pancreas

Arteries

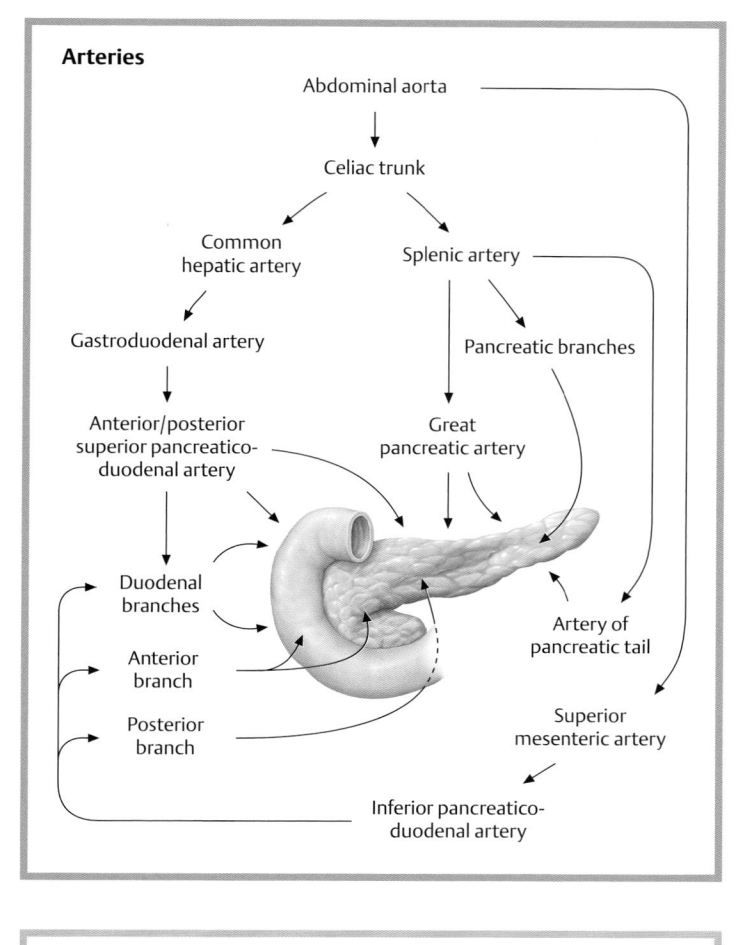

Abdominal aorta

Celiac trunk

Common hepatic artery

Splenic artery

Gastroduodenal artery

Pancreatic branches

Anterior/posterior superior pancreatico-duodenal artery

Great pancreatic artery

Duodenal branches

Anterior branch

Artery of pancreatic tail

Posterior branch

Superior mesenteric artery

Inferior pancreatico-duodenal artery

Veins

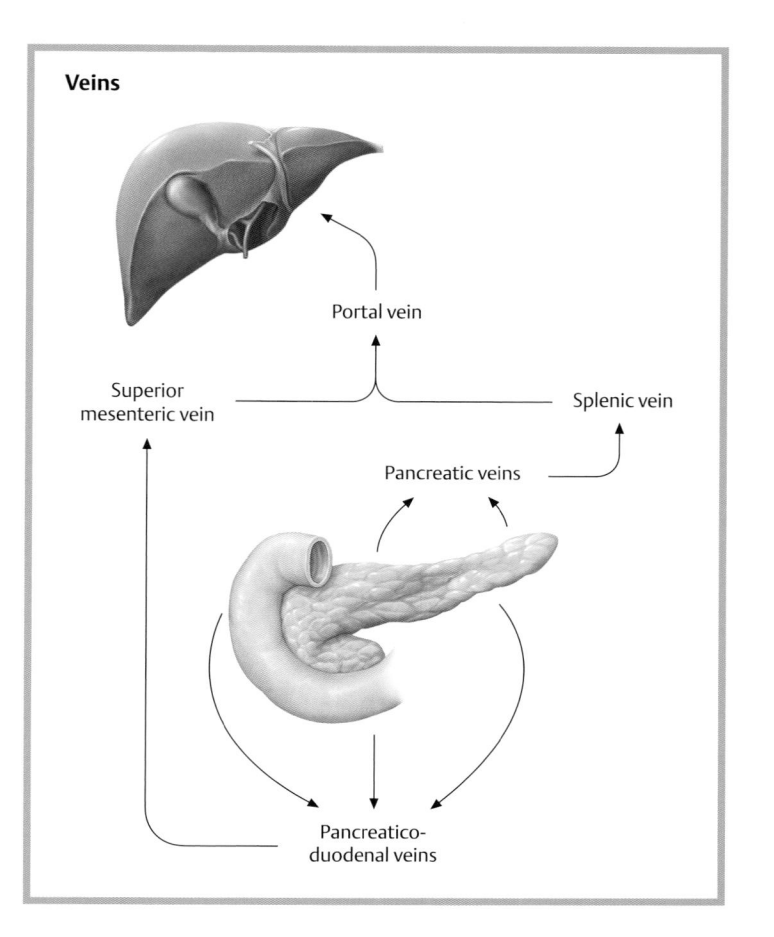

Portal vein

Superior mesenteric vein

Splenic vein

Pancreatic veins

Pancreatico-duodenal veins

Lymph nodes

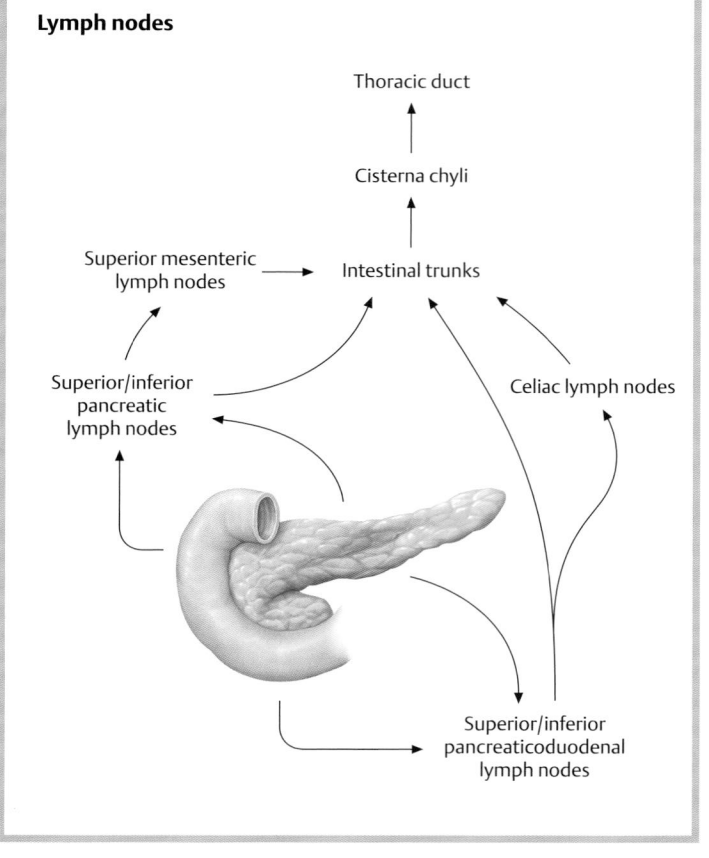

Thoracic duct

Cisterna chyli

Superior mesenteric lymph nodes

Intestinal trunks

Superior/inferior pancreatic lymph nodes

Celiac lymph nodes

Superior/inferior pancreaticoduodenal lymph nodes

Innervation

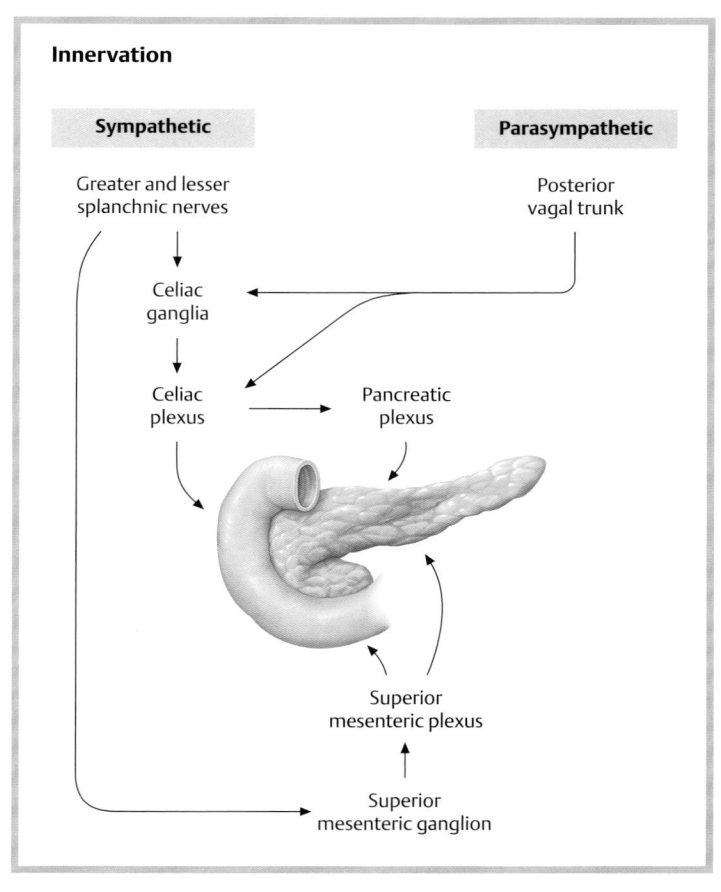

Sympathetic	Parasympathetic

Greater and lesser splanchnic nerves

Posterior vagal trunk

Celiac ganglia

Celiac plexus

Pancreatic plexus

Superior mesenteric plexus

Superior mesenteric ganglion

1.13 Jejunum and Ileum

Arteries

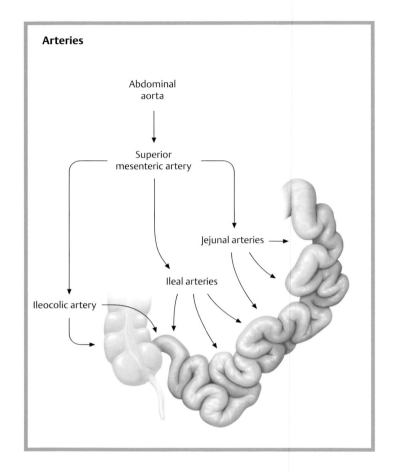

Abdominal aorta
↓
Superior mesenteric artery
↓
Jejunal arteries →
↓
Ileal arteries
Ileocolic artery →

Veins

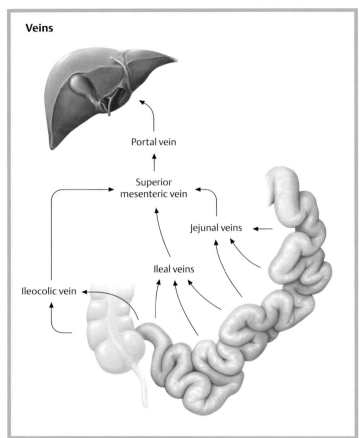

Portal vein
↑
Superior mesenteric vein
← Jejunal veins ←
Ileal veins
Ileocolic vein ←

Lymph nodes

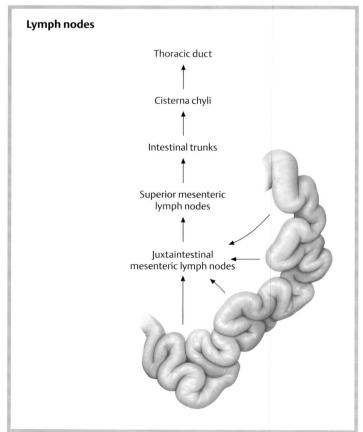

Thoracic duct
↑
Cisterna chyli
↑
Intestinal trunks
↑
Superior mesenteric lymph nodes
↑
Juxtaintestinal mesenteric lymph nodes

Innervation

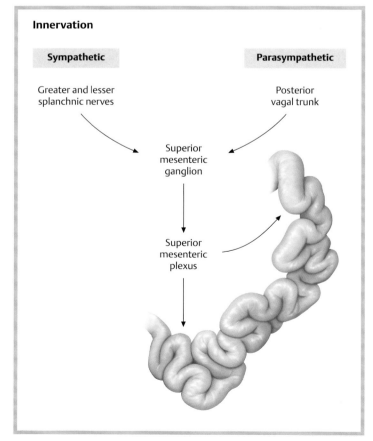

Sympathetic	Parasympathetic

Greater and lesser splanchnic nerves

Posterior vagal trunk

Superior mesenteric ganglion
↓
Superior mesenteric plexus

1.14 Cecum, Vermiform Appendix, Ascending and Transverse Colon

Arteries

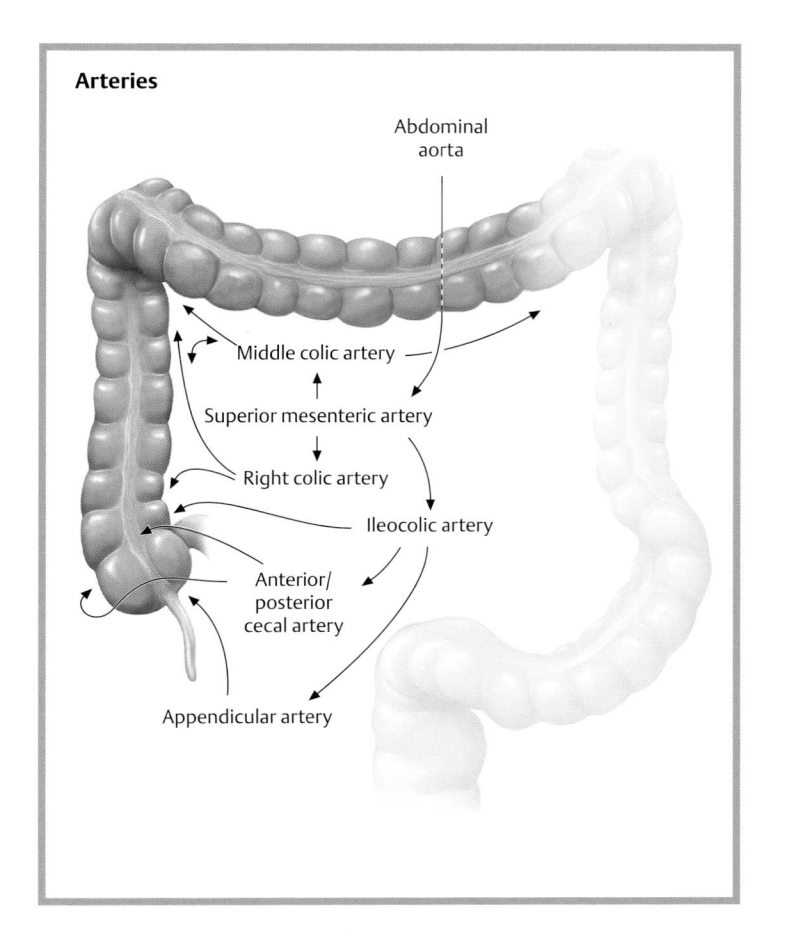

- Abdominal aorta
- Middle colic artery
- Superior mesenteric artery
- Right colic artery
- Ileocolic artery
- Anterior/posterior cecal artery
- Appendicular artery

Veins

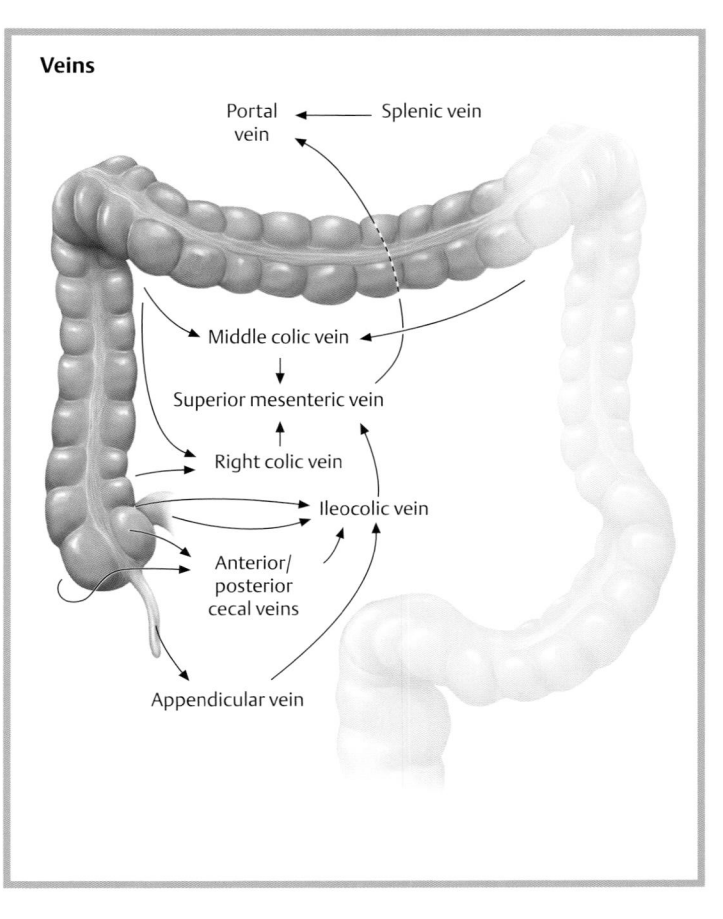

- Portal vein
- Splenic vein
- Middle colic vein
- Superior mesenteric vein
- Right colic vein
- Ileocolic vein
- Anterior/posterior cecal veins
- Appendicular vein

Lymph nodes

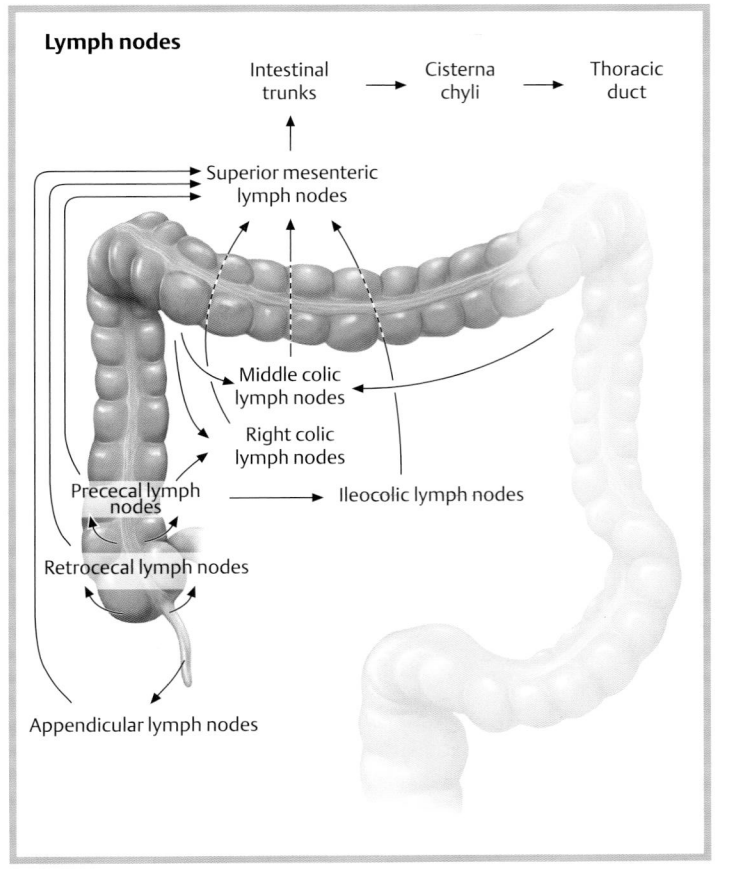

- Intestinal trunks → Cisterna chyli → Thoracic duct
- Superior mesenteric lymph nodes
- Middle colic lymph nodes
- Right colic lymph nodes
- Prececal lymph nodes
- Ileocolic lymph nodes
- Retrocecal lymph nodes
- Appendicular lymph nodes

Innervation

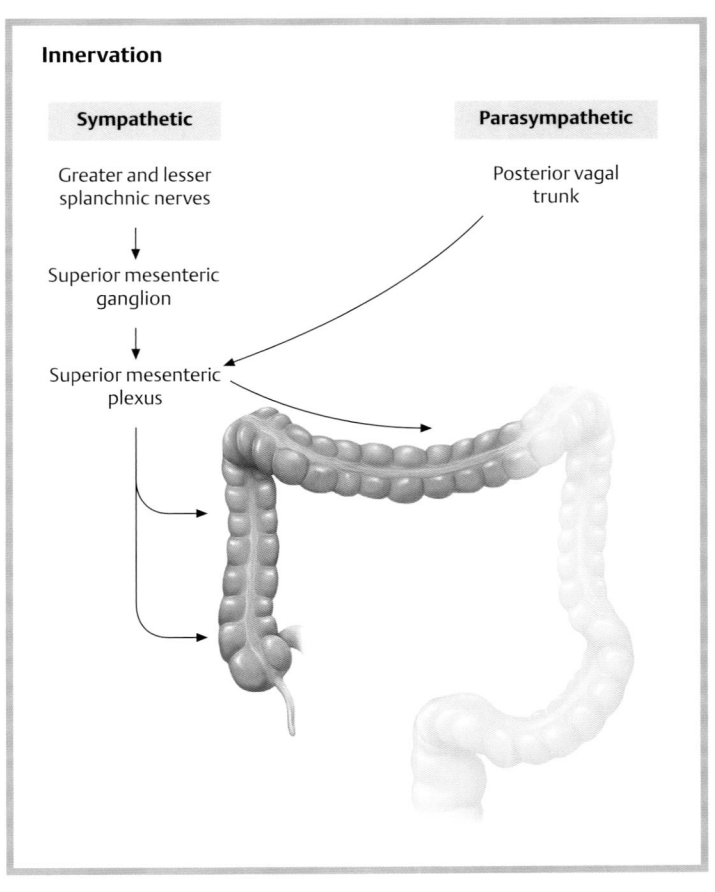

Sympathetic	Parasympathetic
Greater and lesser splanchnic nerves	Posterior vagal trunk
↓	
Superior mesenteric ganglion	
↓	
Superior mesenteric plexus	

1.15 Descending Colon and Sigmoid Colon

Arteries

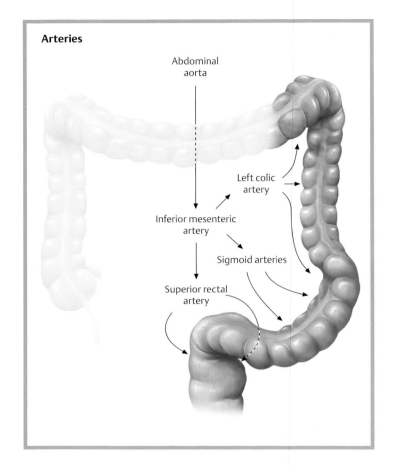

Abdominal aorta

Left colic artery

Inferior mesenteric artery

Sigmoid arteries

Superior rectal artery

Veins

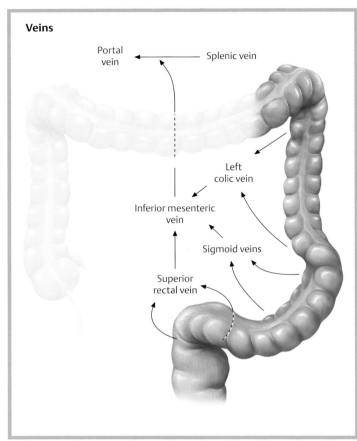

Portal vein ← Splenic vein

Left colic vein

Inferior mesenteric vein

Sigmoid veins

Superior rectal vein

Lymph nodes

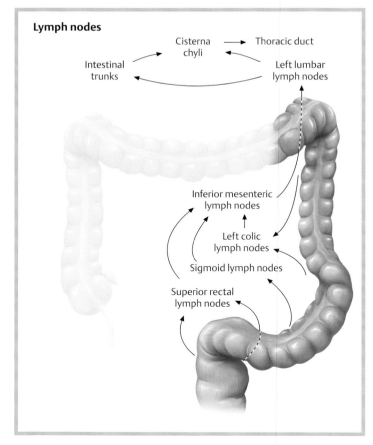

Cisterna chyli → Thoracic duct

Intestinal trunks

Left lumbar lymph nodes

Inferior mesenteric lymph nodes

Left colic lymph nodes

Sigmoid lymph nodes

Superior rectal lymph nodes

Innervation

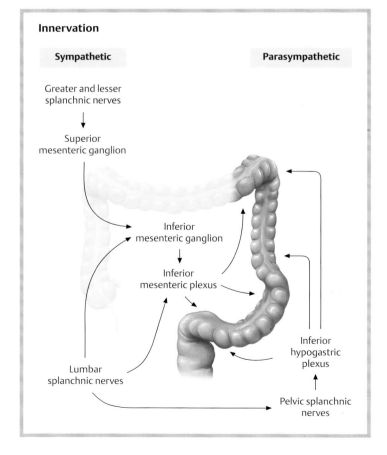

Sympathetic

Parasympathetic

Greater and lesser splanchnic nerves

Superior mesenteric ganglion

Inferior mesenteric ganglion

Inferior mesenteric plexus

Lumbar splanchnic nerves

Inferior hypogastric plexus

Pelvic splanchnic nerves

1.16   Rectum

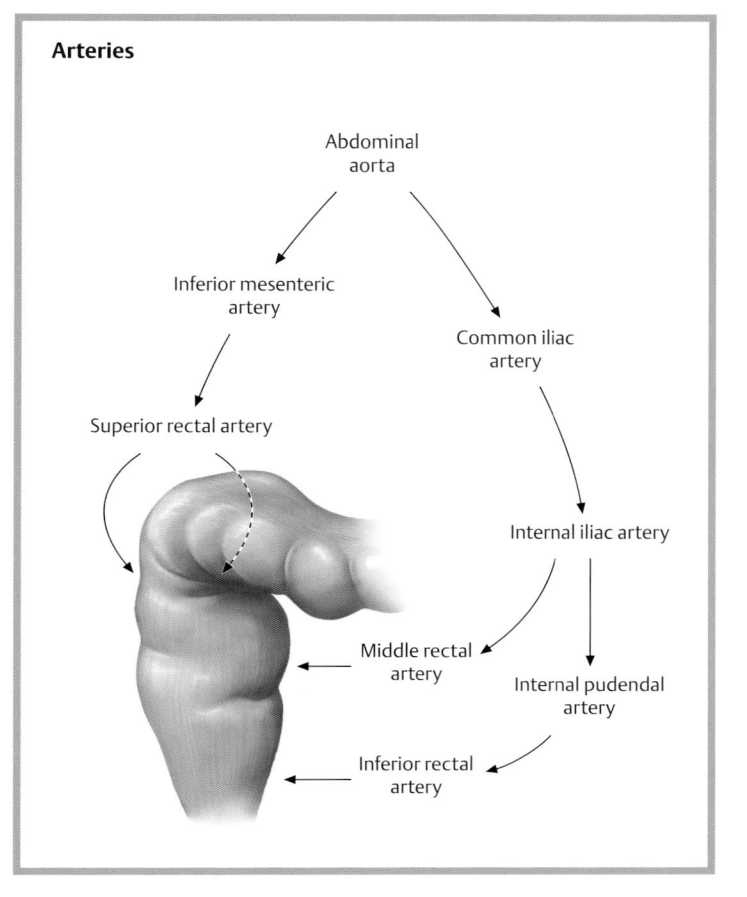

Arteries

Abdominal aorta

Inferior mesenteric artery

Common iliac artery

Superior rectal artery

Internal iliac artery

Middle rectal artery

Internal pudendal artery

Inferior rectal artery

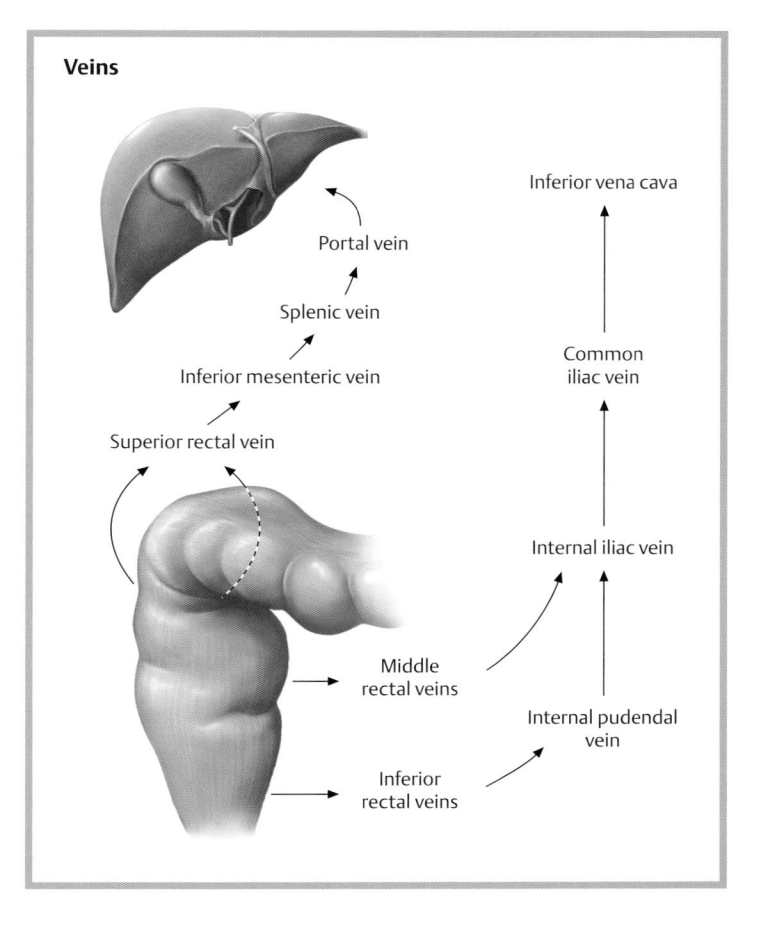

Veins

Inferior vena cava

Portal vein

Splenic vein

Inferior mesenteric vein

Common iliac vein

Superior rectal vein

Internal iliac vein

Middle rectal veins

Internal pudendal vein

Inferior rectal veins

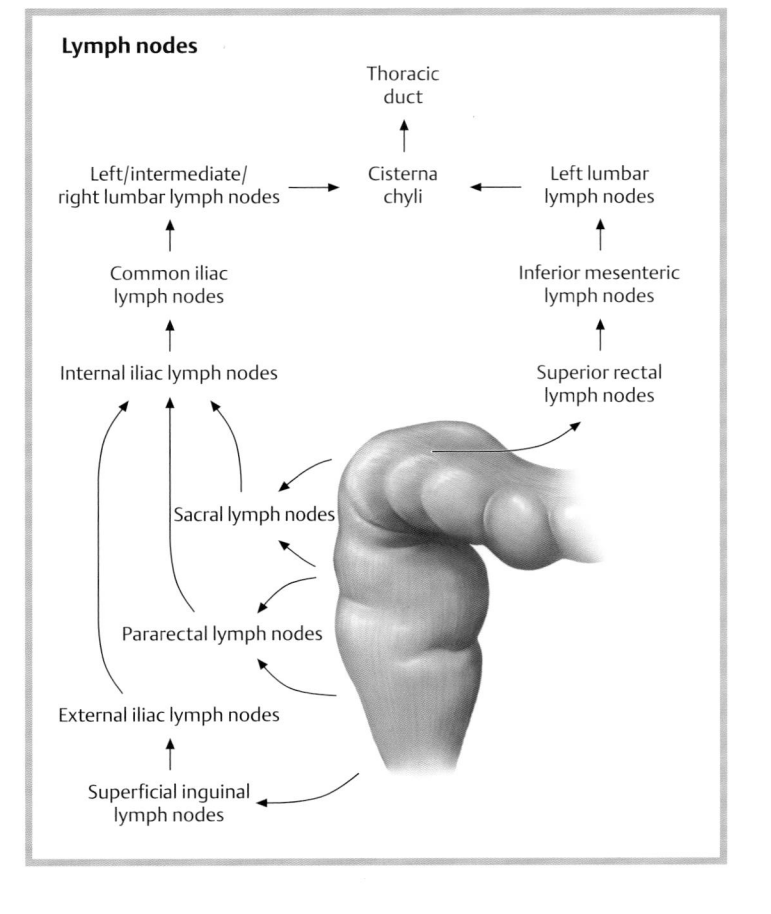

Lymph nodes

Thoracic duct

Left/intermediate/right lumbar lymph nodes

Cisterna chyli

Left lumbar lymph nodes

Common iliac lymph nodes

Inferior mesenteric lymph nodes

Internal iliac lymph nodes

Superior rectal lymph nodes

Sacral lymph nodes

Pararectal lymph nodes

External iliac lymph nodes

Superficial inguinal lymph nodes

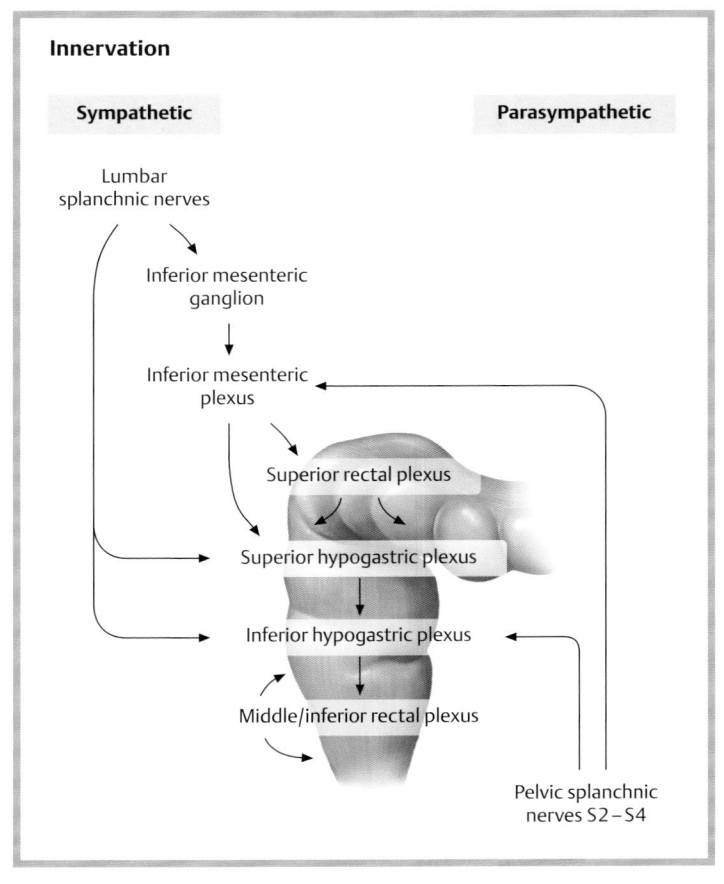

Innervation

Sympathetic   **Parasympathetic**

Lumbar splanchnic nerves

Inferior mesenteric ganglion

Inferior mesenteric plexus

Superior rectal plexus

Superior hypogastric plexus

Inferior hypogastric plexus

Middle/inferior rectal plexus

Pelvic splanchnic nerves S2–S4

1.17 Kidney, Ureter, and Suprarenal Gland

Arteries

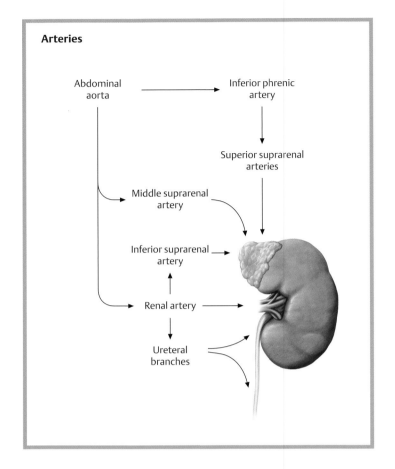

Abdominal aorta → Inferior phrenic artery

↓

Superior suprarenal arteries

Middle suprarenal artery

Inferior suprarenal artery

Renal artery

Ureteral branches

Veins

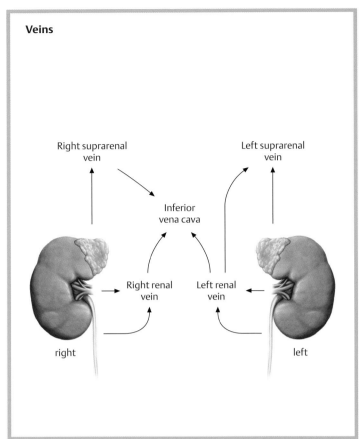

Right suprarenal vein

Left suprarenal vein

Inferior vena cava

Right renal vein

Left renal vein

right

left

Lymph nodes

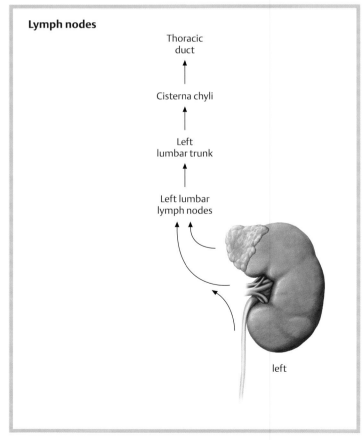

Thoracic duct

↑

Cisterna chyli

↑

Left lumbar trunk

↑

Left lumbar lymph nodes

left

Innervation

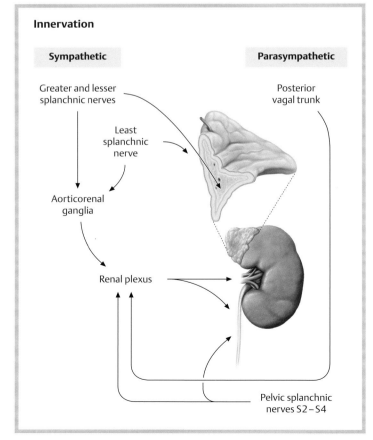

Sympathetic

Parasympathetic

Greater and lesser splanchnic nerves

Least splanchnic nerve

Aorticorenal ganglia

Renal plexus

Posterior vagal trunk

Pelvic splanchnic nerves S2–S4

341

1.18 Bladder, Prostate, and Seminal Vesicle

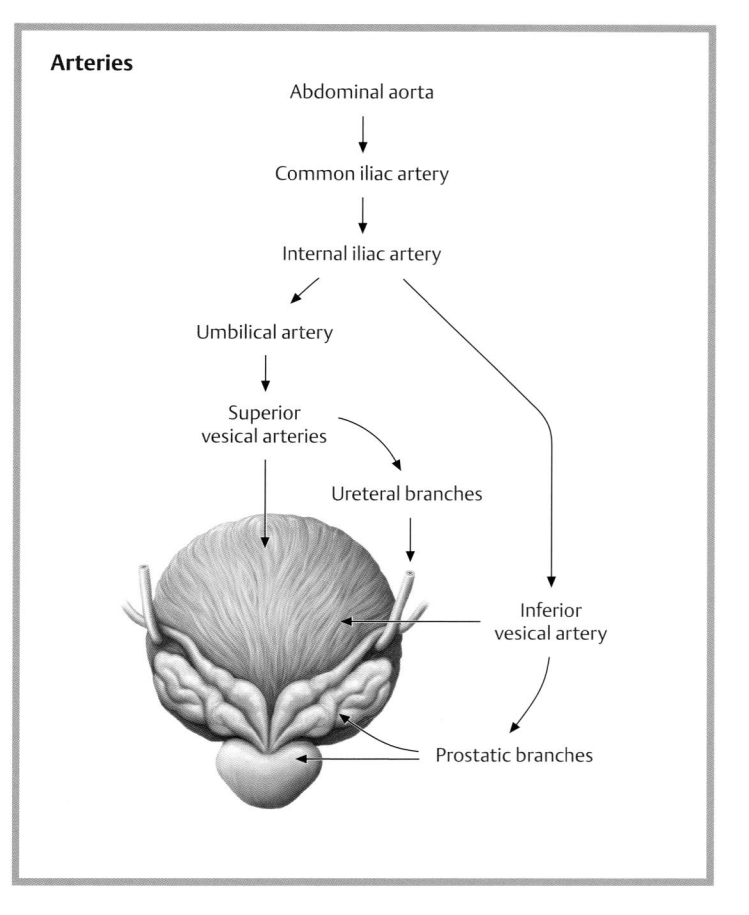

Arteries

Abdominal aorta

↓

Common iliac artery

↓

Internal iliac artery

Umbilical artery

Superior vesical arteries

Ureteral branches

Inferior vesical artery

Prostatic branches

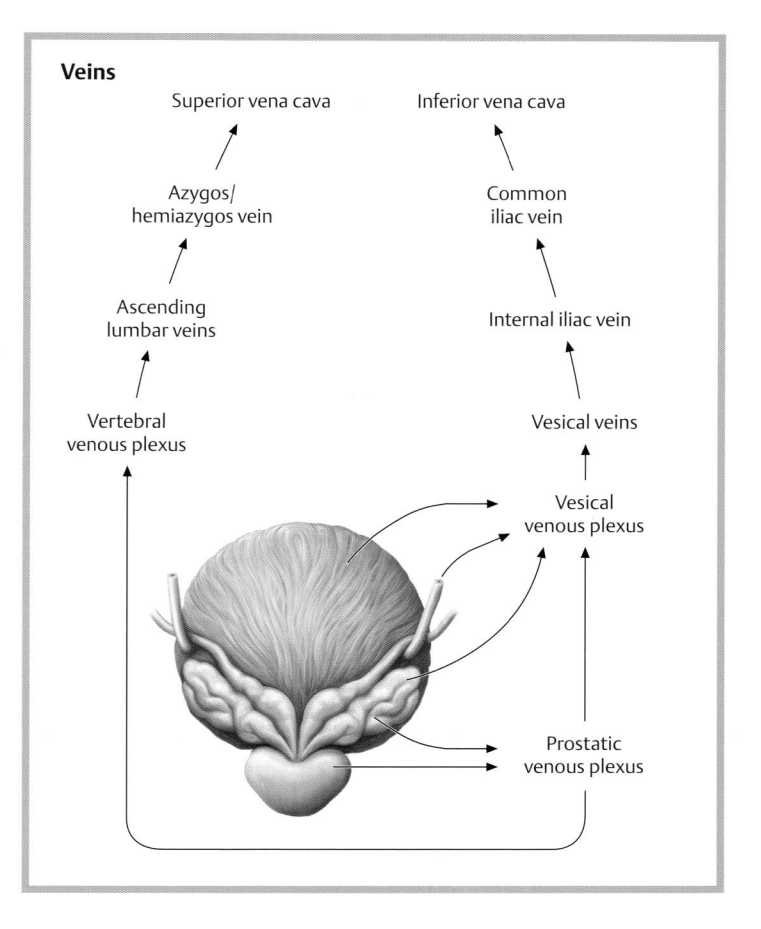

Veins

Superior vena cava

Inferior vena cava

Azygos/ hemiazygos vein

Common iliac vein

Ascending lumbar veins

Internal iliac vein

Vertebral venous plexus

Vesical veins

Vesical venous plexus

Prostatic venous plexus

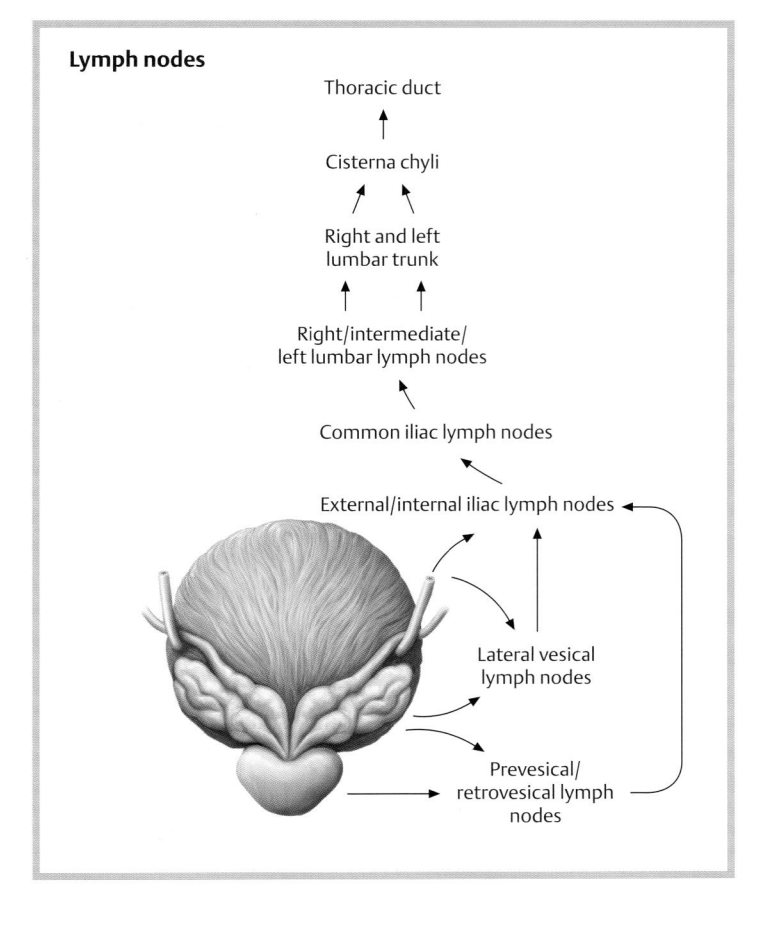

Lymph nodes

Thoracic duct

↑

Cisterna chyli

Right and left lumbar trunk

Right/intermediate/ left lumbar lymph nodes

Common iliac lymph nodes

External/internal iliac lymph nodes

Lateral vesical lymph nodes

Prevesical/ retrovesical lymph nodes

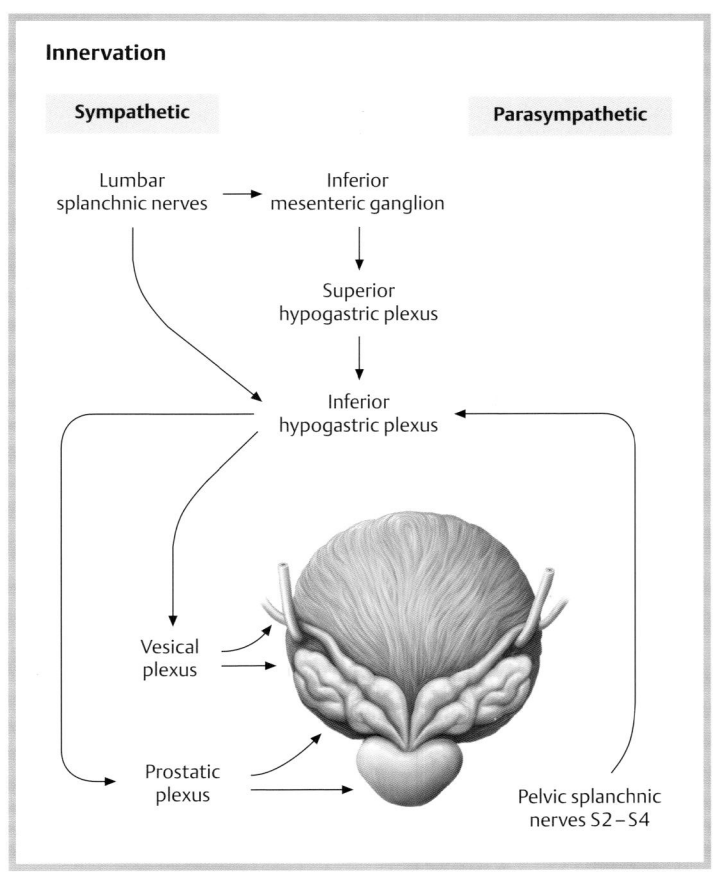

Innervation

Sympathetic	Parasympathetic

Lumbar splanchnic nerves → Inferior mesenteric ganglion

Superior hypogastric plexus

Inferior hypogastric plexus

Vesical plexus

Prostatic plexus

Pelvic splanchnic nerves S2–S4

1.19 Testis, Epididymis, and Vas Deferens

Arteries

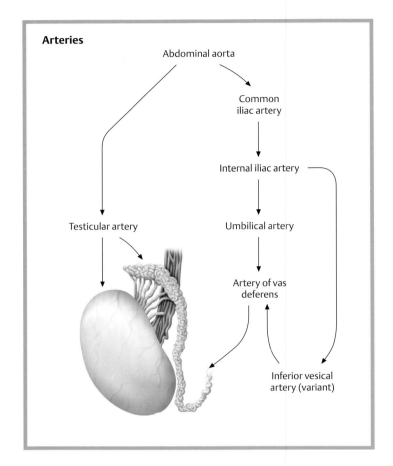

Abdominal aorta

Common iliac artery

Internal iliac artery

Testicular artery

Umbilical artery

Artery of vas deferens

Inferior vesical artery (variant)

Veins

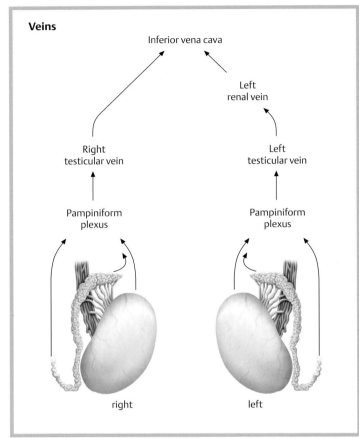

Inferior vena cava

Left renal vein

Right testicular vein

Left testicular vein

Pampiniform plexus

Pampiniform plexus

right

left

Lymph nodes

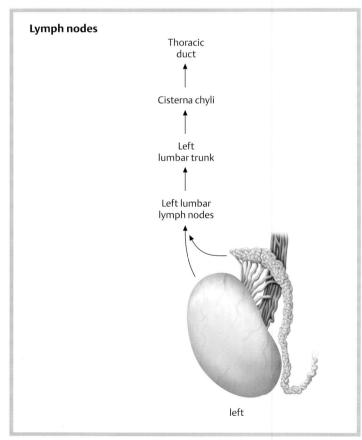

Thoracic duct

Cisterna chyli

Left lumbar trunk

Left lumbar lymph nodes

left

Innervation

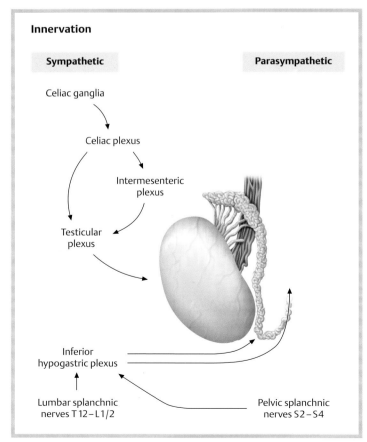

| Sympathetic | Parasympathetic |

Celiac ganglia

Celiac plexus

Intermesenteric plexus

Testicular plexus

Inferior hypogastric plexus

Lumbar splanchnic nerves T 12–L1/2

Pelvic splanchnic nerves S2–S4

343

1.20 Uterus, Fallopian Tube, and Vagina

Arteries

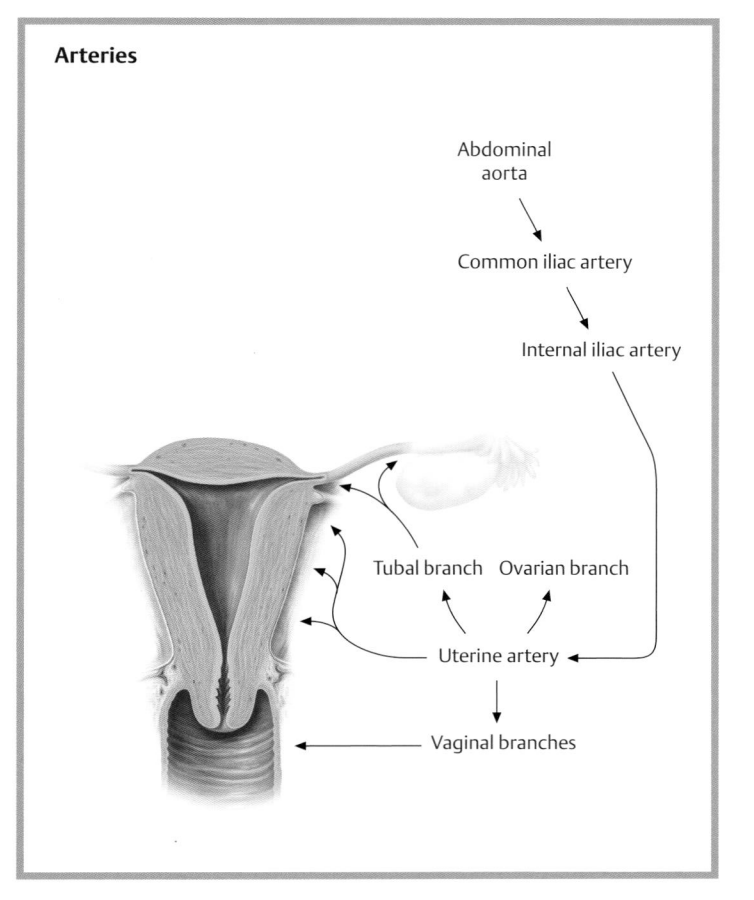

Abdominal aorta

↓

Common iliac artery

↓

Internal iliac artery

Tubal branch   Ovarian branch

Uterine artery

Vaginal branches

Veins

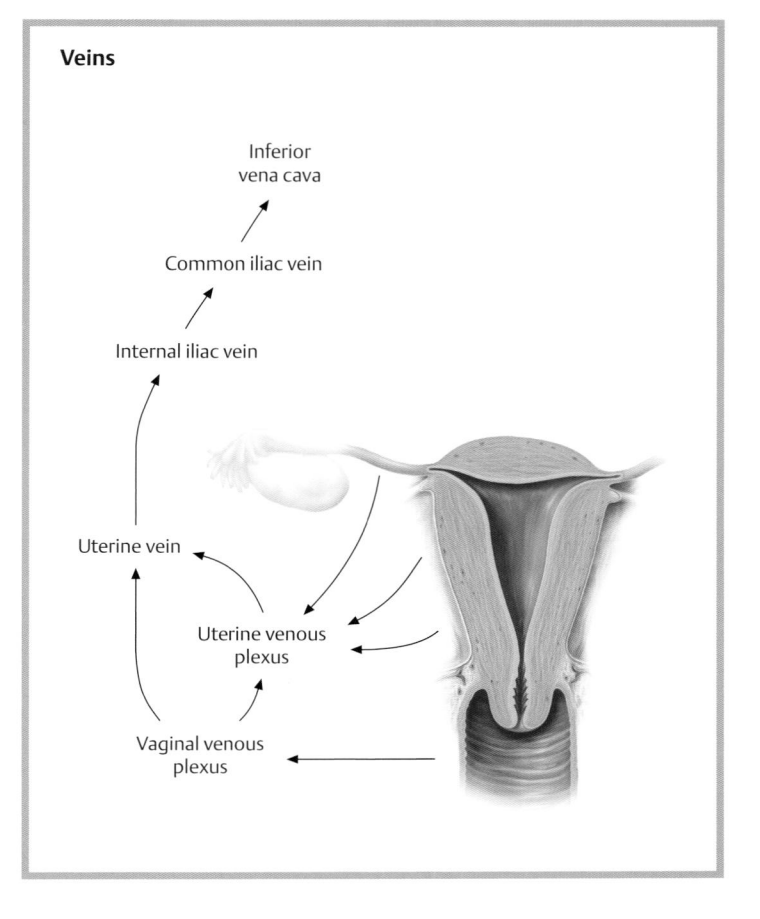

Inferior vena cava

Common iliac vein

Internal iliac vein

Uterine vein

Uterine venous plexus

Vaginal venous plexus

Lymph nodes

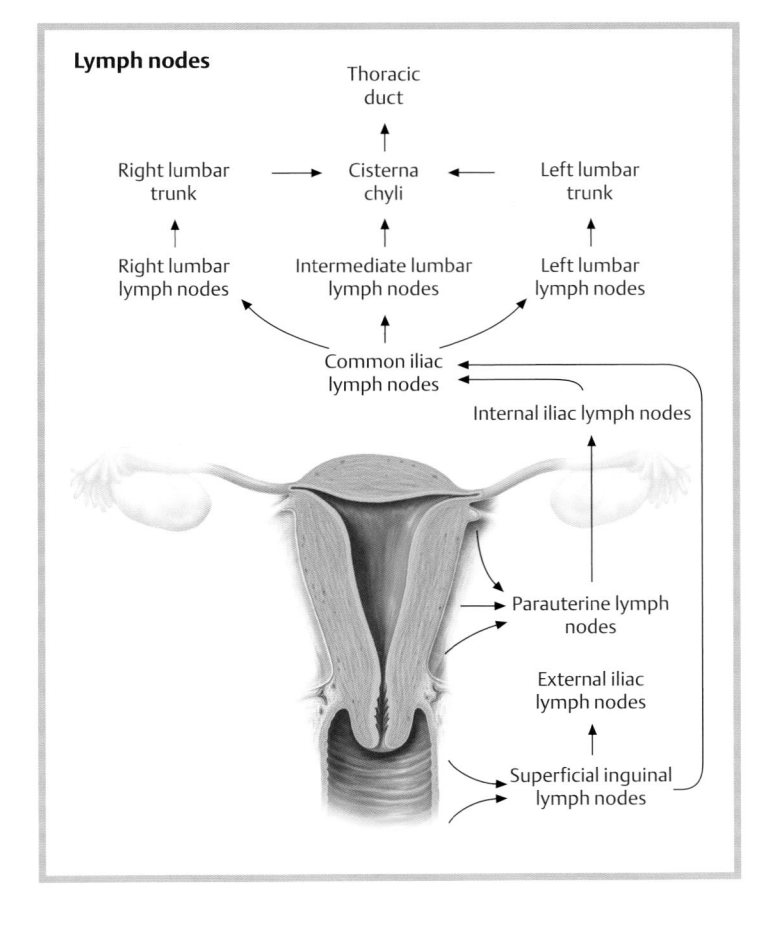

Thoracic duct

Right lumbar trunk → Cisterna chyli ← Left lumbar trunk

Right lumbar lymph nodes   Intermediate lumbar lymph nodes   Left lumbar lymph nodes

Common iliac lymph nodes

Internal iliac lymph nodes

Parauterine lymph nodes

External iliac lymph nodes

Superficial inguinal lymph nodes

Innervation

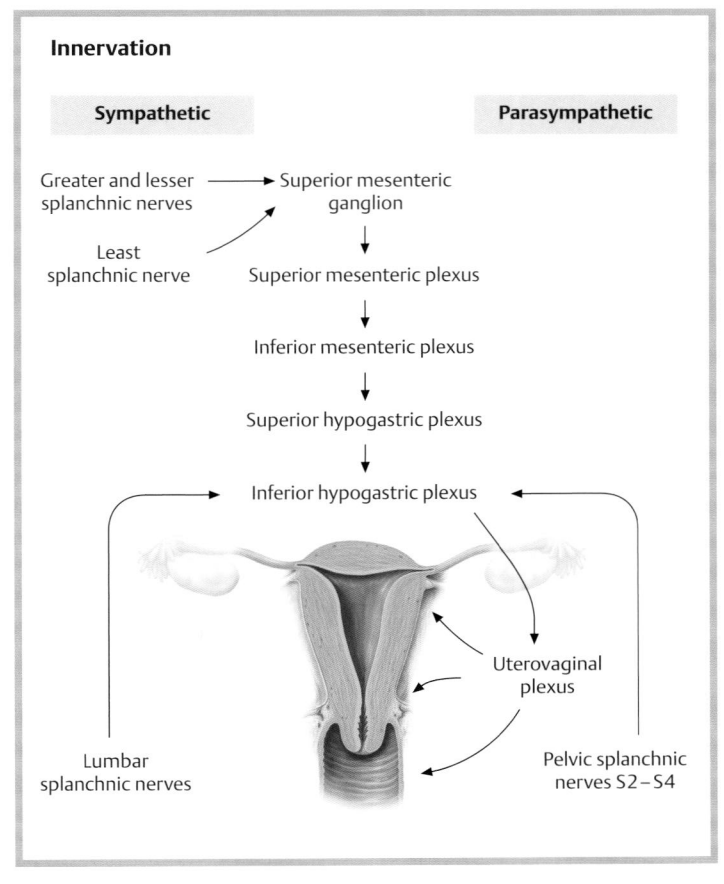

Sympathetic	**Parasympathetic**

Greater and lesser splanchnic nerves → Superior mesenteric ganglion

Least splanchnic nerve

Superior mesenteric plexus

↓

Inferior mesenteric plexus

↓

Superior hypogastric plexus

↓

Inferior hypogastric plexus

Uterovaginal plexus

Lumbar splanchnic nerves

Pelvic splanchnic nerves S2–S4

344

1.21 Fallopian Tube and Ovary

Arteries

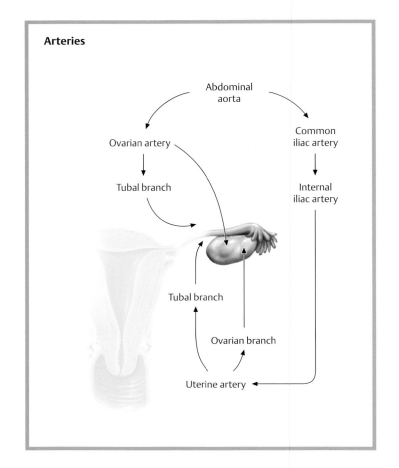

Abdominal aorta

Ovarian artery

Common iliac artery

Tubal branch

Internal iliac artery

Tubal branch

Ovarian branch

Uterine artery

Veins

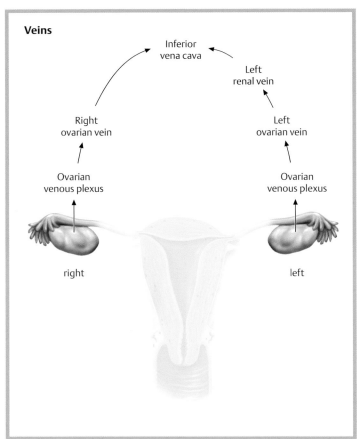

Inferior vena cava

Left renal vein

Right ovarian vein

Left ovarian vein

Ovarian venous plexus

Ovarian venous plexus

right

left

Lymph nodes

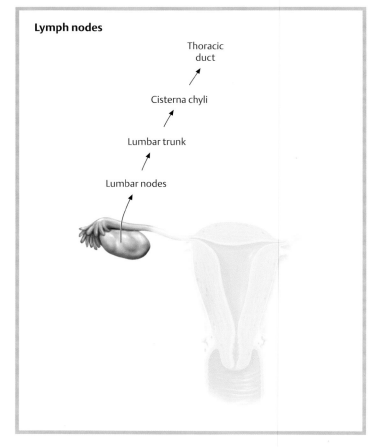

Thoracic duct

Cisterna chyli

Lumbar trunk

Lumbar nodes

Innervation

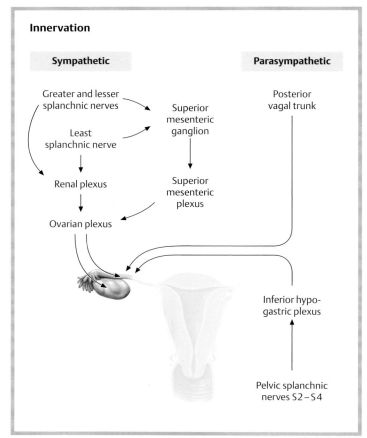

Sympathetic		Parasympathetic

Greater and lesser splanchnic nerves

Superior mesenteric ganglion

Posterior vagal trunk

Least splanchnic nerve

Renal plexus

Superior mesenteric plexus

Ovarian plexus

Inferior hypo-gastric plexus

Pelvic splanchnic nerves S2–S4

Appendix

List of References

Agur, A. M. R.: Grant's Anatomie. Atlas und Lehrbuch. Enke, Stuttgart 1999

Anschütz, F.: Die körperliche Untersuchung, 3. Aufl. Springer, Heidelberg 1978

Bähr, M., M. Frotscher: Duus' Neurologisch-topische Diagnostik, 8. Aufl. Thieme, Stuttgart 2003

Becker, W., H. H. Naumann, C. R. Pfaltz: Hals-Nasen-Ohren-Heilkunde, 2. Aufl. Thieme, Stuttgart 1983

Berghaus, A., G. Rettinger, G. Böhme: Hals-Nasen-Ohren-Heilkunde, Hippokrates, Stuttgart 1996

Block, B., P. N. Meier, M. P. Manns: Lehratlas der Gastroskopie. Thieme, Stuttgart 1997

Block, B., G. Schachschal, H. Schmidt: Der Gastroskopie-Trainer. Thieme, Stuttgart 2003

Dauber, W.: Feneis' Bild-Lexikon der Anatomie, 9. Aufl. Thieme, Stuttgart 2005

Feneis, H., W. Dauber: Anatomisches Bildwörterbuch, 8. Aufl. Thieme, Stuttgart 1999

Flachskamp, F.: Kursbuch Echokardiographie, 2. Aufl. Thieme, Stuttgart 2004

Földi, M., S. Kubik: Lehrbuch der Lymphologie für Mediziner und Physiotherapeuten. G. Fischer, Stuttgart 1989

Frick, H., H. Leonhardt, D. Starck: Allgemeine und spezielle Anatomie. Taschenlehrbuch der gesamten Anatomie, Bd. 1 und 2, 4. Aufl. Thieme, Stuttgart 1992

Fritsch, H., W. Kühnel: Taschenatlas der Anatomie, Bd. 2, 7. Aufl. Thieme, Stuttgart 2001

Graumann, W., D. v. Keyserlingk, D. Sasse: Taschenbuch der Anatomie. G. Fischer, Stuttgart 1994

Hegglin, J.: Chirurgische Untersuchung. Thieme, Stuttgart 1976

Heinecker, R.: EKG in Klinik und Praxis. Thieme, Stuttgart 1975

Kahle, W., M. Frotscher: Taschenatlas der Anatomie, Bd.1, Thieme, Stuttgart 2001

Klinke, R., S. Silbernagl: Lehrbuch der Physiologie, 3. Aufl. Thieme, Stuttgart 2001

Lippert, H., R. Pabst: Arterial Variations in Man. Bergmann, München 1985

Loeweneck, H.: Diagnostische Anatomie. Springer, Berlin 1981

Lüllmann-Rauch, R.: Histologie. Thieme, Stuttgart 2003

Masuhr, K. F., M. Neumann: Neurologie, 5. Aufl. Thieme, Stuttgart 2005

Möller, T. B., E. Reif: Taschenatlas der Röntgenanatomie, 2. Aufl. Thieme, Stuttgart 1998

Moore, K., T. Persaud: Embryologie, 4. Aufl. Schattauer, Stuttgart 1996

Netter, F. H.: Farbatlanten der Medizin. Thieme, Stuttgart 1983–1995

Platzer, W.: Taschenatlas der Anatomie, Bd.1, Thieme, Stuttgart 1999

Platzer, W.: Atlas der topographischen Anatomie. Thieme, Stuttgart 1982

Probst, R., G. Grevers, H. Iro: Hals-Nasen-Ohren-Heilkunde. Thieme, Stuttgart 2000

Rauber/Kopsch: Anatomie des Menschen, Bd. 1–4, Thieme, Stuttgart. Bd. 1., 2. Aufl.: 1997, Bd. 2 u. 3: 1987, Bd. 4: 1988

Rohen, J. W.: Topographische Anatomie, 10. Aufl. Schattauer, Stuttgart 2000

Romer, A. S., T. S. Parson: Vergleichende Anatomie der Wirbeltiere, 5. Aufl. Paul Parey, Hamburg und Berlin 1983

Sadler, T. W.: Medizinische Embryologie, 10. Aufl. Thieme, Stuttgart 2003

Schünke, M.: Funktionelle Anatomie – Topographie und Funktion des Bewegungssystems. Thieme, Stuttgart 2000

Schumacher, G.-H., G. Aumüller: Topographische Anatomie des Menschen, 6. Aufl. G. Fischer 1994

Schumpelick, V., N. Bleese, U. Mommsen: Chirurgie, 4. Aufl. Enke, Stuttgart 1999

Silbernagl, S., A. Despopoulos: Taschenatlas der Physiologie, 6. Aufl. Thieme, Stuttgart 2003

Stelzner, F.: Chirurgie an viszeralen Abschlußsystemen. Thieme, Stuttgart 1998

Stelzner, F.: Der Verschluß der terminalen Speiseröhre. Deutsch. Med. Wochensch. 93 (1968), 1679–1685

Strohmeyer, G., W. Dölle: Ösophagusvarizen: Bedeutung, Ursachen und Behandlung. Med. Klein. 58 (1963), 1649–1653

Tiedemann, K.: Anatomy of the head and neck. Verlag Chemie, Weinheim 1993

Tillmann, B.: Farbatlas der Anatomie Zahnmedizin – Humanmedizin. Thieme, Stuttgart 1997

Thurn, P., E. Bücheler: Einführung in die Röntgendiagnostik, 6. Aufl. Thieme, Stuttgart 1979

von Lanz, T., W. Wachsmuth: Praktische Anatomie, Bd. 2, 6. Teil (hrsg. von Loeweneck u. Feifel), Springer, Berlin 1993

von Lanz, T., W. Wachsmuth: Praktische Anatomie, Bd. 1/2: Hals, Springer, Berlin 1955

Subject Index

Anatomical terms not included in the current *Terminologia Anatomica* are marked with an asterisk (*).

A

Abdomen
– anastomoses, venous 292
– lymphatic trunks 295
– transverse section 166
Abdominal aorta see Aorta, abdominal
Abdominal cavity
– divisions 152
– layers
– – anterior 152
– – middle 152
– – posterior 152
– peritoneal relationships 153, 154
Abdominal layers, organ locations 152
Abdominal levels, organ locations 152
Abdominal pregnancy 254
Abdominal wall, anterior, skin incisions, surgical 151
Abdominal wall, peritoneal relationships 155
Accessory phrenic nerve 146
Acini 217
Acromion 2, 4, 43
Acrosome 259
Action of heart, mechanical 112
Adam's apple 24
Addison's disease 220
Aditus laryngis (laryngeal inlet) 26, 34
Adventitia
– of bladder 239
– of esophagus 72, 74
– of trachea 83
– of ureteral wall 231
– of vas deferens 260
Alcock's canal 288
Allergic reaction, bronchial asthma 87
Alpha (A) cells 217
Alveolar epithelial cells
– type I 88
– type II 88
Alveolus, pulmonary* 86
– lining 88
Ampulla
– hepatopancreatic 213
– – septated 213
– of duodenum 188
– of fallopian tube 246
– of rectum 198
– of urethra 238
– of vas deferens 256
Anal canal 197, 198
– epithelial regions 199

– levels 199
Anastomoses
– arterioarterial, fetal 94
– cavocaval 116, 273, 292
– portosystemic collaterals 75, 95, 119, 274, 278, 289, 292
– portocaval collaterals see Anastomes, portosystemic collaterals
– venovenous, fetal 94
– venous
– – abdomen 292
– – pelvis 292
Anastomoses, arterial, abdominal 271
Anatomical constrictions of the ureter 173, 222, 233
Androgen production 259
Angina pectoris (chest tightness) 127
– radiating pain 144
Angle of His 75
Angle(s)
– inferior scapular, line connecting 58
– of mandible 35
– of sternum 58
Angle, epigastric 92
Anulus/Ring
– [anulus] fibrous
– – left 107
– – right 107
– [ring] inguinal
– – deep 155, 174
– – superficial 155
– [ring] lymphatic, of gastric cardia 135, 298
Ansa
– cervicalis 48
– – deep* 48
– – – root
– – – – inferior 17, 18
– – – – superior 17, 18
– – – thyroid branch 18
– – superficial* 17, 44, 49
– of hypoglossal nerve 18
Anteflexion, of the uterus 171, 175, 251
Anterior cricothyroid muscle see Muscle, cricothyroid
Anterior myocardial infarction, supra-apical 127
Anterior subcostal incision 151
Anterior surface of heart 100
Anteversion, of the uterus 171, 175, 251
Antrum
– follicular 253
– gastric, endoscopic appearance 187
– pyloric 183, 184
Anus 198
Aorta
– abdominal 162 ff, 114, 173, 188, 205, 211, 221, 223, 232,

262, 264, 266 ff, 270, 272, 284, 286
– – in abdominal transverse section 166
– – location 152
– – projection onto skeleton 263
– – sequence of branches 263
– ascending 10, 61, 65, 77, 100, 114
– – projection onto chest wall 114
– branches
– – bronchial 114
– – esophageal 114
– – pericardial 114
– – tracheal 114
– descending 10, 60, 63, 65, 114
– location 115
– – relationship to esophagus 114
– – relationship to trachea 114
– "riding" on left main bronchus 76
– thoracic 63, 79, 114
– – branches
– – – bronchial 122
– – – esophageal 118
– – – tracheal 122
– – descending part 71
– – hiatus in diaphragm 91
– – relationship to esophagus 72
– ventral 20
Aortic aneurysm 115
– left-sided 27
Aortic arch see Arch, aortic
Aortic bifurcation 262
Aortic constriction of esophagus 70
Aortic knob 96
Aortic valve see Valve, aortic
Apex
– cardiac, see Cardiac apex
– of arytenoid cartilage 25
– of bladder 256
– prostatic 257
– pulmonary 59, 79, 80
Apical anterior myocardial infarction 127
Aponeurosis, stylopharyngeal 40
Appendicitis 194
Appendix (-ces)
– epiploic 158, 191
– fibrous, of liver 206
– of bladder 242, 246
– of epididymis 242
– of testis 242
– omental 192
– vermiform 172, 180, 193, 194
– – innervation, sympathetic 315
– – position 152
– – – variants 195
– – projection onto trunk wall 151
– – wall structure 195
Approach
– ischiorectal 196

– perineal 196
– sacral 196
– transanal 196
– transperitoneal, to the rectum 196
Arcades 268
Arch
– costal see costal margin
– iliopectineal 285
– of aorta (aortic arch) 10, 27, 59, 63, 65, 66, 70, 72, 95, 98, 100, 114
– – fetal 94
– – radiographic appearance 96, 98
– – relationship to esophagus 70, 72
– of C7 vertebra 54
– of cricoid cartilage 25
– – viewed with laryngeal mirror 29
– of jugular vein 13, 46
– palatoglossal 36
– palatopharyngeal 34
Arterioles
– glomerular
– – afferent 228
– – efferent 228
– penicillar 219
– straight 229
Artery (arteries)
– abdominal 262
– accompanying the sciatic nerve 285
– angular 11
– appendicular 194, 269
– arcuate 228
– – of kidney 282
– ascending pharyngeal 10, 38
– – tonsillar branches 41
– – variants 38
– azygos, of vagina 285
– basilar 10, 51
– bronchial 120, 122
– bulbar
– – of pelvis 284
– – of vestibule 245, 284
– carotid
– – common 10, 27, 39, 46, 48, 52, 59, 100, 114
– – – esophageal branches 118
– – external 10, 23, 38, 48
– – – branches 10
– – – – anterior, variants 49
– – – variable position 49
– – internal 10, 23, 38
– – – collateral pathways 11
– – – origin of ascending pharyngeal artery 38
– – – stenosis 11
– – – variable position 49
– cecal
– – anterior 194, 268, 270
– – posterior 268, 270
– cervical

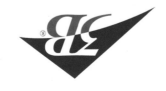

3B SCIENTIFIC —
ANATOMY
IN
3
DIMENSIONS

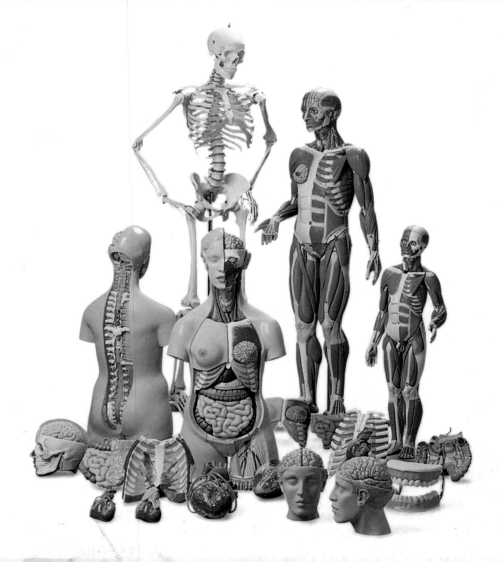